# *Reconstructive*
# Dermatologic Surgery

# *Reconstructive*
# Dermatologic Surgery


***Editors***

**S Brian Jiang** MD
Clinical Professor of Dermatology
Director, Mohs and Dermatologic Surgery
Surgical Director, Dermatology Residency Program
Program Director, Micrographic Surgery and Dermatologic Oncology Fellowship
Department of Dermatology
University of California
San Diego, California, USA

**Arisa E Ortiz** MD
Assistant Clinical Professor of Dermatology
Director, Laser and Cosmetic Dermatology
Department of Dermatology
University of California
San Diego, California, USA


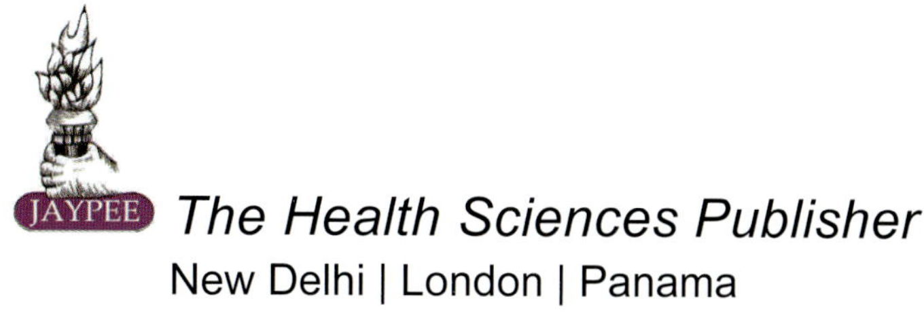



*The Health Sciences Publisher*
New Delhi | London | Panama

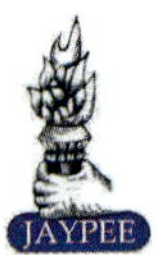


**Jaypee Brothers Medical Publishers (P) Ltd**

**Headquarters**
Jaypee Brothers Medical Publishers (P) Ltd.
4838/24, Ansari Road, Daryaganj
New Delhi 110 002, India
Phone: +91-11-43574357
Fax: +91-11-43574314
E-mail: jaypee@jaypeebrothers.com

**Overseas Offices**
J.P. Medical Ltd.
83, Victoria Street, London
SW1H 0HW (UK)
Phone: +44-20 3170 8910
Fax: +44(0)20 3008 6180
E-mail: info@jpmedpub.com

Jaypee-Highlights Medical Publishers Inc.
City of Knowledge, Bld. 235, 2nd Floor, Clayton
Panama City, Panama
Phone: +1 507-301-0496
Fax: +1 507-301-0499
E-mail: cservice@jphmedical.com

Jaypee Brothers Medical Publishers (P) Ltd.
17/1-B, Babar Road, Block-B, Shaymali
Mohammadpur, Dhaka-1207
Bangladesh
Mobile: +08801912003485
E-mail: jaypeedhaka@gmail.com

Jaypee Brothers Medical Publishers (P) Ltd.
Bhotahity, Kathmandu, Nepal
Phone: +977-9741283608
E-mail: kathmandu@jaypeebrothers.com

Website: www.jaypeebrothers.com
Website: www.jaypeedigital.com





**Inquiries for bulk sales may be solicited at:** jaypee@jaypeebrothers.com

***Reconstructive Dermatologic Surgery***

*First Edition:* **2018**

ISBN 978-93-5152-941-5

*Printed at: Ajanta Offset & Packagings Ltd., Faridabad, Haryana*

# Dedicated to

*My wife, Jeannie, and my son, Max, for their support, patience, and love. My sincere gratitude also goes to my mother Shu Hua, and my father Shii Sheng, for their unwavering willingness to sacrifice their own dreams to provide a better future for my sister Grace, my brother Kevin, and myself.*

*My mentors, colleagues, mentees, staff, and patients who made it all possible for me to have a fulfilling academic career.*

***S Brian Jiang***

*All of my mentors who support me and believe in me, especially Dr Jiang, who gave me this opportunity. My husband, Lucius, for his patience and love throughout this challenging process. My deepest appreciation to Manya and Joe, my loving parents, for always putting my education before anything else. Finally, my adorable, sweet, and bright daughter, Joya, who is the light of my life.*

***Arisa E Ortiz***

# Contributors

**Murad Alam** MD MBA MSCI
Vice-Chair
Department of Dermatology
Professor of Dermatology
Otolaryngology and Surgery
Northwestern University
Chicago, IL, USA

**Sarah Tuttleton Arron** MD PhD
Associate Professor of Dermatology
University of California
San Francisco, CA, USA

**Mathew M Avram** MD
Director, MGH Dermatology
Laser and Cosmetic Center
Boston, MA, USA

**Richard G Bennett** MD
Department of Medicine
(Dermatology), University of
California, Los Angeles
Los Angeles, CA, USA

**Jeremy S Bordeaux** MD MPH
Associate Professor of Dermatology
Director, Dermatologic Surgery
Director, Melanoma Program
University Hospitals
Cleveland Medical Center
Case Western Reserve University
School of Medicine
Cleveland, OH, USA

**Andrew Breithaupt**
Clinical Instructor in
Dermatology, UCLA
Harbor-UCLA Medical Center
West-LA VA Hospital
Los Angeles, CA, USA
Torrance Memorial Hospital
Torrance, CA, USA

**John A Carucci** MD PhD
Professor of Dermatology
Chief, Mohs Micrographic and
Dermatologic Surgery
Program Director, Micrographic
Surgery and Dermatologic Oncology
Fellowship
Section of Dermatologic Surgery
Ronald O Perelman Department of
Dermatology
NYU-Langone Medical Center
New York, NY, USA

**T Minsue Chen** MD FACMS
Dermatology, Houston, TX
Dermatologic Surgery
Chen Skin and Cancer Surgery
Philadelphia, PA, USA

**Suneel Chilukuri** MD
Founder, Refresh Dermatology
Associate Clinical Professor
Baylor College of Medicine
Clinical Faculty, University of
North Texas Health Science Center
Forth worth, TX, USA

**Lisa Chipps** MD MS FAAD
Director of Dermatologic Surgery
Harbor-UCLA Medical Center
Los Angeles, CA, USA

**Steven Chow** MD MS
Department of Dermatology
University of Southern California
Los Angeles, CA, USA

**Brienne Cressey** MD MBA
New York Presbyterian
Hospital Weill Cornell
New York, NY, USA

**Tushar Dabade** MD
Department of Dermatology
Northwestern Medical Center
Chicago, IL, USA

**Consuelo V David** MD
Harbor-UCLA Medical Center
Division of Dermatology
Torrance, CA, USA

**Daihung V Do** MD
Director of Dermatologic Surgery
Beth Israel Deaconess Medical
Center, Harvard Medical School
Boston, MA, USA

**Robert Egbers Jr** MD MSc FAAD
Johns Hopkins University
Baltimore, MD, USA

**Robert Edwin Eilers Jr** MD
Former UCSD Fellow
Riverchase Dermatology
Naples, FL, USA

**Thomas D Griffin Jr** MD FAAD
Attending Dermatologist
Dermatology Associates of
Plymouth Meeting
Philadelphia, PA, USA

**Ezra Hazan** MD
Department of Dermatology
and Cutaneous Biology
Thomas Jefferson University Hospital
Philadelphia, PA, USA

**Jennifer Herrmann** MD
Department of Dermatology
University of California
San Francisco, CA, USA

**Brian Hibler** MD
Memorial Sloan Kettering
Cancer Center
Dermatology Service
Department of Medicine
New York, NY, USA

**Omar A Ibrahimi** MD PhD
Connecticut Skin Institute
Stamford, CT, USA

**S Brian Jiang** MD
Clinical Professor of Dermatology
Director
Mohs and Dermatologic Surgery
Surgical Director, Dermatology
Residency Program
Program Director, Micrographic
Surgery and Dermatologic
Oncology Fellowship
Department of Dermatology
University of California
San Diego, CA, USA

**Joseph Kallini** MD
Clinical Research Fellow
Department of Dermatology
Saint Louis University
St. Louis, MO, USA

**Swati Kannan** MD
Clinical Instructor
Department of Dermatology
University of California in
Los Angeles, CA, USA

**Sailesh Konda** MD
Assistant Clinical Professor
Department of Dermatology
University of Florida
College of Medicine
Gainesville, FL, USA
Adjunct Assistant Professor
Department of Dermatology
Loma Linda University
Medical Center
Loma Linda, CA, USA

**Laura Kruter** MD FAAD
Mariwalla Dermatology
West Islip, NY, USA

**Mary Larijani** MD
Department of Dermatology
Drexel University
Philadelphia, PA, USA

**Patrick K Lee** MD
Professor
Director, Dermatologic Surgery
Co-Director, Micrographic Surgery
and Dermatologic
Oncology Fellowship
Associate Residency Program
Director
Department of Dermatology
University of California
Irvine, CA, USA

**Michelle Levender**
Department of Dermatology
University of California
San Francisco, CA, USA

**Jesse M Lewin** MD
Assistant Professor of Dermatology
Columbia University Medical Center
New York, NY, USA

**Ian A Maher** MD
Assistant Professor
Interim Director of Mohs Surgery and
Cutaneous Oncology
Program Director, Mohs Surgery and
Dermatologic Oncology Fellowship
Department of Dermatology
Saint Louis University
St. Louis, MO, USA

**Bassel H Mahmoud** MD PhD FAAD
Associate Professor of Dermatology
University of Massachusetts
Worcester, MA, USA

**Margaret W Mann** MD
Associate Professor of Dermatology
Director of Aesthetic Dermatology
University Hospitals
Cleveland Medical Center
Case Western Reserve University
Cleveland, OH, USA

**J Ramsey Mellette** MD FAAD FACMS
Professor Emeritus of Dermatology
University of Colorado Health
Sciences Center
Denver, CO, USA

**Christopher J Miller** MD
Associate Professor of Dermatology
Director of Dermatologic Surgery
Hospital of the University
of Pennsylvania
Philadelphia, PA, USA

**Lee M Miller** MD
Mohs Surgery
Dermatology Associates of
Southwest Louisiana
Lake Charles, LA, USA

**Kira Minkis** MD PhD
Department of Dermatology
Weill Cornell Medical College
New York, NY, USA

**Vineet Mishra** MD
Director of Mohs Surgery and
Procedural Dermatology
Assistant Professor of Dermatology
University of Texas
Health Science Center
San Antonio, TX, USA

**Megan Morrison** DO FAAD
Associate Professor of Dermatology
Michigan State University
St Thomas Rutherford Hospital
Stones River Dermatology
Murfreesboro, TN, USA

**Kishwer S Nehal** MD
Director of Mohs and
Dermatologic Surgery
Attending Physician, Memorial Sloan
Kettering Cancer Center
Professor of Dermatology
Weill Cornell Medical College
New York, NY, USA

**Bichchau Michelle Nguyen** MD MPH
Director of Dermatologic Surgery
Assistant Professor of Dermatology
Department of Dermatology
Tufts Medical Center
Boston, MA, USA

**G Richard Nichols** MD FAAD FACMS
President and Director of Cutaneous Surgery
Nichols Mohs and Skin Surgery
Columbia, MO, USA

**Suzanne M Olbricht** MD
Associate Professor of Dermatology
Harvard Medical School
Chief of Dermatology
Beth Israel Deaconess Medical Center
Boston, MA, USA

**Arisa E Ortiz** MD
Assistant Clinical Professor of Dermatology
Director, Laser and Cosmetic Dermatology
Department of Dermatology
University of California
San Diego, CA, USA

**Syril Keena T Que** MD
Fellow
Micrographic Surgery and Dermatologic Oncology
Brigham and Women's Hospital
Harvard Medical School
Boston, MA, USA

**Thomas Rohrer** MD
Director of Dermatologic Surgery
SkinCare Physicians
Chestnut Hill, MA, USA

**Anthony M Rossi** MD FAAD
Memorial Sloan Kettering Cancer Center—Dermatology Service
Assistant Professor, Weill Cornell Department of Dermatology
New York Presbyterian Hospital
Weill Cornell, New York, USA

**Ashley G Rubin** MD
Carlsbad Vista Dermatology
Vista, CA, US

**Nazanin Saedi** MD
Associate Professor
Director, Laser Surgery and Cosmetic Dermatology
Co-Director, Cutaneous Surgery
Department of Dermatology and Cutaneous Biology
Thomas Jefferson University
Philadelphia, PA, USA

**Scott Santilli**
University Hospitals of Cleveland Medical Center
Case Western Reserve University
Cleveland, OH, USA

**Aleta Simmons** MD MS
Dermatology Resident Physician
University Hospitals Cleveland Medical Center
Case Western Reserve University
Cleveland, OH, USA

**Joseph F Sobanko** MD
Assistant Professor of Dermatology
Hospital of the University of Pennsylvania
Philadelphia, PA, USA

**Daniel Y Sugai** MD FAAD
Harvard Medical School/Beth Israel Deaconess Medical Center
Department of Dermatology
Boston, MA, USA

**Sarah M Sung** MD FAAD
Westside Dermatology
Seattle, Washington DC, USA

**Anne Marie Tremaine** MD FAAD
Private Practice
Skin Wellness Physicians
Naples, FL, USA

**Timothy Wang** MD
Department of Dermatology
Johns Hopkins Medicine
Baltimore, MD, USA

**Anne Zhuang**
Department of Dermatology
University of California
Davis, CA, USA

# Preface

*Reconstructive Dermatologic Surgery* offers a practical and comprehensive guide to dermatologic surgical reconstruction. The focus of the textbook is geared towards surgical repair of Mohs Micrographic Surgery defects beginning with basic surgical techniques and covering the breadth and depth of extensive repair options through an image-rich format. The chapters are broken down into fundamentals of reconstruction by flap types and by anatomic region to allow for a quick reference to specific anatomic defects. Other topics covered in the textbook include designing a surgical suite and postoperative management. This practical resource is meant for residents, fellows and experienced surgeons across a wide-range of surgical specialties who want to hone their surgical skills. We have included authors from various academic centers around the United States to represent a cross-section of different philosophies and approaches to surgical repairs culminating many years of experience in the surgical management of skin cancers.

**S Brian Jiang**
**Arisa E Ortiz**

# Acknowledgments

We are extremely grateful to the wonderful authors who helped finalize this textbook. We sincerely appreciate our contributors' time, effort, expertise and dedication to the completion of these outstanding chapters. We would also like to thank the publishing team for their diligence and hard work to make this textbook a reality.

I especially appreciate the constant support and encouragement of Mr Jitendar P Vij (Group Chairman) and Mr Ankit Vij (Group President) of Jaypee Brothers Medical Publishers (P) Ltd., New Delhi, India in helping publish this textbook and also their Associates particularly Ms Chetna Malhotra Vohra (Associate Director–Content Strategy), Ms Kritika Dua (Development Editor) who have been prompt, efficient and most helpful.

# Contents

# CHAPTER 1

# Surgical Space and Equipment

*Lee M Miller, Vineet Mishra*

## INTRODUCTION

The ideal dermatologic surgery office provides an efficient, safe, and comfortable environment for the patients, staff, and the physician. Dermatologic surgery encompasses a wide variety of procedures, which may be performed in various settings. As such, there is no template for the *perfect*—one size fits all—dermatologic surgery office. Rather, each *ideal* office will vary considerably based on the practice's scope as well as current and future needs. The pursuit of such an office can be daunting, as there are many factors to consider. In the beginning, the expenses will heavily outweigh the collections, but these growing pains can be tempered with efficiency and slow, steady growth that meets market demand. Armed with a vision, motivation, appropriate planning, seeking of expert advice, and careful attention to detail, this can prove to be a rewarding venture. The intent of this text is to provide the reader with a basic understanding of the design and planning process and explore other pertinent concepts.

## TYPES OF FACILITIES

There are several different types of outpatient surgical facilities, each with their own benefits. For a general dermatologist practicing primarily medical dermatology with some minor surgical procedures, such as excisional or laser surgery, a dedicated surgical room within a standard medical office will likely be sufficient. This layout while easy to setup and inexpensive to build adds flexibility for the general dermatologist. In a group setting, one surgical room may even be used by multiple physicians in the clinic on an as needed basis. However, this will not be sufficient for a primarily surgical practice.

An office-based surgery practice requires multiple surgical rooms according to the desired size and the number of practitioners. This is often more appropriate for a Mohs micrographic surgery or cosmetic surgical practice. These layouts may vary substantially depending on the physician's ideal configuration. The surgical rooms are often larger in size and fitted with a power surgical table, possibly overhead surgical lighting, and in-room storage of surgical supplies. An office-based surgery practice may be composed entirely of surgical rooms or incorporate smaller examination rooms, which can be used for consultations and follow-up visits. Other areas may be added to this type of practice depending on need such as clean/dirty room, supply stock room, nursing station, laser/medical device storage, and laboratory. If constructing the space from scratch, one may consider the future possibility of upgrading to an ambulatory surgical center (ASC).[1]

An ASC is the most elaborate outpatient surgical facility. Their popularity has increased among some specialties.[2] They may be owned by physicians, hospitals, or some combination thereof. In the context of dermatology, the ASC is often an extension of a surgical dermatology practice, consisting of one or two operating rooms that are used part-time. When partially or completely hospital owned, ASCs tend to be larger, freestanding facilities with many more operating rooms and a full-time staff.[1] Regulations and licensure for ASCs occur at the state level, and vary considerably state by state.[2] In addition to state licensure, these facilities need to be certified by Medicare. Ambulatory surgical centers require extensive planning as the requirements are much more stringent, and may not be feasible for certain practices. Examples include a separate entrance, a separate waiting area, a dedicated recovery room, automatically activated fireproof doors, ceiling sprinkler system, 1-hour firebreaks in walls, 2-hour firebreaks in floors, and a backup emergency power source, just to name a few. Meeting these construction requirements is often much more costly than meeting the standard commercial building code required of a physician's office. The primary advantages of the ASC are the ability to offer a higher level of care and to collect a facility fee.[1]

The final outpatient-surgical facility type is that of a hospital outpatient department. These facilities offer ambulatory services, but are completely owned by a hospital. These are often similar to office-based surgical practices but considered extensions of the hospital. Therefore, hospital outpatient departments are accredited by the Joint Commission on Accreditation of Healthcare Organizations (JCAHO).

## ACCREDITATION

No matter which facility type is chosen, an office-based surgical practice may be accredited or nonaccredited. Accreditation requires evaluation of office policies, procedures, and facilities, demonstrating compliance with nationally recognized standards of excellence.[3] It is independent from the state licensure and medicare certification required of ASCs. It is optional, but may be required for payment from various third-party payers. The Accreditation Association for Ambulatory Health Care and the JCAHO offer office-based surgery accreditation to dermatologists. Compliance is verified for the practice via inspection by a specially trained surveyor. Overall, accreditation demonstrates to the public and the medical community the delivery of high-quality care; though, some believe that the added expense is not justified.[1,3] Some third-party payers will allow facility fees for procedures performed in accredited offices. However, ASC licensure and medicare certification are typically required to collect these fees. State regulation regarding office-based surgery varies with respect to state inspections or accreditation requirements. However, office-based surgery accreditation is currently not required in any state when only local anesthesia is used in the office.[1] The pursuit of accreditation should be considered when opening a practice as it may become more relevant in the future.

## LABORATORY CERTIFICATION

When opening a laboratory, payers will require proof that the laboratory is compliant/registered with Clinical Laboratory Improvement Act. This organization, established in 1988, is responsible for the federal regulatory standards that apply to clinical laboratory testing in the United States, except in clinical trials and basic research. When a laboratory is first opened, a certificate of registration must be obtained. Following the first successful inspection of the laboratory, a certificate of compliance is issued. This must be maintained and usually requires reinspection of the laboratory facility every 2 years. Clinical Laboratory Improvement Act grades specific types of testing as low, moderate, or high complexity based on several criteria, including knowledge; training and experience; reagents and materials preparation; characteristics of operational steps; calibration, quality control, and proficiency testing materials; test system troubleshooting and equipment maintenance; as well as interpretation and judgment. Clinical Laboratory Improvement Act focuses on various components of the laboratory through the inspection process, including but not limited to procedure manual, education and training of the employees, quality assurance, and quality control measures. The processing of fresh tissue samples for microscopic examination, as in Mohs micrographic surgery, qualifies as high complexity and therefore is subject to more stringent regulatory criteria. Careful attention should be paid to these criteria in order to provide for smooth laboratory operations and maintenance of certification.

## UNDERSTANDING THE MARKET

It is important to properly understand local market dynamics, assess the potential, cultivate a referral base, and manage expenses within the location. This begins with awareness of the patients' needs. Services new to the community should be strategically added to the practice. An untested market demographic may not respond to a rapid blitz of marketing and new services. However, smartly offering new services to the area will likely attract patients to the practice.

Proximity to hospitals allows for collaboration with other specialties. However, if multispecialty groups or managed-care clinics are nearby and offer similar services already, referrals may be difficult to garner.[4] This may make cultivating a referral base more difficult for the solo practitioner. Therefore, offering selective new services to the community can assist with attracting new patients.

Although advertising can be helpful, it is important to track the success from advertising on the Internet, on the radio, and in print, in order to streamline one's marketing strategy. A marketing expert can assist with formulating a strategy for advertising and subsequently tracking its success.

## CLINICAL SPACE

Dermatologic surgery offices exist in various sizes and configurations. For the surgeon, building a practice from scratch requires considerable thought. For those adding a dermatologic surgical practice to an existing space, options may be limited. While many clinical spaces and layouts may be sufficient, there are certain basic principles that will help increase the efficiency of the practice.

First off, there must be appropriate square footage for an efficient layout. This implies having procedure rooms large enough to accommodate the necessary personnel and equipment comfortably, as well as a sufficient number of rooms to promote efficient workflow. Due to additional staff and equipment, procedural rooms require more space than examination rooms. A generally accepted minimum procedural room size is 12 × 12 feet.[1] This ought to accommodate a procedural table, cabinetry, and additional equipment as required. Rooms intended for laser treatment may need to be even larger, due to the size of some of these devices. Regarding the number of rooms, one must consider the potential volume of patients to be seen and the amount of time spent in each room. For a Mohs surgery practice, fewer rooms are needed if a waiting room is available where patients may wait while their tissue is being processed. However, when practicing in a group setting, it may not be ideal to mix patients with large surgical defects and bandages with those waiting for a general dermatology appointment. A second waiting room is generally preferred in this setting.

In terms of overall layout, it is often useful to have multiple rooms configured around a frequently used central space such as a clean/dirty room, supply stock room, nursing station, laboratory (in the case of Mohs micrographic surgery), or any combination of the above. This increases efficiency by assuring this frequently used space is always nearby. A surgical practice will need to consider adequate space for an efficient frozen section laboratory, with space for a grossing station, cryostats, a staining area with adequate ventilation, slide storage (for at least 10 years of slides), and a sink for cleaning supplies. A medical architect can assist with planning for various patient traffic and workflow patterns based on the services provided.

Designing an office can be quite complex, particularly if an ASC is to be incorporated. There will be many decisions to be made on a multitude of issues such as climate control, ventilation, lighting, hardware, doors, windows, cabinetry, plumbing, acoustics, flooring, wall coverings, furniture, color themes, window treatments, countertops, and signage. It is also wise to plan for any foreseeable wiring needs such as electrical outlets (including 220 V outlets for lasers), wiring for audio systems, and for computer networks. While wireless hardware is gaining ground, a hardwired computer network is more secure and can be of great value in the event of wireless problems. It is much more expensive to retrofit a wired network than installing upon initial construction. These are but a few examples of the many matters to address when going through the design process. Working with experts in their respective fields, such as medical architects and interior designers, can streamline the process and relieve the physician of much of this burden. They can assist the physician in planning and building the ideal space for the practice style and patient population envisioned.

## LEASING VERSUS OWNING

There are several considerations when deciding whether to rent or to purchase. The first and most obvious is the difference in upfront cost, particularly for a new practice in an untested market, for which revenue may be difficult to forecast. Ideally, the space should allow for the possibility of future expansion and have a renewable lease provided the space meets your needs.

Renting or leasing a medical office has the advantages of requiring less initial capital, less time to prepare, and a smaller commitment overall. In addition, insurance on the building, maintenance costs, and property taxes are also avoided. However, there is no ability to accumulate equity in the building or deduct building depreciation from practice income as a tax incentive. There may also be restrictions on what modifications can be made to the space. It is advisable to contact local hospitals to identify available medical office space in the area. If space is found without using an agent, it may be possible to negotiate a better rate by avoiding the agent's commission.

In contrast, the primary advantages of ownership are deductible building depreciation and the ability to accrue equity in the building, which would otherwise be lost to rent. A single owner-occupied office building has the advantage of complete autonomy and lower total building cost. While, a multitenant, multifloor building will typically have lower construction cost per square foot since only one foundation and one roof are required. Whether deciding to build or lease, the planning process is the foundation for ensuring that final space will meet all of the anticipated needs. While the space, which is designed and purpose-built, will be closest to the ideal, it may be out of the price range of the physician new to practice. An already outfitted rental office will be less costly upfront, allowing the physician time to examine the area closely and determine the optimal place to establish, while immediately providing the physician providing a place to practice upon completion of training.

## EQUIPMENT

A large amount of equipment is required for a dermatologic surgery office to run efficiently. These include computer systems, printers, fax machines, telephone systems, copiers, surgical equipment, and laboratory equipment, just to name a few. In general, it is more economical to purchase smaller office equipment items such as surgical instruments, computers, printers, fax machines, and simple copy machines. Regarding computer and telephone systems, it is reasonable to start small, but wise to maintain the ability to expand to accommodate future growth. For larger, more durable surgical or laboratory equipment, such as powered surgical tables, overhead surgical lights, electrosurgical generators, cryostats, autostainers, and microscopes, outright purchase may be prudent, as these items tend to have long service life and few problems with proper care and maintenance. Although many of these are quite costly if purchased new, second hand equipment may be found and purchased at a substantial savings. Exceptions to this general rule might include equipment whose lease includes a maintenance agreement for regular servicing such as high-capacity copiers or lasers that may become obsolete in a few years.[4]

## SURGICAL BEDS

There are many options to choose from when selecting surgical beds as they typically represent a significant portion of the overall equipment startup cost. Since patients will sometimes spend lengthy periods of time in them, finding a surgical bed that is comfortable for patients, efficient to operate, durable for many years of use, and appropriate for the allocated space is of great importance. There are many high-quality surgical bed models that fit these criteria, and if properly maintained, it will last many years.

If budget allows wireless controls, this can be of wonderful benefit as they allow placement of the controls anywhere in the room without cluttering the floor with wires. This may be particularly important in a practice that will be moving devices such as lasers from room to room on a regular basis. A swiveling base is another useful feature, particularly if treatment rooms are smaller in size, or if multiple devices are to be used in one treatment session. However, having this kind of base may raise the table by a few inches over the base model table and can therefore be slightly more difficult for the weaker patient to access without a footstool.

Lastly, some thought needs to be given to preferred operating positions, and when possible the surgeon should experiment with anticipated operating positions at trade shows or other suitable environment to ensure comfort. If operating in a seated position is planned, the thickness of the table back should be examined as well as the location of the table paper roll, as these may encroach on potential knee/leg space under the table back.

## LIGHTING

Dermatology is an inherently visual specialty. As such, lighting is very important in clinical practice. For the dermatologic surgeon, superb quality lighting is of even higher priority. Supplemental lighting can come in many shapes, sizes, and intensities. These can be in the form of micro head lamps mounted to surgical telescopes, traditional head lamps, fiberoptic head lamps, mobile stand mounted surgical lights, and various types of ceiling mounted surgical lights.

One notable shift in light sources found in the consumer market has been the increased prevalence of light emitting diodes (LEDs) as light sources, and this technology has also spilled over into medical applications. These light sources are incredibly efficient when compared to more traditional incandescent lamps. They are able to produce more light with less heat generation at higher color temperatures (resulting in a "cooler" bluish white light), which better mimics natural sunlight than incandescent light sources.

## SMOKE MANAGEMENT

The use of electrosurgery (including electrocautery, electrodessication, electrofulguration, electrocoagulation, and electrosection) and lasers is associated with the production of surgical smoke. Evidence is mounting that this smoke contains harmful products with the potential for infection, carcinogenesis, and pulmonary damage.[5,6]

Smoke is produced when tissue is rapidly heated above the boiling point and cellular contents are released as fine particles. It is composed of 95% water and 5% particulate matter, including chemicals, viruses, bacteria, and blood and tissue particles.[7] A comprehensive review of the contents of surgical smoke is beyond the scope of this chapter, but there are a few noteworthy components. There are numerous chemicals including hydrocarbons, phenols, nitriles, and fatty acids, found in surgical smoke. Of these, carbon monoxide, benzene, acetylene, butadiene, acrylonitrile, and hydrogen cyanide receive significant attention. Short-term exposure to many of these agents may result in dizziness, nausea, vomiting, headache, and irritation of the eyes, nose, and respiratory tract.[5] Benzene has been linked with the development of blood disorders from anemia to leukemia and has been found in surgical smoke at concentrations of 0.02 ppm. The occupational safety and health administration (OSHA) has established the permissible exposure limit of benzene at 10 ppm.[5] Acrylonitrile is an odiferous liquid that forms hydrogen cyanide, and long-term exposure has been shown to cause cancer in animals and has been linked with a higher incidence of cancer in humans.[8] The level of hydrogen cyanide in surgical smoke has been estimated to be 30 times less than that of directly inhaled smoke from a cigarette.[9] Hydrogen cyanide has been attributed with 89% of the cardiovascular potency of cigarette smoke. Butadiene is also of concern and has been attributed with 45% of the cancer potency. It has been presumed that surgical smoke may present an overall health risk similar to that of chronic second-hand smoke.[10] Adverse pulmonary effects found in rats exposed to surgical smoke included pathologic changes consistent with vascular hypertrophy, alveolar congestion, interstitial pneumonia, bronchiolitis, and emphysema.[11,12] The severity of changes increased proportionately with the duration of exposure. While there is no doubt there are concerning agents present within surgical smoke, it is difficult to determine the concentration of such agents and therefore the true exposure level. In addition, the effect of chronic low-level exposure to these agents is unknown.

In addition to the troubling chemical components found, there are concerns that surgical smoke may have mutagenic effects and even be capable of transmitting viable malignant cells. Gatti et al. found that surgical smoke had mutagenic effects on several strains of Salmonella.[13] Fletcher et al. cauterized murine melanoma tissue and found the surgical smoke was able to carry viable malignant cells after cauterization.[14] The aerosolization of viable malignant cells identified in this in vitro study highlights the importance of respiratory precautions and smoke evacuation during the surgical treatment of cutaneous malignancies such as basal cell carcinoma, squamous cell carcinoma, and melanoma. While these findings raise concern, no known cases of resultant malignant transformation in a human host exist.

Lastly, there is some concern as to the potential infectious nature of surgical smoke, and the literature on this subject has grown. Most of the focus to date has been on the viability of viruses in surgical and laser smoke plumes.[15-20] Intact bovine papillomavirus and human papillomavirus (HPV) have been recovered from the smoke of bovine and human lesions treated with $CO_2$ laser. In 1995, Gloster and Roenigk have shown that $CO_2$ laser surgeons carry a higher risk of developing nasopharyngeal papillomatosis and lower risk of developing plantar, genital, and perianal warts when compared to patients in the community.[19] This is presumably related to inhalation of HPV contained in the laser smoke plume. In 2002, Garden et al. were able to reproduce warts in calves by injecting aerosol collected from the surgical laser plume developed from tissue infected with bovine papillomavirus and treated with $CO_2$ laser at various settings.[17] The tumors produced were shown to be both biochemically and histologically the same virus as present in the laser plume. In addition, there are two reports of healthcare providers developing laryngeal papillomatosis as a result of laser and electrodesiccation of HPV-related anogenital condyloma.[21,22] Though many of these studies use modalities that do not compare with clinical exposure during procedures, they certainly raise concern, warrant further investigation, and reinforce the use of simple protective measures.

Current practice guidelines for protection against surgical smoke exist in some organizations, such as the association for perioperative registered nurses, but are often directed toward the operating room setting rather than an outpatient office setting. Currently, no guidelines are available from OSHA. Rather they state, "Although there has been no documented transmission of infectious disease through surgical smoke, the potential for generating infectious viral fragments, particularly following treatment of venereal warts, may exist. Local smoke evacuation systems have been recommended by consensus organizations, and may improve the quality of the operating field."[23] Despite these consensus warnings, many dermatologists in practice use little to no precaution while using lasers or electrocautery. A worldwide web-based survey examining the surgical smoke practices in North America supports this observation in that 82% and 83% of respondents report "seldom or never" using local exhaust ventilation (including wall suction, smoke evacuator, and respiratory protection) when removing benign and malignant lesions, respectively. Using lasers, 65% and 61% report seldom or never using local exhaust ventilation when removing benign or malignant skin lesions, respectively.[24]

Traditional surgical masks have varying protection from particles ranging from 1 to 9 µm.[25] High filtration masks designed for laser procedures provide greater filtration of particle sizes down to 1.1 µm.[26] However, electrosurgical units and lasers often create particles of ~0.07 and 0.31 µm, respectively.[27] In fact, it has been shown that 77% of particulate matter in surgical smoke is <1.1 µm.[28] While surgical masks offer some protection from larger particles contained in surgical smoke, they may be insufficient as a singular intervention.

Smoke evacuation via either small portable smoke evacuators or wall suction plays a vital role in smoke management as well. There is evidence that use of a smoke evacuator results in a significant reduction in the amount of smoke reaching the level of the surgeon's mask.[29] It can achieve impressive clearance of surgical smoke, but must be used correctly. One study revealed that they are 98.6% effective when placed within 1 cm of the treatment side, but efficacy drops to 50% when the distance is increased to 2 cm.[20] Proper use of smoke evacuation is recommended in combination with high filtration surgical masks for optimal protection from surgical smoke.

## STERILIZATION

In a dermatologic surgical practice, there will undoubtedly be a need to sterilize instruments. This is a process whereby microorganisms, including spores, are removed or destroyed from the instrument. There are a variety of means to accomplish this goal. The best method will vary from practice to practice, based on the size of the practice and a number of other features.

Sterilization via autoclave is one of the most common ways for an office-based practice to sterilize surgical items. These are relatively small countertop units, which use steam under pressure to sterilize instruments and/or surgical drapes. They may be used to sterilize liquids, glass, metal instruments, paper, and cotton. While they are often one of the most amenable to office-based practice, they are capable of damaging heat sensitive items and the repeated exposure to high humidity may dull sharp cutting surfaces of high-grade carbon instruments.[1]

Other means of sterilization include heated chemical vapor, dry heat, gas sterilization, and chemical immersion. Each of these may have certain perceived advantages over autoclave, but are usually more cumbersome for the office-based practice setting. Heated chemical vapor eliminates exposure to humidity, drying time, and decreases sterilization time, but requires alcohol or formaldehyde. These chemicals necessitate the use of protective equipment, adequate ventilation, and safety monitoring. Dry heat avoids both the dulling effects of humidity and toxicity of chemicals but items will be exposed to high temperatures for extended periods of time. This precludes heat sensitive items, adds time to the sterilization process, and demands a cooling period before being handled by staff to avoid burn injuries. Gas sterilization uses prolonged exposure to ethylene dioxide or formaldehyde gas, and may be used to sterilize heat or moisture sensitive items. However, both gases are toxic and known carcinogens and require strict monitoring per OSHA, given their hazardous nature. As such, this method is usually restricted to hospital settings. Lastly, chemical immersion may be used, by soaking instruments in glutaraldehyde or aqueous formaldehyde. However, this method is not reliably sporicidal and thus may be better classified as a cold disinfectant rather than sterilization technique. Following, prolonged immersion times of 6–12 hours, instruments must be handled in sterile fashion, rinsed with sterile water—as both chemicals are toxic—and dried. In order to avoid contamination, they cannot be wrapped and must be used immediately following drying.[1] If one is practicing in a large multispecialty group setting, a larger ASC or hospital setting, some of these methods such as gas sterilization may be available. Otherwise, for the office-based practice, autoclave generally is the most economical, and sterilization of heat-sensitive items may need to be outsourced.

Regarding preparation of a sterile field around the surgical site, one may use sterile paper surgical drapes, disposable sterile cloth surgical towels, or reusable cloth surgical towels. Paper drapes are most economical, but are sometimes frustrating to work with—even with adhesive around the site—, have poor absorption characteristics, and may be uncomfortable to the patient. While reusable towels are more expensive initially, they often feel nicer for patients in the author's experience and are less wasteful. In addition, they decrease the consumables cost for the practice; although, the difference narrows once the man-hours required to wash, fold, and sterilize them are factored. The best choice will likely vary from practice to practice, but if reusable towels are being considered, remember to include a washroom with appropriate electrical, water, and exhaust vent lines for a washer and dryer.

## PERSONNEL

Finding good office personnel is critical to the long-term success of a practice. In the process of seeing one physician, patients will interact with numerous other members of the healthcare team. These individuals often give the first and last impressions to the patients, and can often deeply impact the patients' experience. It is key to find the right personnel who understands and shares the same vision for the practice while striving for service excellence.

The first step is to determine what qualifications are needed for each position. This may vary from state to state, as in some states, there are restrictions as to what level of training is required to perform local anesthesia, etc. The state board of nursing is often helpful with such scope of practice issues. To reach maximum efficiency, all personnel need to be functioning at the highest appropriate level at all times. Once there is a plan as to the number and skill level of employees required, one can begin the search and interview process. Requesting a cover letter with resume provides additional information and may allow for efficient sorting of applications of those who can and cannot draft a succinct letter—thus, avoiding an unnecessary interview. It is highly recommended to interview employees personally, especially for clinical positions and front office, as these will have a great deal of direct interaction with patients. If the physician is pressed for time, consider interviewing finalists, which are preinterviewed by an office manager.

Finding the right personality match for the team is of the utmost importance as skills such as using computer software or assisting in surgery are easier to teach than changing personalities or instructing someone to be pleasant. Also, consider having trusted existing staff interview the applicant, even if informally, as they may gain added insight outside of the formal interview with the physician. Look for above average candidates who are nice, well-rounded individuals based on their impression at the interview and their references. If there is insufficient response to the first cycle of interviews, it is better to place another advertisement for the position than to settle for a marginal candidate from a limited pool of applicants. Just one sub-par employee can potentially wreak havoc on an otherwise outstanding team. A simple test of whether to keep an employee is to ask, "Had I known before hiring what I know now about the employee's performance would I have hired him/her in the first place?" If the answer to this question is "no," the employee should be replaced.[4]

Employees should be provided with job descriptions, which clarify the objectives regularly expected of each employee. While each will have his role, it is also wise to cross train staff to work in multiple areas of the clinic such as front desk, medical records, and/or clinical staff. This provides options as the business expands and continuous coverage in the event an employee is absent. In addition to clear expectations, periodic evaluations are an important part of maintaining a healthy and efficient work environment. This provides feedback on employee performance and an opportunity for improvement in any areas lacking. As the leader of the team, it is the physician's responsibility to compliment exemplary staff performance in the presence of other staff or patients. However, addressing deficient performance should always be done privately, and may be viewed as an "opportunity for improvement." An office manager can assist greatly in organization of the formal evaluation process.

Employees will expect to be compensated fairly for their service. Regional comparative salary and benefit information is available from the medical group management association, as well as other various salary and benefit surveys. In a young practice, it is recommended to use an outside payroll service, which is less costly and simplifies the recordkeeping. They will assist in tracking hours, paid time off, withholdings, pensions, flexible benefit contributions, and tax accounting information for the office administrator.[4]

## CONCLUSION

Dermatologic surgery practices exist in many forms, with varying scope of practice. While they vary in size, layout, and style, each shares the common goals of providing an efficient, safe, and comfortable environment for the patients, staff, and physician. Designing a dermatologic surgery practice is fraught with many issues, which differ greatly from that for which physicians have been extensively trained through residency and/or fellowship. However, there are many resources to assist the physician through this process. With diligent study of the available options, wisdom gained from colleagues having recently been through the process, and consultation with experts in their respective fields, such as interior designers, contractors, and medical architects, decisions can be made confidently regarding building the ideal practice for the physician.

## REFERENCES


1. Robinson J, Hanke CW, Siegel D, et al. Surgery of the Skin, Procedural Dermatology, 3rd edition. St. Louis, MO Elsevier; 2014.
2. Small NC, Bert JM. Office ambulatory surgery centers: creation and management. J Am Acad Orthop Surg. 2003; 11:157-62.
3. Sterling JB, Hanke CW. Office accreditation in dermatology. Semin Cutan Med Surg. 2005;24:128-32.
4. Siegel D. Next Steps in Derm Guide. In: Journal of Drugs and Dermatology. New York, NY. Sanova Works; 2015.
5. Lewin JM, Brauer JA, Ostad A. Surgical smoke and the dermatologist. J Am Acad Dermatol. 2011;65:636-41.
6. Oganesyan G, Eimpunth S, Kim SS, et al. Surgical smoke in dermatologic surgery. Dermatol Surg. 2014;40:1373-7.
7. Gonzalez-Bayon L, Gonzalez-Moreno S, Ortega-Perez G. Safety considerations for operating room personnel during hyperthermic intraoperative intraperitoneal chemotherapy perfusion. Eur J Surg Oncol. 2006;32:619-24.
8. Alp E, Bijl D, Bleichrodt RP, et al. Surgical smoke and infection control. J Hosp Infect. 2006;62:1-5.
9. Moot AR, Ledingham KM, Wilson PF, et al. Composition of volatile organic compounds in diathermy plume as detected by selected ion flow tube mass spectrometry. ANZ J Surg. 2007;77:20-3.
10. Laugesen M, Fowles J. Scope for regulation of cigarette smoke toxicity according to brand differences in published toxicant emissions. N Z Med J. 2005;118:U1401.
11. Baggish MS, Elbakry M. The effects of laser smoke on the lungs of rats. Am J Obstet Gynecol. 1987;156:1260-5.
12. Wenig BL, Stenson KM, Wenig BM, et al. Effects of plume produced by the Nd:YAG laser and electrocautery on the respiratory system. Lasers Surg Med. 1993;13:242-5.
13. Gatti JE, Bryant CJ, Noone RB, et al. The mutagenicity of electrocautery smoke. Plast Reconstr Surg. 1992;89:781-4; discussion 85-6.
14. Fletcher JN, Mew D, DesCoteaux JG. Dissemination of melanoma cells within electrocautery plume. Am J Surg. 1999;178:57-9.
15. Baggish MS, Poiesz BJ, Joret D, et al. Presence of human immunodeficiency virus DNA in laser smoke. Lasers Surg Med. 1991;11:197-203.
16. Ferenczy A, Bergeron C, Richart RM. Human papillomavirus DNA in $CO_2$ laser-generated plume of smoke and its consequences to the surgeon. Obstet Gynecol. 1990;75:114-8.
17. Garden JM, O'Banion MK, Bakus AD, et al. Viral disease transmitted by laser-generated plume (aerosol). Arch Dermatol. 2002;138:1303-7.
18. Garden JM, O'Banion MK, Shelnitz LS, et al. Papillomavirus in the vapor of carbon dioxide laser-treated verrucae. JAMA. 1988;259:1199-202.
19. Gloster HM Jr, Roenigk RK. Risk of acquiring human papillomavirus from the plume produced by the carbon dioxide laser in the treatment of warts. J Am Acad Dermatol. 1995;32:436-41.
20. Sawchuk WS, Weber PJ, Lowy DR, et al. Infectious papillomavirus in the vapor of warts treated with carbon dioxide laser or electrocoagulation: detection and protection. J Am Acad Dermatol. 1989;21:41-9.
21. Calero L, Brusis T. [Laryngeal papillomatosis—first recognition in Germany as an occupational disease in an operating room nurse]. Laryngorhinootologie. 2003;82:790-3. [Article in German]
22. Hallmo P, Naess O. Laryngeal papillomatosis with human papillomavirus DNA contracted by a laser surgeon. Eur Arch Otorhinolaryngol. 1991;248:425-7.
23. OSHA health and safety topics—laser/electrosurgery plume. Available at https://www.osha.gov/SLTC/laserelectrosurgeryplume 2015.
24. Edwards BE, Reiman RE. Results of a survey on current surgical smoke control practices. AORN J. 2008;87:739-49.
25. Chen SK, Vesley D, Brosseau LM, et al. Evaluation of single-use masks and respirators for protection of health care workers against mycobacterial aerosols. Am J Infect Control. 1994;22:65-74.
26. Taravella MJ, Viega J, Luiszer F, et al. Respirable particles in the excimer laser plume. J Cataract Refract Surg. 2001;27:604-7.
27. Ulmer BC. The hazards of surgical smoke. AORN J. 2008;87: 721-34; quiz 35-8.
28. Kunachak S, Sobhon P. The potential alveolar hazard of carbon dioxide laser-induced smoke. J Med Assoc Thai. 1998;81:278-82.
29. Pillinger SH, Delbridge L, Lewis DR. Randomized clinical trial of suction versus standard clearance of the diathermy plume. Br J Surg. 2003;90:1068-71.

# CHAPTER 2

# Surgical Instruments

*Ashley G Rubin, Arisa E Ortiz, S Brian Jiang*

## INTRODUCTION

Various surgical instruments are used in the expanding field of dermatologic surgery. Slight structural variations to these individual instruments allow for differences in functionality so that tools may be best selected for the specific task at hand. This chapter will detail types of instruments most commonly utilized in procedural dermatology. Knowledge of the various tools and materials available will further enhance the skill of the dermatologic surgeon. Proper investment and selection of surgical instruments will influence surgical outcomes by enhancing cosmesis and functionality. Dermatologic surgeons must carefully select tools that will fulfill their needs while also considering quality and cost.

## SCALPEL HANDLES

Scalpel handles are available in a variety of shapes and sizes suited for different surgical needs. The Bard-Parker number (No.) 3 handle is most commonly used in dermatologic surgery (Fig. 2.1, top).[1] This is a flat handle and fits No. 10, 11, and 15 blades.[2] This handle commonly includes a ruler on its side, which is very helpful for operative measurements.[2] Alternatively, the Bard-Parker No. 7 handle, which is preferred by some other surgeons, is thinner and has a slightly rounded and textured shaft. Some surgeons feel this handle offers more control as the operator can slightly roll this handle in his/her fingers to produce fine adjustments while cutting.[3]

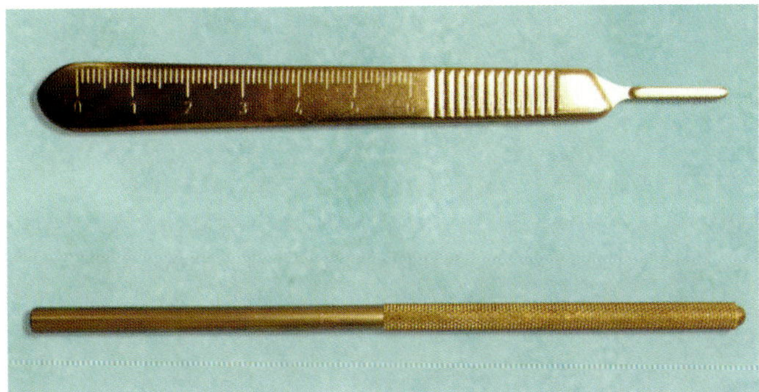

**Fig. 2.1:** Scalpel handles: the most commonly used handle in dermatologic surgery is the No. 3 Bard-Parker handle (top). The rounded Beaver handle (bottom).

The Beaver handle is a scalpel handle that is less frequently used by dermatologic surgeons but has a unique role (Fig. 2.1, bottom). This handle is round or hexagonal and may be useful for delicate work, especially when working in concavities.[1,2] The Beaver handle holds a different set of blades than does the Bard-Parker handle (see below). The surgeon's fingertips may easily roll this handle, increasing fine control with subtle movements.[3]

A third less commonly used system is the Shaw Hemostatic Scalpel. This system may be employed during procedures when hemostasis is more difficult to achieve, for example, in rhinophymatous revision. The handle is attached to a heat source allowing the blade to simultaneously seal vessels and cut tissue. These handles fit standard sized Bard-Parker blades (see below).[1]

## SCALPEL BLADES

The addition of the blade to the scalpel handle completes the scalpel. There are two main groups of blades used in dermatologic surgery: Bard-Parker blades and Beaver blades. Scalpel blades may be comprised of stainless steel or carbon steel. Stainless steel blades are generally preferred due to their affordability, relative to carbon steel blades, and their ability to maintain sharpness.[2,3] Carbon steel blades are sharper initially but dull more quickly with use.[2]

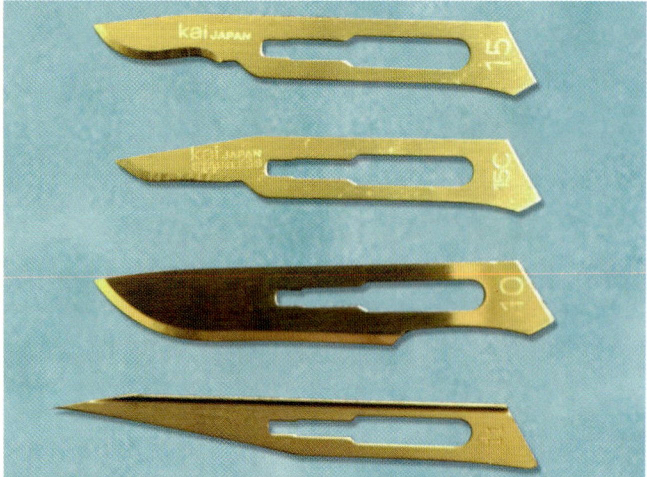


**Fig. 2.2:** Scalpel blades: the most commonly used blades, Bard-Parker blades, fit onto the Bard-Parker scalpel handle. From the top to bottom: Nos. 15, 15C, 10, and 11.

Dermatologists most commonly utilize the numbers 15, 15C, 10, and 11 Bard-Parker blades, which fit onto Bard-Parker handles (Fig. 2.2).[1] The No. 15 blade is the workhorse for dermatologic surgery; it is appropriate for most skin surgeries. This most commonly used blade is slightly curved. In addition to its use in cutaneous procedures, such as excisions and Mohs micrographic surgery (MMS), a No. 15 blade may also be used to perform skin biopsies.[3] The 15C blade is smaller and may be selected for use on thinner skin, such as periocular areas, or in smaller areas, such as the nasal ala.[1,2] The shape of the No. 10 blade is similar to the No. 15 except it is wider and therefore, usually selected for larger excisions on thick skin, such as the back.[1-3] It is important to add that the sharpest part of a curved blade is the belly not the tip.[3] Conversely, the No. 11 blade is tapered to a sharp point and is most appropriate when a puncture or pinpoint incision is desired, such as for an incision and drainage procedure or milia removal.[1-3] Some surgeons also may use this blade when cutting sharp corners of a cutaneous flap during reconstructive procedures.[1,2]

The blade for a Beaver handle is held in place between two jaws.[2] The most commonly used Beaver blades are the Nos. 64, 65, and 67. Beaver blades, in general, are smaller and sharper than standard scalpel blades,[1] but also dull more quickly.[3] The No. 64 blade has a blunt, rounded tip and may be useful during periocular procedures or in concavities, like the conchal bowl.[1-3] The No. 65 blade is similar in shape to the No. 11 blade but smaller. The No. 67 blade is smaller but similar in shape to the No. 15 blade; it is convexly curved with a sharp tip.[1-3] Finally, the tympanoplasty blade may be placed on the Beaver handle and used to obtain MMS layers in areas where beveling of standard scalpel handles would be difficult to achieve. The tympanoplasty blade may be useful during MMS when tumors are located: inside the nares on the nasal mucosa, on certain curved surfaces of the pinna of the ear, and when tumors are advancing into the external auditory meatus (Fig. 2.3).

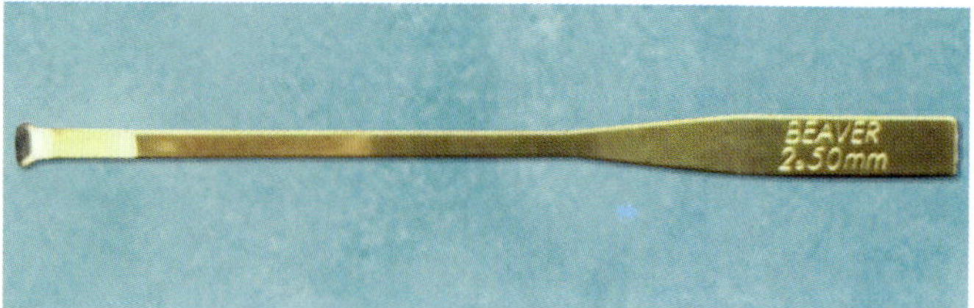


**Fig. 2.3:** The tympanoplasty blade fits onto the Beaver handle.

## NEEDLE HOLDERS

Just like handles and blades, there are various types of needle holders with subtle differences best suiting them for different procedures (Figs. 2.4 and 2.5). Due to the metal-on-metal contact of the needle holder and needle, needle holder selection should reflect the type of needle to be used in the procedure at hand. In general, smaller needle holders are better for smaller needles and larger holders for larger needles. Proper selection will decrease the likelihood of damage; improperly sized holders may damage fine needles and large needles may damage delicate, small holders.[1-3] The jaws of the needle holder may be smooth or serrated (Figs. 2.4 and 2.5); smooth jaws better accommodate fine needles and may be used for more delicate procedures.[1,2] Although smooth jaws are less likely to damage fine needles, they are more likely than serrated jaws to result in slippage.[3] In addition to choosing the appropriate needle holder based on the suture material to be used, anatomical location must also be considered. In general, lightweight needle holders with fine jaws are more appropriate for procedures on facial and hand skin while larger needle holders with more robust jaws will be best used for surgery on the trunk.[3] The addition of tungsten carbide to the needle holder increases its strength and prolongs the life and durability of the holder. The addition of this alloy, which is also included in some scissors, in general, also increases the cost of the product. These instruments may be identified by their gold-plated handles (Fig. 2.6).[1,3]

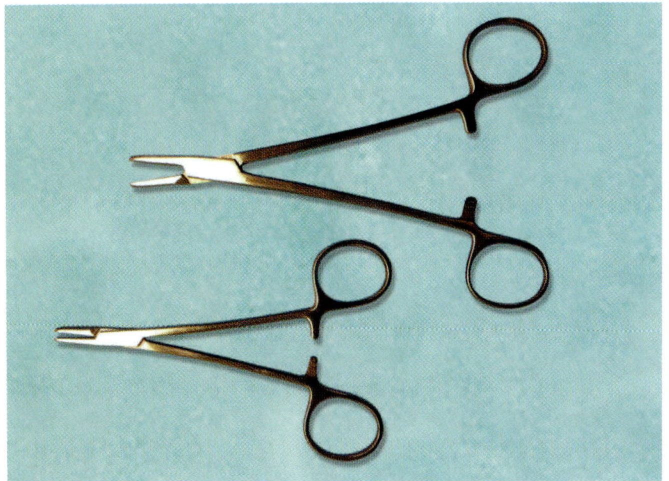

**Fig. 2.4:** The Webster needle holder (bottom) with smooth jaws; the Mayo Hegar needle holder with serrated jaws (top). The Webster needle holder is shorter in length and has smaller jaws.

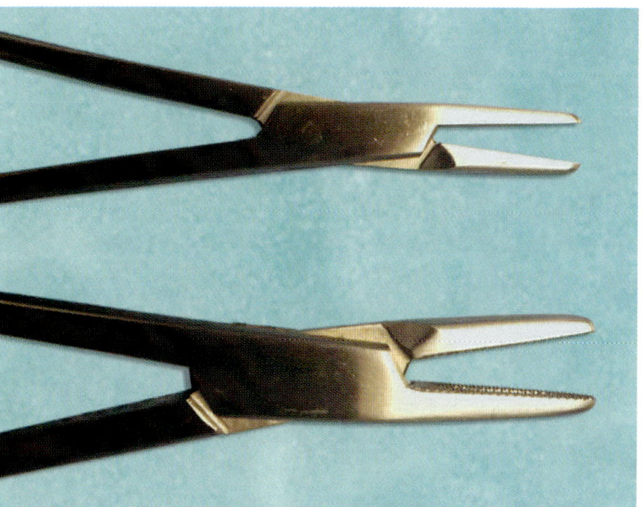

**Fig. 2.5:** Smooth jaws (top) and serrated jaws (bottom) of needle holders.

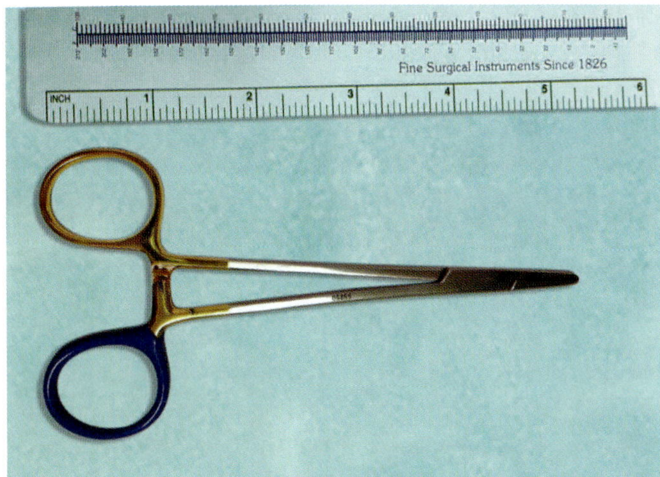


**Fig. 2.6:** Halsey needle holder with gold-plated handles of tungsten carbide.
*Courtesy*: George Tiemann & Company Surgical Instruments, Hauppauge NY.

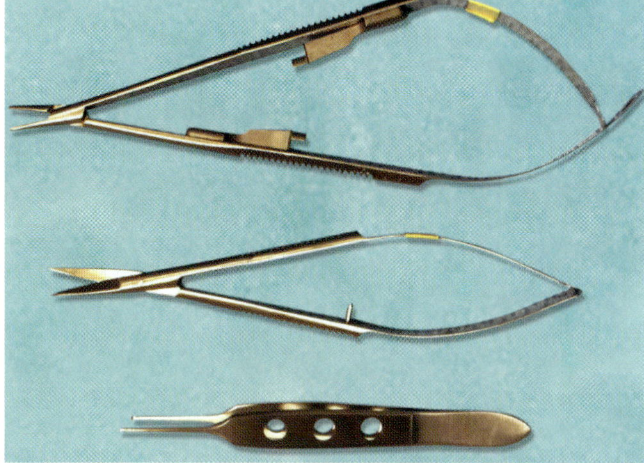

**Fig. 2.7:** "Periocular instrument kit" including (from bottom to top) standard Bishop-Harmon forceps, straight Westcott (Castroviejo) scissors, and Castroviejo needle holder.

There are various types of needle holders that may be encountered in dermatologic surgery. Webster (Figs. 2.4 and 2.5) and Halsey (Fig. 2.6) needle holders are commonly used for facial cutaneous surgery as they have smooth or lightly serrated jaws.[3] The Webster needle holder has short handles and narrow jaws, and therefore, may be used with fine needles and suture materials.[1,2] Use of these delicate instruments for procedures on the trunk could cause damage to the needle holder.[3] Castroviejo needle holders are light in weight and best suited for very delicate procedures such as those on eyelid skin (Fig. 2.7, top). These needle holders are held like forceps and have a spring-lock handle.[1,2] The Castroviejo needle holder is generally more costly and therefore may be unnecessary for the dermatologic surgeon who does not perform periocular procedures.[1] Conversely, Crile-Wood needle holders are more aptly suited for trunk and scalp procedures as they are designed to hold larger needles (Fig. 2.8). These needle holders are long with blunt tips.[1-3] Other suitable choices for procedures on the trunk are Baumgartner and Mayo-Hegar (Figs. 2.4 and 2.5) needle holders as they are strong and durable with serrated jaws. Finally, if working without an

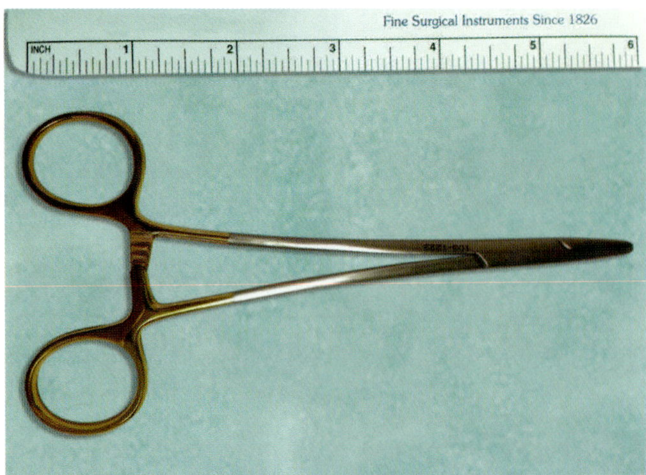


**Fig. 2.8:** Crile-Wood needle holder (with tungsten carbide handles). *Courtesy*: George Tiemann & Company Surgical Instruments, Hauppauge NY.

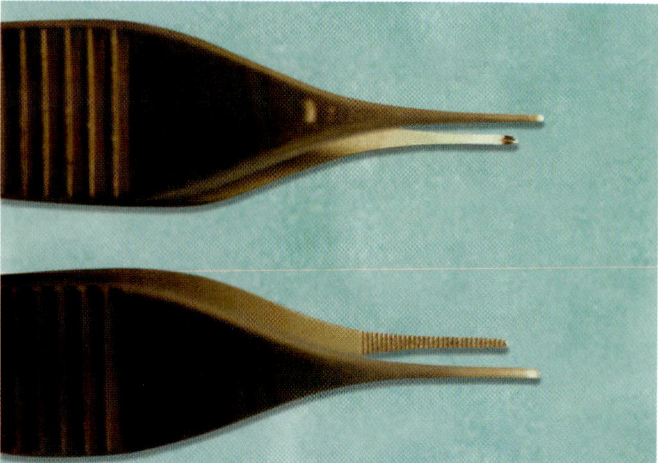

**Fig. 2.9:** Two examples of Adson forceps: toothed (top) and serrated (bottom).

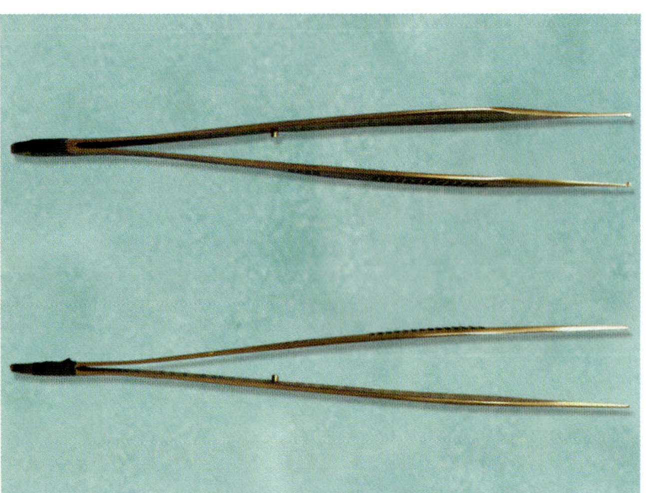

**Fig. 2.10:** Toothed (top) and serrated (bottom) forceps.

assistant, Olsen-Hegar needle holders may be useful as they also include suture-cutting scissors, located behind the jaws.[3]

## FORCEPS

Forceps, also known as "pick-ups," are used in dermatologic surgery to grasp tissue and suture needles. Forceps may be smooth, serrated, or toothed (Figs. 2.9 and 2.10). Although serrated tips allow for a secure grasp, they are generally not preferred, for tissue handling, as they may crush and damage tissue. Alternatively, toothed forceps allow for a firm grasp while minimizing damage to tissue.[1,2] Toothed forceps generally have a single tooth on one end of the instrument, which inserts into two teeth on the opposing end. Toothed forceps may also have additional numbers of teeth allowing for a firmer grasp of the tissue.[1] Additionally, there are forceps available with distal teeth for tissue handling and a proximal elevated platform for stable suture needle grasping.[3] The tips of forceps vary in length with the shortest being the most delicate (at ≤0.6 mm).[3] It is important to note that dermatologic surgeons vary in their use of forceps. Some surgeons exclusively use forceps to handle tissue while others may also employ skin hooks. Skin hooks traumatize tissue less; therefore, some surgeons prefer hooks when handling tissue that is to be sutured and forceps when grasping tissue that is to be removed.[1] Nonetheless, despite the selected tool, gentle handling of tissue is crucial for optimal surgical outcome.

As with other instruments described in this chapter, various types of forceps exist for different functional uses in dermatologic surgery. Adson forceps are the standard forceps for procedural dermatology; they have narrow, tapered tips, and a broad handle (Figs. 2.9 and 2.10). They are available in serrated or toothed versions.[1,2] Brown-Adson forceps have multiple teeth on their tips, and therefore may be utilized when the grasp of tissue is more challenging, such as when handling cartilage or tissue with large amounts of subcutaneous material.[1] Bishop-Harmon forceps are lightweight and have fine tips, making them ideal for delicate procedures such as those on periocular areas (Fig. 2.7, bottom). There are toothed and serrated versions. They are easily identified by the three holes in the handles, making this instrument very lightweight.[1,2]

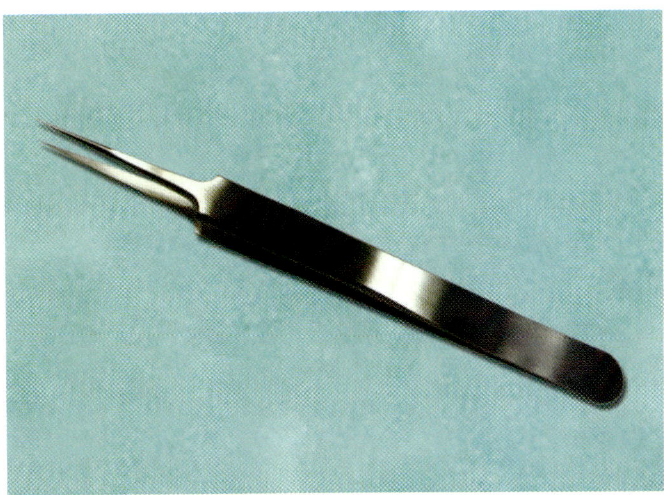

**Fig. 2.11:** Jeweler forceps.
*Courtesy*: George Tiemann & Company Surgical Instruments, Hauppauge NY.

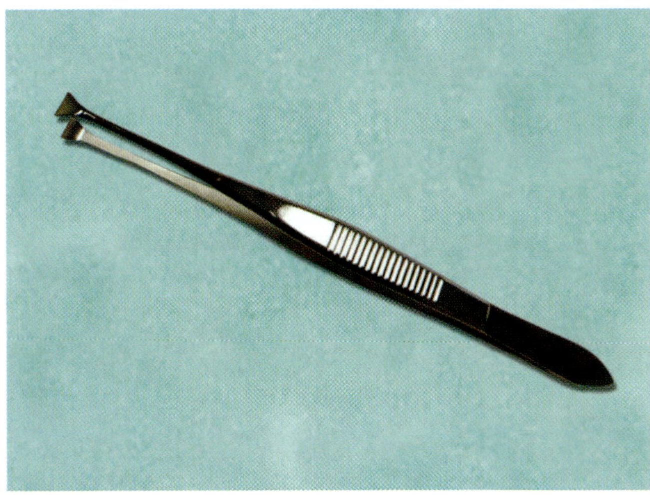

**Fig. 2.12:** Graefe forceps.
*Courtesy*: George Tiemann & Company Surgical Instruments, Hauppauge NY.

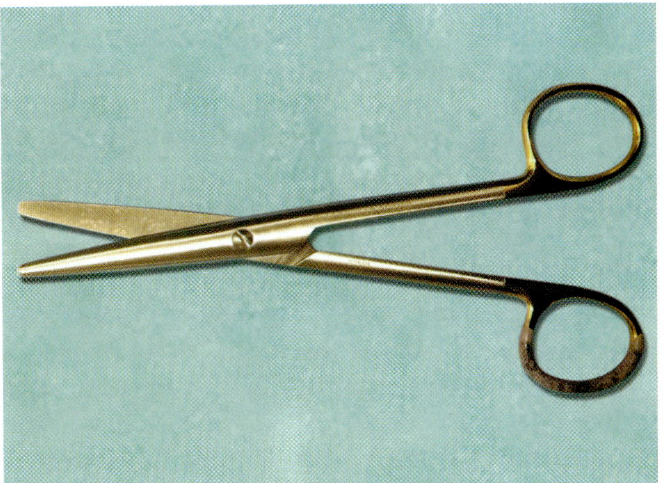

**Fig. 2.13:** Mayo scissors.

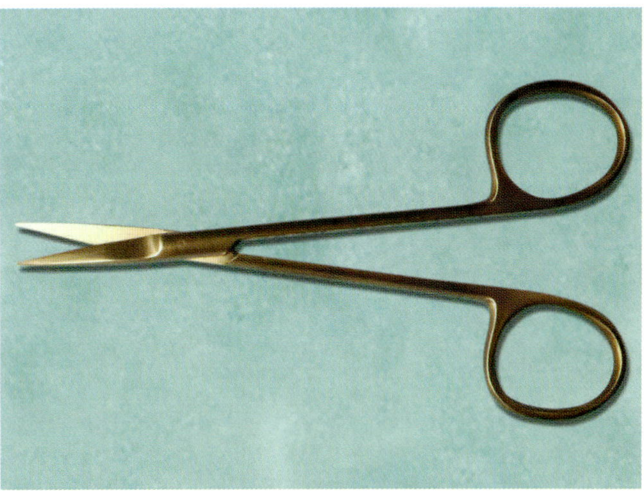

**Fig. 2.14:** Iris scissors; seen here with straight blades.

They should be selected with care as use on thick skin, such as the trunk, could damage these delicate forceps.[3] Other less commonly used forceps are: Jeweler's [small with fine, sharp tips for recovering splinters or suture fragments (Fig. 2.11)], Graefe (Fig. 2.12), and DeJardin (both are toothed with wide jaws for handling cartilage).[1,2] Of note, some offices may prefer to bundle their instruments for use on specific areas. For instance, if a procedure is to be performed on eyelid skin, the surgeon may request their "periocular instrument kit," which may include Bishop-Harmon forceps, Westcott scissors, and Castroviejo needle holders (*see* Fig. 2.7).

## SCISSORS

Various types of scissors exist for different functions; they are used for cutting tissue, dissecting and undermining, thinning grafts, cutting suture, and removing dressings. The structure of the scissor guides its function; therefore knowledge and proper selection are key for the dermatologic surgeon. Scissors may have blunt (Fig. 2.13) or sharp tips (Fig. 2.14). Blunt tipped scissors may be selected to avoid disturbing tissue structures when undermining, while sharp tipped scissors are more appropriate for dissection.[1,2] Scissor blades may be smooth or serrated, straight

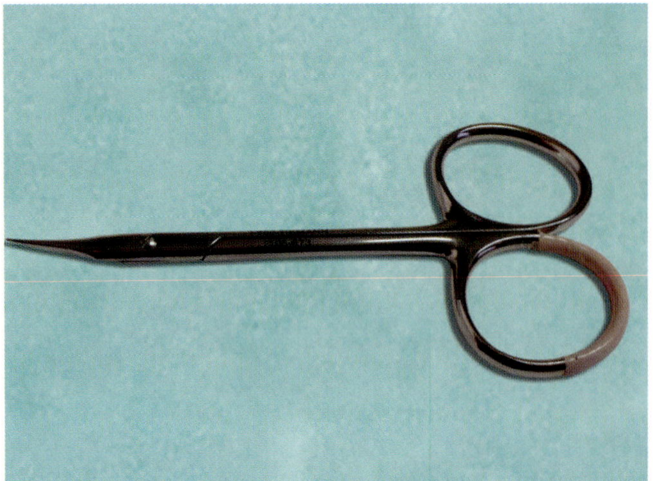

**Fig. 2.15:** Gradle scissors.
*Courtesy*: George Tiemann & Company Surgical Instruments, Hauppauge NY.

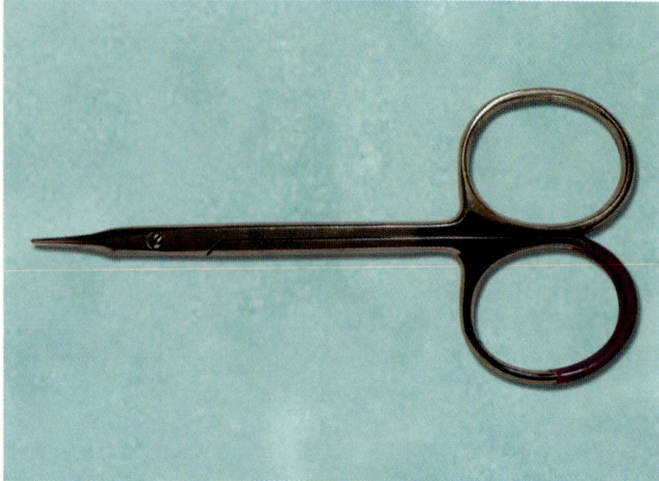

**Fig. 2.16:** Stevens Tenotomy scissors.
*Courtesy*: George Tiemann & Company Surgical Instruments, Hauppauge NY.

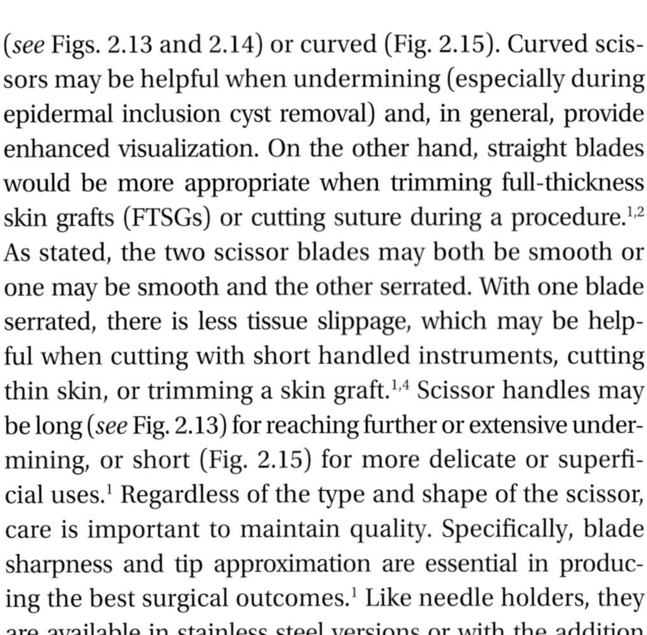

(*see* Figs. 2.13 and 2.14) or curved (Fig. 2.15). Curved scissors may be helpful when undermining (especially during epidermal inclusion cyst removal) and, in general, provide enhanced visualization. On the other hand, straight blades would be more appropriate when trimming full-thickness skin grafts (FTSGs) or cutting suture during a procedure.[1,2] As stated, the two scissor blades may both be smooth or one may be smooth and the other serrated. With one blade serrated, there is less tissue slippage, which may be helpful when cutting with short handled instruments, cutting thin skin, or trimming a skin graft.[1,4] Scissor handles may be long (*see* Fig. 2.13) for reaching further or extensive undermining, or short (Fig. 2.15) for more delicate or superficial uses.[1] Regardless of the type and shape of the scissor, care is important to maintain quality. Specifically, blade sharpness and tip approximation are essential in producing the best surgical outcomes.[1] Like needle holders, they are available in stainless steel versions or with the addition of tungsten carbide for added durability.[3]

Several named scissor types exist. The most delicate scissors used in dermatologic surgery are Westcott scissors (Fig. 2.7, middle). They, like Castroviejo needle holders, are held like forceps; these scissors operate on a spring system and the handles are squeezed to cut. For this reason, they are also known as Castroviejo scissors. They have a pointed tip and are ideal for fine delicate work such as cutting eyelid skin.[1,2] They are commonly used by Ophthalmologic surgeons.[3] Gradle scissors (Fig. 2.15) are small and delicate as well with short handles and a sharp, tapered tip with a fine point.[1,2,5] They are best used when cutting or undermining delicate tissues. Gradle scissors, like Westcott scissors, may be chosen for use on periocular skin.[1,2] They may also be used for skin tag removal.[3] Although not as delicate as Gradle scissors, Iris scissors (*see* Fig. 2.14) are also used for skin cutting and undermining and are the more commonly used scissor for this function. Iris scissors have sharp tips and short handles and are available in straight or curved models with smooth or serrated blades.[1,2] Tenotomy scissors (Fig. 2.16) may also be used for undermining but are usually selected for more superficial delicate undermining. They are similar to Gradle scissors but do not have a sharp tip and therefore more suited for undermining. Metzenbaum scissors (Fig. 2.17) are longer and heavier and may be useful in areas when a long reach is needed or for thicker skin that is more difficult to dissect or cut.[1,2] Some surgeons prefer these scissors when working on the scalp or trunk.[1] They are available in sharp or blunt and curved or straight models.[1,2] Mayo scissors are long, general use scissors; they are heavy and should be avoided in delicate procedures (see Fig. 2.13). Unlike Metzenbaum scissors, the Mayo scissor handle to blade length ratio is roughly 1:1, making them more ideal for coarse dissection.[2] They are uncommonly used in dermatologic surgery.[1] LaGrange scissors (Fig. 2.18) have very curved tips and handles of intermediate length with a reverse curve on the handle shank.[1,2] They have traditionally been employed for harvesting hair transplant donor grafts[1,4] and for the removal of punch biopsy specimen from the punch tool.[2] Scissors designated as "Supercut" scissors have uniquely

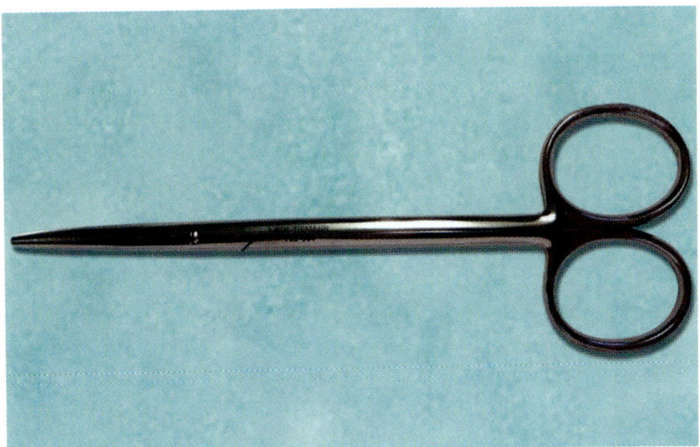

**Fig. 2.17:** Metzenbaum scissors.
*Courtesy*: George Tiemann & Company Surgical Instruments, Hauppauge NY.

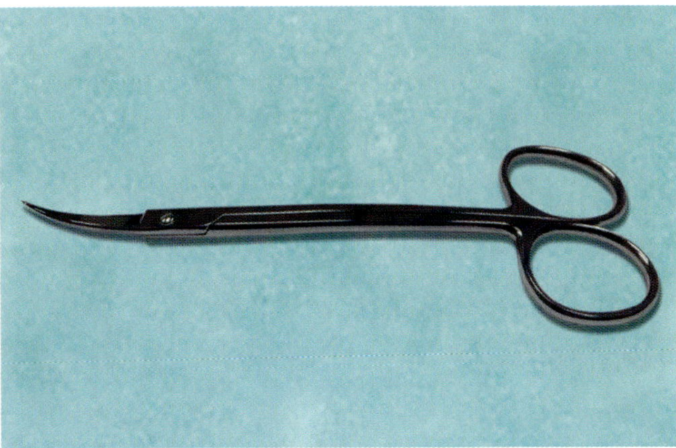

**Fig. 2.18:** LaGrange scissors.
*Courtesy*: George Tiemann & Company Surgical Instruments, Hauppauge NY.

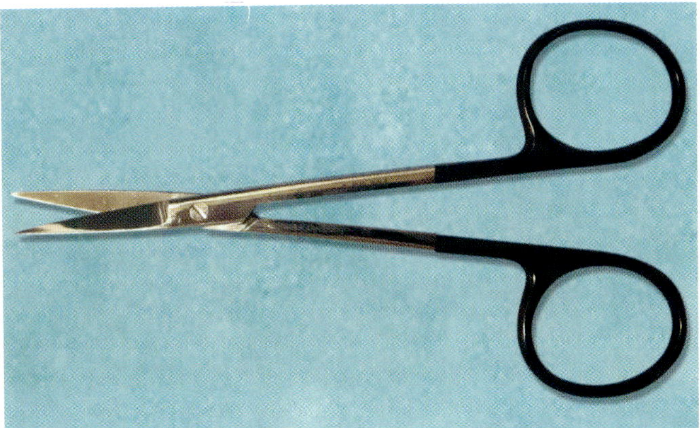

**Fig. 2.19:** Supercut iris scissors often used for preparing full-thickness skin grafts.

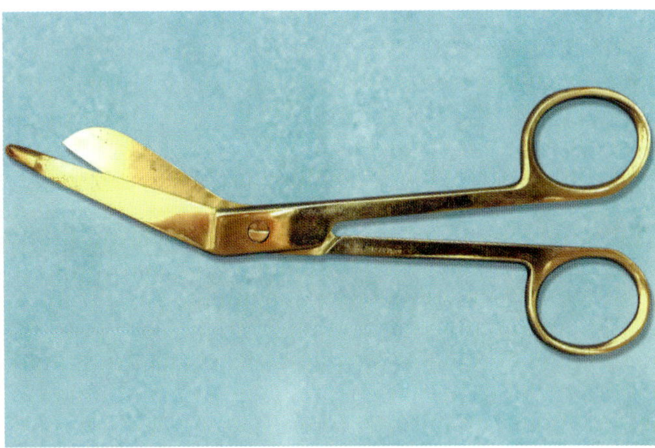

**Fig. 2.20:** Standard bandage scissors.

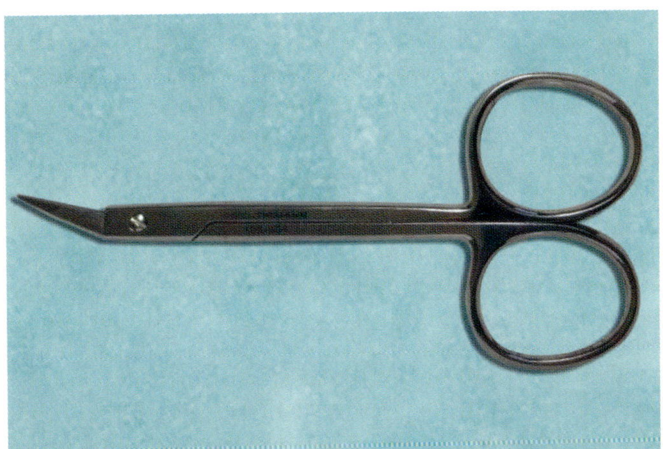

**Fig. 2.21:** O'Brien scissors.
*Courtesy*: George Tiemann & Company Surgical Instruments, Hauppauge NY.

ground razor-like edges for upmost cutting ability (Fig. 2.19). They are available in different scissor types and due to their enhanced sharpness are ideal for thinning FTSGs.[2] Bandage scissors (Fig. 2.20), called Lister scissors, are large with angled, bent blades, and blunt tips; they are perfect for protecting a patient's skin while removing bandages.[3]

Certain general operating scissors should be designated as suture-cutting scissors so that the surgeon's delicate sharp scissors will be preserved for upmost functionality on skin and tissue.[1,2] For example, cutting suture with Westcott or Gradle scissors would quickly damage these delicate instruments.[3] It is appropriate to choose less expensive scissors as designated suture-cutting scissors. O'Brien scissors (Fig. 2.21) have a short and angled blade and may be used to cut suture in tight spaces.[3] Suture-cutting scissors with a curved blade and a notch at the

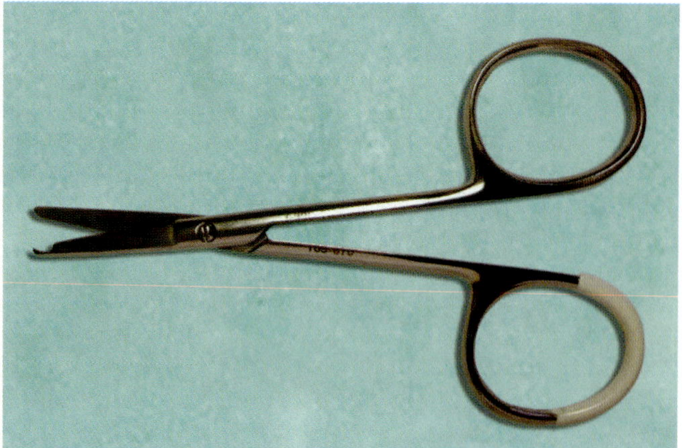

**Fig. 2.22:** Spencer stitch scissors.
*Courtesy*: George Tiemann & Company Surgical Instruments, Hauppauge NY.

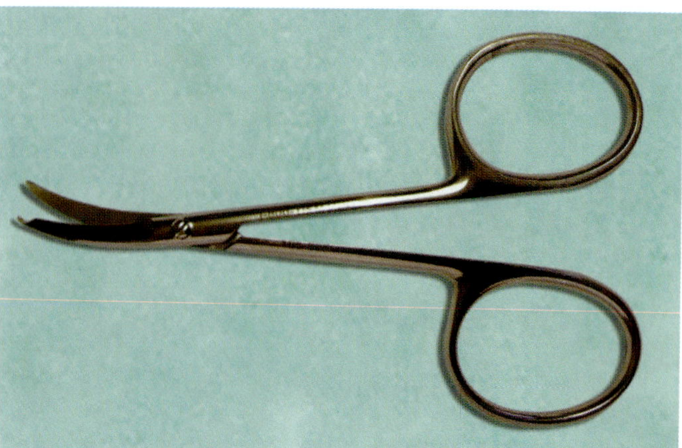

**Fig. 2.23:** Shortbent suture removal scissors.
*Courtesy*: George Tiemann & Company Surgical Instruments, Hauppauge NY.

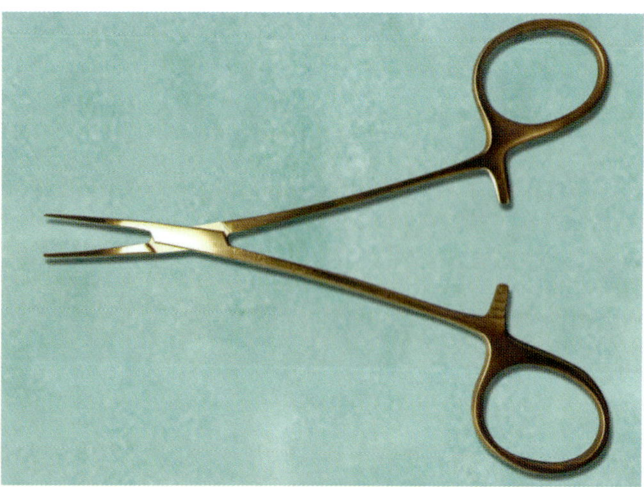

**Fig. 2.24:** Hemostat.

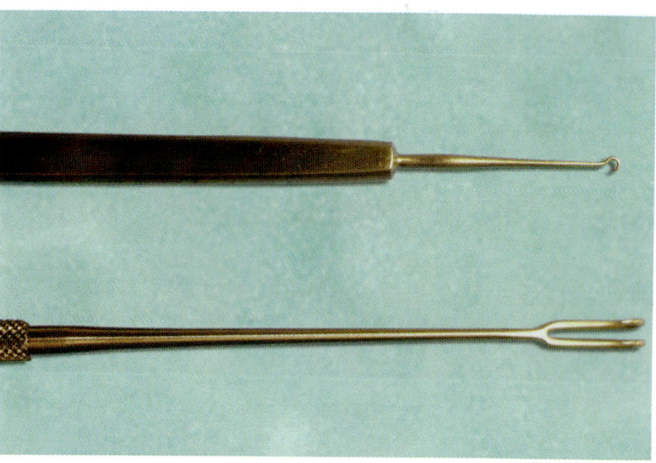

**Fig. 2.25:** A small sized single-pronged skin hook (top); a slightly larger double-pronged skin hook (bottom).

tip of one blade are Spencer (Fig. 2.22) and Shortbent scissors (Fig. 2.23).[1,2] Some practitioners prefer blunt tipped scissors for cutting suture for enhanced safety.[1] Scissor selection is important not only to improve surgical results but also to protect and preserve the individual scissor for its continued function.

## OTHER INSTRUMENTS

Various other instruments with specific functions are commonly used in dermatologic surgery include hemostats, skin hooks, curettes, and towel clamps.

Hemostats, which can be straight or curved, have blunt tips and are ideal for clamping severed vessels to achieve hemostasis (Fig. 2.24). In dermatologic surgery, hemostasis is most commonly reached with electrocautery, but occasionally brisk arterial bleeding is encountered, making the hemostat a valuable tool. Once the culprit vessel is identified and clamped with a hemostat, it can then be addressed with electrocautery or ligated with suture in a controlled fashion. Ideally to enhance function, hemostats should be lightweight and have fine tips.[1] The most popular hemostat in dermatologic surgery is the Halstead Mosquito.[3]

Skin hooks, which are available in a variety of sizes and hook variations, are ideal for handling tissue while producing minimal trauma (Fig. 2.25). They are available in various lengths and may be single, double, or multipronged. As stated above, they may be selected to handle

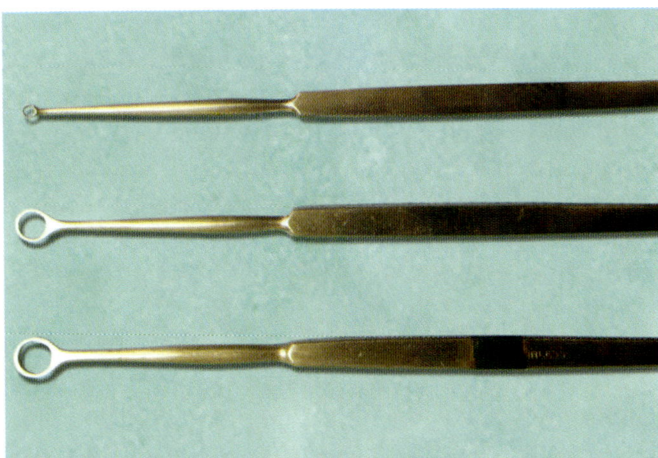

**Fig. 2.26:** Curettes of varying sizes (with round heads).

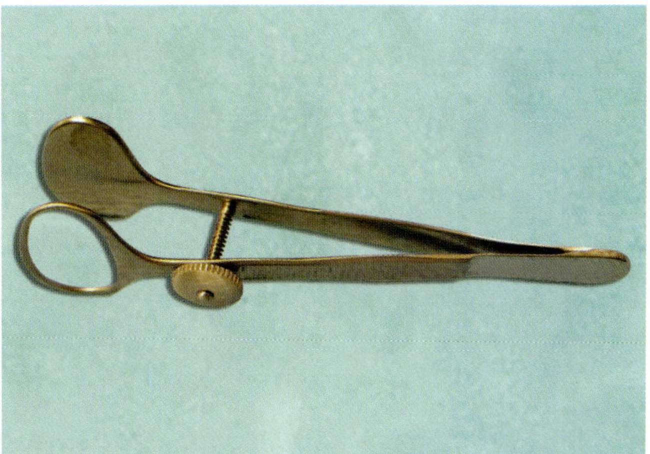

**Fig. 2.27:** Chalazion clamp useful for immobilization and hemostasis.

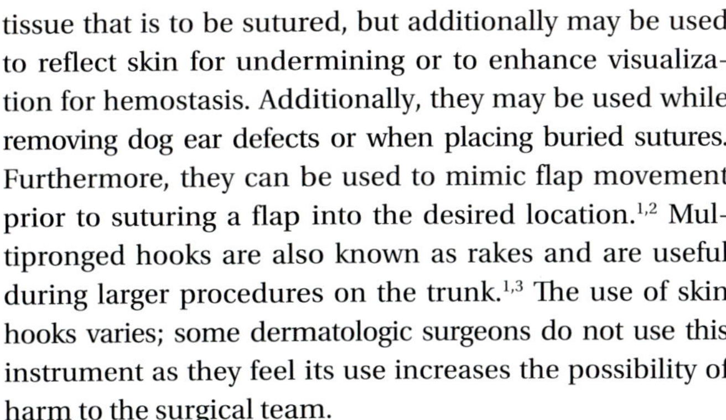

tissue that is to be sutured, but additionally may be used to reflect skin for undermining or to enhance visualization for hemostasis. Additionally, they may be used while removing dog ear defects or when placing buried sutures. Furthermore, they can be used to mimic flap movement prior to suturing a flap into the desired location.[1,2] Multipronged hooks are also known as rakes and are useful during larger procedures on the trunk.[1,3] The use of skin hooks varies; some dermatologic surgeons do not use this instrument as they feel its use increases the possibility of harm to the surgical team.

Curettes are commonly encountered in dermatologic surgery and were among the first dermatologic instruments. They may be utilized during a curettage and electrodesiccation procedure to treat cutaneous carcinomas or in the removal of benign lesions.[1-3] Additionally, they are sometimes employed prior to obtaining the initial layer in MMS in order to eliminate clinically apparent tumor.[1,2] In addition to "debulking" a tumor, prior to the first Mohs layer, lightly curetting the skin also allows the surgeon to better visualize the extent of the tumor.[6] Curettes are available in various sizes and shapes (Fig. 2.26). The curette heads may be round (known as Fox) or oval (Cannon) and are available in a variety of sizes to better suit specific needs. The sizing is based on the aperture of the head and various sizes are usually divided in 1 mm gradations, ranging from 1 to 9 mm.[2,3] In general, smaller heads and lighter handles are more appropriate for more delicate procedures or tissues.[1,2] This tool, like many others, must be sharpened occasionally, but caution should be given to disposable curettes as they may be very sharp and easily cut normal, noncancerous tissue.[3]

Towel clamps are most helpful in preserving a sterile field. They are used to secure electrocautery devices onto the surgical tray or to position towels on the patient.[1,2,7] They are available in various sizes[1] and may also be employed in large scalp procedures to hold skin under tension.[2]

Other less commonly encountered instruments include chalazion clamps, eye shields, Jaeger plates, periosteal elevators, and bone chisels. Chalazion clamps (Fig. 2.27) were designed for incision and drainage of chalazia, but in dermatologic surgery, they are useful in assisting in immobilizing structures and providing hemostasis. They are suited for procedures on mobile areas such as the lips, tongue (as mucosal surfaces are difficult to grasp), and earlobes. The tip of the instrument is oval in shape with an opposing similarly shaped ring; a screw on the shaft is tightened to bring the two tips together.[1] Alternatively, eye shields (Fig. 2.28) may be used to protect the eye during laser procedures or when cutaneous surgery breaches the lid margin. They are available in plastic, Teflon, and metal versions; note that metal eye shields will conduct electricity and should not be used with radiofrequency devices.[3] Similarly, Jaeger eyelid plates (Fig. 2.29) may be placed under the eyelid to stabilize the tissue for scalpel incisions while protecting the globe.[8] Finally, if a tumor is invading bone, periosteal elevators and bone chisels (Fig. 2.30) may be employed to facilitate removal.[1]

## NAIL SURGERY INSTRUMENTS

Nail surgery involves its own specific set of unique instruments. Freer septum elevators (Fig. 2.31) are thin blunt blades with a curved tip, which are used to avulse the nail

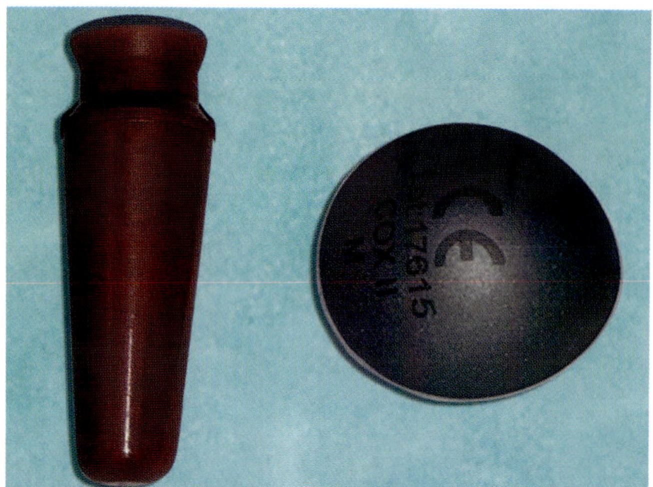

Fig. 2.28: Eye shield (right) with suction based applicator (left).
*Courtesy*: George Tiemann & Company Surgical Instruments, Hauppauge NY.

plate. Double-action nail clippers (Fig. 2.32) are heavy, sturdy clippers designed to cut thick plates. The English nail splitter (Fig. 2.33) allows for longitudinal cutting of the nail plate; opposite to the sharp cutting blade, there is a smooth anvil-like surface. There are also specific forceps for nail pulling (Fig. 2.34), which grasp the nail plate while the surgeon gently rolls the instrument side-to-side to pull the nail in one motion.[9]

## SURGICAL TRAY

Surgical trays should be organized in a repeated fashion for familiarity and, therefore, ease of use for the surgeon. Organization will not only improve usefulness and efficiency but also aids in maintaining safety for the surgical team. Mayo surgical stands may be used along with removable stainless steel trays to display instruments and materials.[2]

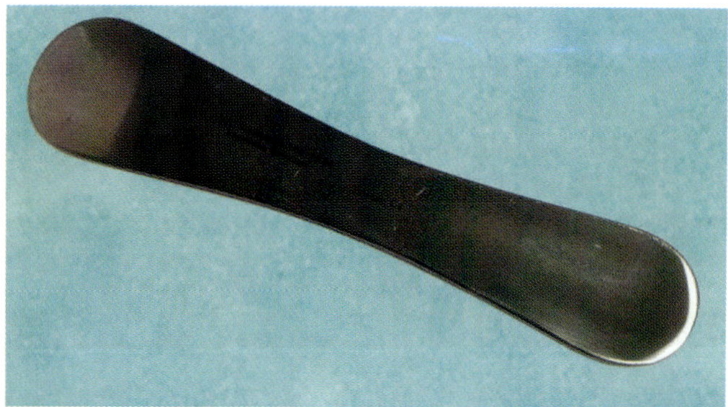

Fig. 2.29: Metal Jaeger lid plate.
*Courtesy*: George Tiemann & Company Surgical Instruments, Hauppauge NY.

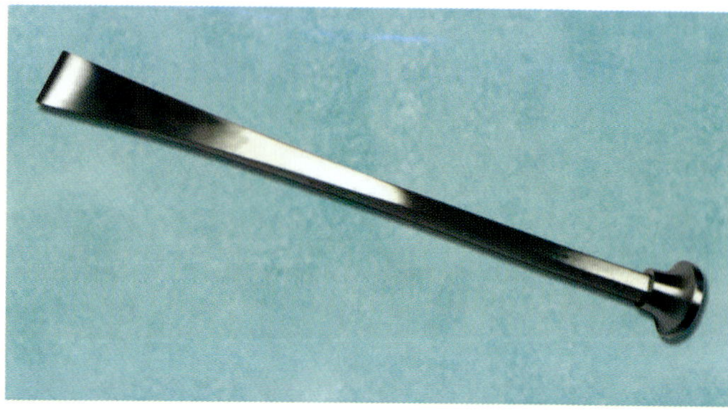

Fig. 2.30: Bone chisel (specifically, the Boston City Osteotome).
*Courtesy*: George Tiemann & Company Surgical Instruments, Hauppauge NY.

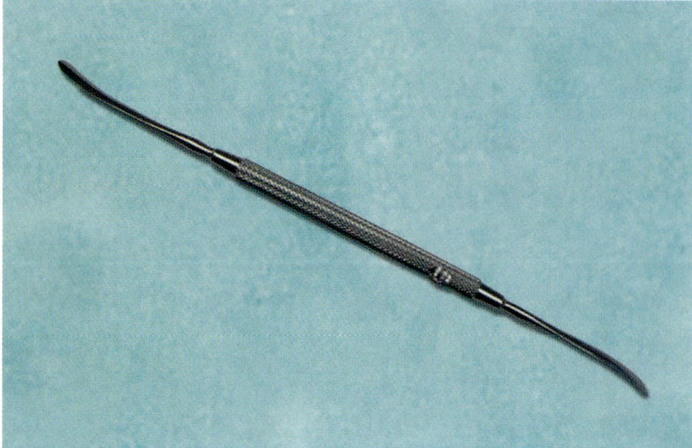

Fig. 2.31: Freer septum elevator.
*Courtesy*: George Tiemann & Company Surgical Instruments, Hauppauge NY.

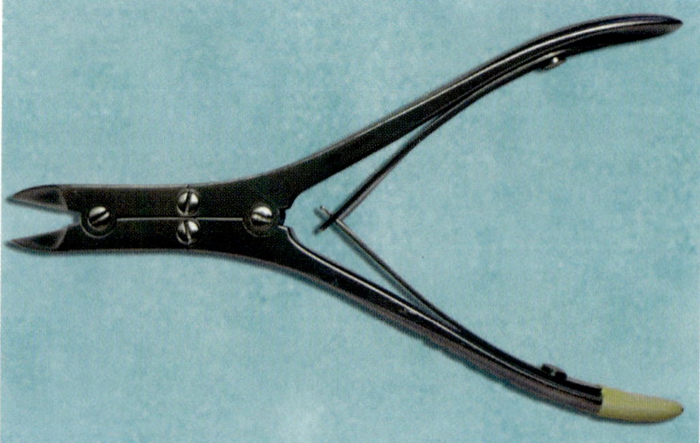

Fig. 2.32: Double action nail clipper.
*Courtesy*: George Tiemann & Company Surgical Instruments, Hauppauge NY.

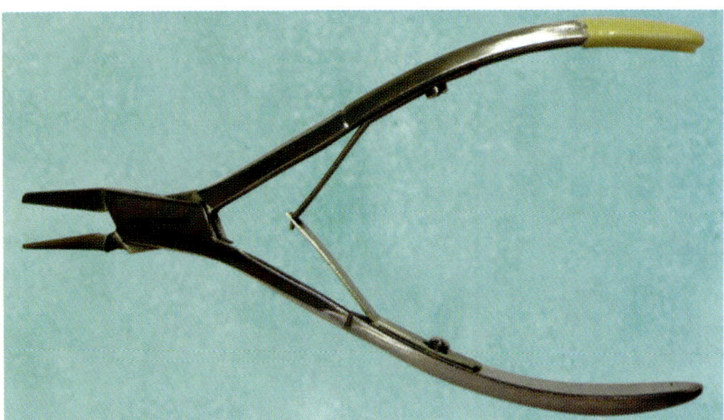

**Fig. 2.33:** English nail splitter.
*Courtesy*: George Tiemann & Company Surgical Instruments, Hauppauge NY.

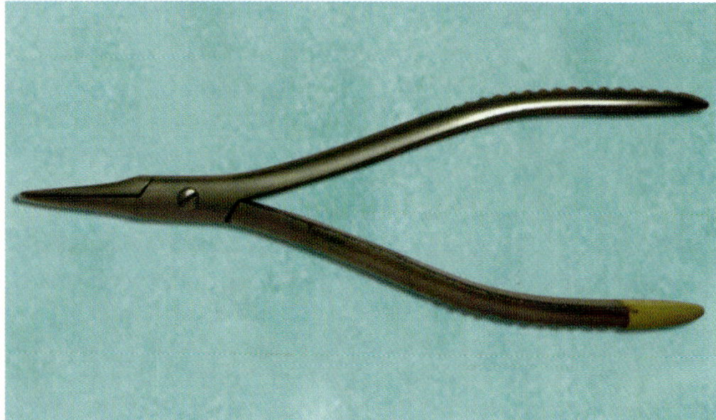

**Fig. 2.34:** Nail pulling forceps.
*Courtesy*: George Tiemann & Company Surgical Instruments, Hauppauge NY.

Removable trays allow for quick transitions between types of surgical tray setups. There are both two-wheeled and four-wheeled versions of the Mayo stand; both of which are adjustable for desired height preferences.[2] In general, trays for dermatologic surgery may include forceps, a scalpel handle and blade (usually the standard No. 3 handle and 15 blade), a needle holder, scissors for tissue, scissors for suture, cotton tipped applicators, gauze, sterile towels, or a paper drape. Variations of tray contents will depend on the procedure. Many surgeons may also desire a towel clamp and a skin hook on their tray. Some surgeons may routinely have hemostats on their trays or these can simply be requested if the need arises. Trays for MMS layers may also include a surgical marking pen or a cup with dye to designate orientation of specimens.[2] Rulers may also be a useful addition to the tray, if not etched on the scalpel blade. If a surgical repair will involve a FTSG, supercut scissors, a receptacle for sterile saline (a small plastic bowl, a petri dish, etc.), and a small punch tool (if needed for grafts over cartilage) may be included on the tray. As stated above, a "periocular instrument kit" (which includes Bishop-Harmon forceps, Westcott scissors, and Castroviejo needle holders) would be appropriate for a surgical tray, which will involve procedures on eyelid skin. In addition, when operating in the periocular area, the tray may also include anesthetic drops, ophthalmic ointment, and perhaps an eye shield.

## SAFETY

Tray organization and mindfulness of sharp instruments and materials is of the upmost importance to the surgeon, healthcare team, and patient. Injury may occur in the form of needle-sticks, lacerations, burns (cautery or laser procedures), and splashes. Common methods of injury occur during suturing, injections, and excisions.[10] To ensure safety, general recommendations include properly fitted gloves, eyewear, closed-toed shoes, masks, good posturing and positioning, and consistent surgical technique.[2,10-12] Furthermore, it is recommended that the surgical tray possesses uniformity so that physicians and assistants are aware of sharp tools and materials and their location. Moreover, as materials such as gauze are used and placed back onto the tray, it is important not to cover sharps to prevent them from being hidden from other members of the healthcare team.[2,12] Once sharps are used, members of the surgical team should be aware of their location. For instance, suture needles may be secured by hooking them on the top of their original packaging or another secure object. Blade extractors are also available for enhanced safety to remove the blade from the scalpel handle.[3] Suture needles should be handled with instruments,[2] fingers should not be used to stabilize tissues, cutting and injecting should be directed away from one's hands, and needles should not be recapped.[10-12] Once the procedure is complete, communication of disposing of sharp materials is imperative. Communication between the surgeon and assistants should be occurring during the procedure, as well. By openly communicating, using proper and consistent technique and positioning, injury can, in most instances, be prevented.

## CONCLUSION

Many different surgical tools exist. Minor variations in structure of these instruments allow the surgeon to select the best tool for a specific function. Knowledge of surgical instruments and materials is important to achieve optimal surgical outcomes. Finally, through communication and consistent technique, injury to the surgeon and assistants may hopefully be avoided.

## REFERENCES


1. Grande DJ, Neuburg M. Instrumentation for the dermatologic surgeon. J Dermatol Surg Oncol. 1989;15:288-97.
2. Bogle MA, Fisher VT, Joseph AK. Instruments and materials. In: Surgery of the Skin: Procedural Dermatology, 2nd edition. Philadelphia, PA: Mosby Elsevier; 2010. pp. 65-72.
3. Ammairati CT, Goldman G. Wound closure materials and instruments. In: Dermatology, 3rd edition. Philadelphia, PA: Elsevier Saunders; 2012. pp. 2353-63.
4. Koranda FC, Kuckasen JR. Instruments and tips for dermatologic surgery. J Dermatol Surg Oncol. 1982;8:451-4.
5. Gibbs RC. A love affair with a gradle scissors. J Dermatol Surg Oncol. 1981;7:771.
6. Johnson TM, Tromovitch TA, Swanson NA. Combined curettage and excision: a treatment method for primary basal cell carcinoma. J Am Acad Dermatol. 1991;24:613-7.
7. Kuwahara RT, Garcia C. Attaching instruments on surgical drapes. Dermatol Surg. 2002;28:542.
8. David LM. The laser approach to blepharoplasty. J Dermatol Surg Oncol. 1988;14:741-6.
9. Rich P. Nail surgery. In: Dermatology, 3rd edition. Philadelphia, PA: Elsevier Saunders; 2012. p. 2437.
10. Center for Disease Control and Prevention. Available at http://www.gov/sharpssafety/pdf/sharpsworkbook_2008.pdf. 2015.
11. Orengo I, Pielop J, Ransdell BL. The use of a "no-touch" technique to reduce the incidence of glove perforation during suture needle adjustment. Dermatol Surg. Dec 2003; 29:1215-16.
12. Trizna Z, Wagner RF. Surgical pearl: preventing self-inflicted injuries to the dermatologic surgeon. J Am Acad Dermatol. 2001;44:520-2.

# CHAPTER 3

# Facial Anatomy

*Thomas D Griffin Jr, Mary Larijani, Ezra Hazan, Nazanin Saedi*

## INTRODUCTION

A thorough understanding of facial anatomy is crucial for dermatologic surgery. Fundamental components of this knowledge include the location and function of individual skeletal bones, muscles, nerves, and vessels. Herein, we review these components as well as discuss other structures and danger zones relevant in dermatologic surgery.

## SURFACE ANATOMY OF THE FACE

The bony architecture of the face determines the facial appearance of an individual and creates anatomic landmarks for structures underlying the skin. The face is composed of the frontal bone, mandible, and the midface.[1] The midface bones consist of the maxillae, palatine bones, nasal bones, lacrimal bones, ethmoid bones, turbinates, zygomatic bones, and zygomatic processes of temporal bones.[1] Many of these bones serve as attachments for overlying muscles—muscles of facial expression and muscles of mastication. Anatomic locations can be seen in Figures 3.1 and 3.2.

From the hairline of the scalp to the chin there are numerous anatomical features that are consistent between individuals. Eyebrows are curvilinear growths of hair overlying the supraorbital ridges formed by the frontal bone.[1] Between the eyebrows is a hairless region that is termed the glabella.[2] Above the eyebrows and extending laterally are the supraciliary arches. The eyelids are mobile folds that overlie the orbit.[3] The medial and lateral canthi are the points at which the superior and inferior eyelids join together. The depressions superior and inferior to the eyelids are called the supra- and infrapalpebral sulci, respectively.[3]

Below the glabella is the beginning of the surface of the nose. The most superior aspect of the nose is termed the root.[1] The root is an indentation where the nasal

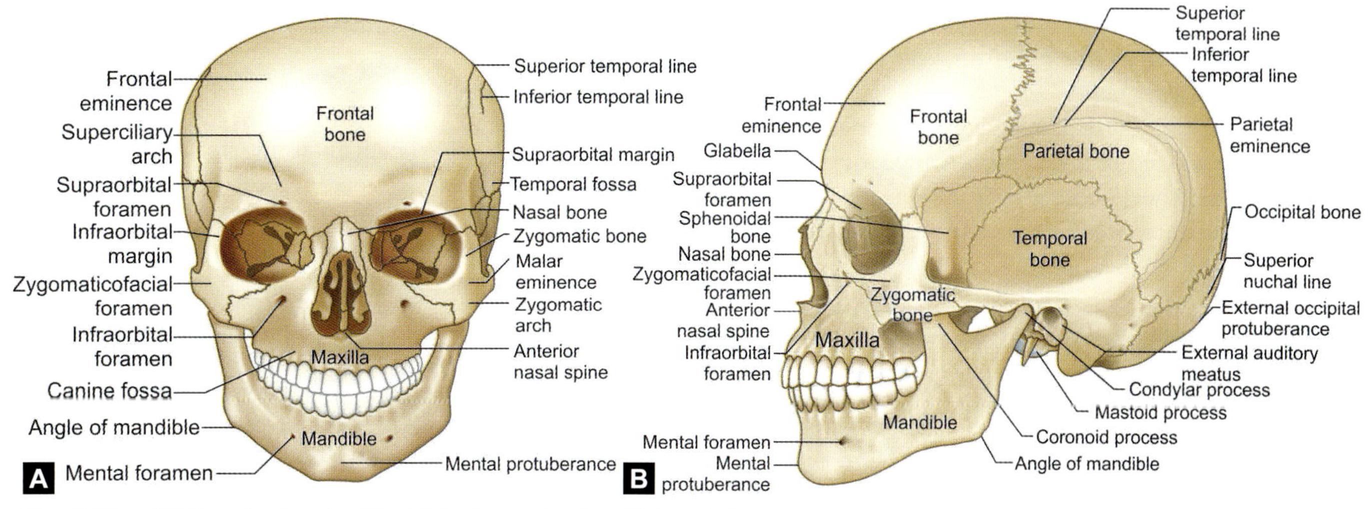


**Figs. 3.1A and B:** Bony landmarks of the skull: (A) anterior view; (B) lateral view.

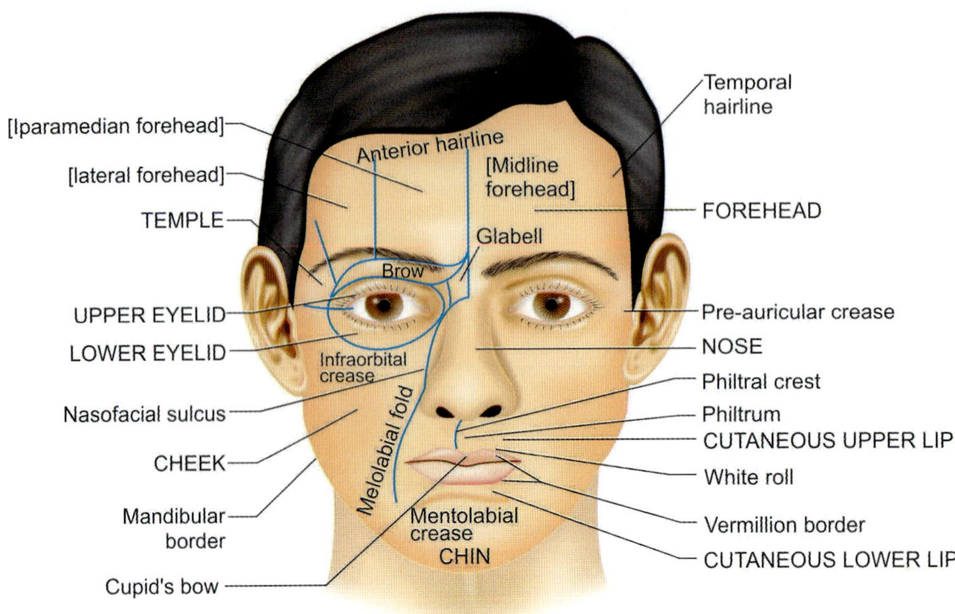


**Fig. 3.2:** Facial cosmetic units (capital letters), forehead subunits [brackets], and junction lines.

bone and frontal bone intersect.[1] The dorsum of the nose connects the root to the nasal tip. Lateral to the nasal dorsum and continuous with the cheeks is the nasal sidewall. The openings of the nose are termed the nares, and they are divided by the columella.[4] The soft triangles are on the underside of the nose anterior to the nares and lateral to the columella.[4] The nasal ala is superior to the nares and lateral to the nasal tip.

The oral fissure is the opening of the mouth. The vermilion border is the transition between the pink mucosa of the lip and the cutaneous lip.[4] The upper and lower lips come together at the corner of the mouth to form the lateral commissure.[4] The philtrum is a vertical groove superior to the upper lip.[4]

The nasolabial fold is a sulcus that extends obliquely between the ala of the nose and the angle of the mouth. It divides the cheeks laterally from the lips medially.[4] The mentolabial crease is a sulcus that divides the mental protuberance from the inferior lip (Fig. 3.2).

## Cosmetic Units and Subunits

Variations in color, texture, thickness, elasticity, pore density and size, hairiness, and amount of sebaceous glands delineate various subunits of skin on the face.[5] These units are referred to as cosmetic units. Major cosmetic units include the forehead, temples, cheeks, eyelids, nose, upper and lower lips, chin, and ears.[5-7] Cosmetic subunits can be appreciated by locating contour or junction lines, which separate various subunits.[5] These include the nasofacial sulcus, melolabial fold, preauricular crease, and mentolabial crease (Figs. 3.2 and 3.3).

Each cosmetic subunit has distinct topical anatomical features that are important for facial reconstructive surgery, as they assist in guiding incisions as well as demarcating the underlying musculature. Additionally, care is taken to ensure that defects generated during facial surgery are reconstructed with tissue from the same cosmetic subunit to optimize tissue match.

## Skin Tension Lines

Facial lines are superficial anatomic features that can enhance the cosmetic appearance of postsurgical scars through camouflaging surgical incisions in the natural contours and lines of the skin.[5,8,9] These include junction lines and skin tension lines. Additional facial lines include wrinkles and lines of facial expression, which are created from the contraction of the underling muscles.[10]

Junction lines demarcate the cosmetic units of the face. These lines are depicted in Figs. 3.2 and 3.3.[5] The junction lines of the upper face include the frontal and temporal hairlines, eyebrows, and glabellar creases. The midface includes the melolabial folds, alar grooves, nasofacial

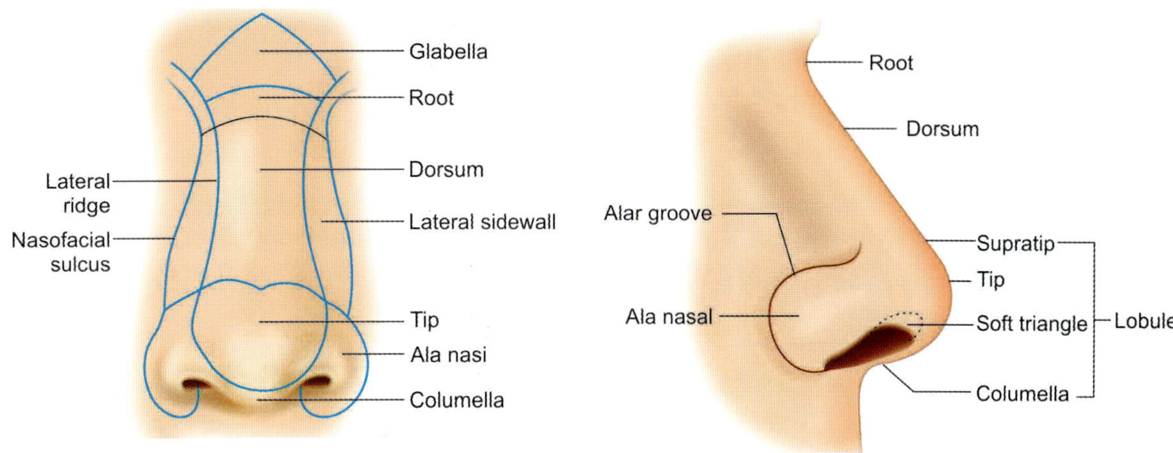


**Fig. 3.3:** Nasal cosmetic subunits and junction lines.

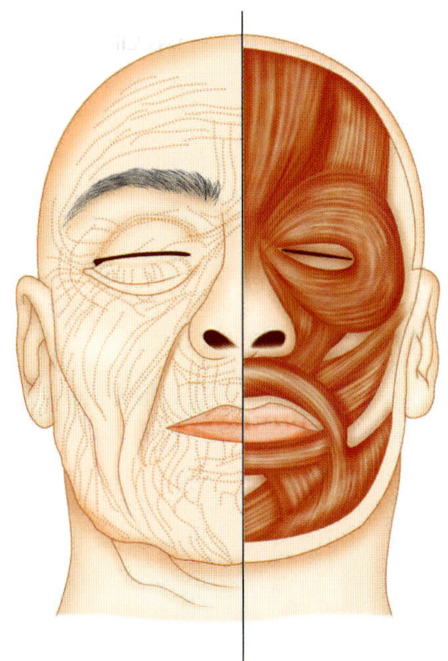

**Fig. 3.4:** Skin tension lines (left) and underlying facial muscles (right).

sulcus, and infraorbital crease.[5,8,9] The lower face includes the philtrum, vermillion-cutaneous junction, and mentolabial crease.[5] Laterally, the preauricular crease acts as an additional junction line for defects in this area[5] (Figs. 3.2 and 3.3).

Unlike junction lines, no single pattern has been described for skin tension lines. The depiction of skin tension lines described by Borges and Alexander in 1962[10] is one that has been commonly used.[5] Borges and Alexander described relaxed skin tension lines as a reflection of underlying tension created by a tenting effect of skin over underlying bony, cartilaginous, and soft tissue structures.[5,10] Skin tension lines run perpendicular to the underlying facial muscles, as is seen in Fig. 3.4,[5] with a more horizontal directionality at the midline and more vertical directionality at the lateral border.[11] In order to find skin tension lines, which are not as clearly visible, one can pinch the skin to detect the natural direction of skin lines[5,8,9] (Fig. 3.3).

## Superficial Musculoaponeurotic System

The superficial musculoaponeurotic system (SMAS) is a fibrous network of collagen fibers, elastic fibers, fat cells, and muscle fibers that serves to connect the facial muscles to the dermis.[12,13] A continuous and organized three-dimensional structure, the SMAS extends from the platysma into the face, temporal area, and onto the forehead as the galea aponeurotica.[12] This facial layer serves a functional role in the coordination of facial expression and contributes to organize facial movement, facial symmetry, and skin tension lines.[14] For the surgeon, the SMAS serves as a convenient and relatively avascular dissection plane and protection for important underlying structures. The SMAS is also an important structure for facelift and rejuvenation procedures where it is utilized for tissue mobilization.[15]

Ghassemi et al. describe two different architectural models for the SMAS. Type 1 is located in the forehead, parotid, zygomatic, and infraorbital areas.[12] It is a meshwork of fibrous septa that envelops fat cells. These septae project perpendicularly between fat lobules and connect to facial muscles or periosteum deep and the dermis

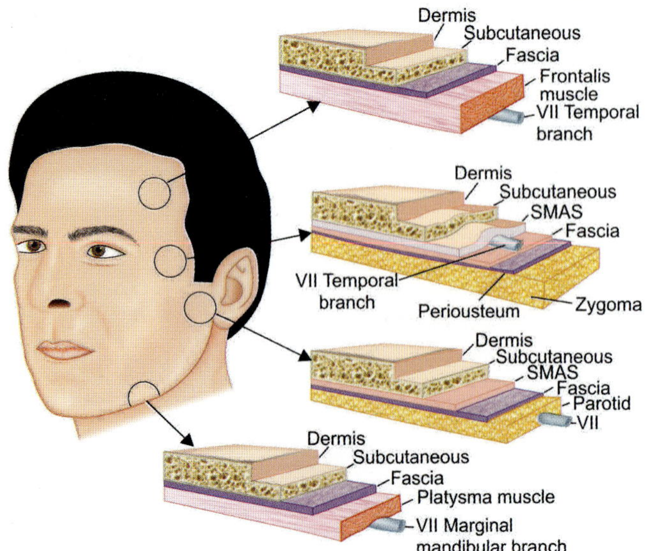


**Fig. 3.5:** Cross-sectional anatomy of facial soft-tissue layers of high-risk areas susceptible to damage during dermatologic surgery in relation to the facial nerve. SMAS, superficial musculoaponeurotic system.

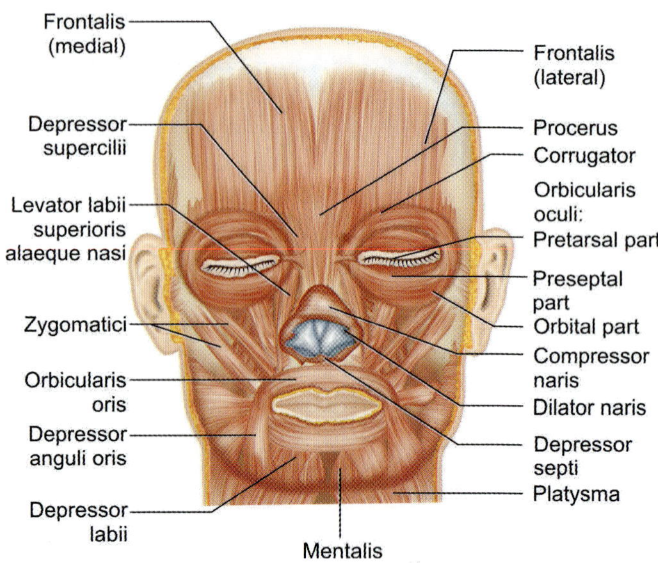


**Fig. 3.6:** Mimetic facial muscles.

superficially. Type II SMAS is found medial to the melolabial fold and in the upper and lower lips.[12] Here, the SMAS is thin and the dense meshwork of collagen, and elastic fibers are entwined with muscle and nerves to help transmit the complex movements of the mouth.

Although the SMAS is considered to be one continuous facial plane, the SMAS of the upper face is discontinuous with the SMAS below the zygoma. There is also considerable regional variation in the thickness and composition of the SMAS.[12] Whereas the SMAS near the mouth is thin, in the temporal area and forehead, where the facial muscles are absent, the SMAS is a thick, inelastic membrane.[12] Over the parotid gland, the SMAS is particularly thick to cover the parotid gland and the facial nerve.[15]

The SMAS lies in a facial plane that divides the subcutaneous fat from the facial muscles. In general, large sensory nerves and axial blood vessels supply the face branch within the SMAS and run in the subcutaneous fat superficial to the SMAS[14] (Fig. 3.5). Motor nerves, on the other hand run deep to the SMAS.[14] Although sensory nerves can be injured, undermining in the subcutaneous fat above the level of the SMAS allows for a safe and relatively avascular dissection plane.[14] However, there are exceptions to this rule. The supraorbital and supratrochlear neurovascular bundles can be injured in the forehead when dissecting to the galea. The superficial temporal vessels and auriculotemporal nerve lie within and above the fascia above the zygomatic arch.[12] Also, the buccal and zygomatic branches of the facial nerve can be injured in the parotid area.[12]

## Facial Musculature

### *Mimetic Muscles*

The facial musculature is composed of the mimetic muscles, also known as the muscles of facial expression, and the masticatory muscles. Mimetic muscles are characteristically thin, flat, and located in the midline of the face.[2,16] These muscles are involved in the expression of thought and feeling, as well as performing a sphincteric action for the eyes and mouth.[2,16]

### *Upper Face*

*Frontalis*: The frontalis muscle originates from the anterior belly of the occipitofrontalis muscle in the epicranium.[2,16,17] It descends vertically to insert into the orbicularis oculi, corrugator supercilii muscles, and dermis over the brows.[2,16,17] The frontalis maintains the resting brow position and elevate the brows, creating horizontal forehead furrows characteristic of a surprised look (Fig. 3.6).[2,16,17]

*Orbicularis oculi*: The orbicularis oculi muscle is a broad muscle composed of concentric striated fibers that encircle the orbital rim.[2,3,17] It is composed of three portions: the orbital, pretarsal, and preseptal. The orbital portion originates in the nasal segment of the frontal bone, the frontal

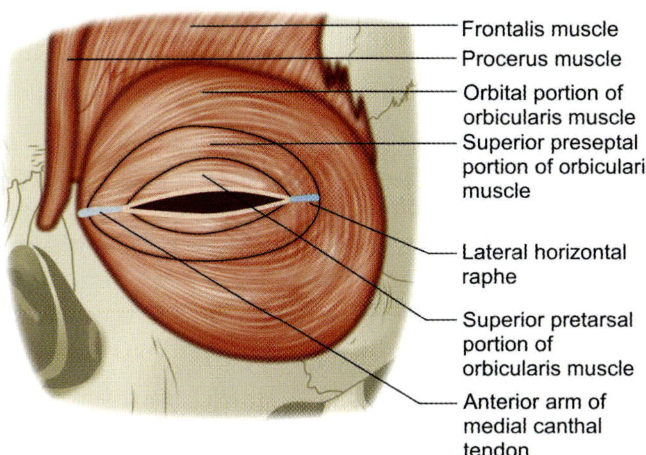


**Fig. 3.7:** Orbicularis oculi muscle anatomy.

process of the maxilla, and the anterior portion of the medial canthal tendon, which serves as a dense area of connective tissue.[2,3] The orbital muscle blends over the frontalis to insert subcutaneously into the lateral canthus and orbital region to cover some of the elevators of the upper lip and ala.[2,17] The orbital portion lowers the upper eyelid and depresses the brow[2] (Fig. 3.7).

The pretarsal portion originates from the upper and lower tarsal plates as well as the innermost medial canthal tendon, and it inserts into the lateral canthal tendon and palpebral raphe.[2,3] The pretarsal portion maintains the canthal angle position, secures the eyelid against the globe, and assists with the blinking reflex and lacrimal pump.[2,3,16]

The preseptal portion originates at the medial canthal tendon.[3,17] It passes over the orbital septum, a fibrous connective tissue encircling the orbit, to insert into the lateral palpebral raphe.[2] The preseptal portion functions similarly to the pretarsal, and produces characteristic "crow's feet" lines at the lateral orbital margin.[17]

*Corrugator supercilii*:The corrugator supercilii muscle originates from the medial end of the superciliary arch of frontal bone and the superomedial aspect of the orbital rim.[2,16] The muscle passes superolaterally to insert into the dermis of the brow deep to the frontalis and orbicularis oculi muscles.[3,16] The corrugator supercilii depresses the brows and contracts the brow medially, producing characteristic vertical lines in the glabellar region known as "frown lines".[2,16,17]

*Depressor supercilii*: The depressor supercilii muscle is a thin muscle that originates from the superomedial fibers of the orbital part of orbicularis oculi.[16] The muscle fibers insert into the medial brow to depress the brow.[16,17] Contraction forms vertical creases in the glabellar and lower medial forehead known as "frown lines".[17]

*Procerus*: The procerus muscle originates from the lower nasal bone. The muscle passes superiorly to insert into the dermis of the glabella between the corrugator muscles and fuses with the corrugator supercilii and medial portion of the orbicularis oculi muscles.[2] The muscle depresses the forehead and produces horizontal creases at the bridge of nose, also known as "glabellar lines".[2,16,17]

## Eyelids

In addition to the orbicularis oculi that surrounds the orbit, there are several muscles that are distinct to the eyelid.

*Levator palpebrae superioris*:The levator palpebrae superioris muscle fibers blend with orbicularis oculi and insert into the lower third of the superior tarsal plate.[3] The tarsal plates serve as a semi rigid support of the eyelid fibroskeleton.[3] The levator palpebrae superioris elevates and retracts the upper eyelid. The mechanism works through anterior-posterior redirection of the levator muscle that is modulated by a fibrous sleeve of tissue intrinsic to the muscle known as the Whitnall ligament.[3]

*Superior tarsal muscle or Müller's muscle*:The superior tarsal muscle, also referred to as Müller's muscle, originates below the levator palpebrae superioris and inserts onto the superior tarsal plate of the upper eyelid.[3] The superior tarsal muscle contributes an extra fewmillimeters of eyelid retraction.[3]

*Lower eyelid retractors*: The lower eyelid retractors originate in the capsulopalpebral head, an extension of the terminal fibers and tendon of the inferior rectus and oblique muscles.[3] These muscle fibers project through the orbicularis oculi to form the transverse eyelid crease visible below the inferior tarsal plate.[3]

## Midface

*Nasalis*: The nasalis muscle is composed of two portions, the upper transverse or compressor naris, and the lower alar portion or dilator naris. The compressor naris portion originates over the canine tooth and passes superomedially to the nasal dorsum where it decussates with fibers from the opposite side.[2,16] The compressor naris compresses the nasal aperture between the vestibule and nasal cavity.[2]

The dilator naris originates from the maxilla, inferomedially to the compressor naris.[2] Muscle fibers insert into the alar cartilage of the nose.[2] The dilator naris muscle functions to depress the ala laterally, causing dilation of the nostrils and opening of the nasal aperture, assisting air entry during exercise or deep inspiration.[17] Excess contraction of these muscles causes the characteristic "bunny lines" on the nasal dorsum.[2]

*Levator labii superioris alaeque nasi*: The levator labii superioris alaeque nasi muscle originates in the frontal process of the maxilla.[2,16,17] The muscle fibers pass inferolaterally to blend with the orbicularis muscle, and insert into the lateral nasal cartilage and the upper lip.[2,16,17] The levator labii superioris alaeque nasi muscle dilates the nasal ala, and everts the upper lip.[17]

*Levator labii superioris*: The levator labii superioris muscle originates lateral to the levator labii superioris alaeque nasi muscle, and superior to the infraorbital foramen.[2] The muscle fibers descend deep to the orbicularis oculi to insert into the upper lip muscular slip lateral to the insertion of the levator labii superioris alaeque nasi fibers.[2,17] The levator labii superioris elevates and everts the upper lip, as well as deepens the nasolabial fold.[2,17]

*Zygomaticus major*: The zygomaticus major muscle originates from the zygomatic bone.[2,17] It passes inferiorly to insert into the modiolus at the corner of the mouth, where the fibers blend with the orbicularis oris and levator anguli oris muscle fibers.[2,17] The modiolus is a dense, fibromuscular interface of muscles that functions as a scaffold for muscles to pull on.[17] The zygomaticus major draws the angle of the mouth superiorly while smiling.[17]

*Zygomaticus minor*: The zygomaticus minor muscle originates medially to the zygomaticus major, on the lateral surface of the zygomatic bone.[17] It passes inferomedially to insert into the upper lip lateral to the levator labii superioris muscle insertion.[2] The zygomaticus minor elevates the upper lip to expose the maxillary teeth while smiling, as well as deepens the nasolabial fold.[2,17]

*Levator anguli oris*: The levator anguli oris originates in the canine fossa of the maxilla below the infraorbital foramen.[16,17] The muscle fibers insert into the upper lip at the modiolus.[17] The levator anguli oris functions to elevate the corners of the mouth.[16]

*Buccinator*: The buccinator muscle originates from the pterygomandibular raphe, the lateral alveolar process of the maxilla, and the mandible.[16] The muscle fibers move toward the modiolus and into the orbicularis oris muscle fibers.[16] The buccinator presses the cheek against the molar teeth to aid in bolus control of chewing and swallowing.[16,17]

*Orbicularis oris*: The orbicularis oris muscle acts as a sphincter for the mouth and is composed of both deep and superficial portions.[2,17] The deep portion, also known as pars peripheralis, connects to each oral commissure at the modiolus to bring the mouth together.[2,17] The superficial portion, also known as pars marginalis, originates deep to the vermilion border and interlaces with other facial muscles to retract the lower lip.[2] The orbicularis oris muscle contraction produces characteristic fine rhytides around the vermilion border.[17]

*Risorius*: The risorius muscle origin is variable, including the zygomatic arch, parotid and masseteric fascia, as well as thickening of the platysma over the lateral cheek.[2,16] The muscle fibers insert into the modiolus at the edge of the oral commissure.[2] The risorius muscle pulls the corners of the mouth laterally during laughing.[2,16]

Depressor septi: The depressor septi muscle originates in the maxilla.[2] The muscle fibers pass superiorly to attach to the inferior surface of the nasal septum cartilage to pull the nasal septum inferiorly.[2]

## Lower Face and Neck

*Depressor labii inferioris*: The depressor labii inferioris muscle originates in the oblique line of the mandible and is found deep to the depressor anguli oris muscle and mental foramen.[2,17] The fibers pass superomedially to the skin and mucosa of the lower lip and into the fibers of the orbicularis oris muscle.[16] The depressor labii inferioris muscle depresses, laterally pulls, and everts the lower lip.[17]

*Depressor anguli oris*: The depressor anguli oris originates from the mental tubercle of the mandible.[16,17] The fibers pass superomedially to converge at the lateral lower lip and modiolus.[17] The depressor anguli oris muscle depresses the lateral corner of the lower lip and everts the lower lip.[2] Increased contraction of this muscle can produce characteristic radially oriented lower lip lines or "marionette lines".[17]

*Mentalis*: The mentalis muscle originates in the incisive fossa of the mandible and inserts into the dermis of the chin.[2,17] The mentalis pulls the chin and lip upward, causing wrinkling of the skin overlying the chin.[17] Excess contraction of this muscle cancause characteristic dimpling of the chin or a "peau d'orange" appearance.[16,17]

*Platysma*: The platysma muscle is a thin, sheet-like muscle that originates from the fascia of the upper parts of the pectoralis major and deltoid muscles.[2,16,17] The muscle fibers ascend superiorly to insert into the inferior border of the mandible, perioral muscles, modiolus, and dermis of the cheek.[16] Laterally, the fibers pass posteriorly at the angle of the mandible, and meet in the midline to form an inverted V at the lower chin region.[2,17] The platysma muscle pulls the angle of mouth laterally and inferiorly acting as a depressor of the lower lip and mandible during deep inspiration.[2]

*Digastric*: The digastric muscle is composed of anterior and posterior bellies. The posterior belly originates in the mastoid notch of the temporal bone.[16] Muscle fibers pass anteriorly and inferiorly to insert into the hyoid bone.[16] The anterior belly originates at the junction of the digastric and intermediate tendons and inserts into the digastric fossa of the mandible near the midline.[16] The digastric muscle depresses and retracts the mandible as well as supports the hyoid bone.[16]

### *Masticatory Muscles*

The masticatory muscles are located on the lateral aspect of the face, deep to the fascia of the midface.[2] They include the temporalis, masseter, medial, and lateral pterygoid muscles.

*Temporalis*: The temporalis muscle originates from the frontal, temporal, sphenoid, and parietal bones on the lateral aspect of the cranium.[2] The muscle passes inferiorly through a gap lateral to the zygomatic arch to insert on the apex of the coronoid process.[2] The temporalis muscle elevates the mandible and retracts the mandible from protrusion.[2]

*Masseter*: The masseter muscle originates from the incisive fossa of the mandible.[16,17] The muscle fibers insert into the dermis of the chin.[16,17] The masseter muscle closes the jaw and retracts the mandible.[2]

*Lateral pterygoid*: The lateral pterygoid is composed of a superior and inferior head. The superior head originates from the infratemporal surface and crest of the greater wing of the sphenoid bone.[2] The inferior head of the lateral pterygoid muscle originates from the lateral plate of the pterygoid process.[2] Both heads insert into the neck of the mandible and capsule of the temporomandibular joint.[2] The lateral pterygoid opens the lower jaw, protrudes the mandible, and moves it from side to side.[2]

*Medial pterygoid*:The medial pterygoid muscle consists of both a superficial and deep head. The superficial head originates from the medial aspect of the lateral pterygoid plate, and the deep head originates from the tuberosity of the maxilla.[2] Fibers from both heads pass posterolaterally to the mandibular foramen into the medial surface of the mandibular ramus.[2] The medial pterygoid muscle elevates the mandible.[2]

## FACIAL INNERVATION

### Sensory Innervation

Sensory innervation to the face is mostly provided by the three trunks of the trigeminal nerve, the fifth cranial nerve (CNV).[16-18] The three trunks are the ophthalmic, maxillary, and mandibular.[4] The great auricular nerve also contributes to facial sensation. Sensory nerves generally travel between the subcutaneous fat and SMAS layers.[12]

The ophthalmic division, V1, enters the orbit through the superior orbital fissure as three branches, lacrimal, nasociliary, and frontal.[4,16,17] The lacrimal branch supplies the lateral part of the upper eyelid.[16,17] The nasociliary branch supplies the glabella, nasal dorsum, and medial part of the upper eyelid.[16,17] The frontal branch supplies the forehead, anterior scalp, and periorbital regions via the supraorbital and supratrochlear nerves, which exit the supraorbital foramen and the more medial supratrochlear notch, respectively.[16]

The maxillary division, V2, supplies the midface.[16,17] The zygomaticotemporal and zygomaticofacial branches supply the skin overlying the zygoma and lateral canthus. The maxillary nerve then travels through the infraorbital canal as it supplies the nasal floor, upper alveolar ridge, gingiva, and palate.[17] Its largest branch, the infraorbital nerve, enters the face through the infraorbital foramen and supplies the lower eyelid, ala of nose, and upper lip.[16]

The mandibular division, V3, in addition to contributing to sensation to the face, provides motor innervation to the muscles of mastication.[4] It provides sensory innervation to the buccal mucosa and cheek skin laterally via the buccal nerve.[16,17] The auriculotemporal nerve innervates the temporal region and preauricular skin. The inferior alveolar nerve passes through its canal and innervates the lower alveolar ridge before exiting the mental foramen to supply the lower lip and chin as the mental nerve.[17] The lingual

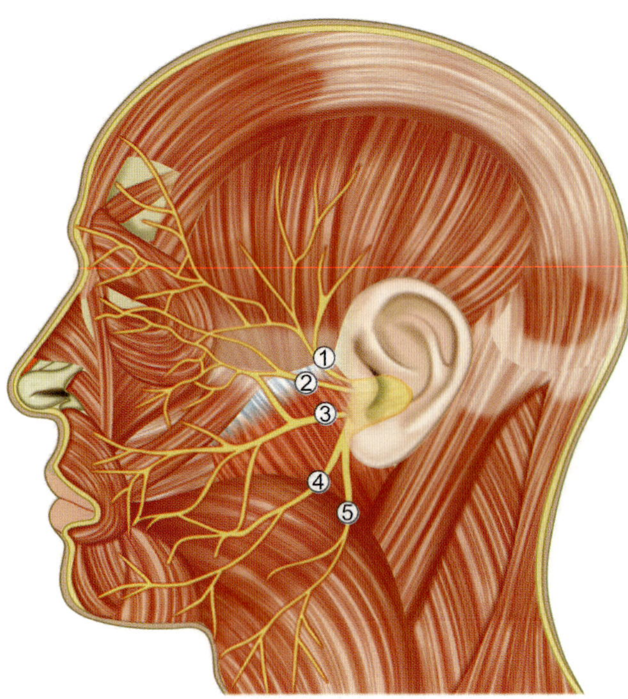


**Fig. 3.8:** Branches of the facial nerve. 1, temporal; 2, zygomatic; 3, buccal; 4, marginal mandibular; 5, cervical.

nerve, derived from V3, provides sensory innervation to the anterior two-thirds of the tongue.[16,17]

The greater auricular nerve, derived from the anterior rami of the second and third cervical nerves, supplies sensory innervation to the skin over the angle of the mandible and the ear.[4] The lesser occipital nerve, derived from the second and third cervical roots as well, provides sensation to the postauricular region.[17] Finally, the greater occipital nerve provides sensation to the posterior scalp.[2]

Sensory nerves, even though they travel more superficially than motor nerves, are not as much of a concern during cutaneous surgical procedures as motor nerves. Transection of sensory nerves generally results in temporary sensation impairment that can last months but usually returns to baseline.[5] Notably, the supraorbital nerve courses superiorly in the deep subcutaneous fat, which is susceptible to injury when undermining in the medial forehead.[5]

## Motor Innervation

Motor innervation to the muscles of facial expression is derived from the facial nerve, the seventh cranial nerve (CNVII) (Fig. 3.8).[16-21] The facial nerve emerges from the skull at the stylomastoid foramen. After giving off three small branches, the main trunk then penetrates the substance of the parotid gland, where it divides into its five terminal branches: temporal branch, zygomatic branch, buccal branch, marginal mandibular branch, and cervical branch.[4] As these branches travel outside the parotid gland, they are protected only by the skin, a variable amount of fat and the SMAS; they enter the deep surface of the muscles they innervate (Fig. 3.5).[18]

The temporal branch leaves the parotid gland superiorly and travels superficially over the zygomatic arch to enter the frontalis muscle.[4,16,17] It also supplies the upper fibers of the orbicularis oculi and the corrugator muscles. The temporal branch is susceptible to injury as it crosses the zygomatic arch and enters the lateral aspect of the frontalis muscle. It travels within the superficial temporal fascia and is covered only by skin and minimal subcutaneous fat.[16] Transection will result in paralysis of the ipsilateral frontalis muscle, which will leave the individual unable to raise that eyebrow or wrinkle the forehead.[5]

The zygomatic branch supplies the frontalis and orbicularis oculi with its upper branch.[4,16,17] Its lower branch supplies the lower orbicularis oculi, zygomaticus major, and other lip elevators. Smaller branches continue medially to supply depressor supercilii and superomedial orbicularis oculi.[16]

The buccal branch leaves the parotid and travels anterior to the buccinator and below and parallel to the parotid duct. It supplies the zygomaticus major and minor, levator labii superioris, levator anguli oris, and the buccinators.[16]

The marginal mandibular nerve leaves the lower parotid gland, travels along the mandible, sometimes below the angle of the mandible, before coursing superiorly and superficially to innervate the orbicularis oris, depressor anguli oris, depressor labii inferioris, and mentalis muscles.[4,16,17] The variable course of the marginal mandibular branch, and the fact that it is only covered by skin, subcutaneous fat, and the thin platysma, leaves it susceptible to injury.[18] Transection will result in ipsilateral flattening, inversion, and elevation of the lip.[5]

The cervical branch travels inferiorly into the neck to supply the platysma muscle.

Transection of nerve fibers in the medial cheek is less likely to result in clinically significant paralysis since there are many anastomosing branches derived from the buccal and zygomatic nerves.[5,18]

## Arterial Supply of the Face

Thorough understanding of the blood supply to the face is important in planning reconstructive procedures and in avoiding surgical complications. Branches of the internal and external carotid arteries supply the face. Branches of the internal carotid supply areas of the scalp, central forehead, eyelids, and dorsal nose. Branches of the external carotid supply the rest of the face[2,4,16,17,22] (Fig. 3.9).

The internal carotid artery enters the skull at the carotid canal. Classically, the internal carotid artery is subdivided into seven segments, C1–C7.[4,16] It is the C6, ophthalmic, segment that gives off the ophthalmic artery that provides arterial blood to the face.[23] From its origin distal to the cavernous sinus, the ophthalmic artery courses anteriorly through the optic canal and into the orbit. Once in the orbit, it gives off multiple branches that have been conveniently grouped into those arteries that supply the eyeball, the ocular group, and those that supply the orbital structures, the orbital group.[23,24] The orbital group includes the supraorbital, supratrochlear, lacrimal, dorsal nasal, and anterior ethmoidal arteries.

Blood supply to the medial forehead is provided by the supraorbital and supratrochlear arteries.[2,4,16,17] They exit the supraorbital rim in their neurovascular bundles through the supraorbital and supratrochlear foramina, respectively.[24] The supratrochlear artery exits and courses medial to the supraorbital artery and supplies the midline forehead and nasal root.[16,24] The supraorbital artery is lateral to the supratrochlear artery and supplies the medial periorbital and scalp tissues of the forehead. The supraorbital and supratrochlear arteries both course in the deep connective tissue, deep to the frontalis muscle and have extensive anastomoses.[16,24]

The nasal dorsum is supplied by the dorsal nasal and anterior ethmoidal arteries.[2,24] The dorsal nasal artery emerges from the orbit above the medial palpebral ligament and supplies the dorsum of the nose and courses medially across the nasal root and anastomoses with the angular artery.[24] The anterior ethmoidal artery courses through the nasal cavity along the inner surface of the nasal bone. After supplying the septum and lateral nasal wall, its terminal branch exits at the interface between nasal bone and cartilage to supply the distal nasal dorsum.

The external carotid artery contributes multiple branches that supply a large portion of the face. These branches include the facial, maxillary, and superficial temporal arteries.[4,16,23,24] The facial artery branches from the external carotid in the neck and in a tortuous course, provides the major arterial supply to the face.[16] After ascending through the neck and close to the submandibular gland, it loops around the inferior and anterior borders of the mandible anterior to the masseter. Here, the facial artery is most superficial and subject to injury, lying just deep to the platysma.[24,25] After crossing the mandible, it courses medially toward the oral commissure where it passes approximately a finger breadth lateral to the angle of the mouth.[25] Here it gives off two branches, the superior and inferior labial arteries. It then courses along the nasolabial fold deep to the zygomaticus major and levator labii superioris muscles and along the side of the nose. At the nasal ala, the facial artery divides into the lateral nasal artery and its terminal branch, the angular artery, before terminating at the medial canthus of the eye. Sources vary on the point at which the facial artery becomes the angular artery, some say that this point is after the superior labial branches, others say it becomes the angular artery after the lateral nasal artery branches.[2,16,17,24]

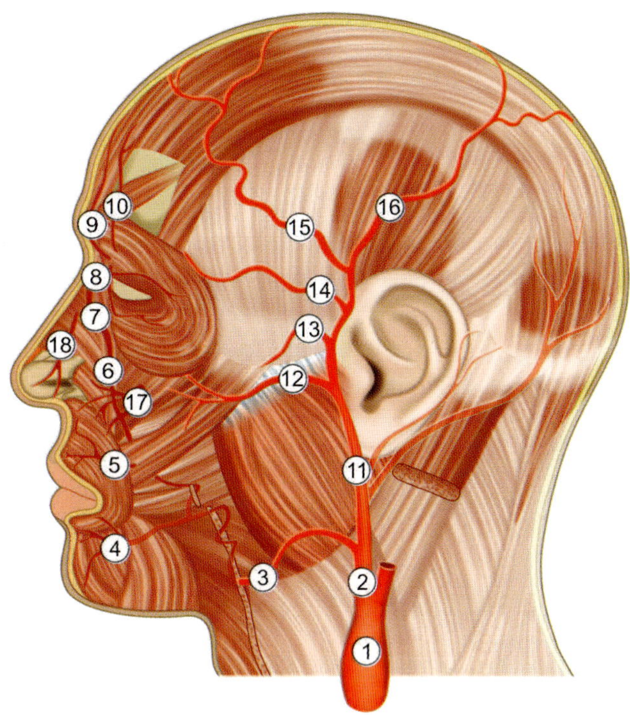


**Fig. 3.9:** Arteries of the face. 1, common carotid artery; 2, external carotid artery; 3, facial artery; 4, inferior labial artery; 5, superior labial artery; 6, lateral nasal artery; 7, angular artery; 8, dorsal nasal artery; 9, supratrochlear artery; 10, supraorbital artery; 11, superficial temporal artery; 12, transverse facial artery; 13, middle temporal artery; 14, zygomatico-orbital artery; 15, frontal branch of superficial temporal artery; 16, parietal branch of superficial temporal artery; 17, infraorbital artery; 18, external nasal artery.

The branches of the facial artery include the inferior labial, superior labial lateral nasal, and angular arteries.[2,16,17,24,26] The inferior labial artery runs medially in the lower lip, deep to the lip mucosa, and supplies the lower lip and chin. The superior labial artery runs medially in the upper lip, deep to the lip mucosa, and supplies the upper lip, alar rim, columella, and membranous septum.[4] The lateral nasal artery runs medially along the alar rim and supplies the nasal dorsum and ala. The angular artery is the terminal branch of the facial artery and runs along the nasal sidewall to the medial canthus, where it anastomoses with the dorsal nasal artery. It supplies the superior medial part of the cheek, inferior eyelid, and nasal dorsum.[4]

The superficial temporal artery is a terminal branch of the external carotid artery and supplies the lateral face, scalp, and forehead.[2,4,16,17] It arises from the external carotid when it bifurcates with the maxillary artery in the parotid gland.[4] It courses superficially to the main facial nerve trunks and gives off the transverse facial artery before exiting the parotid. Running superiorly in the preauricular crease at the level of the subcutaneous fat, the superficial temporal artery crosses the zygomatic arch medial to the tragus of the ear. Here, it lies superficial to the auriculotemporal nerve and together they run superiorly above the SMAS.[12] At the top of the ear, the superficial temporal artery bifurcates into the anterior and parietal branches.

Branches of the superficial temporal artery include the transverse facial, and anterior and parietal branches.[2,4,16,17] The transverse facial artery branches from the superficial temporal artery within the parotid approximately 2 cm below the zygomatic arch and runs medially parallel to the arch.[16] It crosses the face superficial to the masseter muscle and supplies the parotid gland and duct and overlying skin before anastomosing with the facial artery.[4] The anterior and parietal branches of the superficial temporal artery originate at the upper portion of the ear and run above the SMAS to supply the parietal scalp and the anterior lateral scalp.[12] They have many anastomoses that serve to create a rich arterial network in the scalp.

The internal maxillary artery is the second terminal branch of the external carotid artery.[4,16,17,23] It courses medially in the infratemporal fossa deep to the mandibular ramus. It gives off the inferior alveolar, mental, buccal, and infraorbital branches.[4] The inferior alveolar artery runs in the body of the mandible and supplies the lower gingiva before emerging as the mental artery at the mental foramen and supplying the lower lip and chin.[24] The infraorbital branch emerges at the infraorbital foramen and supplies the lower eyelid, cheek, and lateral nose. It anastomoses with branches of the facial, ophthalmic, buccal, and facial arteries. The buccal artery begins at the second part of the maxillary artery, it runs obliquely forward superficial to the buccinator, and supplies the cheek and buccinator before anastomosing with the facial and infraorbital arteries.[24]

## Venous Drainage of the Face

Most of the venous drainage of the face follows the pathways of the arterial circulation running posterior to their corresponding artery.[24] Like their arterial counterpart, veins of the face have many anastomoses creating multiple pathways of flow and possibilities for spread of disease. The supratrochlear and supraorbital veins run with their arteries and pass through the orbit before draining into the cavernous sinus. The angular vein runs parallel to the facial artery and flows into the anterior facial vein. This vein flows over the submandibular glands and into the deep facial vein. This vein ultimately drains into the internal jugular artery along with the retro mandibular vein, which parallels the superficial temporal artery.

## Lymphatics of the Face

The lymphatic drainage of the face is important as it is involved in the spread of infection and malignancy. While the lymphatic drainage is highly variable, the location of individual lymph nodes is consistent between patients, and there is a general drainage pattern that is followed. Drainage is typically found inferolateral to the anatomical location. The upper lateral face including forehead, ear, and upper eyelids drain into the parotid nodes. These nodes then drain into the external or internal jugular vein or jugular nodes. The midface region including the glabella, nose, nasolabial fold, medial cheek, and upper lip drain into the submandibular nodes. These nodes connect to both the submental nodes and the superficial cervical plexus. Ultimately, these nodes drain into the internal jugular chain. The submental nodes collect the drainage from the chin and lower lip, and then drain into the internal jugular chain. The posterior scalp drains into the postauricular nodes, which subsequently drain into the superficial cervical nodes.

## SUMMARY

Dermatologic surgeons have the unique ability to combine therapeutic and cosmetic modalities in the procedures they perform. The anatomy of the affected area is the fundamental basis for these decisions. A dermatologic surgeon must have intimate knowledge of the structures of the face to achieve pleasing results and avoid complications.

## REFERENCES


1. Drake RL, Drake RL, Gray H. Gray's Atlas of Anatomy, 1st edition. Philadelphia, PA: Churchill Livingstone; 2008. xvi P. 558 .
2. Marur T, Tuna Y, Demirci S. Facial anatomy. Clin Dermatol. 2014;32(1):14-23.
3. Harvey DT, Taylor RS, Itani KM, et al. Mohs micrographic surgery of the eyelid: an overview of anatomy, pathophysiology, and reconstruction options. Dermatol Surg. 2013;39(5):673-97.
4. Moore KL, Dalley AF, Agur AMA. Clinically Oriented Anatomy, 7th editon. Philadelphia, PA: Wolters Kluwer/ Lippincott Williams & Wilkins Health; 2014. xxviii, P. 1134.
5. Summers BK, Siegle RJ. Facial cutaneous reconstructive surgery: general aesthetic principles. J Am Acad Dermatol. 1993;29(5 Pt 1):669-81; quiz 682-3.
6. Pepper JP, Baker SP. Local flaps: cheek and lip reconstruction. JAMA Facial Plast Surg. 2013;15(5):374-82.
7. Rapstine ED, Knaus WJ 2nd, Thornton JF. Simplifying cheek reconstruction: a review of over 400 cases. Plast Reconstr Surg. 2012;129(6):1291-9.
8. Borges AF. Relaxed skin tension lines (RSTL) versus other skin lines. Plast Reconstr Surg. 1984;73(1):144-50.
9. Borges AF. Relaxed skin tension lines. Dermatol Clin. 1989; 7(1):169-77.
10. Borges AF, Alexander JE. Relaxed skin tension lines, Z-plasties on scars, and fusiform excision of lesions. Br J Plast Surg. 1962;15:242-54.
11. Summers BK, Siegle RJ. Facial cutaneous reconstructive surgery: facial flaps. J Am Acad Dermatol. 1993;29(6):917-41; quiz 942-4.
12. Ghassemi A, Prescher A, Riediger D, et al. Anatomy of the SMAS revisited. Aesthetic Plast Surg. 2003;27(4):258-64.
13. Menick FJ. Discussion: simplifying cheek reconstruction: a review of over 400 cases. Plast Reconstr Surg. 2012;129 (6):1300-3.
14. Gosain AK, Yousif NJ, Madiedo G, et al. Surgical anatomy of the SMAS: a reinvestigation. Plast Reconstr Surg. 1993;92 (7):1254-63; discussion 1264-5.
15. Mitz V, Peyronie M. The superficial musculo-aponeurotic system (SMAS) in the parotid and cheek area. Plast Reconstr Surg. 1976;58(1):80-8.
16. Prendergast PM. Anatomy of the face and neck. In: Giuseppe AD, Shiffman MA (Eds). Cosmetic Surgery: Art and Techniques. Berlin, NY: Springer; 2012. pp. 29-45.
17. Bentsianov B, Blitzer A. Facial anatomy. Clin Dermatol. 2004;22(1):3-13.
18. Brown SM, Oliphant T, Langtry J. Motor nerves of the head and neck that are susceptible to damage during dermatological surgery. Clin Exp Dermatol. 2014;39(6):677-82; quiz 681-2.
19. Hwang K. Surgical anatomy of the facial nerve relating to facial rejuvenation surgery. J Craniofac Surg. 2014;25(4): 1476-81.
20. Carlson KC, Roenigk RK. Know your anatomy: perineural involvement of basal and squamous cell carcinoma on the face. J Dermatol Surg Oncol. 1990;16(9):827-33.
21. Moskovitz JB, Sabatino F. Regional nerve blocks of the face. Emerg Med Clin North Am. 2013;31(2):517-27.
22. Whetzel TP, Mathes SJ. Arterial anatomy of the face: an analysis of vascular territories and perforating cutaneous vessels. Plast Reconstr Surg. 1992;89(4):591-603; discussion 604-5.
23. Larrabee WF, Makielski KH. Surgical anatomy of the face. New York: Raven Press; 1993. xix, 213 p.
24. Flowers FP, Breza TS. Anatomy of the head and neck. In: Bolognia JL, Jorizzo JL, Schaffer JV (Eds). Dermatology. China: Elsevier; 2012. pp. 2327-41.
25. Pinar YA, Bilge O, Govsa F. Anatomic study of the blood supply of perioral region. Clin Anat. 2005;18(5):330-9.
26. Loukas M, Hullett J, Louis RG Jr, et al. A detailed observation of variations of the facial artery, with emphasis on the superior labial artery. Surg Radiol Anat. 2006;28(3):316-24.

# CHAPTER 4

# Preoperative Considerations

***Margaret W Mann, Megan Morrison, Scott Santilli, Aleta Simmons***

A thoughtful and thorough preoperative evaluation prior to any dermatologic surgery helps to ensure patient safety, optimize surgical outcomes, and minimize complications. Since most dermatologic surgeries are performed in the office with local anesthesia, extensive preoperative evaluation, and perioperative management are often unnecessary. Important clinical history such as allergies (especially to medications used during the procedure), current medications, and relevant medical history (such as immunosuppression and bleeding diatheses) should be noted. In most cases, patients do not need prophylactic antibiotics and can continue their anticoagulants. Complications are infrequent in cutaneous surgery and life-threatening complications are fortunately very rare. Nevertheless, a proper evaluation is essential to anticipate any concerns and establish patient rapport.

This chapter presents three important topics in the preoperative evaluation and management of the dermatologic surgery patients: anesthesia, antibiotic prophylaxis, and anticoagulation. We review current guidelines and highlight at-risk patients in whom special considerations may be necessary.

## ANESTHESIA IN DERMATOLOGIC SURGERY

Effective knowledge and skill of anesthesia are integral to the practice of dermatologic surgery. Dermatologic surgery can typically be performed under local and regional anesthesia, thereby avoiding the risks associated with general anesthesia.[1] The optimal anesthetic requires an understanding of the patient's clinical characteristics, the location, the duration and intensity of anesthesia required, proper dosing, and assessment of anesthetic efficacy before and during the procedure. Patient safety and comfort are maximized when an anesthetic is planned and executed properly.

### Local Anesthetics Structure and Pharmacology

Local anesthetics (LAs) consist of an aromatic ring and an amine group connected by an intermediate chain (Fig. 4.1). Local anesthetics are classified into two broad categories based on their intermediate chain, which is comprised of either an ester or amide linkage. There are two critical distinguishing factors between esters and amides: their metabolic pathway, as well as propensity to cause allergic reaction (Table 4.1). Amides are metabolized in the liver via the *p450* pathway, thus special consideration must be taken when used in patients with liver disease or on medications that inhibit cytochrome *p450* 3A4 (Table 4.2). Esters are hydrolyzed by plasma cholinesterases, producing

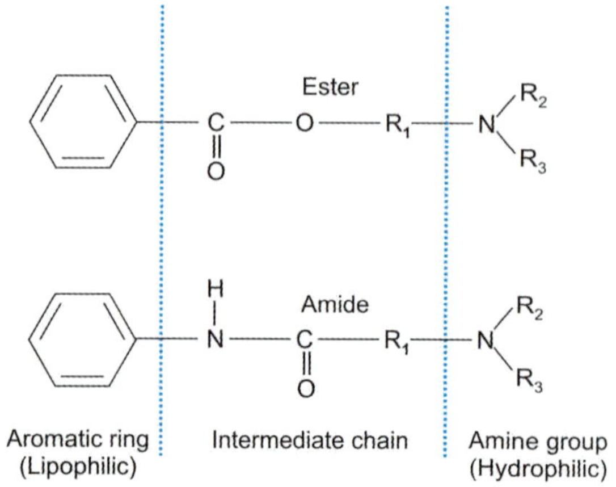

Ester
Amide
Aromatic ring (Lipophilic)
Intermediate chain
Amine group (Hydrophilic)

**Fig. 4.1:** Structure of local anesthetics.

**Table 4.1:** Differences between esters and amides.

| | *Ester* | *Amide (usually contain two "I's")* |
|---|---|---|
| Examples | Procaine, tetracaine | LIdocaIne, bupivacaine |
| Metabolism | Plasma pseudocholinesterase | Liver CYP p450 3A4 |
| Risk for systemic toxicity | Low | High |
| Excretion | Kidney | Kidney |
| Allergic reaction | More common<br>Due to metabolite PABA | Rare<br>Due to preservative methylparaben |

**Table 4.2:** Cytochrome P450 3A4 interaction with amide anesthetics. Commonly used drugs in dermatology are italic.

- Antiarrhythmic agents
  - Amiodarone
  - Quinidine
- Antibiotic agents
  - Chloramphenicol
  - Clarithromycin
  - *Erythromycin*
  - *Tetracycline*
  - *Metronidazole*
- Antidepressant agents (SSRI)
  - Citalopram
  - Fluoxetine
  - Paroxetine
  - Sertraline
- Antiepileptic agents
  - Carbamazepine
  - Valproic acid
- Antifungal agents
  - *Fluconazole*
  - *Itraconazole*
  - *Ketoconazole*
- Antitubercular agents—Isoniazid
- Antiulcer agents—Cimetidine
- Benzodiazepines
- Beta-blockers
- Calcium channel blockers
- HIV protease inhibitors
- Immunosuppressants
  - *Cyclosporine*
  - *Dexamethasone*
  - *Methylprednisolone*

**Table 4.3:** Local anesthetic duration of action.

| | | *Duration (minutes)* | |
|---|---|---|---|
| | | *Without epinephrine* | *With epinephrine* |
| Ester | Procaine | 15–30 | 30–90 |
| | Tetracaine | 120–240 | 240–480 |
| Amides | Lidocaine | 30–120 | 60–400 |
| | Mepivacaine | 30–120 | 30–120 |
| | Bupivacaine | 120–240 | 240–480 |
| | Prilocaine | 30–120 | 60–400 |

para-aminobenzoic acid (PABA), which is associated with a higher incidence of allergic reaction.

The aromatic ring is lipophilic and determines how readily the agent diffuses through the phospholipid membrane of nerve cells. Local anesthetics with greater alkylation of the ring, such as bupivacaine, are more lipophilic and thus more potent due to the fact that they readily cross the nerve cell membrane and are not cleared as rapidly in local circulation. Lipophilicity can also have an effect on onset time: moderately hydrophilic LAs such as lidocaine have a more rapid onset because they are less tissue bound than other hydrophobic LAs, yet still more permeable to membranes than more hydrophilic LAs.[2] The degree of protein binding influences its duration of action; bupivacaine is 96% protein bound thus is longer acting than lidocaine, which is 64% protein bound (Table 4.3).

The tertiary amine group is capable of accepting a proton with weak affinity and thus LAs are weak bases. Its nonionized form is more lipophilic, allowing it to pass through the cell membrane. Once intracellular, the acidic pH environment converts LAs into its more hydrophilic protonated cationic form, which has a higher affinity for the binding site on the inner nerve cell membrane. Thus, the pH of the anesthetic and the surrounding tissue greatly influences its effectiveness. Buffered LAs are more effective due to their increased membrane solubility. On the other hand, infected tissue is acidic and requires more LAs due to poor membrane diffusion in a low pH environment.

## Local Anesthetic Effects on Nerve Action Potential

Transmission of pain occurs via the production of electrical impulses that propagate along the length of the nerve fiber. The normal resting potential of the nerve cell membrane is –70 mV, which is maintained by active sodium ($Na^+$)–potassium ($K^+$) ATPase pumps. In the resting state, $Na^+$ is the primary extracellular ion, while $K^+$ is the primary intracellular ion. Sufficient stimulus opens voltage-gated $Na^+$ channels in the nerve cell membrane, causing an influx of $Na^+$ ions. This leads to depolarization of the membrane and the propagation of the signal, the action potential in an "all-or-none" fashion. Local anesthetics inhibit nerve conduction by reversibly binding and inactivating voltage-gated $Na^+$ channels on the inner nerve cell membrane. This blocks the influx of sodium, preventing depolarization of the nerve, propagation of the nerve impulses, and transmission of pain sensation.

The features that distinguish nerve fibers include their diameter, presence or absence of myelin sheath, conduction velocity, and signal function. These features have important clinical implications for the administration of local anesthetics. In general, larger myelinated fibers are more resistant to blockade, although this is not universally true. In practice, a general rule of thumb indicates that pain and temperature (unmyelinated small fibers) are typically abolished before motor function and sensation of pressure and light touch (larger myelinated fibers). This explains why some patients may feel the sensation of pressure during surgery despite a lack of pain sensation.

## Local Anesthetic Additives

Substances are frequently added to local anesthetic solutions in order to augment their effect and enhance safety. Common local anesthetic additives include epinephrine, sodium bicarbonate, and hyaluronidase.

### *Epinephrine*

Epinephrine has been added to local anesthetics since 1900 and is the most common vasoconstrictor used in practice for local and regional anesthesia. Epinephrine promotes vasoconstriction, which in turn prolongs the intensity and increases the duration of the nerve blockade by reduction of local circulatory clearance of LA and therefore decreases systemic exposure to local anesthetic. Since local anesthetics alone typically induce vasodilation at clinical doses, epinephrine reduces surgical site bleeding by counteracting this effect. Epinephrine will significantly lengthen the duration of block for shorter to medium-acting LAs such as lidocaine. For longer-acting agents such as bupivacaine, the prolongation of block is modest at best.

The effect of epinephrine peaks at 7–15 minutes postinjection. It is available commercially premixed with lidocaine at concentrations of 1:100,000 and 1:200,000. Epinephrine is not stable at alkaline pH, and thus solutions of lidocaine premixed with epinephrine typically contain acidic preservatives that produce painful injection. This can be avoided by freshly preparing the mixture or by the addition of sodium bicarbonate to the mixture to balance the pH.[3] For a fresh preparation of lidocaine with 1:100,000 epinephrine, 0.5 mL of 1:1,000 epinephrine is added to 50 mL of lidocaine solution.

Historically, physicians were taught to avoid epinephrine in local anesthetic use on the fingers toes, penis, nose, and ears due to the risk of necrosis in these sites. Hafner et al. reviewed the use of epinephrine and found no complications in >10,000 surgical procedures on the ear and nose.[4] Krunic et al. reviewed all cases of digital gangrene associated with local anesthetic use and found that most cases were reported in the early part of the 20th century with the use of cocaine and procaine and inaccurate compounded anesthetic mixture. None were associated with the use of commercially prepared lidocaine-epinephrine. They concluded that it is safe to use lidocaine and epinephrine for digital anesthesia.[5] A retrospective review of 1,111 digital and hand surgery cases, with 500 patients receiving 1% plain lidocaine and 611 receiving 1% lidocaine with epinephrine (1:100,000), resulted in no cases of digital gangrene.[6] Contrary to conventional dogma, multiple literature reviews have shown that epinephrine is safe for digits,[5,7,8] penis, nose, and ears.[4] Relative contraindications of epinephrine include patients with a history of vasospastic disorder, peripheral vascular disease, thrombotic conditions, severe uncontrolled hypertension, primary cardiac arrhythmias, hyperthyroidism, and pheochromocytoma.[5,7,9]

### *Sodium Bicarbonate*

Sodium bicarbonate is frequently added to solutions of lidocaine with epinephrine, as it reduces the pain of injection for local infiltration[10] and hastens the onset of the LAs.[11] Sodium bicarbonate acts as a buffer to acidic solutions and thus reduces the pain on injection associated with acidity of the solution. By raising the pH, sodium bicarbonate increases the amount of uncharged LA in its base form, increasing diffusion across the nerve cell membrane resulting in more rapid onset of action. Sodium bicarbonate (8.4%) is added to local anesthetic solution in a 1:10 volume ratio for 1:100,000 epinephrine, or 1:15 ratio for 1:200,000 epinephrine solutions. Addition of sodium bicarbonate will decrease the shelf life of the mixture due to the instability of epinephrine in a more alkaline solution and this should be taken into consideration when preparing LA injections.

### *Hyaluronidase*

Hyaluronidase is an enzyme that degrades hyaluronic acid, a widely distributed component of the extracellular matrix. Hyaluronidase serves to aid in the diffusion of solution through tissue planes and to minimize tissue distortion from the injection of LA solution. Hyaluronidase is useful in the periorbital region to help minimize the number of injection sites and potential ecchymoses. Hyaluronidase-containing solutions are prepared by adding 150 units to 20–30 mL LA solution. Hyaluronidase decreases the duration of action of LA and increases systemic absorption, and thus proper precaution should be considered when planning anesthesia.

## Special Considerations—Pregnant and Nursing Patients

### *Pregnancy*

In pregnancy, the most important consideration is the timing of the procedure. If possible, consider second trimester or postpartum. If it needs to be done immediately, then some special considerations should be taken to maximize safety of the patient and fetus.

Most procedures can be performed under local anesthesia. Changes of pregnancy to be aware of are progesterone-induced sensitivity to local anesthetics. Local anesthetics cross the placenta and enter fetal circulation readily, and thus it is important to be cognizant of dosing.

Lidocaine, etidocaine, and prilocaine are labeled as category B and thus are local anesthetics of choice during pregnancy. Epinephrine is considered as category C due to the theoretical risk of umbilical artery vasoconstriction demonstrated in animal studies. However, it also helps to promote local vasoconstriction and ultimately lowers systemic levels of local anesthetic and therefore fetal exposure. Thus, it may be used, with extra precaution to avoid intravascular injection. Addition of a buffering agent such as sodium bicarbonate should not have any adverse effects.

Bupivacaine and mepivacaine have been shown to cause fetal bradycardia and thus are category C. For longer cases, it is important to plan anesthetics without the use of longer acting local anesthetics.

### *Breastfeeding*

Local anesthetics are excreted in breast milk and thus dosing precautions should be taken. Neonates and infants are capable of metabolizing local anesthetics and a study conducted by Giuliani et al. demonstrated that lidocaine levels in breast milk are safe.[12] Since ester LAs are broken down more quickly than amides, Skidmore et al. suggest consideration of their use in nursing mothers.[13]

## Administration of Local Anesthesia

### *Intralesional Injection*

Intralesional injection is the most common and direct method of achieving local anesthetic effect in dermatologic surgery. Slow injection with a small gauge needle minimizes pain on infiltration. Other methods to decrease pain include distracting the patient and the injection area, buffering with sodium bicarbonate,[10] warming the solution to room temperature,[14] and injecting into the subcutaneous tissue rather than the dermis.[15,16] Techniques to minimize pain with local anesthetic are summarized in Table 4.4.

### *Ring Blocks*

Ring blocks are useful when direct infiltration into the surgical field is undesirable such as in the case of cysts or infected tissue. This technique is also useful when hemostasis is desired such as on the scalp. A series of injections are made circumferentially around the site without actually injecting directly into the surgical area.

### *Nerve Blocks*

Nerve blocks are useful when anesthesia is desired in a large area supplied by a peripheral nerve trunk. It minimizes the number of injections and total amount of anesthesia infiltration needed in the area, thereby minimizing

**Table 4.4:** Practical tips for minimizing pain with local anesthesia.

- Consider topical anesthesia prior to infiltration
- Warming the solution to room temperature 37–42°C
- Buffering lidocaine with 8.4% sodium bicarbonate
- Distract the patient (talkesthesia) and injection site (pinch the skin, icing the area, stroking/vibrating the area)
- Using a small gauge needle (30 gauge)
- Inserting needle through a pore. Reinserting through an area that was previously anesthetized
- Minimize needle punctures by fanning the injection and using a longer needle
- Slow injection
- Inject into the subcutaneous tissue first then into the dermis
- Consider nerve or ring blocks
- Consider the use of longer acting agents for longer procedures

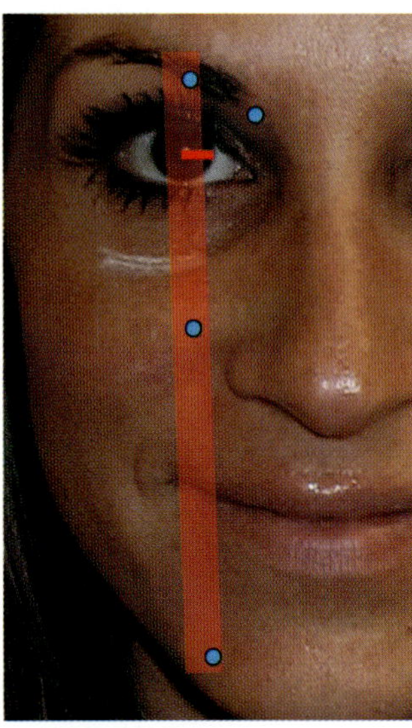

**Fig. 4.2:** Location of the supraorbital, supratrochlear, infraorbital, and mental nerve along the midpupillary line.

discomfort during injection, tissue distortion at the operative site, and the risk of lidocaine toxicity. When done properly, only 1–2 mL of lidocaine are needed at one to two injection points. The major disadvantages of nerve blocks include a delay in onset of anesthetic effect (3–10 minutes after injection), shorter duration of anesthesia, and minimal vasoconstriction effect. In addition, there is a risk of paresthesias due to direct nerve laceration. When performing nerve blocks, one should think of "bathing" the general vicinity of the nerve with anesthetic and not directly injecting into the nerve foramen. Gentle massage helps to disperse

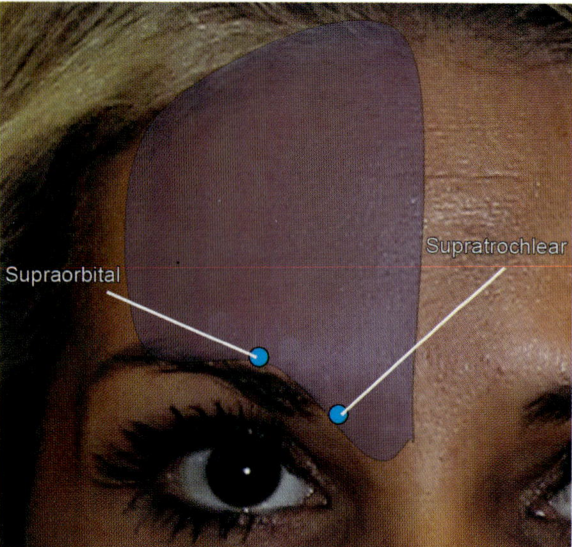


**Fig. 4.3:** The supraorbital and supratrochlear nerves supply sensation to the medial forehead from above the eyebrows to the scalp.

the anesthesia along the nerve. Aspiration prior to injection can minimize intravascular placement and hematoma.[17,18]

Nerve blocks are commonly performed on the branches of the trigeminal nerves of the face and digital nerves. The medial forehead can be anesthetized by blocking the bilateral supraorbital and supratrochlear nerve; the cheek, lower eyelid, nasal sidewall, and upper lip by the infraorbital nerve; and the chin and lower lip by the mental nerve (Fig. 4.2). The entire digit can be anesthetized with a digital nerve block.

## *Supraorbital/Supratrochlear Nerve Block*

The supraorbital and supratrochlear nerves are part of the ophthalmic branch (V1) of the trigeminal nerve, supplying sensation to the medial forehead from above the eyebrow to the hairline (Fig. 4.3). The supraorbital nerve exits through the supraorbital foramen, a notch that can be palpated at the midpupillary line along the supraorbital ridge. The supratrochlear nerve is located along the upper medial corner of the orbit. Both nerves can be anesthetized by placing 1–2 mL of anesthetic solution using a 1½-inch needle starting near the supraorbital foramen and injecting medially toward the bridge of the nose (Fig. 4.4).

## *Infraorbital Nerve Block*

The infraorbital nerve is part of the maxillary branch (V2) of the trigeminal nerve. It innervates the lower eyelid, medial cheek, nasal sidewall, ala, and upper lip. The infraorbital

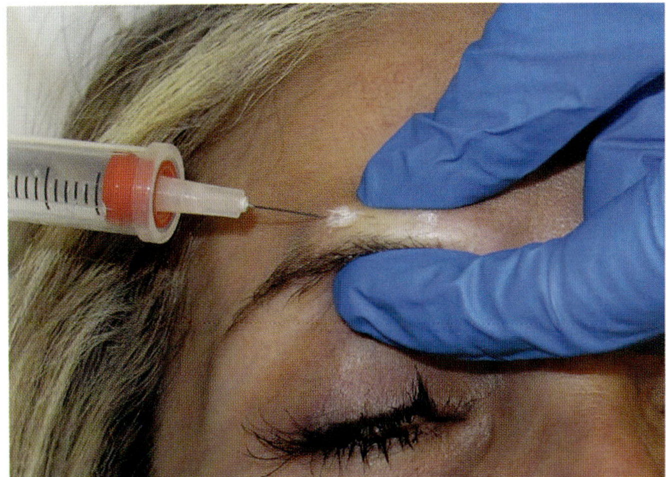

**Fig. 4.4:** Supraorbital and supratrochlear nerves can be anesthetized by placing 1–2 mL of anesthetic solution using a 1½-inch needle starting near the supraorbital foramen and injecting medially toward the bridge of the nose.

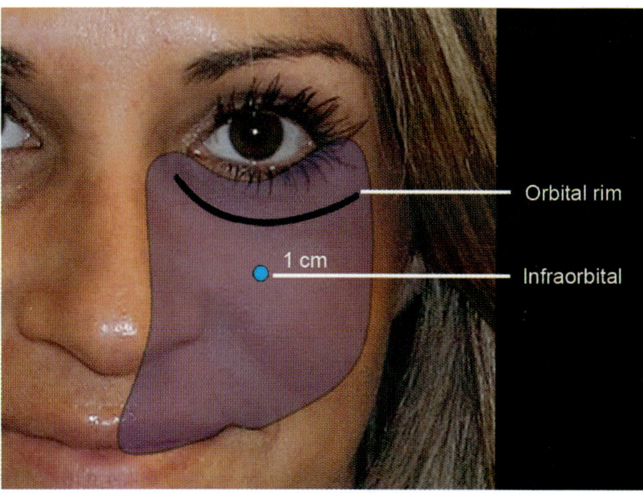


**Fig. 4.5:** The infraorbital nerve innervates the lower eyelid, medial cheek, nasal sidewall, ala, and upper lip. It is located at the infraorbital foramen, 1 cm below the orbital rim at the midpupillary line.

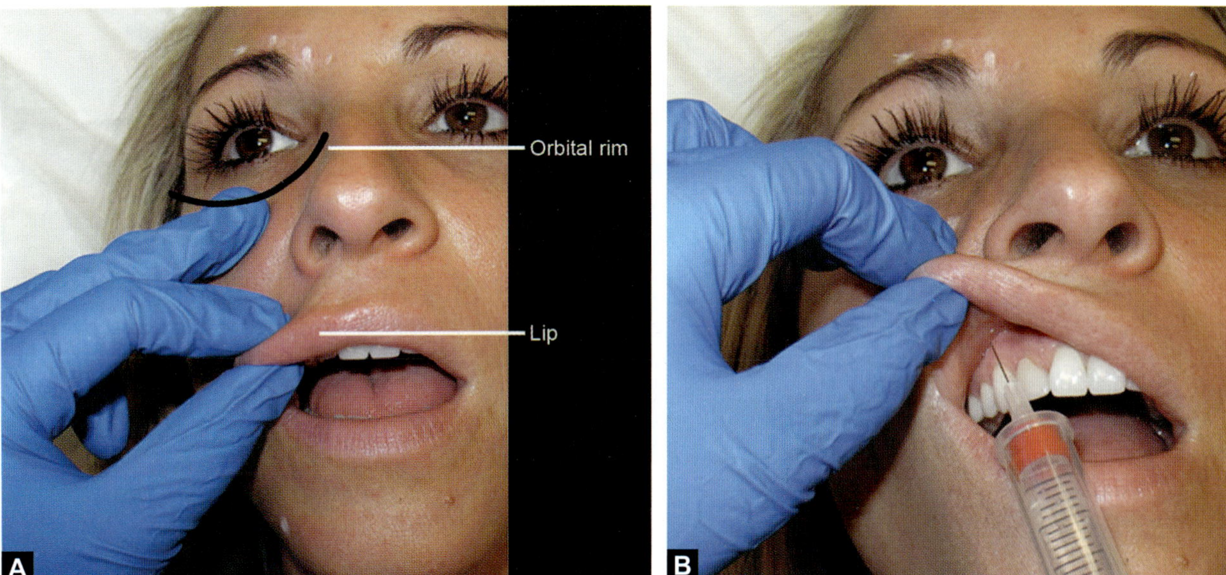


**Figs. 4.6A and B:** (A) Infraorbital nerve block. With the nondominant hand, the thumb and index finger are used to retract the lip, while the third finger is used to locate the infraorbital ridge. (B) The needle should be inserted into the labial sulcus at the first premolar (from midline, the fourth tooth) and advanced ~1 cm toward the direction of the infraorbital foramen using the third finger as a guide.

nerve exits through the infraorbital foramen, which is located along the midpupillary line ~1 cm below the infraorbital ridge (Fig. 4.5). Infraorbital nerve block can be performed percutaneously and intraorally, though the latter is usually less painful and more effective. Topical anesthesia can be applied first along the labial sulcus. With the nondominant hand, the thumb and index finger are used to retract the lip, while the third finger is used to locate the infraorbital ridge. The needle should be inserted into the labial sulcus at the first premolar (from midline, the fourth tooth) and advanced ~1 cm toward the direction of the infraorbital foramen using the third finger as a guide (Figs. 4.6A and B). Care is made not to inject directly into the foramen but to "bathe" the area with 1-2 mL of LA.

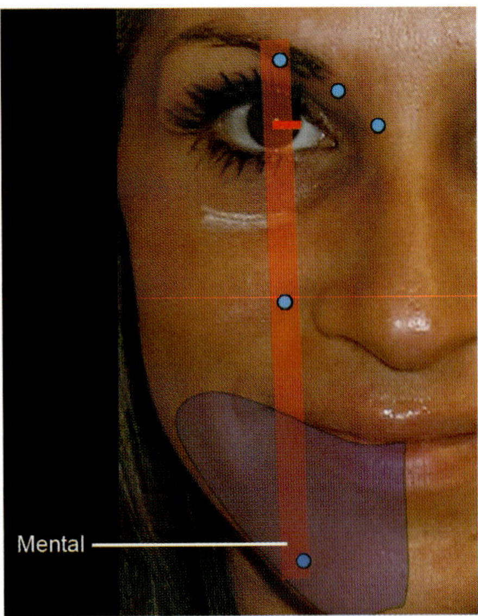


**Fig. 4.7:** The mental nerve provides sensation to the lower lip and chin. It exists the mental foramen along the midpupillary line.

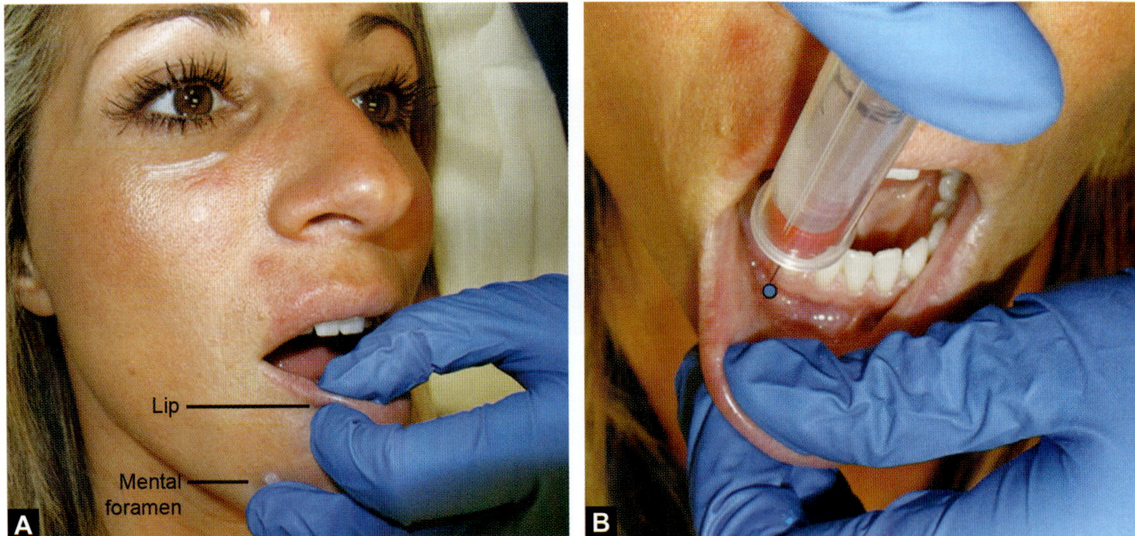


**Figs. 4.8A and B:** (A) Mental nerve block. The nondominant thumb and index finger are used to retract the lip, while the third finger is used to locate the mental foramen. (B) The needle should be inserted into the labial sulcus between the first and second premolar (from midline, the fourth and fifth teeth) and advanced ~5–6 mm toward the direction of the foramen using the third finger as a guide.

## Mental Nerve Block

The mental nerve provides sensation to the lower lip and chin and is part of the mandibular branch (V3) of the trigeminal nerve (Fig. 4.7). It exits through the mental foramen that is located just medial to the midpupillary line on the mandibular bone, though its exact position varies with patient's age due to progressive boney resorption. Topical anesthesia along the inferior labial sulcus can minimize needle insertion discomfort. The nondominant thumb and index finger are used to retract the lip, while the third finger is used to locate the mental foramen. The needle should be inserted into the labial sulcus between the first and second premolars (from midline, the fourth and fifth teeth) and advanced ~5–6 mm toward the direction of the foramen using the third finger as a guide (Figs. 4.8A and B).

## Digital Nerve Block

Two dorsal and two ventral nerves supply sensation to the digit. Several techniques have been described including web space injections, dorsal approach, and the lateral approach. Using a lateral approach, the needle is inserted ~5 mm distal to the metacarpophalangeal joint and a small intradermal injection is performed. The needle is then advanced medially and ventrally while aspirating to prevent intravascular injection. Approximately 1cc is injected while pulling back then the needle is redirected dorsally. The same procedure is performed on the opposite side of the digit.[19]

### *Tumescent Anesthesia*

The delivery of a large volume of diluted local anesthetic is termed tumescent anesthesia (Table 4.5), first described by Klein in 1987 for liposuction.[20] Since then, its use has expanded to laser surgery, facelifts, endovenous ablation, and surgery and reconstructions of large areas, eliminating the need for general anesthesia. The injection of a large volume of solution, from 100 mL to 3 L of 0.05% to 0.1% with 1:1,000,000 epinephrine, causes mechanical compression of the surrounding vascular structures. This tumescent effect enhances hemostasis, resulting in a relatively bloodless field, and prolongs the duration of anesthesia since the lidocaine is sequestrated in the fat compartment and metabolized much more slowly. Thus, it minimizes the risk associated with lidocaine toxicity and reduces the need for general anesthesia. The maximum lidocaine dose is 35–55 mg/kg for tumescent anesthesia, in comparison to 5–7 mg/kg with lidocaine with epinephrine. Due to its slow metabolism, plasma concentrations may peak >8–12 hours after infiltration.[21]

**Table 4.5:** Tumescent anesthesia.

| | *0.1% Lidocaine solution* | *0.05% Lidocaine Klein's solution* |
|---|---|---|
| Normal saline 0.9% | 1 L | 1 L |
| Lidocaine 1% plain | 100 mL | 50 mL |
| Sodium bicarbonate (8.4%) | 10 mL | 10 mL |
| Epinephrine 1:100,000 | 1 mL | 0.5 mL |

## Complications

Local complications are usually due to poor injection technique. Ecchymosis and hematoma formation can occur with inadvertent intravascular puncture, especially in patients who are on anticoagulants. Paresthesia, while rare and usually transient in nature, may happen with peripheral nerve blocks.

Systemic complications are uncommon. Symptoms and management strategies are reviewed in Table 4.6. Syncope can occur secondary to vasovagal reaction particularly in anxious patients. To minimize the risk of syncope or injury from falls, patients should be placed in a supine or sitting position prior to infiltration of local anesthesia. Epinephrine can cause tachycardia, palpitations, and tremors that usually resolve with time and reassurance.

Hypersensitivity/anaphylactic reactions are more common to the ester group (procaine) than the amide group (lidocaine). Allergic reaction to the ester group is usually from its metabolite, PABA, which is highly allergenic.

**Table 4.6:** Systemic complications from local anesthesia.

| *Diagnosis* | *Symptoms* | *Management* |
|---|---|---|
| Vasovagal | Hypotension, bradycardia, diaphoresis, hyperventilation | Trendelenburg, cool compress, and reassurance |
| Epinephrine reaction | Hypertension, tachycardia, palpitations | Reassurance |
| Anaphylactic reaction | Hypotension, tachycardia, bronchospasm, urticaria, angioedema | Stop delivery of anesthetic; airway management; supplemental oxygen; antihistamine; epinephrine 1:1,000 0.3 mL SQ injection |
| Lidocaine toxicity<br>Low (1–5 μg/mL)<br>↓<br>High (20–25 μg/mL) | Lightheadedness, tinnitus, metallic taste, circumoral paresthesia, blurred vision and diplopia<br>Vomiting, tremors, muscle spasms<br>Seizures, bradycardia, hypotension<br>Coma, respiratory and cardiac arrest | Stop delivery of anesthetic; maintain ventilation to decrease $PaCO_2$ below normal levels to decrease the risk of CNS toxicity; supplemental 100% oxygen to raise the threshold for seizure; diazepam for seizure; intravenous lipid emulsion for seizure and cardiac arrhythmia |

(CNS: Central nervous system).

**Table 4.7:** Maximum recommended dose of lidocaine.

| | *Maximum dose* | *Max dose for 70 kg* | *Maximum volume* |
|---|---|---|---|
| Lidocaine without epinephrine | 4.5 mg/kg<br>In children: 1.5–2.5 mg/kg | 300 mg | ~10, 3 cc syringes of 1% lidocaine without epinephrine |
| Lidocaine with epinephrine | 7 mg/kg<br>In children: 3–4 mg/kg | 500 mg | ~16, 3 cc syringes of 1% lidocaine with epinephrine |
| Tumescent Lidocaine* | 35–50 mg/kg | 3,000 mg | 3–5 L of 0.1% lidocaine tumescent solution |

*Tumescent max—assuming aspiration of volume with liposuction.

Patients allergic to esters can safely use amides as the two groups do not cross-react. True allergy to amide LAs is very rare. Most patients who are "allergic" to amides are actually sensitive to the preservative agent methylparaben and less commonly to sodium metabisulfite, though true allergy to lidocaine has been reported. Alternatives to the use of LAs include intralesional diphenhydramine (50 mg/mL) or normal saline (0.9%), which can provide adequate anesthesia for short procedures such as biopsies.

Lidocaine toxicity is rare though it can be life-threatening. To avoid the risk of lidocaine toxicity, one should not reach the maximum safe dose (Table 4.7). Inadvertent intravascular injections especially in highly vascular areas on the head and neck can result in toxicity even at lower doses. Early warning signs include tinnitus, circumoral paresthesia, dizziness, and lightheadedness. If plasma levels continue to rise, patient may develop cardiovascular effects.

## ANTIBIOTIC PROPHYLAXIS IN DERMATOLOGIC SURGERY

The use of prophylactic antibiotics remains an area of controversy in dermatologic surgery. A survey published in 2012 showed that dermatologic surgeons continue to overprescribe prophylactic antibiotics despite our awareness of multidrug resistant bacteria and adverse drug reactions.[22] Historically, recommendations were extrapolated from data in dental and general surgery, which were associated with higher risk of infections. In outpatient cutaneous surgery, infection rates are low and prophylactic antibiotics are rarely warranted. The importance of preventing surgical infection must be balanced against the emergence of bacterial resistance and the risk of unnecessary allergic reactions and systemic side effects.

The aim of this section is to review evidence-based guidelines on the use of antibiotic prophylaxis in cutaneous surgery. While the dermatologic literature lacks high-quality randomized controlled trials on this subject, several guidelines and consensus statements published in the last 10 years have attempted to specifically address dermatologic surgery procedures.[23-26] We will discuss particular scenarios in which the benefits of prophylactic antibiotics outweigh the risks of adverse side effects and antibiotic resistance. In addition, we will explore antibiotic choices for specific anatomic sites and the roles of topical and intralesional antibiotics.

### Goal of Antibiotic Prophylaxis

The goal of antibiotic prophylaxis is to decrease the number of bacterial organisms on the skin below levels required to cause infection. Antibiotic prophylaxis aims to prevent three types of infections: (i) surgical site infection (SSI), (ii) bacterial infective endocarditis (IE), (iii) hematogenous total joint infection. The use of antibiotics should be reserved for patients who are at "high-risk" for developing these infections.

#### *Prevention against Surgical Site Infection*

Surgical site infection is often defined as an infection occurring within 30 days at the operative site involving the skin and subcutaneous tissue. In addition, in a study by Horan et al., their definition of SSI included one of the following: (i) purulent drainage from the surgical wound; (ii) positive bacterial culture aseptically obtained from the wound; (iii) one of the following signs: pain, tenderness, swelling, redness, heat, or incision has been reopened by the surgeon; and (iv) diagnosis of wound infection by the physician.[27] Surgical site infections can be associated with local complications including wound dehiscence, flap necrosis, and poor cosmetic outcome. In addition, SSIs can increase the risk of bacteremia leading to systemic complications such as infectious endocarditis and hematologic

**Table 4.8:** CDC surgical wound classification.

| *Wound class* | | | *Infection rate (%)* | *Antibiotic needed* |
|---|---|---|---|---|
| Class I | Clean | Uninfected wound; sterile procedure; not involving oral mucosa, nasal mucosa, or perineum | 1–4 | None |
| Class II | Clean-contaminated | Uninfected wound involving oral mucosa, nasal mucosa, perineum or axilla; minor breaks in sterile technique | 5–10 | Yes, in high-risk patients |
| Class III | Contaminated | Traumatic wounds; major break in sterile technique; acute, nonpurulent inflammation | 6–25 | Therapeutic antibiotics |
| Class IV | Dirty/infected | Infected wounds, gross contamination or necrotic tissue | >25 | Therapeutic antibiotics |

**Table 4.9:** Factors associated with increased risk of surgical site infection.[24,25,31]

- Surgical locations at higher risk (> 3%)
  - Infected surgical site
  - Oral mucosa
  - Ear
  - Lower extremity, especially below the knee
  - Groin
- Procedures at higher risk (>3%)
  - Wedge excision of lip or ear
  - Skin grafts
  - Flaps on nose
- Patients at higher risk (>3%)
  - Immunosuppressed patients
  - Diabetes
  - Smokers
  - Extensive inflammatory skin disease

total joint infection. Thus, it is imperative to prevent surgical site infections to minimize these complications.

Fortunately, the overall rate of infection in skin surgery is low, with most studies reporting a rate between 1% and 2%.[24,28,29] Dermatologic surgery procedures are class I (clean) or class II (clean-contaminated) wounds according to the CDC classification for surgical wounds (Table 4.8). Maragh et al. prospectively evaluated 1,000 consecutive patients undergoing Mohs micrographic surgery and found an overall infection of 0.7%.[24] Rogers et al. similarly found an infection rate of 0.91%.[30] Dixon et al. performed 5,091 dermatologic surgery procedures without prophylactic antibiotics and found an overall infection rate of 1.47%.[31]

Specific surgical sites, types of procedures, and host factors are associated with higher risks of SSI and warrant consideration for antibiotic prophylaxis (Table 4.9). Dixon et al. noted >5% infection rates with surgery in the groin (10%, 1/10), below the knee (6.92%, 31/448), skin grafts (8.7%, 6/69), and wedge excisions of the lip and ears (8.6%, 3/35).[31] Other high-risk factors include infected surgical sites, flaps on the nose, and any procedures that breach the oral mucosa.[25] The host factors that should be evaluated prior to dermatologic surgery are a history of immunosuppression, human immunodeficiency virus (HIV), diabetes, or extensive inflammatory disease.[24,32]

## *Prevention against Bacterial Endocarditis*

Although relatively uncommon, infective endocarditis can be life-threatening, with a morbidity and mortality rate of 20%.[33] In the past, all "high-risk" patients including those with mitral valve prolapse were routinely prescribed antibiotic prophylaxis for any surgical procedures. The belief that a single preoperative dose of prophylactic antibiotics can prevent endocarditis in "high-risk" patients has never been demonstrated by controlled trials. The development of infective bacterial endocarditis requires a combination of transient bacteremia and turbulent blood flow from a congenital or acquired cardiac condition resulting in bacteria adherence and colonization. While transient bacteremia may result from surgery, it is much more common with daily activities.[34] The incidence of bacteremia with teeth brushing is 24–40%, mastication is 17–24%, and spontaneous bacteremia in healthy adult is 2%. This is in contrast with tooth extraction with a high incidence of 60–90% and outpatient dermatologic surgery with a low incidence of 2–3%.[25,35]

In 2007, the American Heart Association (AHA)/American College of Cardiology revised their guidelines on antibiotic prophylaxis, noting specifically that IE is more

**Table 4.10:** Stratification of cardiac condition for which antibiotic prophylaxis is recommended for the prevention of infective endocarditis based on the American Heart Association 2007 guidelines.[25,26]

| *High-risk patients—antibiotics recommended for surgery in high-risk sites (see Table 4.2)* | *Low risk—antibiotics NOT recommended* |
|---|---|
| Prosthetic heart valves<br>Prior IE<br>Cardiac transplant patients with valvulopathy<br>Repaired congenital heart defect with residual defect | Mitral valve prolapse<br>Rheumatic heart disease<br>Bicuspid valve disease<br>Aortic stenosis |
| | Stable congenital heart defect-ventral septal defect, atrial septal defect, hypertrophic cardiomyopathy<br>CABG<br>Stents<br>Pacemaker<br>Defibrillators |

**Table 4.11:** High-risk factors for prosthetic joint infection.[25]

- Joint replacement within the past 2 years
- Previous prosthetic joint infection
- Patients with high-risk comorbidities with total joint replacement at any time
  - Immunosuppression
    - HIV
    - Malignancy
    - Autoimmune disease
  - Diabetes
  - Malnourishment
  - Hemophilia

likely from random bacteremia from daily activity than from specific dental or surgical procedures. They concluded "only an extremely small number of cases of IE might be prevented by antibiotic prophylaxis even if prophylaxis is 100% effective."[36] Rather, the maintenance of optimal oral hygiene is more important than prophylactic antibiotics in reducing bacteremia and IE. The AHA updated guidelines redefined the "high-risk" group as those who are at the highest risk of adverse outcome from infective endocarditis including patients with prosthetic heart valves, history of infective endocarditis and valvulopathy (Table 4.10). Notably they excluded patients who have a high lifetime risk of infective endocarditis (such as mitral valve prolapse, rheumatic heart disease, bicuspid valve). In addition, prophylaxis is only indicated when "high-risk" patients are undergoing procedures in high-risk locations (such as dental procedures).

Based on the guidelines of the AHA, American Dental Association, and American Academy of Orthopedic Surgeons, Wright et al. issued an advisory statement in 2008 outlining dermatology-specific recommendations for antibiotic prophylaxis. They recommend prophylaxis in high-risk patients that undergo procedures in high-risk locations—breach of the oral mucosa, infected surgical sites, or sites with high-risk of SSI such as the groin or below the knee[25] (Table 4.9). Notably, prophylaxis is not necessary in high-risk patients on low-risk sites (such as routine dermatologic surgery on the cheek or arm). Prophylaxis is also not necessary when these patients undergo minor procedures such as biopsies on intact, noninfected skin in any location.

## Prevention against Prosthetic Joint Infection and Other Implantable Devices

Hematogenous joint infection following dermatologic surgery is rare; nevertheless, it is imperative to prevent such infection given the potential for serious sequelae. Recent updated guidelines by the American Academy of Orthopedic Surgeons and American Dental Association no longer recommend antibiotic prophylaxis in all dental patients with total joint prosthesis. In terms of prosthetic joint infection, at risk populations include patients with a joint replaced within the past 2 years, a previous prosthetic joint infection, and those with high-risk comorbidities with a total joint replacement at anytime. High-risk comorbidities include immunosuppressed patients (HIV, malignancy, patients with autoimmune disease), diabetics, malnourished patients, and hemophiliacs (Table 4.11). Antibiotic prophylaxis is indicated in high-risk patients undergoing procedures in high-risk locations such as infected skin, oral mucosa, groin, lower extremities, ears, and flaps on nose.[23,25]

Prophylaxis is not recommended for cardiac pacemakers and defibrillators per the AHA guidelines. The guidelines are less clear for other implantable devices such as shunts

**Table 4.12:** Prophylactic antibiotics and pathogenic bacteria based on surgical location.[25,26]

| Location | Pathogenic bacteria | Antibiotic prophylaxis (should be given as a single po dose 30–60 minutes prior to surgery or 2 hours after) |
|---|---|---|
| Glabrous skin, nonoral site | *Staphylococcus aureus; Staphylococcus pyogenes* | • Cephalexin 2 g or Dicloxacillin 2 g<br>• Penicillin allergic<br>– Clindamycin 600 mg<br>– Azithromycin 500 mg<br>– Clarithromycin 500 mg |
| Oral and nasal mucosa | *Staphylococcus viridans; S. aureus; S. pyogenes* | • Amoxicillin 2 g<br>• Penicillin allergic<br>– Clindamycin 600 mg<br>– Azithromycin 500 mg<br>– Clarithromycin 500 mg |
| Groin and below the knee | *S. aureus; Escherichia coli; Enterococcus* | • DS TMP-SMX 1 tablet<br>• Levofloxacin 500 mg |
| Ear | *S. aureus; Pseudomonas* | • Ciprofloxacin 500 mg |

(DS TMP-SMX: Double-strength trimethoprim-sulfamethazole).

and neurostimulators. In general, the highest risk of infection and biofilm formation is shortly after implantation, thus antibiotic prophylaxis may be useful in the perioperative period.

## Selection of Oral Antibiotic Prophylaxis

The selection of prophylactic antibiotic should be based on the most likely pathogens found at the specific surgical site (Table 4.12). Ideally, antibiotics should be given 1 hour prior to the start of the procedure, but may be given within 2 hours after the procedure. A single dose is sufficient, in most dermatologic surgeries; a second 6-hour postoperative dose is not necessary.[26] If surgical site infection is suspected, the most appropriate empiric antibiotics should be initiated based on the surgical site while awaiting wound culture results to guide the choice of postoperative antibiotics.

On glabrous skin, the most common pathogens are *Staphylococcus aureus* and *Streptococcus pyogenes.* First-generation cephalosporins such as cephalexin given as a single 2 g dose before surgery would provide adequate coverage. In penicillin allergic patients, clindamycin, azithromycin, or clarithromycin are alternatives. If covering for community-acquired methicillin resistant *Staphylococcus aureus* (CA-MRSA) is a concern, clindamycin is the best option.[24-26]

When considering oral or other mucosal surfaces such as the nose, *Streptococcus viridans* and anaerobes including *Peptostreptococcus* are the pathogenic bacteria. Amoxicillin is the antibiotic of choice for *S. viridans* coverage. Clindamycin, azithromycin, and clarithromycin are options for penicillin-allergic patients. Clindamycin is the drug of choice in patients who are at high-risk for MRSA. An additional option is the combination of double-strength trimethoprim-sulfamethazole (DS TMP-SMX) and penicillin V potassium or clindamycin.[25,26]

In the groin, perineum, and below the knee, the most common pathogens are *Enterococcus* and *Escherichia coli*, as well as *Pseudomonas* and anaerobic gram-negative bacilli. DS TMP-SMX offers the best coverage. On the ears, the most common pathogen is *S. aureus*, but this area can also be infected with *Pseudomonas* and rarely *Serratia marcescens* and gram-negative rods.[26] Second-generation quinolones such as Ciprofloxacin are the treatment of choice for *Pseudomonas*. These antibiotics will cover gram-negative rods and certain gram-positive bacteria. Third-generation quinolones such as levofloxacin provide broad-spectrum coverage against gram-negative rods and gram-positive cocci.[26]

### *Prevention Strategies*

Physician-directed intraoperative strategies could be helpful in preventing SSI and subsequent risk of prosthetic joint infection or infective endocarditis.[37] Good hand washing hygiene has been shown to minimize the risk for SSI.[38] Similarly, the use of an antiseptic solution prior to surgery is a well-recognized strategy to decrease bacterial flora on the skin. Both chlorhexidine and povidone-iodine have been studied, neither is superior to the other.[37] A Cochrane review by Webster et al. did not find any significant reduction in wound infection with the use of preoperative chlorhexidine bath or shower when compared to regular soap.[39] A meta-analysis by Tanner et al. concluded that routine hair removal at the surgical site does not reduce the risk of surgical site infection. In fact, shaving with a razor is associated with higher rates of infection when compared to hair clipping or depilatory creams.[38,40]

### Use of Topical and Intralesional Antibiotics

Topical antibiotics have not been found to be effective in reducing SSI compared to plain white petrolatum[26,41-43] and increase the risk of allergic contact dermatitis.[42,44,45] In 2005, bacitracin was the sixth most prevalent contact allergens according to the North American Contact Dermatitis Group due to its frequent use in the general population.[46]

Intralesional antibiotics have been found to reduce SSI in dermatologic surgery when administered as a single dose preoperatively with local anesthetics.[47-49] Intralesional administration increases the concentration of the antibiotics at the surgical site. Theoretically, this route may make it more effective than systemic antibiotics while reducing the potential for gastrointestinal side effects, interactions with other medications and antibiotic resistance. A prospective, blinded, randomized, placebo-controlled study showed significantly fewer *S. aureus* infections when patients were given intralesional nafcillin (0.5 mg/mL of 1% lidocaine) compared to control.[48] Similar findings were seen in a prospective, blinded, randomized, placebo-controlled study with the use of intralesional clindamycin (0.408 mg/mL).[49]

## ANTICOAGULATION MANAGEMENT IN DERMATOLOGIC SURGERY

With an increasing number of patients on anticoagulation medications and herbal supplements, dermatologic surgeons are challenged on whether to discontinue antithrombotic agents prior to surgical treatment. The decision to suspend antithrombotic agents to reduce the risk of bleeding complications during surgery must be balanced with the increased risk of a thromboembolic event. This section will review the types of anticoagulation therapy commonly encountered in the dermatologic patient, the risk of bleeding complications and thromboembolic events in cutaneous surgery, and current recommendations regarding discontinuing anticoagulants.

### Antithrombotic Agents

Antithrombotic therapy is often prescribed for patients for the prevention and treatment of acute coronary syndrome, cardiac valve disease and mechanical heart valve, atrial fibrillation, and venous thromboembolism (Table 4.13). An estimated 38% of dermatologic surgery patients are on monotherapy antiplatelet or anticoagulant medication while 8% are on two or more.[56] The most common antithrombotic agent used is aspirin as observed in 28–34% of patients and the most commonly used combination regimen is aspirin and warfarin in 3.2% of patients.[57] Additionally, an estimated 65–70% of patients taking one or more dietary supplements do not report it to their physician prior to surgery.[58,59] Many of these supplements have effects on coagulation when taken alone, in combination with each other, or in combination with prescription and over the counter medications.

Antithrombotic agents can be divided into two groups: antiplatelet agents and anticoagulant agents.

*Antiplatelet agents* consist of aspirin (ASA), dipyridamole, nonsteroidal anti-inflammatory drugs (NSAIDs), clopidogrel, prasugrel, and ticagrelor. Aspirin decreases platelet aggregation by irreversibly inhibiting cyclooxygenase. Nonsteroidal anti-inflammatory drugs are reversible inhibitors of cyclooxygenase. The most commonly used NSAIDs are ibuprofen, naproxen, and indomethacin. Dipyridamole is a reversible phosphodiesterase inhibitor. Clopidogrel, prasugrel, and ticagrelor are irreversible P2Y12 inhibitors that inhibit platelet aggregation and fibrinogen binding to platelets.[50] Prasugrel is associated with more life-threatening bleeding as compared with clopidogrel, although there is no difference in mortality.[60] Irreversible inhibitors, such as ASA and clopidogrel, last for the entire lifespan of platelets (an average of 7–10 days). Theoretically, they should be discontinued 10 days prior to surgery to ensure sufficient time for new platelet production.

*Anticoagulant agents* consist of heparin, warfarin, dabigatran, rivaroxaban, and apixaban. Heparin binds to antithrombin III, which inactivates several coagulation factors, namely thrombin and factor Xa. Warfarin is a vitamin K antagonist, which leads to production of nonfunctional coagulation factors thereby preventing the formation of the fibrin clot.[57] Dabigatran is a direct thrombin inhibitor, which acts by binding competitively and reversibly to factor IIa. It was determined to be superior to warfarin for prevention of venous thromboembolism in patients with atrial fibrillation with an equal or reduced bleeding risk based on dose.[51-53,61] Rivaroxaban, apixaban, and edoxaban

**Table 4.13:** Commonly prescribed antithrombotic agents.[50-55]

| *Medication* | *Mechanism of action* | *Monitoring* | *Discontinuation* | *Reversal* |
|---|---|---|---|---|
| *Antiplatelet* | | | | |
| Aspirin | Irreversibly selectively inhibits cyclooxygenase 1 at low doses (75–81 mg/day) and nonselectively inhibits cyclooxygenase 1 and 2 at intermediate doses (650 mg–4 g/day), which decreases platelet aggregation | Platelet function assay, serum drug levels | Prophylactic aspirin with no prior history of myocardial infarction or cerebral vascular event should be discontinued 10–14 days preoperatively and restarted 3 days after surgery | ddAVP—off-label |
| Clopidogrel | Irreversible thienopyridine P2Y12 inhibitor—inhibits platelet aggregation | Platelet function assay | Discontinuation not recommended | ddAVP—off-label |
| Dipyridamole | Reversible phosphodiesterase inhibitor—increases platelet cyclic adenosine monophosphate and inhibits platelet cyclic guanine monophosphate | Platelet function assay | Discontinuation not recommended | ddAVP—off-label |
| NSAIDs | Reversible inhibitor of cyclooxygenase-1 and 2, which decreases platelet aggregation | Platelet function assay | Discontinue 3–5 days preoperatively and restart 3 days postoperatively | |
| Prasugrel | Irreversible thienopyridine P2Y12 platelet receptor inhibitor, which inhibits platelet aggregation | Platelet function assay | No specific recommendations | ddAVP—off-label |
| Ticagrelor | Reversible and direct inhibitor of P2Y12 platelet receptor, which inhibits platelet aggregation | Platelet function assay | No specific recommendations | ddAVP—off-label |
| *Anticoagulant* | | | | |
| Heparin | Binds to antithrombin III, which inactivates several coagulation factors, namely thrombin and factor Xa | Check aPTT and a CBC with platelets 1 week prior to surgery | Discontinuation not recommended | 1 mg of protamine sulfate for every 100 units of heparin in vivo |
| Warfarin | Vitamin K antagonist, which leads to production of nonfunctional coagulation factors, thereby preventing the formation of the fibrin clot | INR should be checked at least 1 week prior to surgery and should be maintained in the therapeutic range 2–3.5 | Discontinuation not recommended | Fresh frozen plasma, prothrombin complex concentrates, recombinant Factor VIIa, or parenteral vitamin K can be used |
| Dabigatran | Direct thrombin inhibitor, acts by binding competitively and reversibly to factor IIa (thrombin), thereby preventing the formation of the fibrin clot. | Thrombin clotting time and ecarin clotting time (not widely available) | Discontinuation not recommended | Hemodialysis, recombinant factor VIIa, aDabi-Fab (not commercially available) |

Contd...

*Contd...*

| | | | | |
|---|---|---|---|---|
| Rivaroxaban | Direct thrombin inhibitor, which inhibits factor Xa/factor Va complex (prothrombinase) activity, preventing conversion of prothrombin to thrombin | Chromogenic anti-Xa assay (not widely available) | Discontinuation not recommended | PCC, recombinant factor VIIa |
| Apixaban | Direct thrombin inhibitor which inhibits factor Xa | Chromogenic anti-Xa assay (not widely available) | Discontinuation not recommended | PCC, recombinant factor VIIa |

(INR: International normalized ratio; PCC: Prothrombin complex concentrate; ddAVP: Desmopressin; aDabi-Fab: Humanized dabigatran-specific antibody fragments).

**Table 4.14:** Commonly prescribed herbal supplementation that interacts with coagulation.[58,59,62]

| *Supplement* | *Uses* | *Side effects* |
|---|---|---|
| Gingko bilobe | Enhances memory, improves circulation, intermittent claudication | Inhibits platelet aggregation and function, decreases plasma viscosity |
| Garlic | Hypercholesterolemia, hypertension, antibacterial properties, immunity stimulant, infections, toothaches, hyperlipidemia | Inhibits platelet aggregation, increases clotting time, decreases plasma viscosity |
| Vitamin E | Antioxidant | Decreases platelet aggregation and adhesion |
| Ginseng | Stress reduction, improves vitality | Inhibits platelet aggregation, contains coumarins |
| Chamomile | Dyspepsia, anxiety | Contains coumarins |
| Feverfew | Migraines, arthritis, fever | Inhibits platelet aggregation |
| Ginger | Nausea, arthritis | Inhibits platelet function |
| Omega-3-fish oil | Hypertriglyceridemia | Decreases platelet adhesion and aggregation |

are direct thrombin inhibitors, which act through inhibition of factor Xa preventing conversion of prothrombin to thrombin.

The most commonly used *herbal medications* that interact with coagulation are garlic, *Ginkgo biloba*, St Johns Wort, ginseng, ginger, vitamin E, and omega-3-fish oil (Table 4.14).[58,59,62] These supplements have anticoagulant effects when taken alone, which are perpetuated when taken in combination with prescription antiplatelet and anticoagulant medications. Supplements that are reported to interact with warfarin include coenzyme q10, danshen, devil's claw, dong quai, ginseng, green tea, papain, and vitamin E.[54] Supplements that contain coumarins or coumarin derivatives may cause potential bleeding complications. An example of a few coumarin-containing supplements is chamomile, ginseng, alfalfa, celery, horseradish, licorice, parsley, red clover, and sweet clover. Supplements containing high concentrations of salicylates may produce similar effects to aspirin and NSAIDs. These supplements are meadowsweet, poplar, and willow bark. Supplements with antiplatelet effects are bromelain, clove, onion and turmeric.[58]

## Bleeding Risk in Cutaneous Surgery

During major surgery, such as intra-abdominal, cardiothoracic, and intracranial procedures, antithrombotic agents are often discontinued to prevent life-threatening intra- and postoperative bleeding. Historically, dermatologic surgeons routinely discontinued anticoagulation based on general surgery guidelines. Furthermore, some patients stop anticoagulants based on advice given for previous surgeries or on the recommendations of their primary care physicians. A 2005 survey of 271 dermatologic surgeons revealed that 87% discontinue prophylactic aspirin, 37% discontinue medically necessary aspirin, 44% discontinue medically necessary warfarin, 77% discontinued NSAIDs, and 77% discontinued vitamin E therapy perioperatively.[63]

Cutaneous surgery, including Mohs surgery, excision, and most flaps are generally associated with low risk of bleeding. Minor bleeding complications such as postoperative oozing may require a patient to apply direct pressure at home and result in prolonged ecchymosis. Moderate bleeding complications are characterized by superficial sloughing and dehiscence (< 2 mm) of the closure. Severe bleeding complications may necessitate a procedure due to the potential significant threat to the wound or patient, including hematoma, flap/graft necrosis, wound infection and dehiscence (> 2 mm). In absence of anticoagulants, the overall risk of major bleeding complications in dermatologic surgery is < 1–2%.[56,64] Rates of bleeding complications in patients receiving antithrombotic medications range from 0.89% to 4.58%.[56,64,65]

A multivariate analysis by Dhiwakar et al. revealed aspirin and local flap reconstruction to be independent risk factors for total postoperative hemorrhage (defined as hemorrhage lasting longer than 4 hours despite external pressure). Surgical patients taking aspirin who also underwent local flap reconstruction were at a 124-fold increased risk of postoperative hemorrhage compared to cases with neither risk factor.[66] A multivariate analysis by Bordeaux et al. also revealed significant association with bleeding complications when a flap, graft, or partial closure was used.[56] A univariate analysis by Cook-Norris et al. found a 12% risk of severe complications when a graft repair was used, while the postoperative surgical defect size was also associated with severe complications.[67] In summary, the use of flaps, grafts, and partial closures, or having larger defects is significantly associated with bleeding complications.[57]

## Warfarin Versus Control

Multiple studies have compared the overall rate of complications in patients taking antithrombotic agents with control patients not on antithrombotics. One prospective study compared 47 patients taking warfarin with 49 control patients and found that there were significantly more minor bleeding complications in the warfarin group (26%) than the control group (6%). None of the patients in either group had severe complications.[68] Another study comparing 16 patients receiving warfarin with 77 patients receiving no anticoagulant therapy showed there to be no significant bleeding differences between the two groups.[69] A retrospective chart review by Otley et al. on 12,000 procedures showed the rate of severe complications while taking warfarin or platelet inhibitors was 1.6%, while the control subjects was 0.7%.[70] Severe complications were defined as potential significant threats to wound or patient. A prospective study comparing warfarin and control patients showed 23.8% major complications in the warfarin group with 0% in the control group.[71] Major complications included persistent bleeding, loss of skin graft, and wound infection. A meta-analysis by Nast et al. reviewed six prospective studies on warfarin with a total of 189 patients and 2,548 control patients.[72] Within the warfarin group there was a 12% risk of mild-to-moderate bleeding, and a 0.6% risk of mild-to-moderate bleeding in the control group. In summary, bleeding complications in coagulated patients on warfarin or antiplatelet inhibitors ranges from 1.6% to 26%, while nonanticoagulated control patients ranges from 0% to 6%.

## Antiplatelets Versus Control

Aspirin and NSAIDs have a lower risk of bleeding than warfarin. A prospective study comparing aspirin and control patients showed no difference between the aspirin and control group and no major complications.[71] In a meta-analysis by Lewis et al., 81 patients taking aspirin or NSAIDs while undergoing dermatologic surgery showed a twofold increase in moderate-to-severe postoperative complications as compared to 51 control subjects (4.1% vs 2.0%).[73] Another meta-analysis done by Nast et al. reviewed six trials with a total of 479 patients taking aspirin and 2,681 control patients. In the control group, the frequency of mild-to-moderate bleeding was 0.9%, with a 3.1% risk of severe bleeding. In patients with aspirin, there was no increase in mild, moderate, or severe bleeding.[72] A retrospective study by Bartlett of 52 aspirin users and 119 aspirin nonusers showed significant complications in 3.8% of the aspirin users, and 4.2% in the aspirin nonusers.[52] A similar retrospective study of 974 patients by Dhiwakar et al. demonstrated only 1.6–2.2% of patients taking aspirin experienced postoperative hemorrhage.[66] In summary, moderate-to-severe bleeding complications in coagulated patients on aspirin ranges from 0% to 4.1%, while nonanticoagulated control patients ranges from 0% to 6.5%.

Overall, there is a seven- to ninefold increased risk of moderate-to-severe bleeding in patients receiving warfarin compared to controls,[73] while the risk of bleeding in patients receiving clopidogrel is six- to eightfold.[51,56,67,73] Patients are 40 times more likely to have bleeding complications when taking clopidogrel and warfarin in combination.[56] No studies have been done to measure the risk of hemorrhagic complications in patients using prasugrel or ticagrelor in dermatologic surgery. Although there have been no studies measuring risk in cutaneous surgery, it has been found that patients receiving rivaroxaban have a higher rate of gastrointestinal bleeding, but a significantly lower rate of fatal and serious bleeding events compared to high-risk patients with atrial fibrillation patients on warfarin.[74] Also, incidence of major bleeding is lower in patients receiving apixaban compared with patients with atrial fibrillation and at least one additional risk factor for stroke receiving warfarin.[74]

Over the counter blood thinners such as vitamin E, fish oil, and *G. biloba* have not been associated with bleeding complications in surgery.[51,56,57]

### Antithrombotic Continuation Versus Discontinuation

Few studies have been done comparing hemorrhagic complications between those who hold their antithrombotics versus those who continue them. A retrospective chart review looking at Mohs surgery and excisions compared patients who continued their warfarin and aspirin or NSAIDs to those patients that withheld them. Patients undergoing Mohs surgery had no severe complications whether they continued their warfarin or held their warfarin. There was also no difference in severe complications (2%) observed between patients who continued their aspirin or NSAIDs and those who held their aspirin or NSAIDs, each having a severe complication rate of 2%. The unmedicated control group had a 1% rate of severe complications. In the excisional surgical procedure group, the risk of severe complications in patients continuing warfarin was 8%, whereas those who held their warfarin had a severe complication rate of 2%. The rate of severe complications between those who continued versus held their aspirin or NSAIDs was minimal at 1% and 0%, respectively. The unmedicated control group had no severe complications.[70] Another prospective study looking specifically at warfarin showed no significant difference in the rate of postoperative bleeding between those that continued or withheld their medication.[75] In summary, there is no significant difference in hemorrhagic complications between those who continue or withhold their antithrombotic medication. In fact, study by West et al. showed that dermatologic surgeons are often unable to accurately identify patients who are on anticoagulants based on visual inspection of intraoperative bleeding.[76]

## Thrombotic Risk in Cutaneous Surgery

While continuation of anticoagulants may increase the risk of bleeding complications, withholding anticoagulants may result in life-threatening, albeit rare, thrombotic events. In fact, temporary cessation of anticoagulants such as warfarin may induce a transient hypercoagulable state, putting patients at higher risk of thrombosis. Thrombotic complications most commonly seen after warfarin cessation occurred at a median of 2 days postoperatively. These complications were stroke, cerebral embolism, deep venous thrombosis, and pulmonary embolism. Thrombotic complications seen after aspirin cessation occurred at a median of 2.5 days postoperatively and consisted mainly of myocardial infarction and transient ischemic attack.[77]

A 2003 survey of 168 Mohs micrographic surgeons reported 46 patients with thromboembolic events after perioperative discontinuation of anticoagulants, including 3 deaths, 24 strokes, 8 transient ischemic attacks, 3 cerebral emboli, 5 myocardial infarctions, 3 deep vein thrombosis, 2 pulmonary emboli, and 1 retinal artery occlusion. Fifty-four percent of thrombotic complications occurred when warfarin was withheld, 39% when aspirin was withheld, and 4% when both aspirin and warfarin were withheld. The authors estimated the risk for thrombotic complications at ~1 event per 12,816 operations, 1 event in 6,219 operations when the use of warfarin is discontinued, and 1 in 21,448 when aspirin was discontinued. They suggest that 50% of dermatologic surgeons would experience at least one thrombotic event in their career.[77]

## Preoperative and Intraoperative Management

As an alternative to discontinuation of anticoagulation therapy, hemorrhagic complications can be avoided with careful surgical technique and early recognition and management of those at risk for perioperative bleeding.

### Preoperative Management

- Routine blood tests such as international normalized ratio (INR), bleeding time, and platelet levels on all patients are usually not helpful. In patients who had a recent warfarin dose adjustment or undergoing a complex reconstruction, INR can be screened at least 1 week prior to surgery and should be maintained in the therapeutic range 2–3.5.[50,78,79] There is a sharp increase risk of bleeding once the INR is above 4.5.
- Screen for underlying bleeding tendencies such as spontaneous bleeding, alcoholism, and chronic liver disease. Patients with heritable coagulation defects such as Von Willebrand's disease and hemophilia should undergo preoperative consultation with a hematologist.

### Intraoperative and Postoperative Techniques to Minimize Bleeding

1. Wait 15 minutes after injection of lidocaine with epinephrine (1:100,000 or 1:200,000) to maximize vasoconstrictive effects of the epinephrine
2. Use of tumescent effects of anesthesia to aid in the compression of the blood vessels
3. Avoiding complex closures, such as grafts and flaps, and minimize undermining
4. Meticulous intraoperative control of bleeding with spot electrosurgery
5. Clamping and suture-ligation of large vessel bleeders
6. Use of hemostatic agents such as Gelfoam or Surgicel in open wounds or during closure of surgical sites with uncontrollable persistent slow bleeding
7. Application of a well-constructed pressure dressing
8. Encourage patient-applied pressure and ice postoperatively
9. Limit postoperative physical activity.

## SUMMARY

A clear relationship exists between antibiotic overuse and multidrug resistance bacteria. In the last 10 years, there has been a shift to limit prophylactic antibiotic use to situations in which the benefits outweigh the risks of adverse side effects and antibiotic resistance. Fortunately, the rate of infection is low for cutaneous surgery, and in most cases with proper surgical technique, antibiotic prophylaxis is not necessary. A review of the literature and updated guidelines recommend against routine antibiotic prophylaxis for the prevention of SSI, endocarditis, and hematogenous joint infection. Prophylactic antibiotic is warranted only in high-risk patients when undergoing surgery in high-risk locations.

Dermatologic surgery can be safely and painlessly performed with the use of local anesthetic. Additives such as epinephrine can assist in hemostasis and bicarbonate can reduce pain of infiltration. Careful attention should be paid to injection technique and maximum dosage use. Special techniques such as tumescent anesthesia and nerve blocks allow for anesthesia of large areas while minimizing the risk of lidocaine toxicity.

Patients on warfarin or clopidogrel, or any combination of 2 anticoagulants have a higher risk for bleeding complications. Nevertheless to date in cutaneous surgery there have been no lethal of life-threatening bleeding events reported. In contrast, there have been a few thrombotic events reported shortly after cutaneous surgery for which antithrombotic agents were withheld. A review of the literature suggests that withholding antithrombotic agents perioperatively increases the risk of adverse thrombotic events, without significantly reducing the risk of bleeding complications. The overall consensus is to continue medically necessary anticoagulants during cutaneous surgery, while at the same time, limit the risk of bleeding complications intraoperatively by obtaining meticulous hemostasis and limiting the extent of surgical repairs.

The safety of outpatient dermatologic surgery has been confirmed through large multicenter prospective study and data from mandatory reporting databases.[80] The rate of adverse events in dermatologic surgery is 2% and usually due to infection and postoperative bleeding.[64,81] Alam et al. reviewed adverse events associated with 20,821 cases of Mohs surgery in a multicenter prospective cohort study and found only 149 cases of adverse events, the majority due to infection, dehiscence, and bleeding.[82] Thus with proper preoperative management, complications from anesthesia, bleeding, and infection can be minimized.

## REFERENCES

1. Starling J, Thosani MK, Coldiron BM. Determining the safety of office-based surgery: what 10 years of Florida data and 6 years of Alabama data reveal. Dermatol Surg. 2012;38:171-7.
2. Berde C. Developing better local anesthetics. Anesth Analg. 2015;120:718-20.
3. Hruza G. Anesthesia. In: Bolognia JL (Ed). Dermatology. New York: Elsevier Science; 2003. pp. 2233-42.
4. Hafner HM, Rocken M, Breuninger H. Epinephrine-supplemented local anesthetics for ear and nose surgery: clinical use without complications in more than 10,000 surgical procedures. J Dtsch Dermatol Ges. 2005;3:195-9.
5. Krunic AL, Wang LC, Soltani K, et al. Digital anesthesia with epinephrine: an old myth revisited. J Am Acad Dermatol. 2004;51:755-9.
6. Chowdhry S, Seidenstricker L, Cooney DS, et al. Do not use epinephrine in digital blocks: myth or truth? Part II. A retrospective review of 1111 cases. Plast Reconstr Surg. 2010;126:2031-4.
7. Thomson CJ, Lalonde DH, Denkler KA, et al. A critical look at the evidence for and against elective epinephrine use in the finger. Plast Reconstr Surg. 2007;119:260-6.
8. Denkler K. A comprehensive review of epinephrine in the finger: to do or not to do. Plast Reconstr Surg. 2001;108:114-24.
9. Que SK, Whalen J. A systematic review of the uses and contraindications of epinephrine in local anesthesia in the dermatologic setting. JAAD. 2015;72(Suppl 1):AB259.

10. Stewart JH, Cole GW, Klein JA. Neutralized lidocaine with epinephrine for local anesthesia. J Dermatol Surg Oncol. 1989;15:1081-3.
11. McKay W, Morris R, Mushlin P. Sodium bicarbonate attenuates pain on skin infiltration with lidocaine, with or without epinephrine. Anesth. Analg. 1987;66:572-4.
12. Giuliani M, Grossi GB, Pileri M, et al. Could local anesthesia while breast-feeding be harmful to infants? J Pediatr Gastroenterol Nutr. 2001;32:142-4.
13. Skidmore RA, Patterson JD, Tomsick RS. Local anesthetics. Dermatol Surg. 1996;22:511-22; quiz 23-4.
14. Brogan GX, Giarrusso E, Hollander JE, et al. Comparison of plain, warmed, and buffered lidocaine for anesthesia of traumatic wounds. Ann Emergency Med. 1995;26:121-5.
15. Strazar AR, Leynes PG, Lalonde DH. Minimizing the pain of local anesthesia injection. Plast Reconstr Surg. 2013;132: 675-84.
16. Randle HW. Reducing the pain of local anesthesia. Cutis 1994;53:167-70.
17. Davies T, Karanovic S, Shergill B. Essential regional nerve blocks for the dermatologist: part 1. Clin Exp Dermatol. 2014;39:777-84.
18. Grekin RC, Auletta MJ. Local anesthesia in dermatologic surgery. J Am Acad Dermatol. 1988;19:599-614.
19. Albom M. Surgical gems: Digital Block Anesthesia. J Dermatol Surg Oncol. 1976;2:366-7.
20. Klein J. Tumescent technique for liposuction surgery. Am J Cosmetic Surg. 1987;4:263-7.
21. Burk 3rd RW, Guzman-Stein G, Vasconez LO. Lidocaine and epinephrine levels in tumescent technique liposuction. Plast Reconstr Surg. 1996;97:1379-84.
22. Yoon-Soo CA, Liang CB. Perioperative antibiotic use of dermatologic surgeons in 2012. Dermatol Surg. 2012;39: 1592-601.
23. Bae-Harboe YS, Liang CA. Perioperative antibiotic use of dermatologic surgeons in 2012. Dermatol Surg. 2013;39: 1592-601.
24. Maragh SL, Otley CC, Roenigk RK, et al. Antibiotic prophylaxis in dermatologic surgery: updated guidelines. Dermatol Surg. 2005;31:83-91.
25. Wright TI, Baddour LM, Berbari EF, et al. Antibiotic prophylaxis in dermatologic surgery: advisory statement 2008. J Am Acad Dermatol. 2008;59:464-73.
26. Rossi AM, Mariwalla K. Prophylactic and empiric use of antibiotics in dermatologic surgery: a review of the literature and practical considerations. Dermatol Surg. 2012;38: 1898-921.
27. Horan TC, Gaynes RP, Martone WJ, et al. CDC definitions of nosocomial surgical site infections, 1992: a modification of CDC definitions of surgical wound infections. Infection control and hospital epidemiology 1992;13:606-8.
28. Sabetta JB, Zitelli JA. The incidence of bacteremia during skin surgery. Arch Dermatol. 1987;123:213-5.
29. Halpern AC, Leyden JJ, Dzubow LM, et al. The incidence of bacteremia in skin surgery of the head and neck. J Am Acad Dermatol. 1988;19:112-6.
30. Rogers HD, Desciak EB, Marcus RP, et al. Prospective study of wound infections in Mohs micrographic surgery using clean surgical technique in the absence of prophylactic antibiotics. J Am Acad Dermatol. 2010;63:842-51.
31. Dixon AJ, Dixon MP, Askew DA, et al. Prospective study of wound infections in dermatologic surgery in the absence of prophylactic antibiotics. Dermatol Surg. 2006;32:819-26; discussion 26-7.
32. Messingham MJ, Arpey CJ. Update on the use of antibiotics in cutaneous surgery. Dermatol Surg. 2005;31:1068-78.
33. Dajani AS, Taubert KA, Wilson W, et al. Prevention of bacterial endocarditis. Recommendations by the American Heart Association. JAMA. 1997;277:1794-801.
34. Nishimura RA, Otto CM, Bonow RO, et al. 2014 AHA/ACC guideline for the management of patients with valvular heart disease: executive summary: a report of the American College of Cardiology/American Heart Association Task Force on Practice Guidelines. J Am Coll Cardiol. 2014;63: 2438-88.
35. Eskinazi D, Rathbun W. Is systematic antimicrobial prophylaxis justified in dental patients with prosthetic joints? Oral Surg Oral Med Oral Pathol. 1988;66:430-1.
36. Wilson W, Taubert KA, Gewitz M, et al. Prevention of infective endocarditis: guidelines from the American Heart Association: a guideline from the American Heart Association Rheumatic Fever, Endocarditis, and Kawasaki Disease Committee, Council on Cardiovascular Disease in the Young, and the Council on Clinical Cardiology, Council on Cardiovascular Surgery and Anesthesia, and the Quality of Care and Outcomes Research Interdisciplinary Working Group. Circulation 2007;116:1736-54.
37. Fife D. Evidence-Based Procedural Dermatology. New York, NY: Springer; 2012.
38. Mangram AJ, Horan TC, Pearson ML, et al. Guideline for Prevention of Surgical Site Infection, 1999. Centers for Disease Control and Prevention (CDC) Hospital Infection Control Practices Advisory Committee. Am J Infect Control. 1999;27:97-132; quiz 33-4; discussion 96.
39. Webster J, Osborne S. Preoperative bathing or showering with skin antiseptics to prevent surgical site infection. Cochrane Database Syst Rev. 2015;2:CD004985.
40. Tanner J. Surgical hand antisepsis: the evidence. J Perioper Pract. 2008;18:330-4, 39.
41. McHugh SM, Collins CJ, Corrigan MA, et al. The role of topical antibiotics used as prophylaxis in surgical site infection prevention. J Antimicrob Chemother. 2011;66:693-701.
42. Levender MM, Davis SA, Kwatra SG, et al. Use of topical antibiotics as prophylaxis in clean dermatologic procedures. J Am Acad Dermatol. 2012;66:445-51.
43. Smack DP, Harrington AC, Dunn C, et al. Infection and allergy incidence in ambulatory surgery patients using white petrolatum vs bacitracin ointment. A randomized controlled trial. JAMA. 1996;276:972-7.
44. Lipsky BA, Hoey C. Topical antimicrobial therapy for treating chronic wounds. Clin Infect Dis. 2009;49:1541-9.
45. Sheth VM, Weitzul S. Postoperative topical antimicrobial use. Dermatitis 2008;19:181-9.
46. Zug KA, Warshaw EM, Fowler JF, et al. Patch-test results of the North American Contact Dermatitis Group 2005-2006. Dermatitis 2009;20:149-60.

47. Rosengren H, Heal C, Smith S. An update on antibiotic prophylaxis in dermatologic surgery. Curr Derm Rep. 2012; 155-63.
48. Griego RD, Zitelli JA. Intra-incisional prophylactic antibiotics for dermatologic surgery. Arch Dermatol. 1998;134: 688-92.
49. Huether MJ, Griego RD, Brodland DG, et al. Clindamycin for intraincisional antibiotic prophylaxis in dermatologic surgery. Arch Dermatol. 2002;138:1145-8.
50. Henley J, Brewer JD. Newer hemostatic agents used in the practice of dermatologic surgery. Dermatol Res Pract. 2013; 2013:279289.
51. Brown DG, Wilkerson EC, Love WE. A review of traditional and novel oral anticoagulant and antiplatelet therapy for dermatologists and dermatologic surgeons. J Am Acad Dermatol. 2015;72:524-34.
52. Bartlett GR. Does aspirin affect the outcome of minor cutaneous surgery? Br J Plast Surg. 1999;52:214-6.
53. Plovanich M, Mostaghimi A. Novel oral anticoagulants: what dermatologists need to know. J Am Acad Dermatol. 2015; 72:535-40.
54. Heck AM, DeWitt BA, Lukes AL. Potential interactions between alternative therapies and warfarin. Am J Health Syst Pharm. 2000;57:1221-7; quiz 28-30.
55. Palamaras I, Semkova K. Perioperative management of and recommendations for antithrombotic medications in dermatological surgery. Br J Dermatol. 2015;172:597-605.
56. Bordeaux JS, Martires KJ, Goldberg D, et al. Prospective evaluation of dermatologic surgery complications including patients on multiple antiplatelet and anticoagulant medications. J Am Acad Dermatol. 2011;65:576-83.
57. Shimizu I, Jellinek NJ, Dufresne RG, et al. Multiple antithrombotic agents increase the risk of postoperative hemorrhage in dermatologic surgery. J Am Acad Dermatol. 2008; 58:810-6.
58. Collins SC, Dufresne RG Jr. Dietary supplements in the setting of Mohs surgery. Dermatol Surg. 2002;28:447-52.
59. Kaye AD, Clarke RC, Sabar R, et al. Herbal medicines: current trends in anesthesiology practice—a hospital survey. J Clin Anesth. 2000;12:468-71.
60. Yousuf O, Bhatt DL. The evolution of antiplatelet therapy in cardiovascular disease. Nat Rev Cardiol. 2011;8:547-59.
61. Schmitt AR, Zender CA, Bordeaux JS. A new oral anticoagulant in the setting of dermatologic surgery. J Am Acad Dermatol. 2013;68:869-70.
62. De J, Souza SS, Silva JE. Use of herbal medicines by elderly patients: a systemic review. Arch Gerontol Geriatr. 2014; 59:227-33.
63. Kirkorian AY, Moore BL, Siskind J, et al. Perioperative management of anticoagulant therapy during cutaneous surgery: 2005 survey of Mohs surgeons. Dermatol Surg. 2007;33:1189-97.
64. Cook JL, Perone JB. A prospective evaluation of the incidence of complications associated with Mohs micrographic surgery. Arch Dermatol. 2003;139:143-52.
65. Billingsley EM, Maloney ME. Intraoperative and postoperative bleeding problems in patients taking warfarin, aspirin, and nonsteroidal antiinflammatory agents. A prospective study. Dermatol Surg. 1997;23:381-3; discussion 84-5.
66. Dhiwakar M, Khan NA, McClymont LG. Surgical resection of cutaneous head and neck lesions: does aspirin use increase hemorrhagic risk? Arch Otolaryngol Head Neck Surg. 2006;132:1237-41.
67. Cook-Norris RH, Michaels JD, Weaver AL, et al. Complications of cutaneous surgery in patients taking clopidogrel-containing anticoagulation. J Am Acad Dermatol. 2011;65:584-91.
68. Syed S, Adams BB, Liao W, et al. A prospective assessment of bleeding and international normalized ratio in warfarin-anticoagulated patients having cutaneous surgery. J Am Acad Dermatol. 2004;51:955-7.
69. Alcalay J. Cutaneous surgery in patients receiving warfarin therapy. Dermatol Surg. 2001;27:756-8.
70. Otley CC, Fewkes JL, Frank W, et al. Complications of cutaneous surgery in patients who are taking warfarin, aspirin, or nonsteroidal anti-inflammatory drugs. Arch Dermatol. 1996;132:161-6.
71. Kargi E, Babuccu O, Hosnuter M, et al. Complications of minor cutaneous surgery in patients under anticoagulant treatment. Aesthetic Plast Surg. 2002;26:483-5.
72. Nast A, Ernst H, Rosumeck S, et al. Risk of complications due to anticoagulation during dermatosurgical procedures: a systematic review and meta-analysis. J Eur Acad Dermatol Venereol. (JEADV) 2014;28:1603-9.
73. Lewis KG, Dufresne RG Jr. A meta-analysis of complications attributed to anticoagulation among patients following cutaneous surgery. Dermatol Surg. 2008;34:160-4; discussion 64-5.
74. Becattini C, Vedovati MC, Agnelli G. Old and new oral anticoagulants for venous thromboembolism and atrial fibrillation: a review of the literature. Thromb Res. 2012;129: 392-400.
75. Lam J, Lim J, Clark J, et al. Warfarin and cutaneous surgery: a preliminary prospective study. Br J Plast Surg. 2001;54:372-3.
76. West SW, Otley CC, Nguyen TH, et al. Cutaneous surgeons cannot predict blood-thinner status by intraoperative visual inspection. Plast Reconstr Surg. 2002;110:98-103.
77. Kovich O, Otley CC. Thrombotic complications related to discontinuation of warfarin and aspirin therapy perioperatively for cutaneous operation. J Am Acad Dermatol. 2003;48:233-7.
78. Blasdale C, Lawrence CM. Perioperative international normalized ratio level is a poor predictor of postoperative bleeding complications in dermatological surgery patients taking warfarin. Br J Dermatol. 2008;158:522-6.
79. Stables G, Lawrence CM. Management of patients taking anticoagulant, aspirin, non-steroidal anti-inflammatory and other anti-platelet drugs undergoing dermatological surgery. Clin Exp Dermatol. 2002;27:432-5.
80. Hansen TJ, Lolis M, Goldberg DJ, et al. Patient safety in dermatologic surgery: part I. Safety related to surgical procedures. J Am Acad Dermatol. 2015;73:1-12; quiz 13-4.
81. O'Neill JL, Lee YS, Solomon JA, et al. Quantifying and characterizing adverse events in dermatologic surgery. Dermatol Surg. 2013;39:872-8.
82. Alam M, Ibrahim O, Nodzenski M, et al. Adverse events associated with Mohs micrographic surgery: multicenter prospective cohort study of 20,821 cases at 23 centers. JAMA Dermatol. 2013;149:1378-85.

CHAPTER

5

# Postoperative Considerations

***Anne Zhuang, S Brian Jiang***

## BANDAGING

### General Bandaging Considerations

Bandaging is a crucial aspect of postoperative care, and there are many factors in bandaging that contribute to optimal wound healing. Although maintaining a clean and dry wound was historically thought to promote healing, this paradigm has shifted over the past several decades. Moist wound environments have been shown to hasten re-epithelialization and reduce pain from wound desiccation.[1] Furthermore, wound occlusion can augment collagen synthesis and promote angiogenesis through a relative reduction in the oxygen content of the healing wound.[2,3] As a result, one of the primary goals of the modern dressing is to preserve a moist wound environment via wound occlusion. Modern dressings may be either fully occlusive (impermeable to fluids, gas, and water vapor) or semi-occlusive (impermeable to fluids but partially permeable to gas and water vapor) and have been produced from a wide array of synthetic and natural products. Although moisture is an important factor in wound healing, the successful dressing must be able to prevent overhydration of wounds, as retained wound exudate can lead to maceration and delayed re-epithelialization.[4]

Currently, there is a vast array of dressing options available for postoperative bandaging, and finding the appropriate bandage can be quite daunting for the dermatologic surgeon. Most surgical wounds resulting after Mohs Micrographic Surgery (MMS) can be left to heal by secondary intention or repaired with linear closure, flap, or with skin graft. Although there are numerous ways to achieve the ideal environment for wound healing, gauze-based dressings are an easy and cost-effective bandage often used in the postoperative period following MMS. To achieve the optimal moisture environment, an emollient is usually first applied over the surgical site to keep the wound surface clean and lubricated. Petrolatum-based ointments such as white petrolatum and Aquaphor (Beiersdorf Inc, Wilton, CT, USA) are most frequently used due to a lower risk of allergic contact dermatitis compared to topical antibiotics.[5] Next, a gauze-based pressure dressing can be applied on top of the topical emollient to promote hemostasis and absorb any wound exudate. Nonstick gauze such as Telfa (Covidien Ltd, Mansfield, MA, USA) can be used to prevent adherence of the dressing to the surgical wound and thus improve patient comfort during bandage changes. These dressings can be changed every few days by the patient, depending on the amount of wound exudate, until the wound edges have re-epithelialized.

### Bandages and Considerations of Special Sites

#### *Eyelid*

As in other surgical sites, tissue stability after reconstruction of eyelid defects is important for successful wound healing. Many eyelid wounds can be dressed with a simple, compressive, nonadherent bandage that is then temporarily sutured to the surrounding skin. However, these dressings can be bulky, difficult to apply, and obstruct the visual field. The ocular stick, a thin roll of compressed gauze that distributes pressure evenly across an entire wound bed, is a useful alternative in these situations. These dressings are usually sutured in placed and removed after a few days.[6]

For larger eyelid defects where a substantial portion of the cornea is exposed, dressings must be able to provide adequate moisture to the cornea so as to avoid corneal desiccation and abrasion, a condition termed exposure keratopathy. This is especially important in situations when repair is delayed. Commercially available eye pads such as Pro-Ophta (Lohman & Rauscher, Neuwied, Germany), in combination with ophthalmic ointments, are useful for this purpose. Foster et al. described a similar dressing that can be made from commonly available supplies—woven gauze wrapped in Tegaderm (3M, St. Paul, MN, USA) and coated with ophthalmic ointment—that can be used to dress large eyelid defects without fear of corneal abrasion.[7]

Various topical antibiotic and antibiotic-steroid combination eyedrops and ointments have been used in the postoperative care of eyelid surgical wounds; however, there is no general consensus about their use. Moreover, their impact on wound healing and prevention of surgical site infections of eyelid defects is unclear. Despite these considerations, over 85% of oculoplastic surgeons worldwide use topical antibiotics in the immediate postoperative period and also at home after routine, elective eyelid surgery.[8]

### *Nose*

The nose can be very vascular, and in the immediate postoperative period, hemostasis may be an issue for surgical wounds involving the nose or nasal mucosa. Although compressive dressings may help with postoperative bleeding, external pressure dressings can be difficult to place on the nose if this causes collapse of the nostril. As a result, various forms of nasal packing have been used to prevent bleeding complications and to serve as a bolster against which an external dressing can be placed.

Biodegradable and nonbiodegradable intranasal dressings are both available. Examples of conventional, nonbiodegradable intranasal dressings include dental rolls, cotton balls, and synthetic polymers such as Merocel (Medtronic Xomed, Jacksonville, FL, USA). Some of the more sophisticated dressings have a built-in airway to allow patency of the involved nostril. Merocel nasal stents are comprised of a synthetic foam polymer of hydroxylated polyvinyl alcohol wrapped around a plastic tube that can expand to fill the nasal cavity and compress bleeding vasculature after rehydration.[9] These nasal stents are often lubricated prior to insertion, however, removal of these packing materials may still cause significant discomfort and disruption of the nasal mucosa. Biodegradable dressings such as Nasopore (Polyganics, Groningen, the Netherlands), a synthetic polyurethane foam, have been of interest in the otolaryngology literature. They have been used after endoscopic sinus surgery due to their ability to more rapidly resorb and, thus, result in improved quality of life during the immediate postoperative period and at packing removal.[10]

### *Ear*

Bandaging of surgical wounds on the auricle can be challenging due to the ear's complex anatomy. The optimal dressing is one that protects the surgical wound while avoiding any structural distortion of the ear. For smaller ear wounds or defects, especially on the helical rim or posterior ear, a simple dressing of ointment, nonstick gauze, and tape can be used. Full-thickness skin grafts may benefit from a bolster. For larger wounds, there are several bandaging techniques described in the literature that are cost-effective and avoid bulk. These include a "pocket sandwich" dressing described by Schmidtberger et al. and a "trapdoor" bandage from Wasserman et al.[11,12] These and other similar dressings reflect a shift away from bulky pressure dressings, as there is evidence of increased bruising and local skin irritation in patients treated with pressure bandages after uncomplicated ear surgery.[13]

In certain circumstances, it may be advantageous for the patient and surgeon to allow the wound to heal by second intention. In these situations, and in dealing with chronic, slow-healing wounds, it is more critical to understand the available dressing options as well as their properties, so as to choose one that is most appropriate. When considering what type of dressing to apply, important considerations include both the features of the wound—its depth, the amount of exudate, and location—and those of the patient—whether the patient and/or his support is able to perform frequent dressing changes. The major types of dressings, including biologic dressings, will be discussed in the following sections (Table 5.1).

## DRESSINGS AND BANDAGES

### Gauze

The term gauze encompasses a wide range of products that have been used since ancient Egypt. Gauze is inexpensive and versatile—it can be used as a primary dressing in clean and dry wounds or as a secondary dressing in an exudative wound. The classic type of gauze is formed from natural cotton fibers, interlaced together to form

**Table 5.1:** Major types of dressings.

| | *Advantages* | *Disadvantages* | *Examples* |
|---|---|---|---|
| Gauze | Inexpensive | Does not retain moisture | Avant Gauze (Medline, Mundelein, IL, USA) |
| | Ease of application | No barrier to external bacteria | Curity gauze sponges (Covidien, Mansfield, MA, USA) |
| | | | Telfa (Covidien) |
| Film | Can be a primary or secondary dressing | Nonabsorbent | Bioclusive (Systagenix, London, UK) |
| | Barrier to external bacteria | Fluid-trapping | Kendall Polyskin II (Covidien) |
| | Transparent | Strong adhesive may strip epidermis | Mepore Film (Molnlycke Health Care, Gothenburg, Sweden) |
| | | | Opsite (Smith & Nephew) |
| | | | Tegaderm (3M) |
| | | | Transeal (DeRoyal, Powell, TN, USA) |
| Hydrogel | Can rehydrate a dry wound | Limited absorptive capacity | Aquasorb (DeRoyal) |
| | Pain relief for dry or necrotic wounds | Requires a secondary dressing | Carrasyn (Carrington Laboratories, Irving, TX, USA) |
| | Easy removal | | Elasto-Gel (SW Technologies or Southwest Technologies, North Kansas City, MO, USA) |
| | | | Hypergel (Molnlycke Health Care) |
| | | | Kendall Curafil (Covidien) |
| | | | Nu-gel (Systagenix) |
| | | | SoloSite (Smith & Nephew) |
| Hydrocolloid | Absorbent | Can become malodorous | Duoderm (ConvaTec) |
| | Stimulate autolytic debridement | May require a secondary dressing | Comfeel (Coloplast, Minneapolis, MN, USA) |
| | Long wear time | | Cutinova (Smith & Nephew) |
| | | | Procol (DeRoyal) |
| | | | Replicare (Smith & Nephew) |
| | | | Tegasorb (3M) |
| Foam | Provides cushion over bony prominences | May require a secondary dressing | Allevyn (Smith & Nephew) |
| | Absorbent | Can become malodorous | Aquacel Foam (ConvaTec) |
| | | | Biatain (Coloplast) |
| | | | Kendall Foam Island (Covidien) |
| | | | Lyofoam (Molnlycke Health Care) |
| | | | Mepilex (Molnlycke Health Care) |
| Alginate | Highly absorbent | Dressing changes can be painful | Algisite (Smith & Nephew) |
| | Provides pain relief | Requires a secondary dressing | Nu-Derm (Systagenix) |
| | Hemostatic | | Kaltostat (ConvaTec) |
| | | | Melgisorb (Molnlycke Health Care) |
| | | | SeaSorb (Coloplast) |
| | | | Sorbsan (UDL Laboratories, Rockford, IL, USA) |

*Contd...*

*Contd...*

| | *Advantages* | *Disadvantages* | *Examples* |
|---|---|---|---|
| Silver impregnated | Can treat superficial infection | Local skin irritation | Acticoat (Smith & Nephew) |
| | | Argyria | Actisorb Silver 220 (Systagenix) |
| | | | Aquacel Ag (ConvaTec) |
| | | | Silverlon (Cura Surgical, Geneva, IL, USA) |
| | | | Silvercel (Systagenix) |
| | | | Silver sulfadiazine (generic) |

an absorbent sheet. Newer versions are composed of synthetic fibers that are biodegradable, adhere less to the wound bed, and are less likely to release lint compared to their traditional counterparts. However, these synthetic types are less absorbent.[14] Regardless of its composition, the primary purpose of gauze is to allow evaporation of wound exudate and prevent entry of bacteria. Gauze-based dressings often require frequent dressing changes to prevent maceration of the wound bed and formation of a nidus for infection. Furthermore, unless the gauze is coated, it can cause desiccation of the wound, adhere to the wound bed, and cause mechanical debridement and significant patient discomfort with dressing changes.

Impregnated gauze typically consists of a gauze sheet with a coating that limits adherence to the wound bed and, as a result, mechanical debridement. There are a variety of coating materials, including water, petrolatum, saline, zinc oxide, silver, paraffin, and iodine, among others, and some serve additional antimicrobial purposes. However, the coating decreases the absorbency of the gauze material and is thus not recommended for highly exudative wounds.[15]

## Semipermeable Films

Films are synthetic sheets of polyurethane that are transparent and have self-adhesive properties. They are elastic, easily conform to any wound, and allow direct wound visualization. The material is typically semiocclusive, allowing for passage of gas and water vapor while forming a protective barrier against external bacteria and other contaminants. However, film dressings have no absorptive capabilities and should not be used alone for exuding wounds, as moisture build-up can quickly lead to fluid-trapping and maceration. Furthermore, the adhesive nature of film dressings may lead to stripping of normal or new epidermis during dressing changes. Given these characteristics, films are most often used as a secondary dressing to secure a nonadhesive primary dressing or as a primary dressing for superficial wounds such as those after phlebotomy.[16]

## Hydrogels

Hydrogel dressings are water-based products that maintain wound moisture during wound healing and are best used for dry, low-exuding wounds. They are made from synthetic polymers such as polymethacrylates and polyvinylpyrrolidine and can exist in many physical states, including gels, solid sheets, or film. These polymers retain a significant amount of water and, as a result, cannot absorb as much wound exudate or suppuration. This can result in maceration and bacterial growth in highly exudative wounds. When in the form of a solid sheet or film, hydrogels allow passage of gas and water vapor through their semipermeable backing, enhancing autolytic debridement of the wound bed. Due to their high-water content, hydrogel dressings are often soothing and have analgesic properties for dry or necrotic wounds. However, hydrogel dressings are usually nonadherent and require a secondary dressing.[17]

## Hydrocolloids

Most hydrocolloids are composite dressings, comprising of a gel-forming agent such as gelatin or carboxymethylcellulose and other additives such as adhesives and other starches. They are available as powders, solid sheets, or pastes. These dressings provide more hydration than alginate dressings, thus promoting autolytic debridement, but are not as absorptive. On intact skin, hydrocolloids are impermeable to water vapor, thus eliminating the risk of transepidermal water loss and serving as an occlusive barrier to bacterial infection.

When a hydrocolloid dressing makes contact with wound exudate, it turns into a gel that allows free passage of gas and water vapor. This gel provides a certain amount of cushion to a healing wound and may be useful around bony prominences. However, hydrocolloid dressings may require frequent dressing changes, especially for heavily exudative wounds. Furthermore, continued occlusion from this type of dressing can prevent adequate oxygenation of the wound bed and wound healing. Hydrocolloid dressings also tend to form a brown, malodorous exudate that can be troubling for the patient and mistaken for wound infection. Most hydrocolloid dressings contain an adhesive border; as a result, frequent dressing changes can cause de-epithelialization of the wound periphery.[18,19]

In a randomized clinical trial comparing the time to re-epithelialization of split-thickness skin graft donor sites when various dressings were applied, hydrocolloid dressings resulted in the fastest wound healing times compared to hydrofiber, gauze, alginate, film, and silicone dressings.[20]

## Foams

Foams are semiocclusive dressings best for moderately draining wounds. They are typically composed of an outer membrane surrounding a silicone or polyurethane center. The outer layer is permeable to water vapor and thus serves to thermoregulate and maintain the moisture homeostasis of the wound bed, while the center portion provides the absorptive properties of the dressing. These dressings can be nonadherent and may require a secondary dressing. Foam dressings can be used to cushion the wound bed and redistribute pressure, making these useful over bony prominences and in conditions such as diabetic foot ulcers and pressure sores. However, it is important to note that foam dressings are not meant as a substitute for pressure-relieving devices. Like hydrocolloids, these dressings can become malodorous and require frequent dressing changes.[19]

## Alginates

Alginate dressings are highly absorbent dressings that can hold as much as 20 times their dry weight in fluid and are used for highly exudative wounds. They are composed of seaweed or kelp polysaccharides and alginic acid and often require a secondary dressing. The calcium ions in alginate dressings form an absorbent gel upon contact with the sodium ions from an exuding wound bed, allowing these dressings to maintain an optimal wound healing environment. The dressing fibers are biodegradable and easily removed with saline, allowing for easy and pain-free dressing changes. Furthermore, the calcium ions within alginate dressings can help with hemostasis by affecting platelet activation.[21]

However, alginate dressings should be avoided in dry or mildly exudative wounds, as they can quickly desiccate the wound bed and delay healing.[22] Moreover, alginate dressings tend to absorb fluid and rehydrate evenly across the entire wound surface, a phenomenon known as lateral wicking. This can result in maceration of intact skin if placed over periwound skin.[23]

Given their high absorptive capacity, these dressings have been used most often in chronic, highly exudative wounds on the lower extremity as well as pressure ulcers.[16] Despite anecdotal and theoretical advantages of alginate dressings in these situations, several Cochrane database reviews have reported no significant difference in healing of diabetic foot ulcers or chronic venous leg ulcers when alginate dressings were used, compared to other types of dressings.[24,25]

## Impregnated Dressings

### *Silver*

Silver has antibacterial properties against a number of pathogens, including gram-positive bacteria, methicillin-resistant *Staphylococcus aureus*, and vancomycin-resistant enterococci. Silver ions bind and disrupt bacterial cell membranes and cause bacterial DNA and RNA to denature, among other antimicrobial functions, resulting in cell death.[26] Some disadvantages of silver dressings include local skin irritation and deposition of silver ions in tissues (argyria), although the latter is quite rare. In vitro, silver ions can be cytotoxic to keratinocytes; however, no in vivo studies have demonstrated an adverse effect of silver on wound healing.[27] There are numerous dressings that have incorporated silver, including gauzes, hydrocolloids, alginates, and foams, so the use of silver-containing dressings can be customized to the characteristics of the wound.

### *Other*

Iodine is another agent used in wound dressings that has antimicrobial properties. It is often complexed with cadexomer, which promotes absorption of exudate from the wound bed while controlling release of iodine. Examples include Iodosorb and Iodoflex (Smith & Nephew, London, UK).

**Table 5.2:** Biologic dressings.

| | *Uses* | *Examples* |
|---|---|---|
| Epidermal grafts | Severe partial or full-thickness burns | Epicel (Genzyme Biosurgery) |
| Dermal xenografts | Severe partial or full-thickness burns<br>Chronic ulcers<br>Surgical wounds | OASIS Wound Matrix (Smith & Nephew)<br>EZ Derm (Molnlycke Health Care)<br>Integra (Integra NeuroSciences)<br>Biobrane (Smith & Nephew) |
| Dermal allografts | Diabetic ulcers<br>Dystrophic epidermolysis bullosa | Alloderm (LifeCell)<br>GraftJacket (Wright Medical)<br>Dermagraft (Organogenesis) |
| Composite grafts | Chronic ulcers | Apligraft (Organogenesis)<br>OrCel (Ortec International) |

## Biologic Dressings

Biologic dressings are becoming more prevalent and commercially available (Table 5.2). With advances in tissue culture and tissue engineering, cultured keratinocytes and fibroblasts can now be incorporated into synthetic scaffolds and placed into healing wounds. These dressings are an attractive alternative to traditional dressings, as they essentially simulate an autologous skin graft without the need to remove donor tissue. There are several biologic dressings on the market, and each can be placed in one of three categories based on the aspect(s) of normal skin they replace—epidermis, dermis, or a combination of both. Biologic dressings have been most studied in treating chronic wounds from burns, venous stasis or diabetic foot ulcers, and dystrophic epidermolysis bullosa.[28]

Epidermal grafts are comprised primarily of cultured keratinocytes. The Epicel system requires the patient to donate a small piece of normal skin, from which the patient's keratinocytes are cultured, placed on a scaffold of petrolatum gauze, and subsequently transferred back to the host.[29] However, the lack of a dermal component to these dressings has been shown to result in scar fragility. Furthermore, the lengthy wait and cost of this system make it less applicable for most patients.

Dermal grafts are made from collagen and other components of the extracellular matrix, including fibroblasts and growth factors. They can be allografts (derived from neonatal foreskin or cadaveric dermis) or xenografts (of bovine or porcine origin). These grafts have been studied to be useful in deep, chronic ulcers, burns, and wounds from dystrophic epidermolysis bullosa.[30]

Composite grafts are dual-layered systems consisting of an epidermal layer of keratinocytes and a dermal layer of collagen and fibroblasts. Apligraf is an example of a composite system that has been used for chronic venous ulcers, diabetic foot ulcers, and, in one study, wounds after skin cancer surgery. In a study by Eaglstein et al., Apligraf was applied over acute, partial, or full-thickness excisional wounds and resulted in reasonable graft persistence at the 1-week follow-up. However, graft persistence fell at subsequent follow-up visits. Furthermore, the aesthetic results were not impressive—over half of the wounds became hypopigmented and more than 90% were hairless.[31]

# CONCLUSION

Postoperative bandaging and wound care play key roles in successful wound healing after MMS and, as a result, can significantly impact patient satisfaction. It is important that the dermatologic surgeon understands the mechanics and uses of different dressing types so as to choose the correct bandage for each situation.

## REFERENCES


1. Kannon GA, Garrett AB. Moist wound healing with occlusive dressings. A clinical review. Dermatol Surg. 1995;21: 583-90.
2. Alvarez OM, Mertz PM, Eaglstein WH. The effect of occlusive dressings on collagen synthesis and re-epithelialization in superficial wounds. J Surg Res. 1983;35:142-8.
3. Knighton DR, Silver IA, Hunt TK. Regulation of wound-healing angiogenesis—effect of oxygen gradients and inspired oxygen concentration. Surgery. 1981;90:262-70.
4. Cutting KF, White RJ. Avoidance and management of periwound maceration of the skin. Prof Nurse. 2002;18: 33-6.
5. Smack DP, Harrington AC, Dunn C, et al. Infection and allergy incidence in ambulatory surgery patients using white petrolatum ointment vs bacitracin ointment. A randomized controlled trial. JAMA. 1996;276:972-7.
6. Farace F, Faenza M, Bulla A, et al. The ocular stick as wound dressing in lower-eyelid reconstruction. Aesthetic Plast Surg. 2013;37:480-1.
7. Foster KW, Roberts D, Goodwin CR, et al. Surgical pearl: preventing perioperative exposure keratopathy. J Am Acad Dermatol. 2005;53:707-8.
8. Fay A, Nallasamy N, Bernardini F, et al. Multinational comparison of prophylactic antibiotic use for eyelid surgery. JAMA Ophthalmol. 2015;133(7):778-84.
9. Haas AF, Vargo N. Surgical pearl: use of nasal packing with airway after reconstruction of deep nasal defects. J Am Acad Dermatol. 1997;36:1007-8.
10. Yan M, Zheng D, Li Y, et al. Biodegradable nasal packings for endoscopic sinonasal surgery: a systematic review and meta-analysis. PLoS One. 2014;9(12):e115458.
11. Schmidtberger L, El Tal AK, MacFarlane DF. "Pocket sandwich" dressing in auricular surgery. Int J Dermatol. 2015;54: 92-4.
12. Wasserman DI, Tucker D, Zeltser R, et al. "Trapdoor" ear dressing for auricular surgery. Dermatol Surg. 2008;34:567-70.
13. Castelli ML, Di Llisi D, Marcato P, et al. Is pressure dressing necessary after ear surgery? Ann Otol Rhinol Laryngol. 2001;110:254-6.
14. Jones VJ. The use of gauze: will it ever change? Int Wound J. 2006;3:79-88.
15. Boateng JS, Matthews KH, Stevens HNE, et al. Wound healing dressings and drug delivery systems: a review. J Pharm Sci. 2008;97:2893-2923.
16. Skorkowska-Telichowska K, Czemplik M, Kulma A, et al. The local treatment and available dressings designed for chronic wounds. J Am Acad Dermatol. 2013;68:e117-26.
17. Lay-Flurrie K. The properties of hydrogel dressings and their impact on wound healing. Prof Nurse. 2004;19: 269-73.
18. Thomas S. Hydrocolloid dressings in the management of acute wounds: a review of the literature. Int Wound J. 2008; 5:602-13.
19. Fonder MA, Lazarus GS, Cowan DA, et al. Treating the chronic wound: a practical approach to the care of non-healing wounds and wound care dressings. J Am Acad Dermatol. 2008;58(2):185-206.
20. Brölmann FE1, Eskes AM, Goslings JC, Niessen FB, et al. Randomized clinical trial of donor-site wound dressings after split-skin grafting. Br J Surg. 2013;100(5):619-27.
21. Sayag J, Meaume S, Bohbot S. Healing properties of calcium alginate dressings. J Wound Care. 1996;8:357-62.
22. Piacquadio D, Nelson DB. Alginates: a "new" dressing alternative. J Dermatol Surg Oncol. 1992;18:992-5.
23. Agren MS. Four alginate dressings in the treatment of partial thickness wounds: a comparative experimental study. Br J Plast Surg. 1996;49:129-34.
24. O'Meara S, Martyn-St James M, Adderley UJ. Alginate dressings for venous leg ulcers. Cochrane Database Syst Rev. 2015;8:CD010182.
25. Dumville JC, O'Meara S, Deshpande S, et al. Alginate dressings for healing diabetic foot ulcers. Cochrane Database Syst Rev. 2013;6:CD009110.
26. Wright JB, Lam K, Burrell RE. Wound management in an era of increasing bacterial antibiotic resistance: a role for topical silver treatment. Am J Infect Control. 1998;26:572-7.
27. Lam PK, Chan ES, Ho WS, et al. In vitro cytotoxicity testing of a nanocrystalline silver dressing (Acticoat) on cultured keratinocytes. Br J Biomed Sci. 2004;61:125-7.
28. Broussard KC, Powers JG. Wound dressings: selecting the most appropriate type. Am J Clin Dermatol. 2013;14: 449-59.
29. Rheinwald JG, Green H. Formation of a keratinizing epithelium in culture by a cloned cell line derived from a teratoma. Cell. 1975;6:317-30.
30. Ehrenreich M, Ruszczak Z. Update on tissue-engineered biological dressings. Tissue Eng. 2006;12:2407-24.
31. Eaglstein WH, Alvarez OM, Auletta M, et al. Acute excisional wounds treated with a tissue-engineered skin (Apligraf). Dermatol Surg. 1999;25(3):195-201.

# CHAPTER 6

# Suturing Techniques

Robert Edwin Eilers Jr, Arisa E Ortiz, S Brian Jiang

## INTRODUCTION

Proper suturing technique is essential during the repair of surgical defects to prevent postoperative complications and to maximize wound healing and cosmetic outcomes. This chapter provides a comprehensive review of both the preoperative and operative considerations given toward proper suture selection and technique.

## LOADING THE NEEDLE

The needle is composed of three parts: the eye, the body, and the point. The eye connects the needle to the suture. The eye of the needle used in dermatologic surgery is swaged, or crimped, which allows the needle to pass through tissue atraumatically.[1] The body of the needle is the greatest component of the needle and is the area grasped by the needle-driver. The point of the needle is the leading edge that passes through tissue.

The needle should be grasped with the needle driver from one-fourth to halfway along the body of the needle from the eye to the point, as this is the strongest point of the needle.[1] Loading the needle correctly into the needle driver allows for more consistent and predictable needle turnout from the tissue. Needles that are grasped toward the proximal aspect of the needle make it difficult for the surgeon to drive the suture through tissue and leads to higher occurrences of bent needles.

## HANDLING THE NEEDLE AND SUTURE

The surgeon should handle the needle and suture material in a consistent manner throughout every repair. The reasons for this are twofold. First, correct and consistent handling of the needle and suture material minimizes the chances of accidental needle-sticks to the surgeon. Care should be taken to always handle the needle with tissue forceps and the needle driver and never with gloved fingers. Second, proper technique promotes ease of movement of the needle and the suture material through the tissues, thereby minimizing trauma to the tissue and improving surgical cosmetic outcomes.

Attention to a long suture tail reduces the risk of wound infection by minimizing the chance that the suture tail comes into contact with nonsterile areas outside of the surgical field.

## HANDLING THE TISSUE

Tissue should be handled with extreme care throughout the procedure.

Mohs micrographic surgery reconstructions frequently require surgeons to manipulate tissue when securing flaps and grafts with sutures. Many surgeons manipulate wounds with tissue forceps when placing both deep and epidermal sutures. Gentle pressure is essential when handling tissue with forceps to minimize trauma to tissue and allow for proper wound healing. Skin hooks are also commonly used to manipulate skin edges, often at the apices of wounds, when placing sutures. Regardless of how the tissue is stabilized and handled, attention to the preservation of wound edges will lead to greater functional and cosmetic outcomes.

## THE SIMPLE INSTRUMENT TIE

The instrument tie is the most fundamental suture knot used in dermatologic surgery. It is employed to both anchor and tie off the majority of the more complex sutures outlined in this chapter and, therefore, will be reviewed at this time. Instrument ties usually involve three or four separate throws to secure the knot.

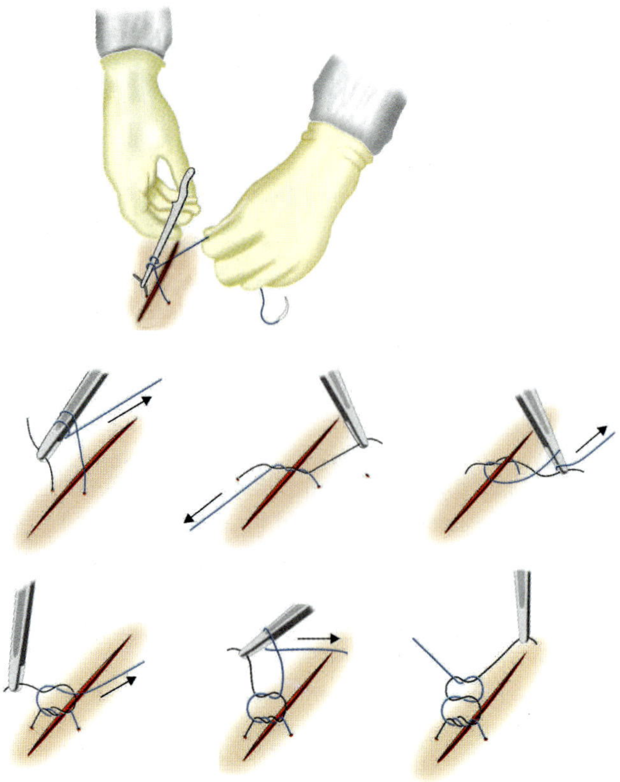

**Fig. 6.1:** Simple instrument tie.

The steps to perform an instrument tie are as follows (Fig. 6.1):

1. With the thumb and second finger of the nondominant hand, pull the leading edge of the suture through the deficit until the tail of the suture measures several centimeters in length and resides near the wound edge.
2. Position the closed needle driver in line with the axis of the deficit, between the two strands of suture.
3. With the nondominant hand, wrap the leading strand of suture counter-clockwise around the closed needle driver twice.
4. Open the teeth of the needle driver and grasp the short tail of the suture.
5. In a crossing motion, gently pull the short tail and the leading strand of suture toward the opposite sides of the deficit, laying the knot flat against the epidermis.
6. Upon completion of this first throw, place the needle driver between the two strands of suture, parallel to the axis of the deficit.
7. Wrap the long strand of suture clockwise around the closed needle driver once, then grasp the short tail of the suture with the needle driver teeth and pull gently in the opposite direction.
8. Repeat the above step for one or two more throws alternating counter-clockwise and clockwise to secure the instrument tie.

## PREOPERATIVE CONSIDERATIONS

Prior to initiating a repair, the surgeon must decide whether to close the defect primarily or let it heal by secondary intention. This initial decision often depends on the patient's age, the durability of the surrounding skin, the anatomic location of the defect, the patient activity level, and the ability of the patient to follow-up postoperatively.

Selection of appropriate suture material is of the utmost importance if the wound is to be closed primarily. This decision is most often dictated by the anatomic location of the defect and the type of repair to be performed.

### Needle Selection

Surgical needles come in a large variety of shapes and sizes. The body of the needle determines the overall size and shape of the needle. For superficial skin closure, the most common needle shape used is the three-eighth circle needle.[2] When properly loaded into the needle driver, the broad arc of this needle allows for closure of relatively large cutaneous wound edges with a simple pronation of the surgeon's wrist. This needle is less suited for use in more confined spaces for these same reasons. The most commonly used needle shape for use in more confined spaces is the half circle needle. The arc of this needle is greater and more ideal for use within deep, confined wound defects. More pronation or supination of the surgeon's wrist is required to manipulate this needle.[2] If a smaller needle is not available, one can simply load the needle more distally on the body to accommodate for confined spaces.

In addition to needle size, needles are classified based on the cross-section of the point. When the point of the triangle points inside the needle curve, it is called a conventional-cutting needle. When the point of the triangle points outside the needle curve, it is called a reverse-cutting needle.[2] For the majority of cutaneous reconstructions, the reverse-cutting needle is preferred because it is less likely to tear through tissue while suturing.

### Suture Material Selection

The ideal suture material for any repair is one that is easy to handle, has high tensile strength, forms secure knots,

**Table 6.1:** Characteristics of suture materials.

| *Absorption* | | *Composition* | | *Configuration* | |
|---|---|---|---|---|---|
| **Absorbable** | **Nonabsorbable** | **Natural** | **Synthetic** | **Monofilament** | **Multifilament** |
| Polyglactin 910 | Nylon | Silk | Polyglactin 910 | Nylon | Polyglactin 910 |
| Poliglecaprone 25 | Polypropylene | Surgical gut | Poliglecaprone 25 | Polypropylene | Silk |
| Polyglyconate | Silk | Chromic gut | Polyglyconate | Polyglyconate | Surgical gut |
| Polydioxanone | | | Polydioxanone | Polydioxanone | Chromic gut |
| Surgical gut | | | Nylon | Poliglecaprone 25 | |
| Chromic gut | | | Propylene | | |

and has the ability to stretch and retract with associated wound edema.[3] Sutures are classified by numerous factors including absorption, composition, and configuration (Table 6.1).[3]

## Absorption

Absorbable sutures are defined as sutures that lose the majority of their tensile strength after 60 days.[4] They are most frequently used as deep dermal sutures to close dead space and provide support and strength to a layered closure. However, some absorbable sutures may also be used as epidermal sutures in patients who are not able to return to the office for suture removal.

The most common subcutaneous absorbable sutures used in cutaneous surgery are polyglactin 910 (Vicryl) and poliglecaprone 25 (Monocryl).[5] Other common subcutaneous absorbable sutures include polyglyconate (Maxon) and polydioxanone (PDS).[1] As a general rule, absorbable sutures placed deeper in the dermis are less likely to be extruded than absorbable sutures placed more superficially. Regan et al. found that poliglecaprone 25 (Monocryl) sutures were extruded (spitting suture) to a significantly lesser degree than polyglactin 910 (Vicryl) sutures.[6]

Absorbable sutures were traditionally considered to cause redness, transepidermal elimination, and track mark formation when used as epidermal sutures.[7] For this reason, nylon (Ethilon) and polypropylene (Prolene) sutures remain the most frequently used epidermal sutures for two-layered closures in dermatologic surgery. However, in a small pilot study, Gabel et al. found no significant difference in redness, infection, dehiscence, scar hypertrophy, or patient satisfaction when comparing absorbable polyglactin 910 (Vicryl) and nonabsorbable (Nylon) sutures for closure of small 3-mm punch biopsy wounds.[8] In another study, Rosenzweig et al. compared poliglecaprone 25 (Monocryl) with polypropylene (Prolene) sutures used in primary closure on the face after Mohs micrographic surgery, and they also did not find significant differences in cosmetic outcome or other complications.[9] The editor (SBJ) routinely uses poliglecaprone 25 (Monocryl) for deep and superficial sutures to close donor sites for skin grafts. Other absorbable sutures used for epidermal closure of layered wounds include fast absorbing surgical gut, chromic gut, and fast absorbing polyglactin 910 (Vicryl Rapide).[1]

## Composition

Sutures may be composed of either natural or synthetic material. Natural suture materials include Silk, which is nonabsorbable, and surgical or chromic gut, which is absorbable.[5] These natural sutures tend to have a higher inflammatory reaction than synthetic sutures and have lower tensile strength.[1] Silk sutures are often chosen for use on mucosal surfaces and chromic gut is commonly used for attaching skin grafts.[1]

Synthetic suture materials tend to have less tissue reactivity, higher tensile strength, and high infection resistance as compared to the natural Silk or gut sutures.[1] The most common synthetic suture materials used in dermatologic surgery include polyglactin 910 (Vicryl), poliglecaprone 25 (Monocryl), polyglyconate (Maxon), polydioxanone (PDS), nylon (Ethilon), and polypropylene (Prolene).

## Configuration

The configuration of suture material is another important consideration. Suture configurations are divided into monofilamentous and multifilamentous. As the name suggests, monofilamentous sutures have a smooth, single-fiber design, reminiscent of a fishing line. Multifilamentous sutures, on the other hand, have multifiber designs reminiscent of a climbing rope.

Monofilamentous sutures have high tensile strength and smooth surfaces, allowing them to pass through tissue with low tissue reactivity and inflammation.[1] A disadvantage

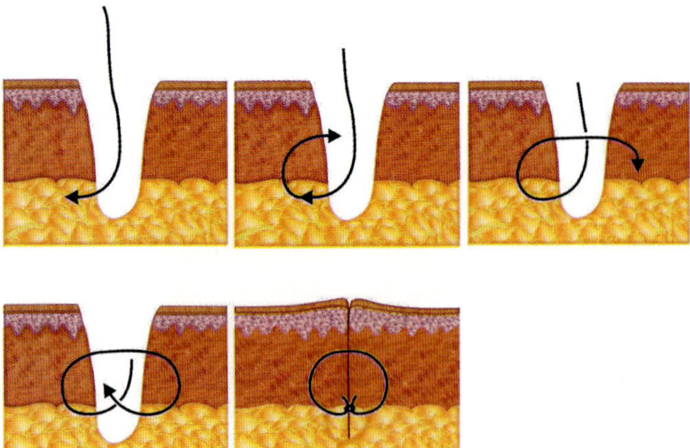

**Fig. 6.2:** Interrupted buried dermal suture.

of these sutures is that they have a higher memory, meaning they are stiffer than multifilamentous sutures and retain the shape they were packaged in. As a result, these sutures are more difficult to handle.[1] Furthermore, these sutures tend to have inferior knot security as compared to multifilamentous sutures given their stiffness and smooth surfaces. Commonly used monofilamentous sutures include nylon (Ethilon), polypropylene (Prolene), polyglyconate (Maxon), polydioxanone (PDS), and poliglecaprone 25 (Monocryl).[5]

Multifilamentous sutures, in contrast, have a braided texture. These sutures have less memory, are easier to handle during a procedure, and allow for greater knot security.[1] However, the braided texture of these sutures leads to higher amounts of friction and inflammation when passing through tissue. The increased capillarity of the suture also predisposes to higher rates of infection. Commonly used multifilamentous sutures include polyglactin 910 (Vicryl), Silk, surgical gut, and chromic gut.[5]

## SUTURE TECHNIQUES

### Deep Dermal Sutures

Deep dermal sutures are often the first sutures placed in the repair of a cutaneous surgical defect following meticulous hemostasis and wound edge undermining. These sutures serve to both close dead space previously occupied by the tumor and to provide the majority of the strength of the layered closure. The suture materials used in these deep sutures are typically made of absorbable material, such as poliglecaprone 25 (Monocryl) or polyglactin 910 (Vicryl), which slowly dissolve over a period of weeks to months as the wound reepithelializes.

### Interrupted Buried Dermal Suture

The interrupted buried dermal suture is the simplest of deep dermal sutures that are used in two-layered closures. The suture is employed both in wide local excisions as well as a host of flaps. When placing the interrupted buried dermal suture, a component of eversion is also attained. Epidermal, nonabsorbable sutures are typically then used to approximate the wound edges once the interrupted buried dermal sutures are placed.

The steps to place an interrupted buried dermal suture are as follows (Fig. 6.2):

1. Enter the deep, undermined subcutaneous surface of the wound edge then arc the needle upward toward the epidermis, taking care to remain deep to the dermal–epidermal junction.
2. Exit the same wound edge at the level of the superficial papillary dermis.
3. Carefully reload the needle and enter the superficial papillary dermis of the wound edge directly across from the wound cavity.
4. Arc the needle parallel to the dermal–epidermal junction initially, then downward into the deep dermis and subcutaneous tissue, where it exits into the wound cavity.
5. Ensure that the leading edge of the suture and the suture tail are on the same side of the suture that was just placed.
6. Secure the interrupted buried dermal suture with an instrument tie. The knot should lie in the deep dermal and subcutaneous tissue.

### Buried Vertical Mattress Suture

The buried vertical mattress suture is the most common deep dermal suturing technique utilized by dermatologic surgeons. It affords prolonged wound eversion in addition to apposing wound edges.

The steps to place a buried vertical mattress suture are as follows (Fig. 6.3):

1. Enter the deep, undermined subcutaneous surface of the wound edge and arc the needle upward toward the superficial dermis.
2. Continuing the arc, exit the same wound edge at the level of the mid-dermis.
3. Carefully reload the needle and enter the mid-dermis of the wound edge directly across the wound cavity.
4. Arc the needle upward toward the upper reticular dermis, and continue the curve downward to exit the wound cavity.

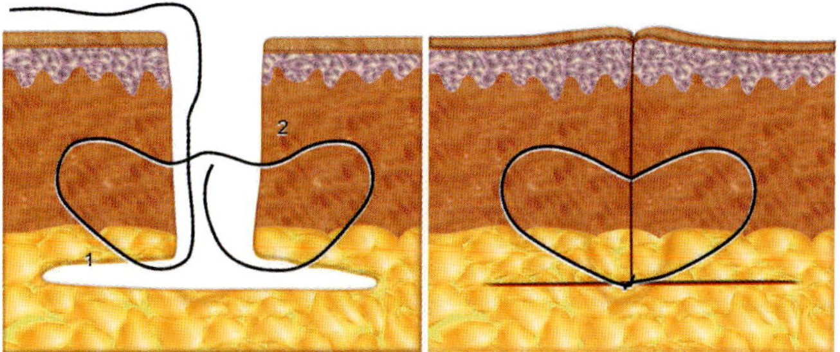


**Fig. 6.3:** Buried vertical mattress suture.

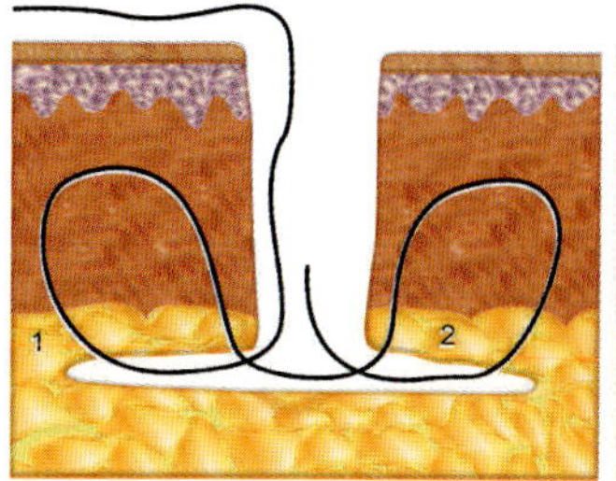


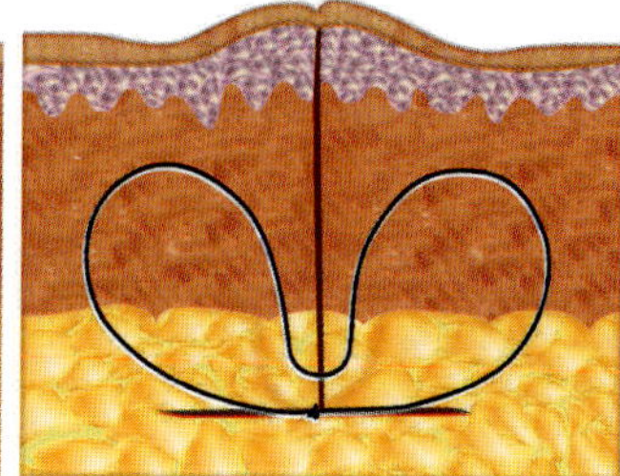

**Fig. 6.4:** Buried butterfly suture.

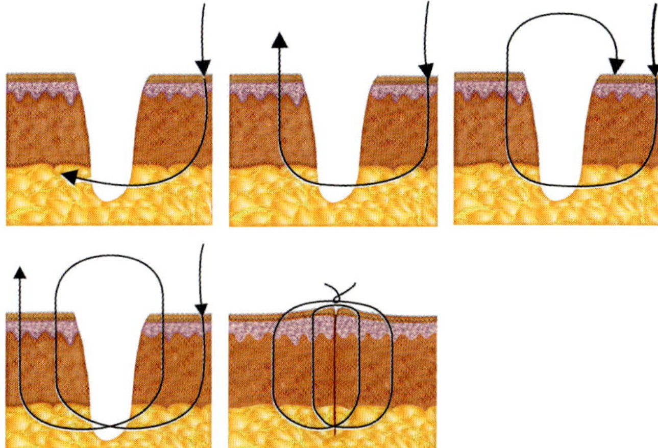

**Fig. 6.5:** Epidermal pulley suture.

5. Ensure that the leading edge of the suture and the suture tail are on the same side of the suture that was just placed.
6. Secure the buried vertical mattress suture with an instrument tie.

## Buried Butterfly Suture

For even greater wound eversion than the buried vertical mattress suture, a buried butterfly suture may be employed. This suturing technique distributes the tension away from the wound edge to the surrounding skin. Dimpling in the surrounding skin may be apparent due to the exaggerated eversion of the epidermal edges. This technique improves cosmesis by alleviating tension from the wound edge, resulting in a finer scar.

The steps to place a buried butterfly suture are as follows (Fig. 6.4):

1. Enter the undersurface of the undermined flap and arc the needle upward toward the reticular dermis.
2. Continuing the arc, exit the undersurface of the flap in the subcutaneous tissue.
3. Carefully reload the needle and enter the undersurface of the flap directly across from the wound cavity.
4. Arc the needle upward toward the dermis, and exit the wound cavity lateral to the wound edge from the entry point.
5. Secure the buried butterfly suture with an instrument tie.

## Pulley Sutures

An epidermal pulley suture is used in situations where there is a significant amount of tension on a full thickness wound, such as on the scalp, back, or legs. This suture serves to both decrease the tension on the wound, facilitating placement of deep dermal and epidermal sutures, and to slowly promote tissue expansion. The epidermal suture may be removed following placement of the deep dermal sutures or may be left in place and removed when the epidermal sutures are removed at the patient's postoperative visit. A variation of the epidermal pulley suture, the dermal buried pulley suture, has been described and offers similar resistance to the spread of wounds under tension.[10]

The steps to place an epidermal pulley suture are as follows (Fig. 6.5):

1. Enter the epidermis 5 mm lateral to the wound edge, arcing the needle downward and exiting into the wound cavity at the level of the deep subcutaneous tissue.
2. Carefully reload the needle and enter the deep subcutaneous tissue on the opposite side of the wound cavity.
3. Arc the needle upward and exit the epidermis 2–3 mm lateral to the wound edge.
4. Carefully reload the needle and enter the epidermis 2–3 mm lateral to the wound edge, in line with the wound cavity and the initial suture.
5. Arc the needle downward and exit into the wound cavity at the level of the deep subcutaneous tissue.

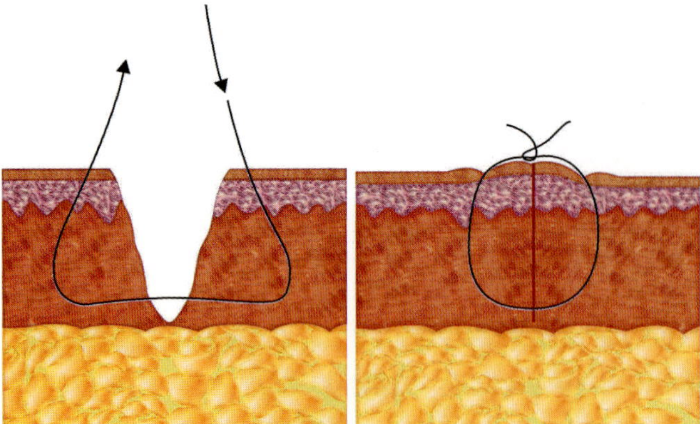

**Fig. 6.6:** Simple interrupted epidermal suture.

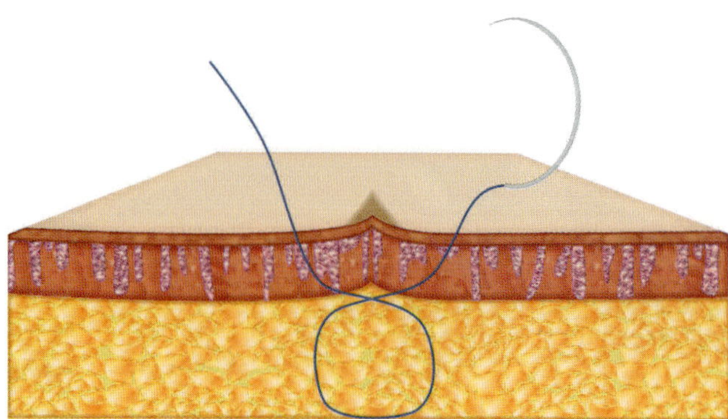

**Fig. 6.7:** Figure of eight suture.

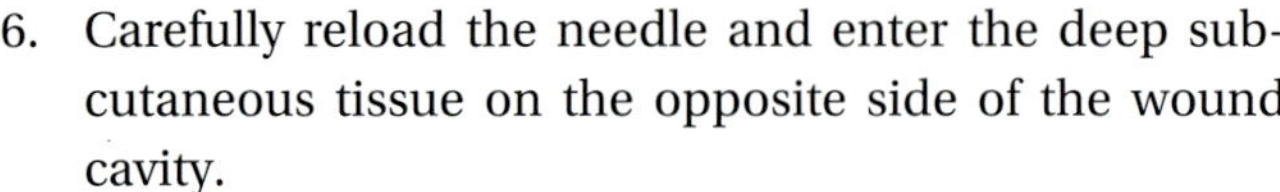

6. Carefully reload the needle and enter the deep subcutaneous tissue on the opposite side of the wound cavity.
7. Arc the needle upward and exit the epidermis 5 mm lateral to the wound edge, in line with the previous suture on this side of the wound cavity.
8. The entire suture should lie on a single axis perpendicular to the wound cavity.
9. Secure the suture with an instrument tie.

## Epidermal Sutures

### *Simple Interrupted Suture*

The simple interrupted suture is a common epidermal suture used to both approximate epidermal wound edges and to provide structural support to a layered closure. The individual interrupted epidermal sutures are preferred to close wounds that are under greater tensile stress. This allows wound tension to be spread across a number of individual, independent sutures. Each simple interrupted suture is secured with a single instrument tie, typically with three to four throws. Caution should be taken with all epidermal sutures to closely approximate the wound edges, but to leave enough laxity in the suture to account for wound expansion secondary to edema. The sutures should not be tied so tight as to cause tissue strangulation or necrosis.

The steps to place a simple interrupted suture are as follows (Fig. 6.6):

1. Enter the epidermis 3–5 mm lateral to the wound edge, arcing the needle downward and exiting into the wound cavity at the level of the deep reticular dermis.
2. Enter the deep reticular dermis on the opposite side of the wound cavity and arc the needle upward through the epidermis, exiting the epidermis 3–5 mm lateral to the wound edge.
3. Secure the suture with an instrument tie.

### *Figure of Eight Suture*

The figure of eight suture is most commonly utilized to close small punch biopsy sites. Nonabsorbable suture is typically used and the suture is characterized as an epidermal suture. The figure of eight suture employs two suture throws that are reminiscent of a "figure of eight" pattern, which is then secured with a simple instrument tie. The suture provides efficient closure of dermal dead space as well as epidermal approximation.

The steps to place a figure of eight suture are as follows (Fig. 6.7):

1. Enter the epidermis 2–3 mm lateral to the wound edge, arcing the needle downward and exiting into the wound cavity at the level of the deep reticular dermis.
2. Enter the deep reticular dermis on the opposite side of the wound cavity and arc the needle upward through the epidermis, exiting the epidermis 2–3 mm lateral to the wound edge.
3. Carefully reload the needle and, on the same side of the wound cavity, re-enter the epidermis 2–3 mm lateral to the previous suture.
4. Arc the needle downward, almost in a perpendicular fashion to the previous suture throw, and exit into the wound cavity at the level of the deep reticular dermis.
5. Enter the deep reticular dermis on the opposite side of the wound cavity and arc the needle upward through the epidermis, exiting the epidermis 2–3 mm lateral to the entry point of the initial suture.
6. Secure the suture with an instrument tie.

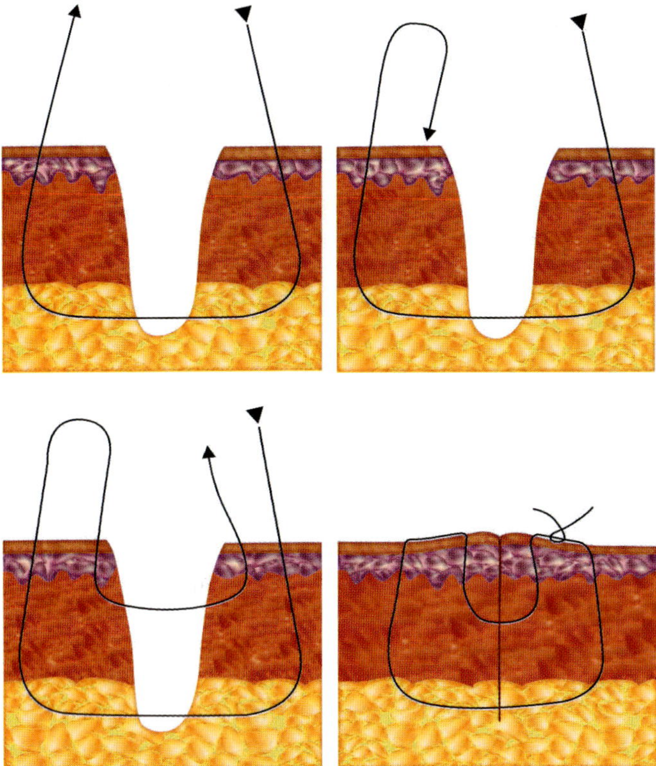

**Fig. 6.8:** Vertical mattress suture.

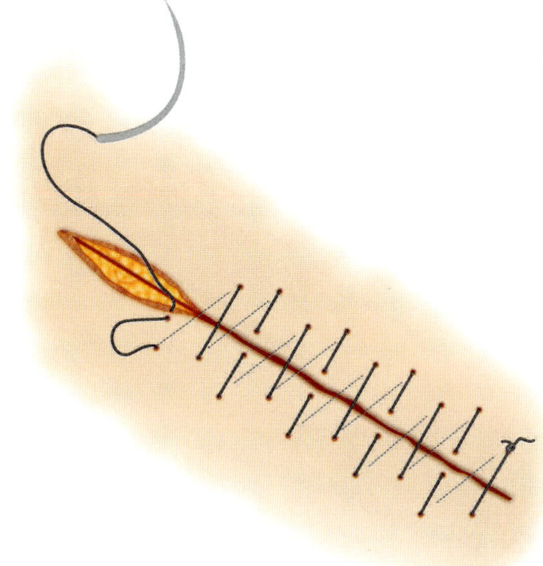

**Fig. 6.9:** Running combined simple and vertical mattress suture.

## *Vertical Mattress Suture*

Vertical mattress sutures are used frequently to provide eversion to wound edges.[11] As wounds tend to contract as they heal, the eversion provided by the vertical mattress sutures allows for a more aesthetically pleasing surgical outcome.[12] As seen in the diagram, this suture uses a "far-far, near-near" approach and allows a substantial amount of tissue to be secured within each suture, allowing for greater closure strength and wound distribution of wound tension than a simple interrupted suture.[12] The suture is ideal for wounds with edges that tend to invert, such as those that occur on a concave surface.[13] The suture also provides adequate dead-space closure and hemostasis, though not to the degree of a horizontal mattress suture, which is discussed later in the chapter.

The steps to place a vertical mattress suture are as follows (Fig. 6.8):

1. Enter the epidermis 5 mm lateral to the wound edge, arcing the needle downward and exiting into the wound cavity at the level of the deep subcutaneous tissue.
2. Carefully reload the needle and enter the deep subcutaneous tissue on the opposite side of the wound cavity.
3. Arc the needle upward and exit the epidermis 5 mm lateral to the wound edge.
4. Carefully reload the needle and again enter the epidermis 2–3 mm lateral to the same wound edge, in line with the wound cavity and the previous suture.
5. Arc the needle downward and exit into the wound cavity at the level of the deep reticular dermis.
6. Carefully reload the needle and enter the deep reticular dermis on the opposite side of the wound cavity.
7. Arc the needle upward and exit the epidermis 2–3 mm lateral to the wound edge, in line with the initial suture on this side of the wound cavity.
8. The entire suture should lie on a single axis perpendicular to the wound cavity.
9. Secure the suture with an instrument tie.

A variation of this technique performed as a running vertical mattress alternating with simple running has also been reported by Krunic et al. and it may be useful to increase efficiency and facilitate suture removal (Fig. 6.9).[14]

## *Half-Buried Vertical Mattress Suture*

The half-buried vertical mattress suture is an adaptation of the vertical mattress suture in which one side of the suture is placed entirely in a subcuticular manner. Although the strength provided by this buried adaptation of the vertical mattress is less than the original, the subcuticular placement of the suture makes it ideal for suturing along the hairline.

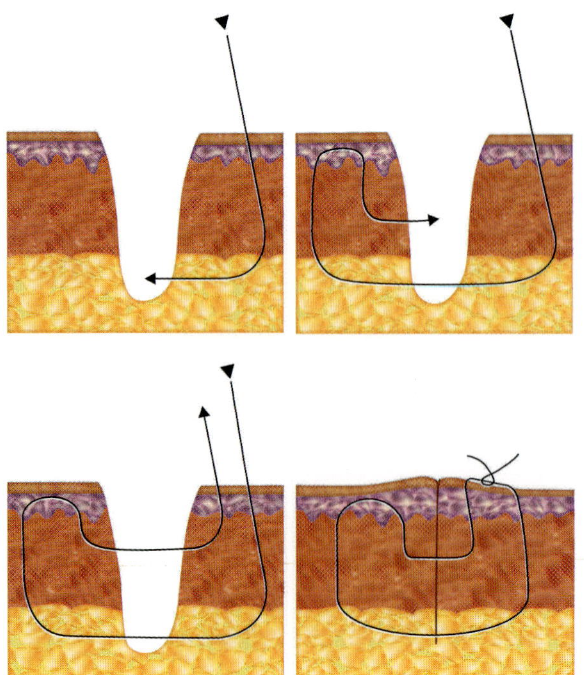

Fig. 6.10: Half-buried vertical mattress suture.

The steps to place a half-buried horizontal mattress suture are as follows (Fig. 6.10):

1. Enter the epidermis 5 mm lateral to the wound edge, arcing the needle downward and exiting into the wound cavity at the level of the deep subcutaneous tissue.
2. Carefully reload the needle and enter the deep subcutaneous tissue on the opposite side of the wound cavity.
3. Through pronation of the wrist, arc the needle upward toward the epidermis, taking care to remain deep to the dermal-epidermal junction.
4. Exit the same wound edge at the level of the deep reticular dermis.
5. Carefully reload the needle and enter the deep reticular dermis on the opposite side of the wound cavity.
6. Arc the needle upward and exit the epidermis 2–3 mm lateral to the wound edge, in line with the initial suture on this side of the wound cavity.
7. The entire suture should lie on a single axis perpendicular to the wound cavity.
8. Secure the suture with an instrument tie.

## Horizontal Mattress Suture

Horizontal mattress sutures are extremely effective hemostatic sutures that are primarily utilized for the hemostasis they provide to a wound edge. They are commonly used in vascular areas, such as the scalp.[12] The significant hemostasis achieved with the horizontal mattress suture is due to the large amount of tissue contained within the suture material. The horizontal mattress suture, like the vertical mattress suture, also provides eversion to the wound edge. Another advantage of these sutures is that they spread tension along the wound edges, making it an ideal suture for elderly patients and for closing wound edges composed of fragile skin.[15] Care should be taken to ensure the epidermal component of the suture is not too tight as to prevent tissue necrosis and strangulation.

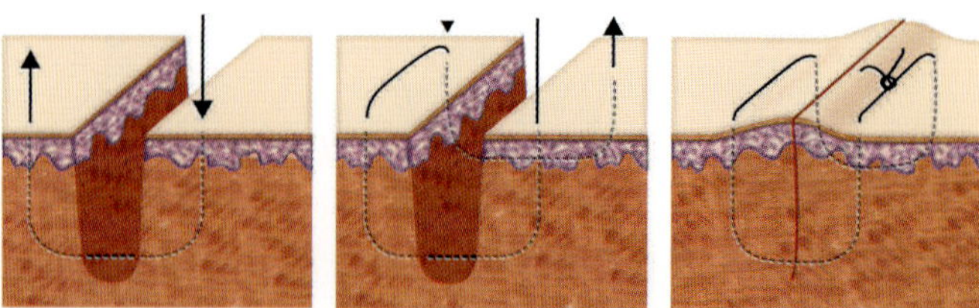

Fig. 6.11: Horizontal mattress suture.

Alam and Goldberg have described a completely buried variant of the horizontal mattress suture which, when used with a running nonabsorbable suture, provides a two-layered closure with excellent cosmetic outcomes.[16] The authors note that this suture allows for strong wound edge eversion while eliminating the epidermal component of the horizontal mattress, thus eliminating the risk of epidermal track marks.[16]

The steps to place a horizontal mattress suture are as follows (Fig. 6.11):

1. Enter the epidermis 3–5 mm lateral to the wound edge, arcing the needle downward and exiting into the wound cavity at the level of the deep subcutaneous tissue.
2. Carefully reload the needle and enter the deep subcutaneous tissue on the opposite side of the wound cavity.
3. Arc the needle upward and exit the epidermis 3–5 mm lateral to the wound edge.
4. Carefully reload the needle and, on the same side of the wound cavity, re-enter the epidermis 2–3 mm lateral to the previous suture.
5. Arc the needle downward and exit into the wound cavity at the level of the deep reticular dermis.
6. Carefully reload the needle and enter the deep reticular dermis on the opposite side of the wound cavity.
7. Arc the needle upward and exit the epidermis 5 mm lateral to the wound edge, in line with the initial suture on this side of the wound cavity.
8. Secure the suture with an instrument tie.

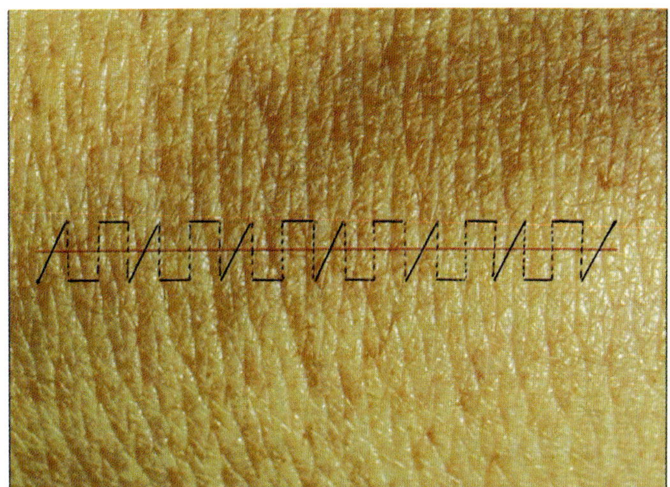

Fig. 6.12: Horizontal running mattress suture alternating with simple running.

A variation of this technique performed as a horizontal running mattress suture alternating with simple running sutures has also been reported by Chacon et al. and it may be useful to increase efficiency and facilitate suture removal (Fig. 6.12).[17]

### 3-Point Corner Tip Stitch

The 3-point corner tip stitch is a variant of the horizontal mattress suture. It is used to secure flap tips, typically those that are triangular shaped, into corners of wounds. Essentially, the suture begins and finishes just like a classic horizontal mattress suture, but on the far side of the wound cavity, the suture passes entirely subcutaneously through the apex of the wound tip. This effectively anchors the flap tip into the corner of an existing wound. The epidermal component of the suture, including the knot, resides entirely outside of the apex of the flap tip.

The steps to place a 3-point corner tip stitch are as follows (Fig. 6.13):

1. Enter the epidermis 3–5 mm lateral to the apex of the wound defect, arcing the needle downward and exiting within the deep reticular dermis within the wound defect.
2. Grasp the flap tip gently with forceps and navigate the needle through the apex of the tip at the level of the deep reticular dermis.
3. Re-enter the deep reticular dermis on the opposite side of the wound defect and arc the needle upward through the epidermis, exiting the epidermis 3–5 mm lateral to the opposite apex of the wound defect.
4. Secure the suture with a simple instrument tie.

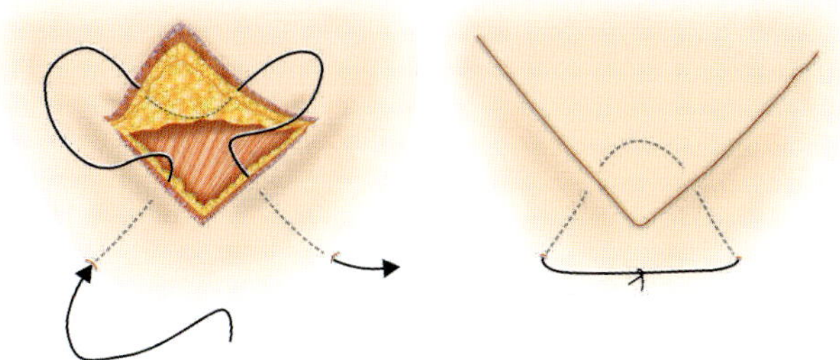

Fig. 6.13: Sutures 3-point corner tip stitch.

## Running Epidermal Sutures

### Subcuticular Suture

The subcuticular suture is used as a running suture in two-layered closures to approximate wound edges. As the suture is completely subcutaneous, it eliminates any risk of track marking from epidermal sutures and maximizes cosmesis. An additional advantage of using this suturing technique is that one can use absorbable sutures so that patients do not have to return for suture removal. Streams and Jiang reported that using buried subcuticular running sutures with fast absorbing gut on facial repairs yielded equivalent cosmetic outcomes as using simple interrupted nylon sutures.[18] Alam et al. also found that bilayered closures of elliptical excisions on the trunk and extremities had better overall appearance and less erythema with use of subcuticular running polyglactin 910 (Vicryl) sutures as compared to simple running epidermal closures of the same sites 9 months postoperatively.[19] In addition, Cordova et al. have observed significant aesthetic results and patient satisfaction when using a subcuticular running poliglecaprone (Monocryl) suture in bilayered closures of elliptical excisions on the trunk and extremities.[20]

The steps to placing a nonabsorbable subcuticular suture are as follows (Fig. 6.14):

1. At one apex of the wound cavity, enter the epidermis 3–5 mm distal to the apex of the wound defect, arcing the needle downward and exiting within the deep reticular dermis within the wound defect. Secure the end of the suture with a hemostat.
2. Enter the superficial papillary dermis and pronate the wrist to arc the needle in a horizontal fashion,

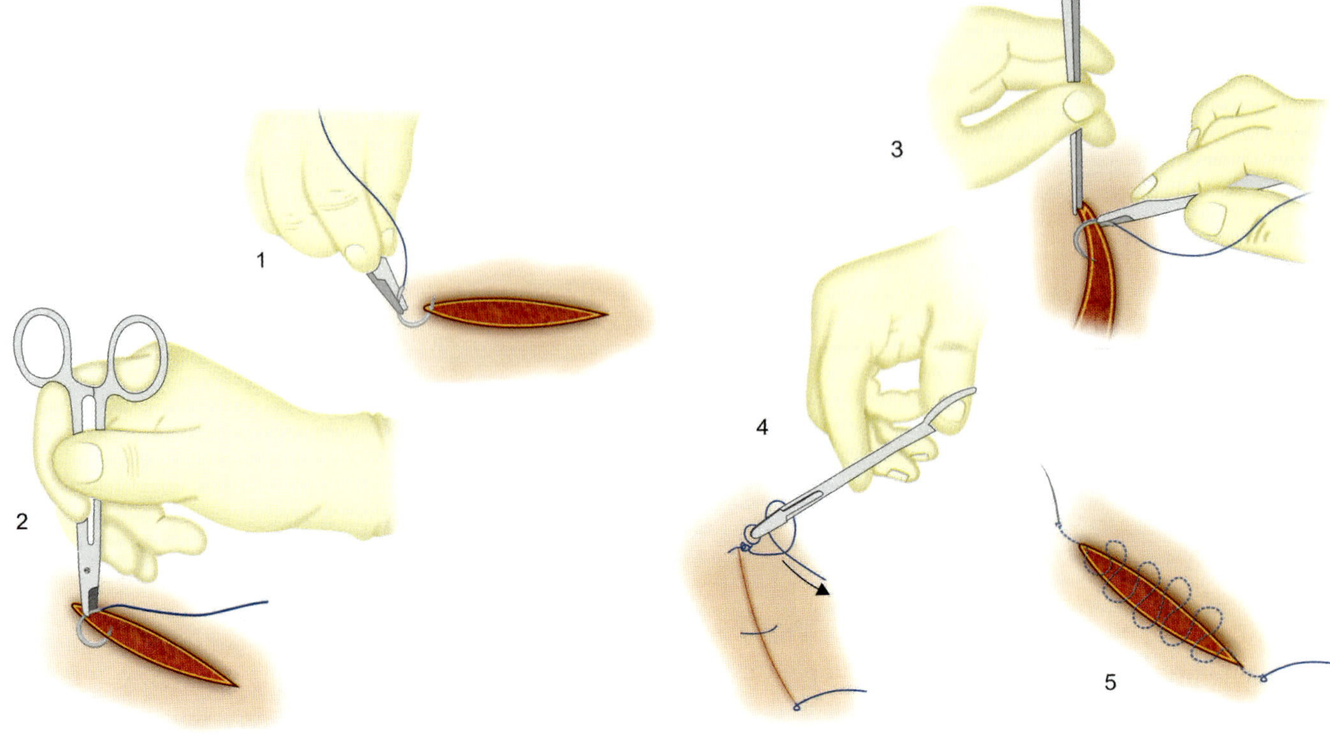


**Fig. 6.14:** Nonabsorbable subcuticular suture.

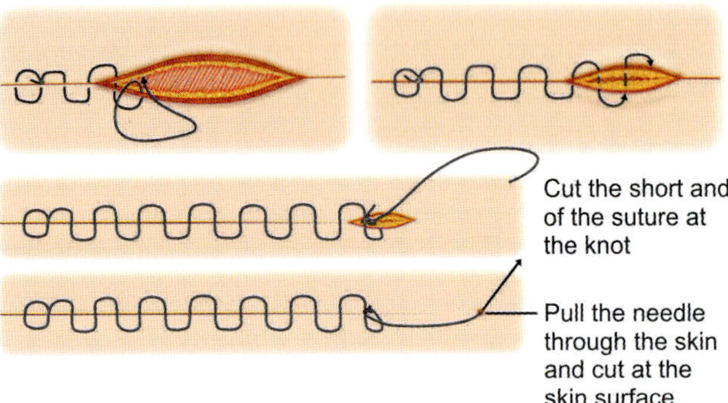


**Fig. 6.15:** Absorbable buried subcuticular suture.

parallel to the level of the epidermis, until the needle reappears in the wound cavity at the level of the superficial papillary dermis.

3. Carefully reload the needle and enter the superficial papillary dermis on the opposite side of the wound cavity.
4. Pronate the wrist to arc the needle in a horizontal fashion, parallel to the level of the epidermis, until the needle once again reappears in the wound cavity at the level of the superficial papillary dermis.
5. Repeat this suturing motion, alternating sides of the wound cavity that each throw, and continue to take horizontal bites. Taking care to enter and exit the wound cavity at the same level of the superficial papillary dermis, ensuring that the epidermis is closely and securely approximated.
6. Once the suture reaches the opposite apex of the wound cavity, exit the skin in line with the incision axis 3–5 mm distal to the apex of the wound.
7. Pull the two ends of the suture until the wound closes without overlap. Tie the free ends to themselves with an instrument tie or tape them onto the skin with tape or steri-strips.

The steps for placing an absorbable buried subcuticular suture are as follows (Fig. 6.15):

1. At one apex of the wound cavity, place a single interrupted dermal suture to serve as an anchoring knot. Cut the short tail of the suture only.
2. Enter the superficial papillary dermis and pronate the wrist to arc the needle in a horizontal fashion, parallel to the level of the epidermis, until the needle reappears in the wound cavity at the level of the superficial papillary dermis.

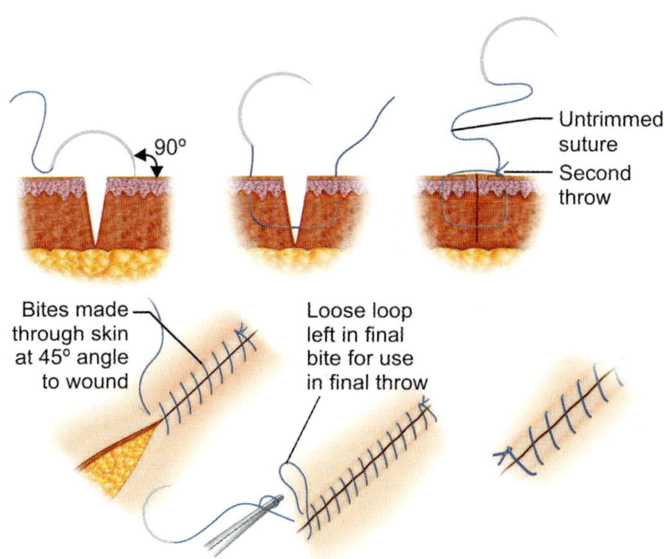


**Fig. 6.16:** Simple running epidermal suture.

3. Carefully reload the needle and enter the superficial papillary dermis on the opposite side of the wound cavity.
4. Pronate the wrist to arc the needle in a horizontal fashion, parallel to the level of the epidermis, until the needle once again reappears in the wound cavity at the level of the superficial papillary dermis.
5. Repeat this suturing motion, alternating sides of the wound cavity with each throw, and continue to take horizontal bites. Taking care to enter and exit the wound cavity at the same level of the superficial papillary dermis, ensuring that the epidermis is closely and securely approximated.
6. Once the suture reaches the opposite apex of the wound cavity, leave slack in the trailing edge of the suture and throw a deep instrument tie within the wound cavity to secure the suture.
7. Once the deep suture is secured, place the needle into the wound cavity, taking a large subcutaneous bite, in line with the incision axis, exiting the skin in line with the incision axis, and pulling the suture taught.
8. Cut the suture at the level of the epidermis to completely bury the suture.

## *Simple Running Suture*

The running epidermal suture is one of the most common epidermal sutures used in layered closures. This suture is most often used to approximate wound edges in closures that are not under a great deal of tension. An advantage of this suture is that it can be placed fairly quickly to provide close approximation of wound edges once deep subcutaneous sutures have been placed. However, the simple running suture is not ideal for wounds under tension as the wound tension is spread over the single running suture. High-tension wounds are better closed with a number of simple interrupted sutures, allowing wound tension to be spread over a larger number of individual sutures.

The steps for placing a running epidermal suture are as follows (Fig. 6.16):

1. Place a single interrupted suture at one apex of the wound cavity to serve as an anchoring suture. Cut the short tail of the suture only.
2. Enter the epidermis 3–5 mm lateral to the wound edge on one side of the wound, pronating the wrist and exiting the epidermis 3–5 mm lateral to the wound edge on the opposite side of the wound edge.
3. Carefully reload the needle and continue this suturing motion along the length of the wound cavity.
4. Once the suture reaches the far apex of the wound cavity, leave slack in the trailing edge of the suture and throw an instrument tie to secure the suture.

## *Running Locked Suture*

The running locked suture is utilized when hemostasis is a priority. The suture is a variation of the running epidermal suture and is commonly used to close wounds in highly vascular areas, such as the scalp. The surgeon must take care to ensure the suture is not placed too tightly as to avoid tissue strangulation and necrosis.

The steps for placing a running locked suture are as follows (Fig. 6.17):

1. Place a single interrupted suture at one apex of the wound cavity to serve as an anchoring suture. Cut the short tail of the suture only.
2. Enter the epidermis 3–5 mm lateral to the wound edge on one side of the wound, pronating the wrist and exiting the epidermis 3–5 mm lateral to the wound edge on the opposite side of the wound edge.
3. Repeat the above step but, prior to throwing this next suture, pass the needle behind the previous suture, thus effectively "locking" the suture.
4. Carefully reload the needle and continue this suturing motion along the length of the wound cavity.
5. Once the suture reaches the opposite end of the incision, leave slack in the trailing edge of the suture and throw an instrument tie to secure the suture.

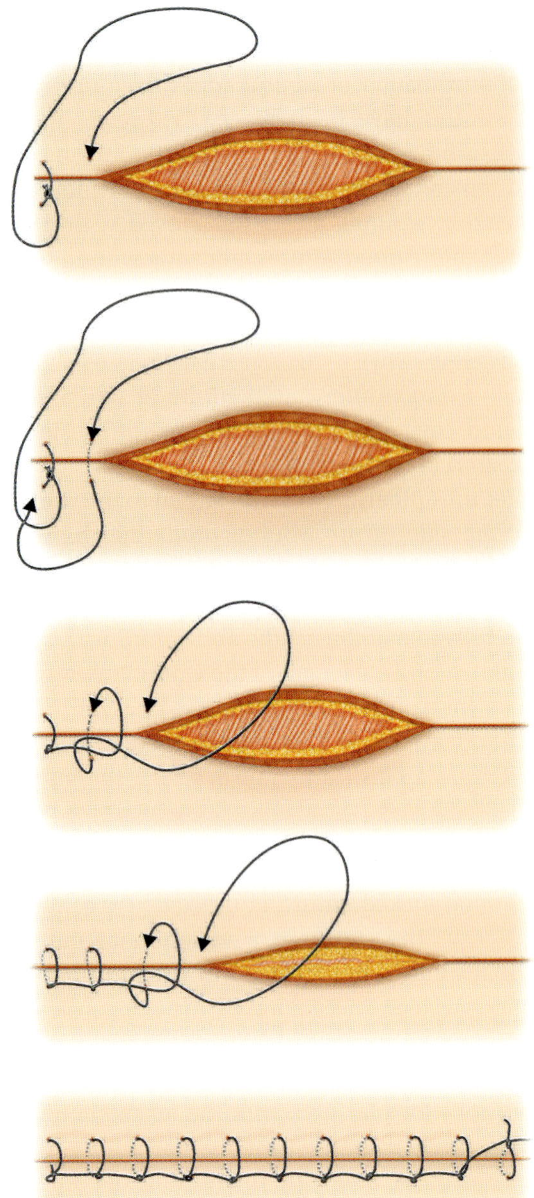

**Fig. 6.17:** Running locked suture.

## Purse-String Suture

The purse-string suture is used to close large circular or oval-shaped surgical defects, often in areas where there is fragile, thin skin or in areas where there is not significant skin laxity.[21] The purse-string suture can be used in place of or in conjunction with skin grafts to expedite healing.[21] The suture effectively shrinks the size of the surgical wound and, thus, can help to expedite the healing. Furthermore, the purse-string suture is rather simple to execute, as described below. This suture commonly uses epidermal sutures, but a variant utilizing intradermal sutures can also be used. However, a recent study by Joo et al. demonstrated that the purse-string suture results in similar cosmetic outcomes, scar size, and pain level compared with secondary intention healing for circular or oval wounds on the trunk and extremities.[22]

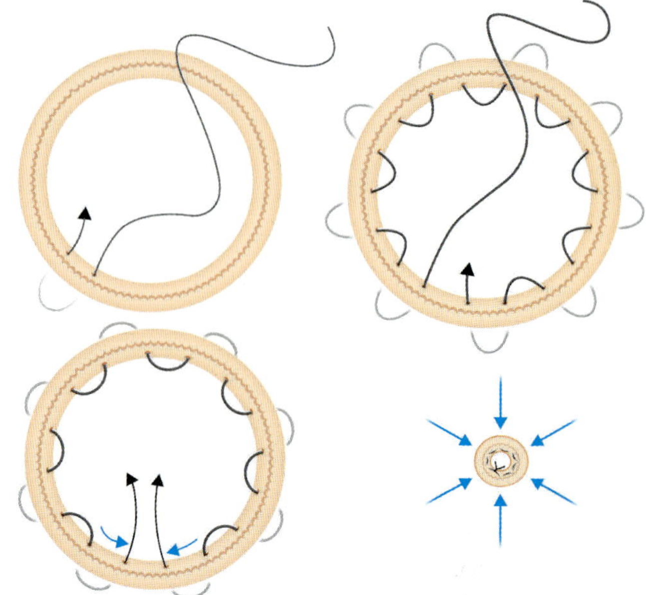

**Fig. 6.18:** Epidermal purse-string suture.

The steps for placing an epidermal purse-string suture are as follows (Fig. 6.18):

1. Enter the epidermis 3–5 mm lateral to the edge of the wound defect.
2. Through pronation of the wrist, take a bite with the suture parallel to the edge of the wound defect, exiting the epidermis again 3–5 mm lateral to the edge of the wound defect.
3. Continue this suturing motion circumferentially around the entire wound defect.
4. Once the circumference of the wound is sutured in this manner, pull the suture taught to decrease the wound diameter and secure the suture with an instrument tie.

## REFERENCES


1. Yag-Howard C. Sutures, needles, and tissue adhesives: a review for dermatologic surgery. Dermatol Surg. 2014;40: S3-S15.
2. Dunn DL. Ethicon, Inc. Wound Closure Manual 2007. [Accessed January 25, 2015]. http://www.uphs.upenn.edu/surgery/Education/facilities/measey/Wound_Closure_Manual.pdf

3. Moy ML, Waldman B, Hein DW. A review of sutures and suturing techniques. J Dermatol Surg Oncol. 1992;18:785-95.
4. Moy RL, Kaufman JA. Clinical comparison of polyglactic acid (Vicryl) and polytrimethylene carbonate (Maxon) suture material. J Dermatol Surg Oncol. 1991;17:667-9.
5. Adams B, Levy R, Rademaker AE, et al. Frequency of use of suturing and repair techniques preferred by dermatologic surgeons. Dermatol Surg. 2006;32:682-9.
6. Regan T, Lawrence N. Comparison of poliglecaprone 25 and polyglactin-910 in cutaneous surgery. Dermatol Surg. 2013;39:1340-4.
7. Kudur MH, Pai SB, Stripathi H, et al. Sutures and suturing techniques in skin closure. Indian J Dermatol Venerol Leprol. 2009;75:425-34.
8. Gabel EA, Jiminez GP, Eaglstein WH, et al. Performance comparison of nylon and an absorbable suture material (polyglactin 910) in the closure of punch biopsy sites. Dermatol Surg. 2000;26:750-3.
9. Rosenzweig LB, Abdelmalek M, Ho J, et al. Equal cosmetic outcomes with 5-0 poliglecaprone-25 versus 6-0 polypropylene for superficial closures. Dermatol Surg. 2010;36(7):1126-9.
10. Whalen JD, Difrense RG, Collins SC. Surgical pearl: the modified buried dermal suture. J Am Acad Dermatol. 1999;40:103-4.
11. Krunic AL, Weitzul S, Taylor S. Running combined simple and vertical mattress suture: a rapid skin-everting stitch. Dermatol Surg. 2005;31:1325-9.
12. Zuber TJ. The mattress sutures: vertical, horizontal, and corner stitch. Am Fam Physician. 2002;66:2231-6.
13. Stasko T. Advanced suturing techniques and layered closures. In: Wheeland RG (Ed). Cutaneous Surgery. Philadelphia, PA: Saunders; 1994. pp. 304-17.
14. Krunic A, Weitzul S, Taylor R. Running combined simple and vertical mattress suture: a rapid skin-everting stitch. Dermatol Surg. 2005;31:1325-9.
15. Coldiron BM. Closure of wounds under tension. The horizontal mattress suture. Arch Dermatol. 1989;125:1189-90.
16. Alam M, Goldberg LH. Utility of fully buried horizontal mattress suture. J Am Acad Dermatol. 2004;50:73-6.
17. Chacon A, Shiman M, Strozier N, et al. Horizontal running mattress suture modified with intermittent simple loops. J Cutan Aesthet Surg. 2013;6(1):54-6.
18. Streams BN, Jiang SB. A modified running subcuticular suturing technique for the closure of defects after Mohs micrographic surgery. Dermatol Surg. 2003;29(11):1118-21.
19. Alam M, Posten W, Marini M, et al. Aesthetic and functional efficacy of subcuticular running epidermal closures of the trunk and extremity. Arch Dermatol. 2006;142:1272-8.
20. Cordova K, Sweeney S, Jellinek N. The elegant ellipse-running subcuticular closures. Dermatol Surg. 2013;39(5):804-7.
21. Harrington A, Montemarano A, Welch M, et al. Variations of the purse-string suture in skin cancer reconstruction. Dermatol Surg. 1999;25:277-81.
22. Joo J, Custis T, Armstrong A, et al. Purse-string suture vs second intention healing, results of a randomized, blind clinical trial. JAMA Dermatol. 2015;151(3):265-70.

# CHAPTER 7

# Flap Classification and Design/ Biomechanics of Skin

**Andrew Breithaupt, Patrick K Lee**

## INTRODUCTION

Reconstruction of surgical defects using flaps is an essential component of dermatologic surgery. Given the complex interplay of anatomy, vascular supply, and tissue dynamics, a fundamental understanding of flaps is best approached from the ground up.

A flap is defined as the transfer of tissue from one site (donor) to another (recipient) with an intact blood supply. This broad ranging definition translates to a wide variety of flaps from simple local tissue movement to distant free flaps requiring delicate microvascular reanastomosis.

Given a particular skin defect, options for management include second-intention healing, primary closure, skin grafting, and flap closure. The same defect can often be reasonably managed by a number of different options. The optimal choice depends on several factors including defect size, location, the medical conditions of the patient, and patient preferences (Table 7.1).

### History of Flaps

The first recorded account of flap surgery dates back as far as 600 BC to the Sanskrit text *Sushruta Samhita* describing the use of cheek flaps to reconstruct nasal wounds from war or punishment.[1] The word flap itself originated in the 16th century from the Dutch word *flappe*, meaning anything that hangs broad and loose fastened only on one side.[2]

In 1597, Italian Renaissance surgeon Tagliacozzi described the use of upper arm tissue to reconstruct the nose. His flap is still occasionally practiced today and the figure of this flap is very popular in many reconstruction books.[3]

While progress on flaps continued to be refined in Europe throughout the 18th and 19th centuries, it was not until World War I that the use of the tubular pedicle was developed, and ushered in the modern era of flap reconstruction.[4] Throughout the first half of the 20th century, the majority of flaps were axial and pedicle flaps, based on named arteries requiring a staged approach. With increased understanding of the blood supply to flaps, more and more advanced flaps including free tissue transfer became possible.

**Table 7.1:** Factors influencing reconstructive decision.

| *Defect* | *Patient* |
|---|---|
| Location (including proximity to free margins) | Age |
| Size (width and depth) | Immune status |
| Type of underlying tissue exposed | History of radiation |
| Surrounding skin characteristics | Smoking status |
| | Risk of tumor recurrence |

### Flap Terminology (Table 7.2)

All local flaps contain two basic components. The *body* of a flap is the portion of tissue being transferred to repair the defect. The *pedicle* is the portion of the flap that contains the blood supply and remains intact to provide circulation to the flap during the intraoperative and early postoperative period.

The portion of tissue to be covered by a flap is referred to as the *primary defect*. The *secondary defect* (or *donor site defect)* is the site from which the flap is harvested. *Primary flap movement* is the movement necessary to place the flap into the primary defect. *Secondary flap movement* is the movement needed to close the secondary defect created by the movement of the flap into the primary defect.

**Table 7.2:** Flap terminology.

| *Term* | *Definition* |
|---|---|
| Body | The portion of tissue being transferred to repair the defect |
| Pedicle | The portion of the flap that contains the blood supply and remains intact to provide circulation to the flap during the intraoperative and early postoperative period |
| Primary defect | The portion of tissue to be covered by a flap |
| Secondary defect | The site from which the flap is harvested |
| Primary flap movement | The movement necessary to place the flap into the primary defect |
| Secondary flap movement | The movement needed to close the secondary defect created by the movement of the flap into the primary defect |
| Primary tension vector | The counterforce created by the movement of the flap into place |
| Secondary tension vector | The force resulting from closure of the secondary defect |

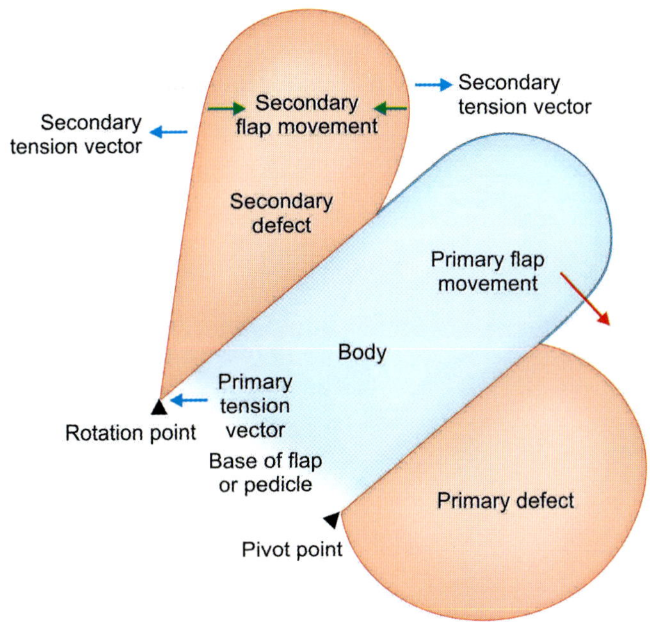


**Fig. 7.1:** Flap components.

These movements result in two vectors of tension: the *primary tension vector* created by the counterforce to the movement of the flap into place, and the *secondary tension vector* resulting from closure of the secondary defect (Fig. 7.1).

## Classification of Flaps

Flaps are characterized based on three basic components: vascular supply, tissue composition, and donor site location (Table 7.3).[5] The types of flaps most commonly used in dermatology, local flaps, are further subdivided based on movement (Table 7.4).

**Table 7.3:** Flap classification.

| *Vascular* | *Tissue composition* | *Donor site location* | *Movement* |
|---|---|---|---|
| Random | Cutaneous | Local | Advancement |
| Axial | Fascial | Distant—pedicle | Rotation |
| | Muscular | Distant—free | Transposition |
| | Osseous | | Interpolation |
| | Visceral | | Combination |
| | Fasciocutaneous | | |
| | Myocutaneous | | |
| | Osteocutaneous | | |
| | Tendocutaneous | | |

### *Vascular Supply*

A proper understanding of the vascular supply of flaps is essential to the correct flap selection and execution. Without a viable blood supply, a flap will not survive. Flaps can be divided into two major categories based on vascular supply: random and axial (Fig. 7.2).

Random flaps are fed by the unnamed vessels of the subdermal plexus in the tissue below. Many of the local flaps used in dermatologic reconstruction fall into this category. These flaps are sensitive to drops in perfusion pressure due to the limited blood supply.[6] Thus, care must be taken during design to give adequate blood flow for the amount of tissue being transferred to ensure flap survival.[7]

Axial flaps receive their blood supply by specific named cutaneous or musculocutaneous arteries. Due to their robust blood supply, increased flap lengths are possible

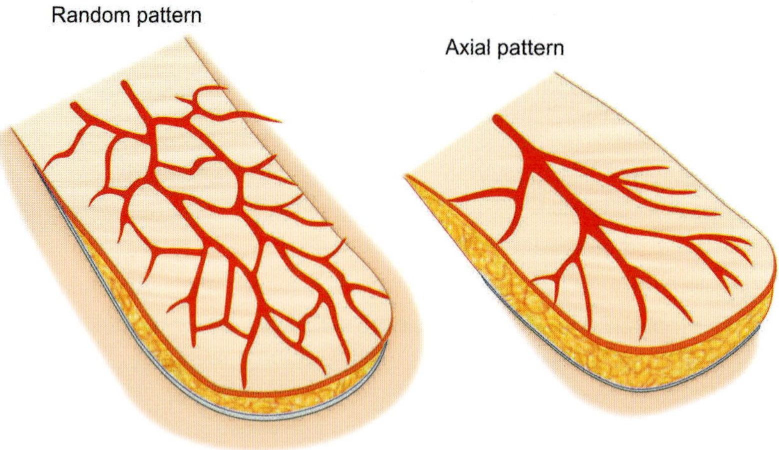


**Fig. 7.2:** Illustration of blood supply: random versus axial flap.

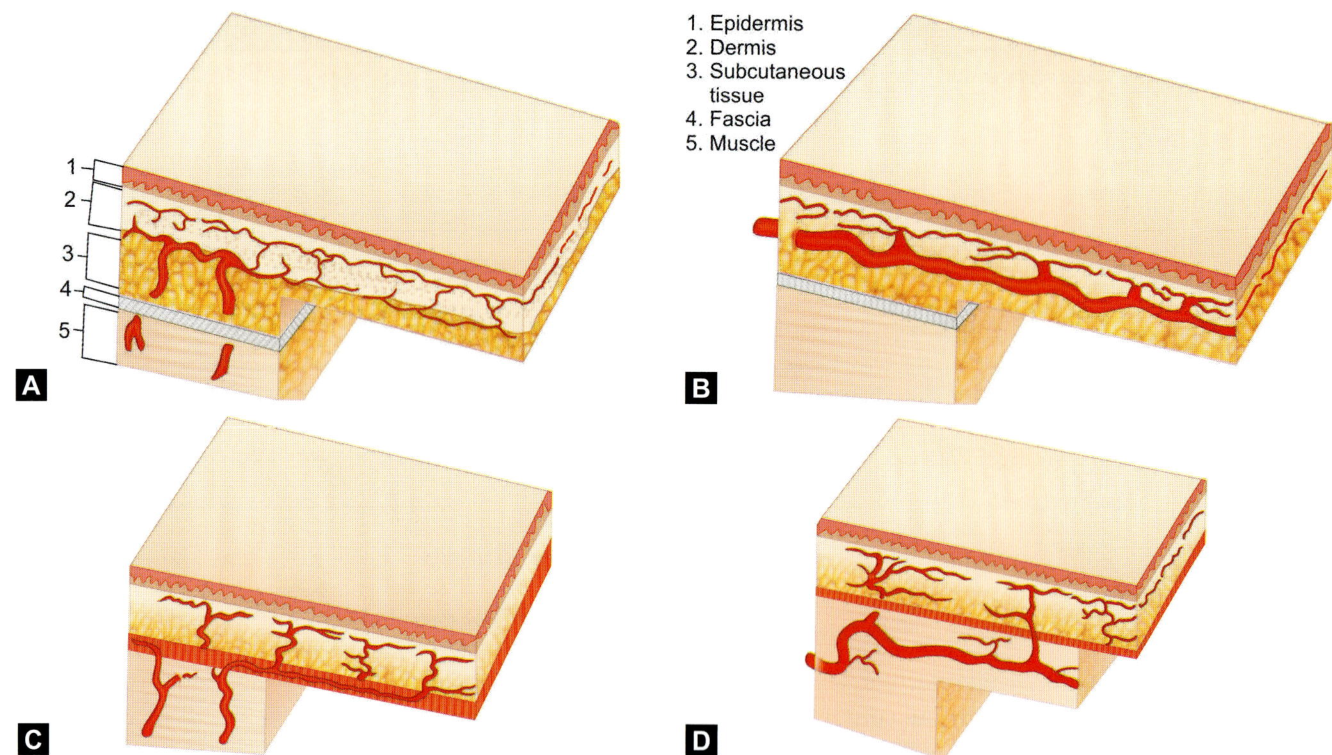


**Figs. 7.3A to D:** Flap classification based on tissue compositions. (A) Cutaneous random pattern. (B) Cutaneous, axial pattern. (C) Fasciocutaneous. (D) Myocutaneous.

when compared to random flaps. Several flaps rarely encountered in dermatologic reconstruction including regional flaps and free flaps also fall into this category.

## *Tissue Composition*

Flaps are additionally classified based on the type or types of tissue being transferred (Figs. 7.3A to D). Flaps can be comprised of one or multiple types of tissue. Flaps composed of a single tissue type include cutaneous, fascial, muscular, osseous, and visceral. Composite flaps include fasciocutaneous, tendocutaneous, myocutaneous, chondrocutaneous, and osteocutaneous flaps.

The choice of flap is most often determined by the composition of the defect and the tissue needed to restore

**Table 7.4:** Local flaps.

| *Advancement* | *Rotation* | *Transposition* | *Interpolation* | *Combined* |
|---|---|---|---|---|
| Unipedicle or U flap | Classic | Classic rectangular/ finger flap | Paramedian forehead flap | Spear flap |
| Bipedicle or H flap | Bilateral rotation or O-to-Z flap | Note flap | Melolabial interpolation | "Shark" island-pedicle flap |
| Burow's advancement flap | Dorsal nasal rotation or Rieger/hatchet/glabellar turn-down | Rhombic flap Limberg/Webster/ Dufourmentel | Nasofacial interpolation | Hinge flap |
| Helical rim advancement flap | Mustarde | Bilobed flap | Retroauricular interpolation flap | Tunneled island flaps |
| Bilateral advancement flaps A to T | Cervicofacial flap | Trilobed flap | Hughes tarsoconjunctival flap | |
| V to Y or island pedicle | Modified Tenzel | Nasolabial transposition flap | Abbe or lip-switch flap | |
| | | Z-plasty | | |

functionality and cosmesis. The majority of flaps used in dermatologic reconstruction are cutaneous, fasciocutaneous, or myocutaneous flaps.

## Donor Site Location

Tissue transferred to a defect from an adjacent area is classified as a local flap while transfer of tissue from a noncontiguous anatomic site is a distant flap.

Local flaps are commonly used in dermatologic reconstruction. They are further subclassified based on the flap design and tissue movement. Local flaps include advancement, rotation, transposition, and interpolation flaps (Table 7.4).

Distant flaps are typically used for larger and more complex reconstructions. Pedicle flaps remain attached to their original blood supply during transfer and are divided and inset at a later date. Free flaps are completely detached from their blood supply during transfer and reattached to vessels at the recipient site through microsurgical anastomosis.

## Movement

The most common method to classify flaps used in reconstructive dermatology is based on the flap design and movement. When a flap is cut, elevated, and placed into the recipient site, various movements of tissue result. The primary flap movement is used to define the flap. The three classic types of primary tissue flap movement are advancement, rotation, and transposition.

It should be noted that flaps often incorporate more than one type of movement. The experienced dermatologic surgeon will often design flaps with components of more than one basic flap type to provide the ideal reconstruction tailored to a particular patient and defect.

## Advancement Flaps

In a pure advancement flap, primary tissue movement is along a linear axis from donor site to defect site. Secondary movement occurs directly opposite the primary movement vector (Fig. 7.4). The point of maximal tension of the flap is at the midpoint of the most distal portion of the flap arm.

The main advantage of advancement flaps is that they allow displacement of redundant tissue or "dog-ears" to more favorable sites. While tissue redundancy is often excised at the most proximal portion of the flap, it can in fact be removed anywhere along the length of the flap allowing for some creativity in hiding incisions. Advancement flaps do not significantly decrease the closure tension of a defect when compared to primary closure.[8] They are not the repair of choice for large defects lacking surrounding laxity and do carry a risk of free margin distortion from the secondary tension vector. They are best used in areas where tissue is relatively pliable and incisions can be hidden in linear skin creases.

The most basic advancement flap is a unilateral, double-tangent design in which a rectangular piece of tissue is linearly advanced into the defect site. There are numerous variants on this basic design including the bilateral, single-tangent advancement flap (Burow's flap) (Fig. 7.5),

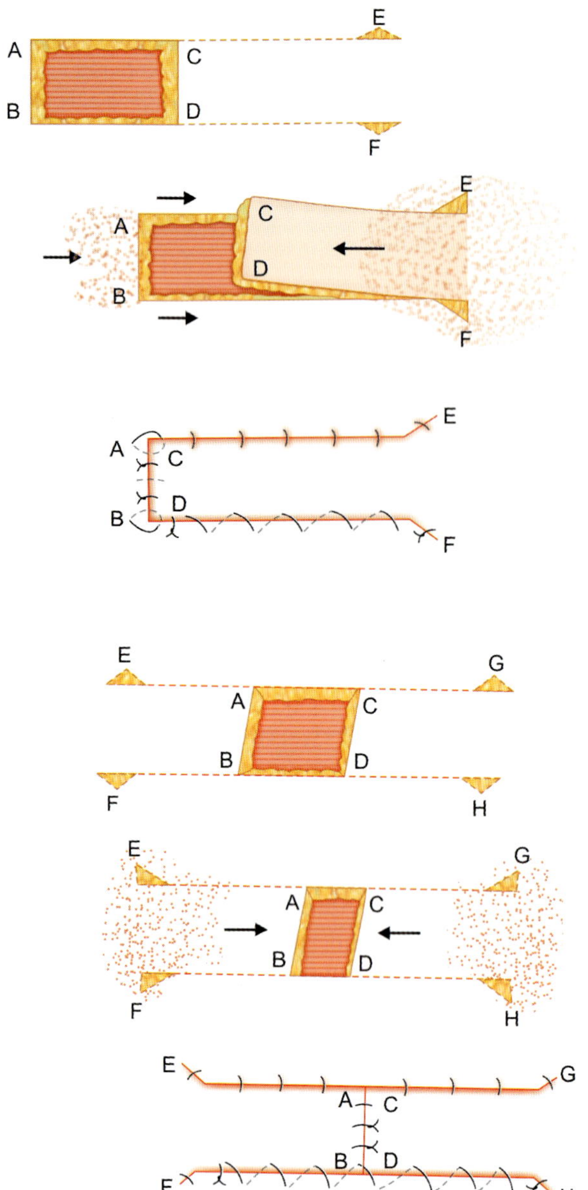


Fig. 7.4: Basic advancement flap (unilateral or bilateral).

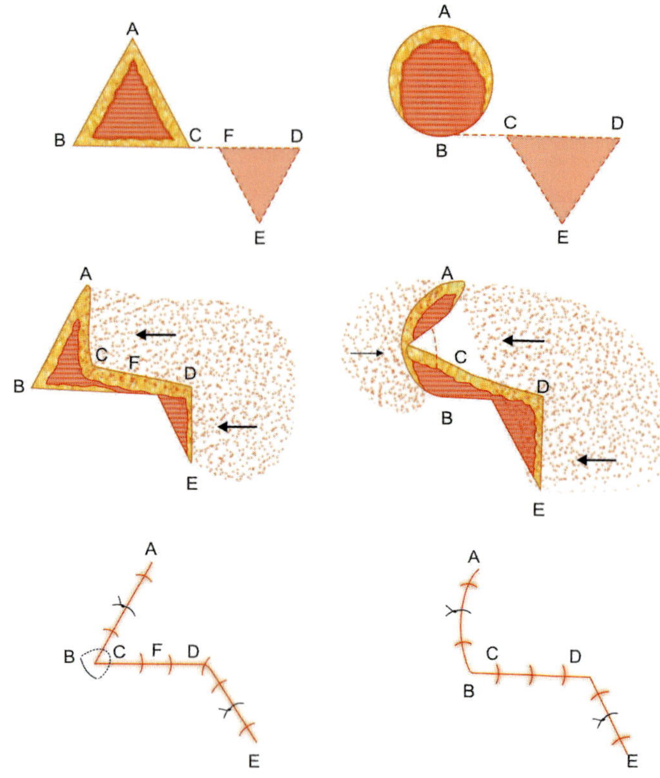


Fig. 7.5: Burrow's advancement flap.

"A to T" or "O to T," and the helical rim advancement flap (Fig. 7.6).

The island pedicle flap (or "V-to-Y" advancement flap) also falls into this classification (Figs. 7.7A and B). This versatile flap has a number of advantages and applications that will be discussed in detail in later chapters.

## Rotation Flaps

Rotation flaps are moved in an arc around a fixed point at the base of the flap. The primary tissue movement is in a half-circle arc defined by the defect and the length of the flap.[9] Secondary movement occurs opposite this vector. The point of maximal tension is at the most distal tip of the flap (Fig. 7.8). Most rotation flaps are designed to move along an arc of 30° or less. The arc radius is approximately two to three times the defect diameter and the arc length is approximately four to five times the defect diameter.[10]

Rotation flaps are most advantageous when their resulting curvilinear scars can be hidden along natural creases or cosmetic subunits. Unlike pure advancement flaps, rotation flaps redistribute some portion of tension from the primary defect to the secondary defect.[11] As the length of the flap is increased, the tension in the primary defect closure decreases.

Tissue redundancy results from flap movement and is most often removed at the leading and trailing edges of the flap. A "back-cut" may be made into the trailing portion of the flap to increase flap mobility and reduce wound tension. Care should always be taken with this modification as it reduces the vascular pedicle of the flap and increases the risk of flap failure.

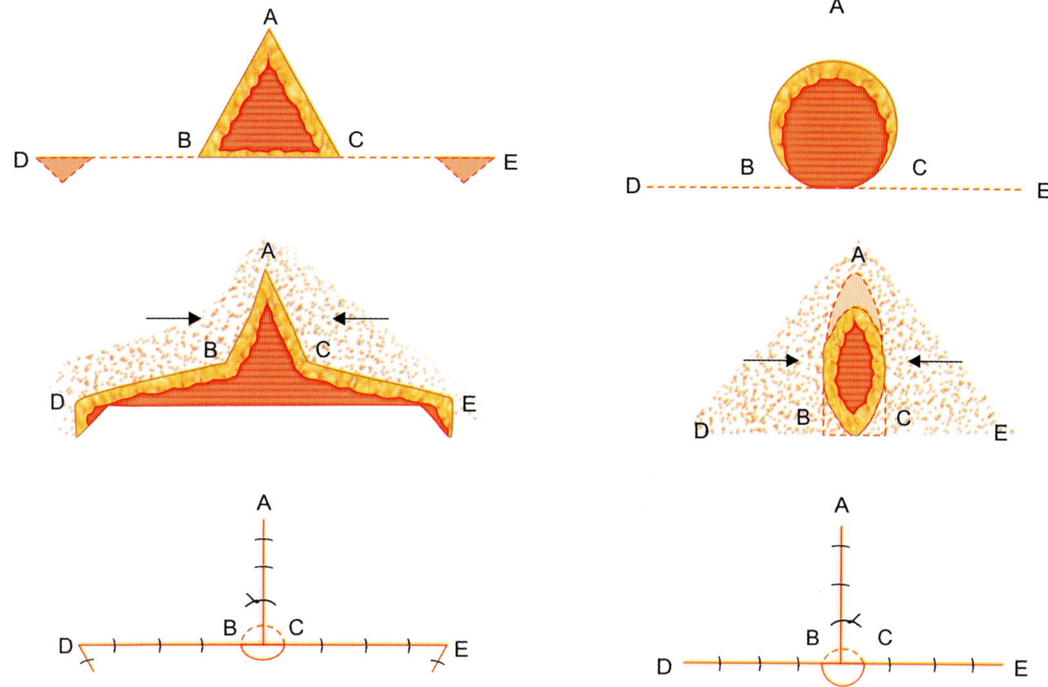


**Fig. 7.6:** A-to-T bilateral advancement flap.

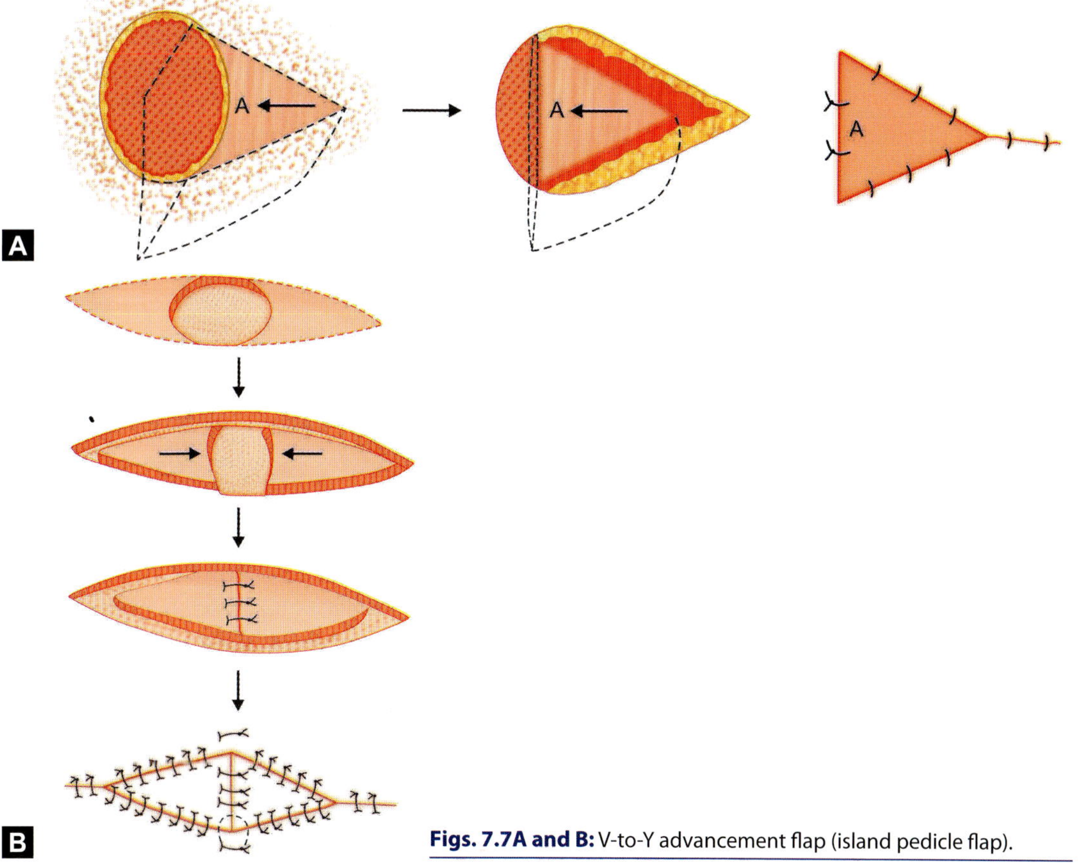


**Figs. 7.7A and B:** V-to-Y advancement flap (island pedicle flap).

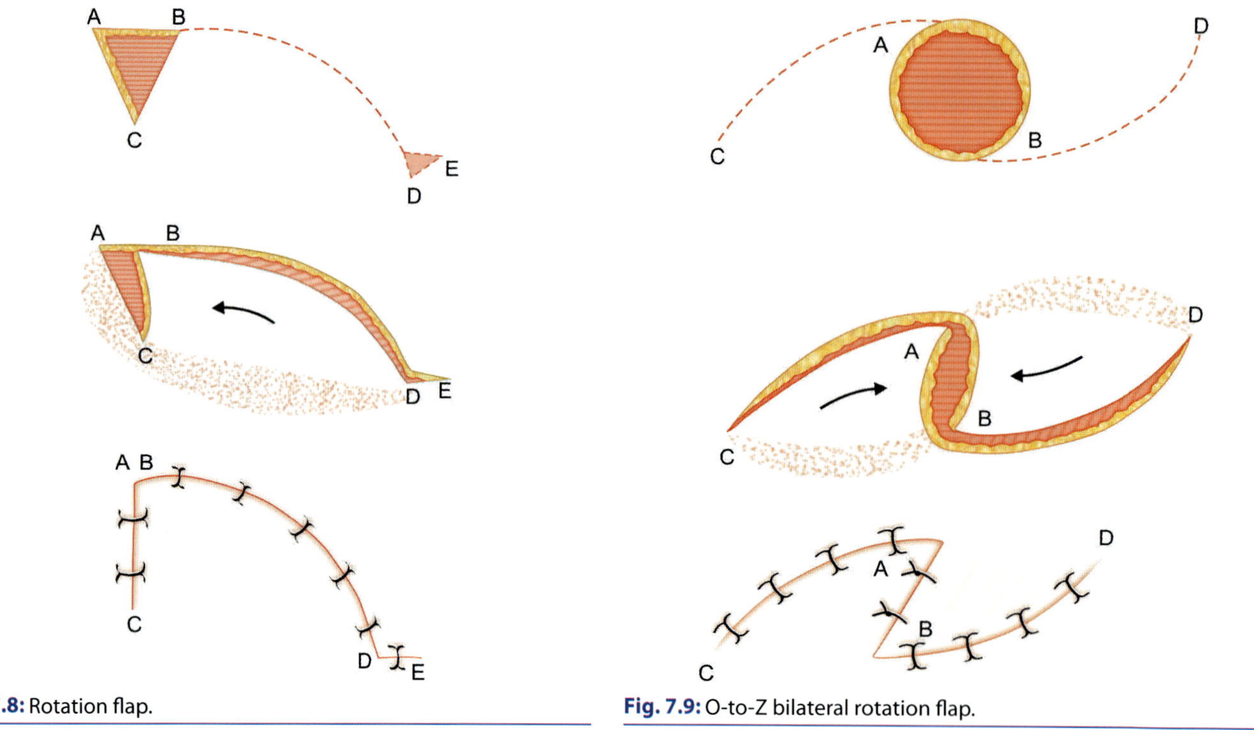


Fig. 7.8: Rotation flap.

Fig. 7.9: O-to-Z bilateral rotation flap.

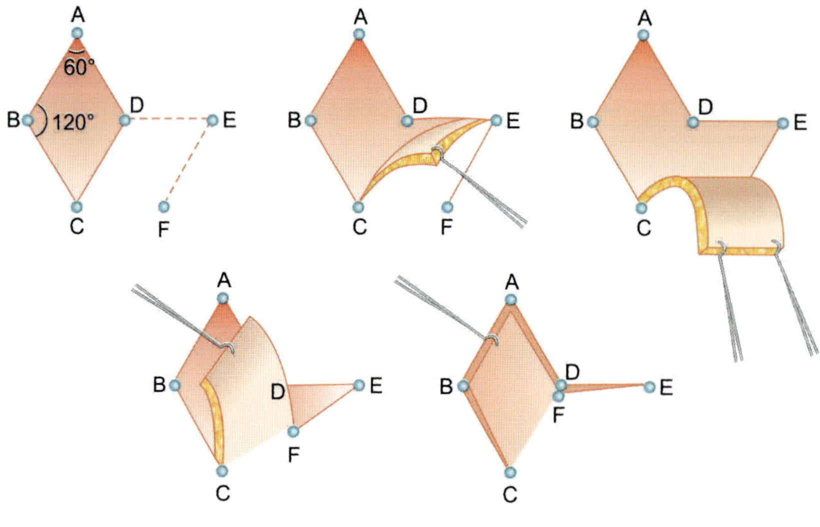


Fig. 7.10: Rhombic flap.

Variants of rotation flaps are found throughout reconstructive dermatology and include the "O-to-Z" flap (Fig. 7.9), the dorsal nasal rotation flap (also referred to as a Rieger flap, hatchet, and glabellar turn-down flap), the Mustarde flap, and the modified Tenzel flap.

## Transposition Flaps

Perhaps the most versatile type of flap used in reconstructive dermatology, transposition flaps move donor tissue over an intervening bridge of intact skin to cover the defect site. This creates a rotation type of primary tissue movement while allowing for redirection of tension vectors to a distant, secondary site. These flaps are more efficient at moving tissue compared to advancement and rotation flaps, and can mobilize relatively distant reservoirs of skin while still remaining small.[8]

The classic transposition flap is the rhombic flap as originally described by Limberg in 1963 (Fig. 7.10).[12] In it,

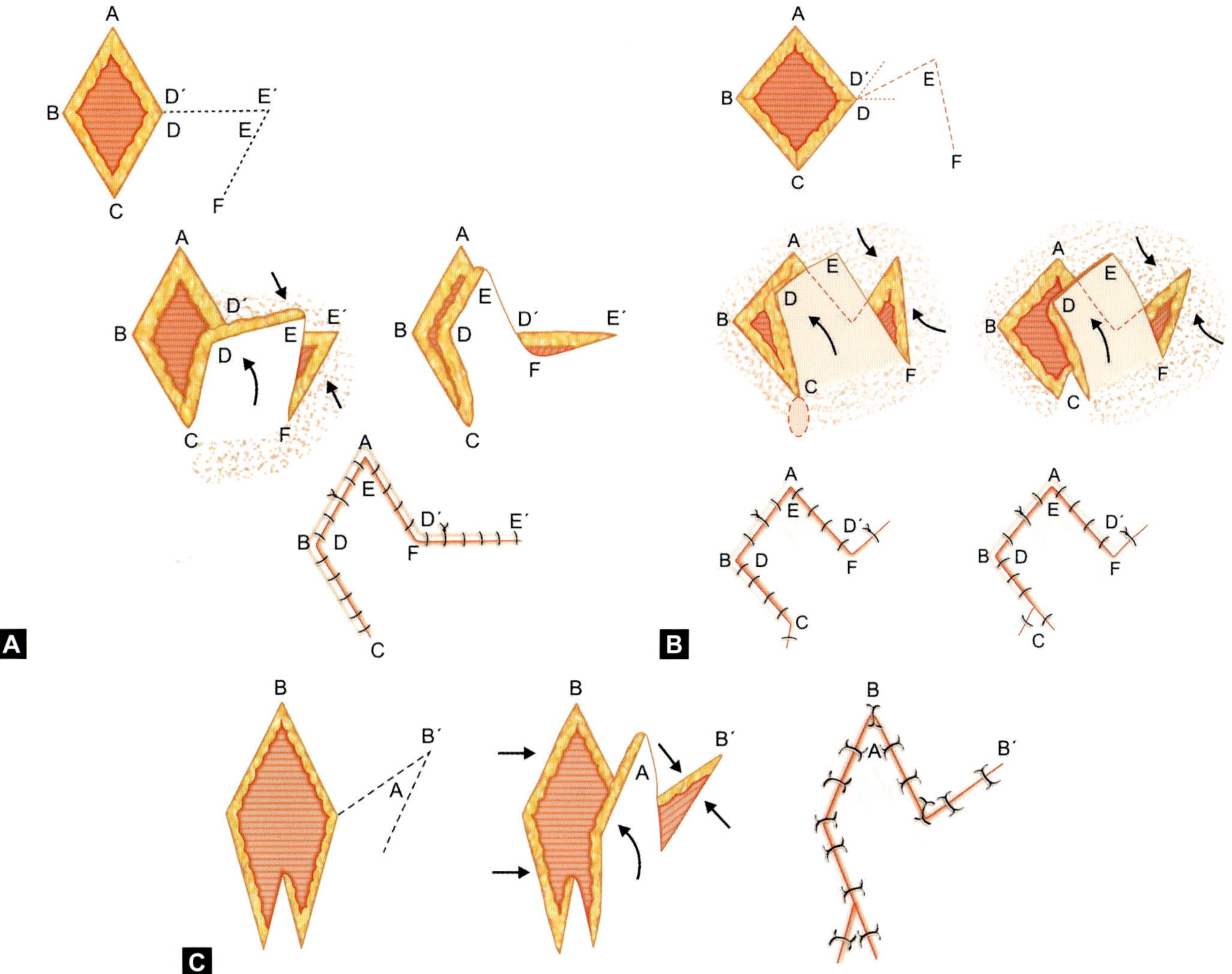


**Figs. 7.11A to C:** Different types of rhombic (Limberg, Webster, Dufourmental).

a triangular piece of tissue is cut and lifted over a healthy bridge of skin into the defect. The secondary defect created by the flap is closed first with the resulting tension vector oriented perpendicular to the primary tension vector. This redirection of tension allows the primary defect to be closed under minimal tension.

The ability of transposition flaps to both reorient tension and mobilize distant tissue reservoirs makes them very useful in reconstruction. This can be especially true around free margins where minimal tension can result in distortion leading to functional and aesthetic impairment.

Owing to its versatility, a number of variants on the transposition flap have been designed including the Dufourmental modification to the rhombic flap, the Webster modification to the rhombic flap (Figs. 7.11A to C), the bilobed and trilobed flaps, the Z-plasty, and the nasolabial transposition flap.

## Interpolation and Combined Flaps

Like transposition flaps, interpolation flaps also cross over intervening intact tissue. However, the base of interpolation flaps is not contiguous with the base of the defect, as it is in transposition flaps. Because of this difference, this flap requires two stages where the pedicle is divided and inset at a later date.

Interpolation flaps are often based on an axial blood supply and can be useful in larger and more complex reconstructions requiring greater amounts of viable tissue. The classic interpolation flap is the paramedian forehead

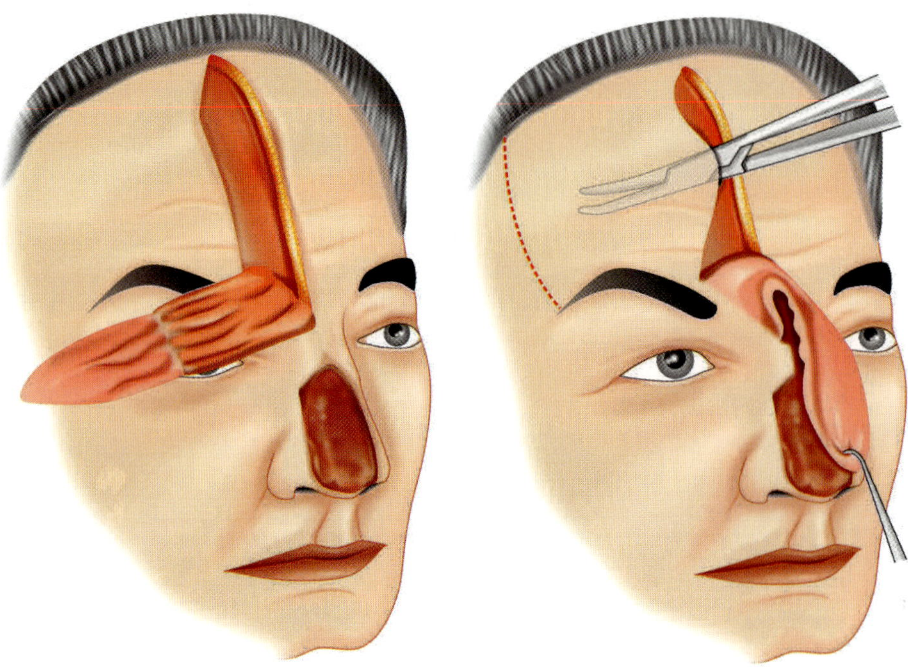

**Fig. 7.12:** Paramedian forehead flap.

flap, used to reconstruct large nasal defects (Fig. 7.12). Other examples of interpolation flaps including the melolabial interpolation flap, nasofacial interpolation flap, mastoid or retro-auricular interpolation flap, Hughes or tarsoconjunctival flap, and Abbe or lip-switch flap.

In practice, many flaps used by the dermatologic surgeon combine elements of two or more tissue movements. While these are generally classified according to the predominant movement, a few combined flap types deserve mention.

The "shark" island pedicle flap uses an advancement pedicle that is subsequently rotated 90°.[13] The combined movement can be useful for simultaneously repairing the alar-facial sulcus and nasal ala. The Spear flap, originally described in 1987, uses a nasolabial transposition flap that is then flipped over, and can be used to reconstruct both the interior and exterior nasal ala in a single stage.[14]

## BIOMECHANICS OF SKIN FLAPS

### Introduction

As the previous section discusses, anatomical and vascular supply considerations are paramount in the design of viable cutaneous flaps. Appropriate planning of where to place the secondary defect and its subsequent influence on surrounding tissue varies with location, size, patient profile, etc. of equal, importance are the characteristics of the skin itself. Skin has complex properties that directly influence the biomechanics of its movement, affecting blood supply and flap integrity. These mechanical properties of the skin contribute to the ability to mobilize tissue and directly influence reconstruction options. A complete appreciation and understanding of the biomechanics of skin is necessary for expert flap design and execution.

### Mechanical Properties of Skin

#### *Structural Components*

Skin has multiple biochemical components that affect its mechanical integrity. These include collagen fibers, elastin fibers, capillaries, lymphatic vessels, and ground substance. Thick and thin collagen bundles make up the bulk of the connective tissue and are randomly distributed throughout the skin as a network of loosely connected fibers. Elastic fibers are attached at multiple points to the collagen strands and help them to return to their original orientation after movement has caused deformation. It is the unique interplay within this network that dictates skin's reaction to movement and tension.

During initial force on skin with movement, randomly oriented collagen and elastic fibers are stretched in the direction of the applied force. Collagen fibers do not bear a significant burden until the bundle is completely straight in the direction of the applied force.[15] Therefore, initial resistance is low. However, as force and deformation increase, additional collagen fibers are recruited into a load-bearing role and resistance rises. Finally, at a high stress load, almost all dermal collagen fibers are aligned in the direction of the applied force. At this point, no further deformation is possible because of the inextensible nature of fully oriented collagen. These wholly oriented collagen fibers, with the support of elastin fibers, preserve the structural integrity of skin by limiting deformation during accidental or applied stresses.

## Tension

Tremendous variability exists among patients as to how much resistance an individual's skin will tolerate when subjected to outside stresses or forces. The resultant tension will induce varying deformation based on location on the patient. Specific areas on the face, such as the melolabial folds and the cheeks, can have greater laxity and, therefore, minimal tension with deformation. However other areas, such as the convexity of the nasal tip or chin, will have significant tension with deformation. This is due in part to a lack of excess tissue availability and laxity.

Directional forces dictated by underlying muscle groups help define the relaxed skin tension lines (RSTL) and illustrate the spectrum of tissue resistance when planning reconstructions (Fig. 7.13). Previous data indicate that the degree of tension in a wound is greatest parallel to the RSTL in that area.[16] Also, the dynamic qualities of RSTL are directly related to the interaction between the collagen and elastin fibers, as described previously.[17] An incision made parallel to the RSTL will have little dynamic force applied and can close under minimal tension. While an incision made perpendicular to the same RSTL may spread widely, from the tension vectors brought to bear on the same area, often leading to a hypertrophic scar. The reconstructive surgeon will be served in these considerations by planning flap closures in which the secondary defect repair is placed parallel to the RSTL.

Aging properties also affect tension vectors. Physiologic aging of the skin can progressively lead to laxity, and photoaging greatly accelerates and potentiates this phenomenon. The underlying collagen fibers are heavily denatured by ultraviolet damage, and there is also a reduction in new collagen formation in photodamaged skin. The elastin fiber network is grossly disrupted and there are significant degenerative changes in the ground substance.[18] The clinical application for the reconstructive surgeon is to identify areas with more lax and pliable skin which can be moved with relatively little tension, particularly in those areas of higher tissue availability and laxity.

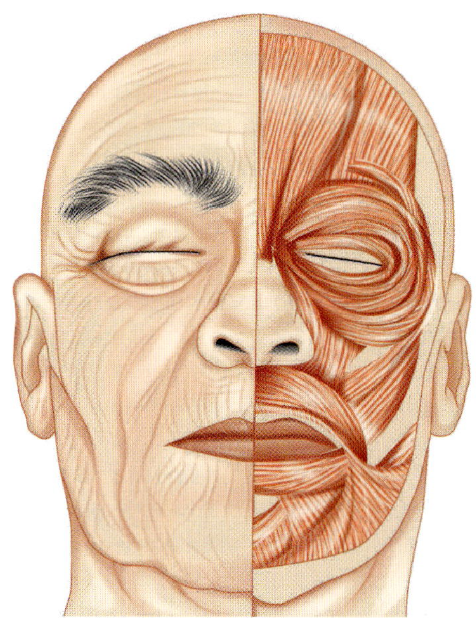

**Fig. 7.13:** Illustration showing relaxed skin tension lines (RSTL) running perpendicular to the underlying muscles.

## Biochemical Responses

Physical alterations of the skin can lead to changes at the cellular level. Folkman and Moscona grew cells in culture in which they were able to manipulate cell shape and cell tension; they found that varying cell shape and tension led to differences in DNA synthesis and proliferation.[19] This phenomenon in which mechanical forces can influence cellular activity was termed mechanotransduction.

Mechanotransduction can be direct or indirect. In direct mechanotransduction, cells convert mechanical stimuli into biochemical signals. They perform this activity by the use of cellular adhesion molecules such as integrins. Integrins connect the extracellular matrix to the cytoskeleton and transmit mechanical changes directly into the cell. This communication regulates a number of cellular activities, such as apoptosis and gene expression, and may be significant in wound healing and scar formation.[20] In addition, some cells possess mechanosensitive ion channels that respond to mechanical forces with either the activation or inactivation of an ion flux such as that seen in a mechanosensitive calcium ion channel.[21]

In one study in which stretching-induced hyperproliferation in cultured keratinocytes, a calcium channel blocker almost completely inhibited hyperproliferation after being cultured with the cells, illustrating the presence and significance of this mechanism.[22]

Indirect mechanotransduction occurs when a cell-detected mechanical change causes release of proteins and other chemical mediators, leading to biochemical changes. The skin possesses mechanoreceptors and nociceptors that sense pain as well as mechanical forces. These receptors and nociceptors can then cause the release of neuropeptides, such as substance P, which then regulate vasodilation, cytokine production, and vascular flow, among other changes.[23,24] These changes can then influence the response of the skin to stress, tension, and movement, and this release of neuropeptides in reaction to mechanical manipulation has implications for wound healing and scar formation.[25]

## Surgical Implications of Skin Biomechanics

### *Wound Tension and Blood Flow Alterations*

The skin demonstrates ample intrinsic versatility to the application of external tension, but the reconstructive surgeon will often apply further tension in wound closures, and that is after already compromising the blood supply with incisions. Animal models have revealed the effect of wound closure tension on the blood supply to surgically manipulated tissue, such as in flap preparation: in a pig model, blood flow was inversely proportional to the distance from the base of the flap and it decreased steadily with increasing tension until a critical value of 200–250 g was reached.[26] Further, this study showed that 3 cm wide flaps longer than 6 cm underwent some necrosis, while other flaps, also 3 cm wide, shorter than 1.5 cm remained viable, irrespective of wound closure tension. Flaps of intermediate length were sensitive to the effects of tension. Flaps closed with less than 250 g of tension tended to survive, and those closed under greater tension tended to have areas of necrosis. This reiterates that, once the skin has reached its limit in stress, blood flow plays the next most major role in surviving tension.

### *Flap Design and Elevation*

Proper flap design takes all properties of skin into consideration and exploits the characteristics of the skin's mechanics. A well-designed flap will use areas of maximal skin availability and laxity, close with minimal tension because its lines fall parallel to RSTL, and will maintain good vascular integrity. Minor variations in flap design can lead to poor perfusion and tissue necrosis. For example, pig models have demonstrated that rectangular advancement flaps should have at least a length:width ratio of 1:1; otherwise, excess wound tension can compromise blood flow to the distal tip of the flap. Similarly, facial flaps benefit from a ratio of 1:1 or 2:1, while further lengthening offers little advantage. Likewise, extending rotation flaps beyond 90° offers no mechanical benefit.[27] In addition, elevation of a flap at the appropriate level for the defect directly impacts its viability and survival: a musculocutaneous flap carries additional tissue which brings its own blood supply and increases the ability for the flap to sustain additional tension and manipulation; and an axial flap, while carrying its own artery, essentially brings its own blood supply, directly feeding the distal end of the flap and raising the perfusion and chances of survival.

### *Undermining*

Finally, undermining allows the reduction of tension at the leading edge of the flap. The resistance offered at the edge of the flap varies with the laxity and location of the defect. Undermining is the separation of the deep dermis from the underlying tissues, while in some locations, undermining occurs at the subcutaneous fat-fascial plane. The separation releases the skin to slide unrestricted over the deeper tissue, and as more tissue is undermined, the stress at the leading edge of the flap is reduced, allowing more skin to be available and the closure of the primary defect to occur with less wound tension. Most of the benefit from undermining is achieved within the first 1–2 cm. Undermining beyond a short distance risks injury to surrounding structures and may compromise blood flow.[28]

# FLAP PHYSIOLOGY

## Introduction

The creation of local flaps for reconstruction places significant stressors on what is otherwise healthy tissue. In order to properly execute a flap, the reconstructive surgeon should have a complete understanding of the physiologic changes that occur during flap creation, placement, and healing. This section will also address the complications that can arise with flaps and how to best avoid them.

## Anatomy

A thorough knowledge of the neurovascular anatomy of skin provides the basis for understanding flap physiology.

As described in earlier chapters, the skin has two vascular plexuses: the deep (or subdermal) and superficial vascular plexuses.

This vascular supply serves two functions: nutritional support and thermoregulation. Due to its thermoregulatory function, the rate of blood flow is one of the most variables in the body and under normal circumstances is almost ten times more than is required for nutritional support.[29] Thermoregulation is achieved through arteriovenous shunts under sympathetic control.[30] Nutritional support is mostly regulated by precapillary sphincters that dilate in response to local hypoxia or increased metabolic byproducts.[31]

Most local flaps used in dermatologic reconstruction are based on a random-pattern blood supply as described in the classification section. The small-caliber vessels supplying these flaps are subject to nutritional and thermoregulatory control and the stresses applied to the tissue during flap creation and movement can result in significant physiologic responses.

The survival of a randomly patterned flap can be unpredictable. It was originally thought that a length-to-width ratio of 1:1 was required for survival, but random flaps with ratios upward of 4:1 can survive with proper execution.[32] The belief that increasing the width of a flap will increase perfusion and thus survival is often misleading. The small vessels perfusing the flap are fed by the nearest local cutaneous arterial perforator. The surviving length of the flap is determined by the perfusing pressure of this vessel being greater than the intravascular resistance of the small vessels along the length of the flap. Increasing the width of the flap only adds to the number of vessels with the same perfusion pressure and resistance, thus keeping the length of the surviving tissue the same.[33,34]

Axial patterned flaps typically show improved survival relative to randomly patterned flaps, and this is attributable to the high perfusion pressure of the direct cutaneous vessel incorporated into the flap. However, these flaps are still subject to the same interplay of perfusion pressure and vascular resistance as described for randomly patterned flaps.

## Physiologic Changes

### *Vascular*

The process of incising and raising a skin flap immediately cuts off a portion of the neurovascular supply of the tissue. This results in a local decrease in perfusing pressure. The fact that flaps survive at all is in part due to the excessive blood flow of healthy skin in relation to the minimal nutritional requirements of skin survival. When perfusion in one area is decreased, adjacent vascular territories can provide additional low-pressure circulation through the subdermal plexus.[35] If tissue perfusion can remain above these minimal requirements through flap creation, movement, and healing, complete flap survival occurs.[36]

In a surviving flap, neovascularization occurs and will gradually increase the blood flow to the tissue. Flap neovascularization begins 3–7 days after the procedure.[37,38] The process continues to increase during the second week of healing especially in the distal portions of the flap despite already having an adequate nutritional supply.[39]

Reduced venous outflow also occurs with flap elevation and may in fact be more damaging to flap survival than inadequate arterial supply.[40] Venous outflow can occur through both the subdermal plexus and the large venous channel that accompanies the feeding arteries of the flap. Recognition of significant vascular congestion in the immediate postoperative period should trigger the surgeon to be wary of possible flap necrosis.

### *Neurologic*

Flap incision severs both cutaneous and sympathetic nerve fibers. When a sympathetic fiber is transected, catecholamines release from the terminal and reuptake is inhibited.[41] This results in a temporary local hyperadrenergic state that produces vasoconstriction. This vasoconstriction can have significant effects on flap perfusion and survival.[42] The released neurotransmitters are usually depleted within 24–48 hours and blood flow increases steadily with the declining concentration of norepinephrine.[43]

While transection of cutaneous nerve fibers may lead to a loss of sensation, this is often temporary, with injured nerve fibers slowly regenerating over a period of weeks to months.[44]

### *Inflammatory*

The trauma associated with flap creation results in both an immediate and delayed inflammatory response. This response is critical in preparing the tissue for the healing process. As part of the early response, histamine, serotonin, and kinins are released into the extracellular space, increasing vascular permeability.[36] This response contributes to the healing and survival of the flap, but the resulting edema, if severe, may compromise flap survival. Following

**Table 7.5:** Potential causes of flap failure.

| *Cause* | *Prevention* |
|---|---|
| Poor flap design | Ensure adequate size and blood supply prior to incision |
| Excess tension | Increase flap size<br>Wider undermining<br>Addition of back cuts<br>Addition of Z-plasties |
| Hematoma | Meticulous hemostasis<br>Early evacuation if hematoma forms |
| Infection | Strict sterile procedure<br>Prophylactic antibiotics when indicated |
| Smoking | Eliminate or minimize smoking during the postoperative period |
| Diabetes | Strict glucose control |
| Hypertension | Strict adherence to antihypertensive regimen |
| Mechanical compression | Proper postoperative wound dressing and patient instructions |

the release of these immediate mediators, prostaglandin synthesis occurs and facilitates both the late inflammatory stages and early stages of tissue repair.

### *Reperfusion*

During the first hours of flap creation, a significant ischemic state exists due to the combined influences of reduced vascular supply and both exogenous and endogenous catecholamines.[36] With reduction of neurotransmitter concentration and ongoing inflammatory response, blood flow reaches a maximum approximately 24 hours later as demonstrated in animal models.[43,45] As increased oxygen becomes available, free radical byproducts are created that can damage the flap at cellular and subcellular levels.

## Flap Failure

As described above, the physiologic changes occurring within a flap are numerous and complex. This interplay of influences will determine whether or not a flap survives. Poor flap design is one of the most common reason for failure.[46] The surgeon must carefully design a flap to ensure that it has adequate size and blood supply to withstand all the changes that occur with flap movement and healing (Table 7.5).

Placing excess tension on a flap, especially the distal portion, increases the microvascular resistance and decreases subsequent flap perfusion. This is a common reason for either partial or total flap necrosis in dermatologic surgery. Tension on flaps can be decreased through increasing the flap size, wider undermining, or the addition of "back-cuts" or Z-plasties.

Hematoma formation can also lead to flap failure through two apparent mechanisms. First, the direct pressure from the underlying hematoma increases wound tension and decreases perfusion. Second, there appears to be a direct toxic effect of hematoma byproducts that contributes to flap necrosis, likely through the release of active vasoconstrictive compounds.[47] The achievement of meticulous hemostasis and early evacuation of hematomas can help minimize the likelihood of this complication.

Postoperative infection can also lead to flap failure. The inflammation associated with bacterial or fungal infection can easily lead to the necrosis of what is already tenuous tissue. Strict sterile procedures should be used for all flap surgeries and prophylactic antibiotics may be warranted in certain situations (e.g., mucosal flaps or flaps on the nose).

Additional factors that may decrease the blood supply to a flap include smoking, diabetes, hypertension, and mechanical compression of the flap pedicle. Patients should be instructed to discontinue or minimize smoking during healing and adhere to all of their routine medicines used to manage any comorbidities.

## REFERENCES


1. Sushruta Samhita. An English translation of the Sushruta Samhita, based on original Sanskrit text. Calcutta: Bose; 1907.
2. Flaps. In: Hayes M (Ed). Practical Skin Cancer Surgery. Elsevier Health Sciences; London, 2014.
3. Mendelson BC, Masson JK. Cervical and clavicular tubed skin flaps. In: Grabb's Encyclopedia of Flaps, 3rd edition. Lippincott Williams & Wilkins; Philadelphia 2009.
4. Shastri-Hurst N. Sir Harold Gillies CBE, FRCS: the father of modern plastic surgery. Trauma. 2012;14:179-87.
5. Baker SR. Local cutaneous flaps. Otolaryngol Clin North Am. 1994;27:139-59.
6. Cutting C, Ballantyne D, Shaw W, et al. Critical closing pressure, local perfusion pressure, and the failing skin flap. Ann Plast Surg. 1982;8:504-9.
7. Baker SR. Local Flaps in Facial Reconstruction, 3rd edition. Philadelphia, PA: Saunders/Elsevier; 2014.
8. Dzubow LM. Flap dynamics. J Dermatol Surg Oncol. 1991; 17:116-30.

9. McGregor IA, McGregor AD. Techniques of Plastic Surgery and Their Surgical Applications, 9th edition. Churchill Livingston; London 2010.
10. Papel ID. Facial Plastic and Reconstructive Surgery, 2nd edition. Thieme; Stuttgart 2002.
11. Summers BK, Siegle RJ. Facial cutaneous reconstructive surgery—general aesthetic principles. J Am Acad Dermatol. 1993;29:669-81.
12. Gibson T (Ed). Modern Trends in Plastic Surgery. London: Butterworths; 1964.
13. Cvancara JL, Wentzell JM. Shark island pedicle flap for repair of combined nasal ala-perialar defects. Dermatol Surg. 2006;32:726-9.
14. Spear SL, Kroll SS, Romm S. A new twist to the nasolabial flap for reconstruction of lateral alar defects. Plast Reconstr Surg. 1987;79:915-20.
15. Daly CH, Odland GF. Age-related changes in the mechanical properties of human skin. J Invest Dermatol. 1979;73:84-7.
16. Borges AF. Relaxed skin tension lines. Dermatol Clin. 1989; 7:169-77.
17. Pierard GE, Lapiere CM. Microanatomy of the dermis in relation to relaxed skin tension lines and Langer's lines. Am J Dermatopathol. 1987;9:219-24.
18. Fisher GJ, Kang S, Varani J, et al. Mechanisms of photoaging and chronological skin aging. Arch Dermatol. 2002; 138:1462-70.
19. Folkman J, Moscona A. Role of cell shape in growth control. Nature. 1978;273:345-9.
20. Hynes RO. Integrins: bidirectional, allosteric signaling machines. Cell. 2002;110:673-87.
21. Sachs F, Morris CE. Mechanosensitive ion channels in nonspecialized cells. Rev Physiol Biochem Pharmacol. 1998; 132:1-77.
22. Yano S, Komine M, Fujimoto M, et al. Mechanical stretching in vitro regulates signal transduction pathways and cellular proliferation in human epidermal keratinocytes. J Invest Dermatol. 2004;122:783-90.
23. Chin MS, Lancerotto L, Helm DL, et al. Analysis of neuropeptides in stretched skin. Plast Reconstr Surg. 2009;124: 102-13.
24. Ogawa R. Mechanobiology of scarring. Wound Repair Regen. 2011;19 (Suppl 1):s2-9.
25. Akaishi S, Ogawa R, Hyakusoku H. Keloid and hypertrophic scar: neurogenic inflammation hypotheses. Med Hypotheses 2008;71:32-8.
26. Larrabee WF Jr, Holloway GA Jr, Sutton D. Wound tension and blood flow in skin flaps. Ann Otol Rhinol Laryngol. 1984; 93(Pt 1):112-5.
27. Larrabee WF Jr, Sutton D. The biomechanics of advancement and rotation flaps. Laryngoscope. 1981;91:726-34.
28. Cox KW, Larrabee W Jr. A study of skin flap advancement as a function of undermining. Arch Otolaryngol 1982;108: 151-5.
29. Guyton AC. Textbook of Medical Physiology. Saunders; Philadelphia 1976.
30. Gullane PJ, et al. Regional Flaps of the Head and Neck. Wahsington, DC: American Academy of Otolaryngology—Head and Neck Surgery Foundation; 1982.
31. Granger HJ, Goodman AH, Granger DN. Role of resistance and exchange vessels in local microvascular control of skeletal muscle oxygenation in the dog. Circ Res. 1976; 38:379-85.
32. Connor CD, Fosko SW. Local skin flap anatomy and physiology. Facial Plast Surg Clin North Am. 1996;4:447-54.
33. Daniel RK, Cunningham DM, Taylor GI. The deltopectoral flap: an anatomical and hemodynamic approach. Plast Reconstr Surg. 1975;55:275-82.
34. Milton SH. Pedicled skin-flaps: the fallacy of the length: width ratio. Br J Surg. 1970;57:502-8.
35. Cutting C, Ballantyne D, Shaw W, et al. Critical closing pressure, local perfusion pressure, and the failing skin flap. Ann Plast Surg. 1982;8:504-9.
36. Chu EA, Byrne PJ, Odland RM, et al. Skin flap physiology and wound healing. In: Flint PW, Haughey BH, Lund LJ, et al. (Eds). Cummings Otolaryngology: Head & Neck Surgery, 5th edition. Philadelphia, PA: Mosby Elsevier; 2010.
37. Tsur H, Daniller A, Strauch B. Neovascularization of skin flaps: route and timing. Plast Reconstr Surg. 1980;66:85-93.
38. Gatti JE, LaRossa D, Brousseau DA, et al. Assessment of neovascularization and timing of flap division. Plast Reconstr Surg. 1984;73:396-402.
39. Cummings CW, Trachy RE. Measurement of alternative blood flow in the porcine panniculus carnosus myocutaneous flap. Arch Otolaryngol. 1985;111(9):598-600.
40. Su CT, Im MJ, Hoopes JE. Tissue glucose and lactate following vascular occlusion in island skin flaps. Plast Reconstr Surg. 1982;70:202-5.
41. Pearl RM. A unifying theory of the delay phenomenon—recovery from the hyperadrenergic state. Ann Plast Surg. 1981;7(2):102-12.
42. Jurell G. Adrenergic nerves and the delay phenomenon. Ann Plast Surg. 1986;17:493-7.
43. Pang C, Neligan PC, Forrest C, et al. Hemodynamics and vascular sensitivity to circulating norepinephrine in normal skin and delayed and acute random skin flaps in the pig. Plast Reconstr Surg. 1986;78:75-84.
44. Manek S, Terenghi G, Shurey C, et al. Neovascularisation precedes neural changes in the rat groin skin flap following denervation: an immunohistochemical study. Br J Plast Surg. 1993;46:48-55.
45. Sasaki GH, Pang CY. Hemodynamics and viability of acute neurovascular island skin flaps in rats. Plast Reconstr Surg. 1980;65:152-8.
46. Lamberty BGH, Healy C. Flaps: physiology, principles of design, and pitfalls. In: Cohen M (Ed). Mastery of Plastic and Reconstructive Surgery, Vol 1. Boston, MA: Little, Brown and Co; 1994. pp. 56-70.
47. Hillelson RL, Glowacki J, Healey NA, et al. A microangiographic study of hematoma-associated flap necrosis and salvage with isoxsuprine. Plast Reconstr Surg. 1980; 66:528-33.

# CHAPTER 8

# Advancement Flaps

*Laura Kruter, Thomas Rohrer*

The advancement flap is the oldest type of tissue transfer described, first postulated by Celsus in ancient Rome, nearly 2,000 years ago. Geometrically, when compared to rotation and transposition flaps, which by definition involve a pivoting motion and change in orientation, the advancement flap has the advantage of being simpler to envision and design. Its relative simplicity, however, does not undermine its utility and power in appropriate anatomic areas that can aesthetically accommodate the long, straight lines that result.

The classic advancement flap is defined as tissue transfer that slides into a surgical defect in one direction. Both the flap and its underlying pedicle move jointly in a single linear vector. The primary tissue movement consists of the advancement of the flap into the defect, led by the flap's advancing tip. Secondary tissue movement involves skin peripheral to the defect, which is pulled to the center of the primary defect upon closure.[1]

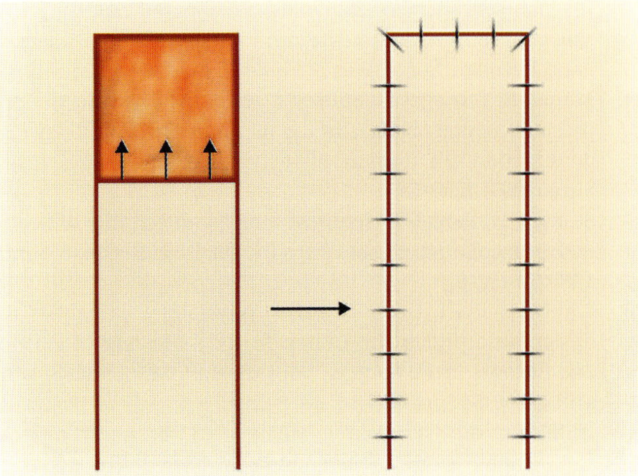

**Fig. 8.1:** Diagram of classic advancement flap, or U-plasty.

Also known as a U-plasty, or unilateral advancement flap, the classic advancement flap shape is rectangular (Fig. 8.1). As such, the incisions result in two parallel straight lines bordered by a connecting line. These linear scars are aptly masked in areas with unidirectional muscle pull, such as the eyebrow or forehead, where the frontalis muscle produces natural horizontal lines, or linear cosmetic unit junctions, such as the upper lip, dorsal nose, or helical rim.[2]

By design, the length of the advancement flap is shorter than the distance it travels, which includes the diameter of the defect. Thus, redundancy forms along the total length of the peripheral tissue. Not unlike a fusiform closure, this redundancy can be managed with excision of dog-ears either at the base or along the sides of the flap, or can be "sewn" away using the rule of halves. The flexibility of dog-ear placement allows for creativity and options in designing incision lines that rest in cosmetically favorable lines.

## FLAP DESIGN AND CONSIDERATIONS

Biomechanically, the maximal length to width ratio that allows sufficient blood flow to the flap tip is 3–4:1.[3] Flap perfusion is largely based on tension, the quality of pedicle vasculature, and its dimensions.[4] When planning the length of an advancement flap, it is critical to determine whether surrounding tissue laxity will allow for the intended movement. Laxity is clinically evaluated with careful pinching and manipulation of the surrounding skin, and anatomic areas permitting sufficient stretching are ideal for this type of motion. As such, less mobile areas, such as the scalp, often introduce excessive tension to allow for flap viability.

A useful gauge to estimate surrounding mobility prior to flap incision is to undermine around the surgical defect.

If laxity is deemed appropriate and a longer flap is required, larger caliber vessels in deeper tissues can be recruited, as blood flow is proportional to the vessel's diameter.[5] Flap thickness should match the defect depth and should gradually thicken as it extends toward the pedicle base to allow for larger vessel recruitment.[1] The pedicle should contain a portion of the upper subcutaneous fat and at minimum, subdermal vascular plexus.

Judicious undermining can assist in determining the feasibility of an advancement flap for a determined anatomical site (Table 8.1). The entire perimeter of the flap should be undermined to allow for maximal movement with greatest redistribution of forces of contraction. This may limit potential pincushioning as an adverse outcome.[6] Though undermining deep at the base of the pedicle is necessary to free flap motion, care must be taken to avoid excessive disruption of the vascular pedicle, which perfuses the flap.

Distortion of anatomic symmetry involving a free margin can cause significant functional and cosmetic compromise, and its avoidance should be a priority when planning reconstructions. This is of prime importance when determining the utility of an advancement flap, wherein the resulting tension vector is linear. When a free margin is in the vicinity of the defect, the tension vector should be oriented parallel to it—and if not feasible, another reconstruction option, such as a rotation flap, should be considered.

**Table 8.1:** Plane of undermining in specific anatomic sites.

| | |
|---|---|
| Zygoma/mandible | Upper subcutaneous fat |
| Forehead (small defect) | Subcutaneous fat |
| Forehead (large defect) | Subgaleal |
| Hair bearing areas | Subcutis deep to hair papillae |
| Nose | Submuscular |
| Ear | Above perichondrium |

At every step of reconstruction planning and execution, re-evaluations should be performed to judge whether the current plan remains the ideal one. After placing the key suture at the advancing edge, excess tension may be relieved by further undermining, elongation of the flap or conversion to a bilateral advancement.[7] Excision of standing cones after closure of the primary defect closure allows the surgeon to design incision lines deliberately rather than in a formulaic fashion. Similarly, widening the defect to include resting skin tension lines (RSTLs) or cosmetic unit junctions or squaring the defect versus rounding the flap tip are tools that optimize flap biomechanics and cosmesis.

## Bilateral Advancement Flap

Also known as an H-plasty, the bilateral advancement flap is composed of mirror images of two opposing unilateral advancements, forming two Us, or an H-shaped incision (Figs. 8.2A and B). These need not be identical—after the first limb is mobilized, laxity and need for additional defect coverage determine the length of the second limb. Bilateral flaps redistribute tension to two opposing sides, and are useful where it is prudent to avoid unilateral pull, such as in areas in proximity to the midline wherein distortion

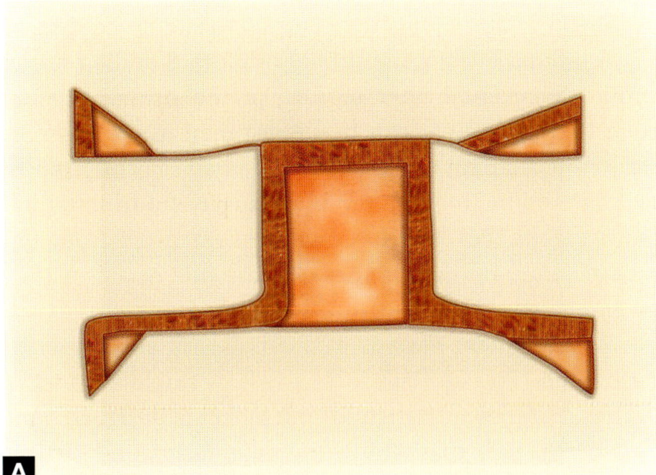


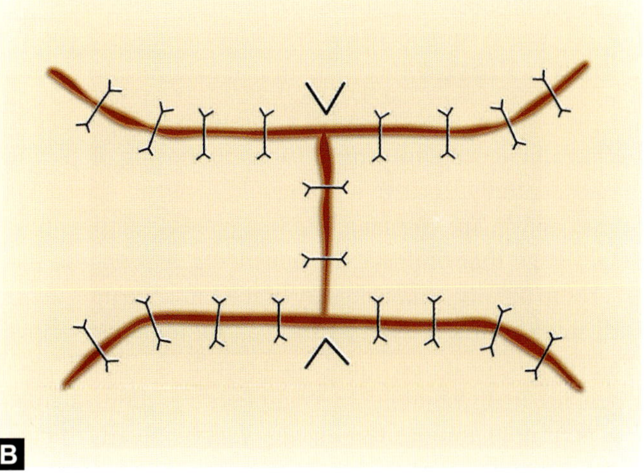


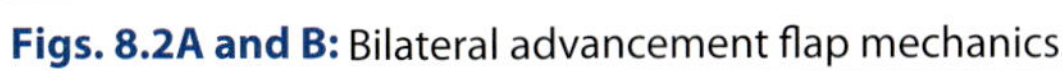

**Figs. 8.2A and B:** Bilateral advancement flap mechanics.

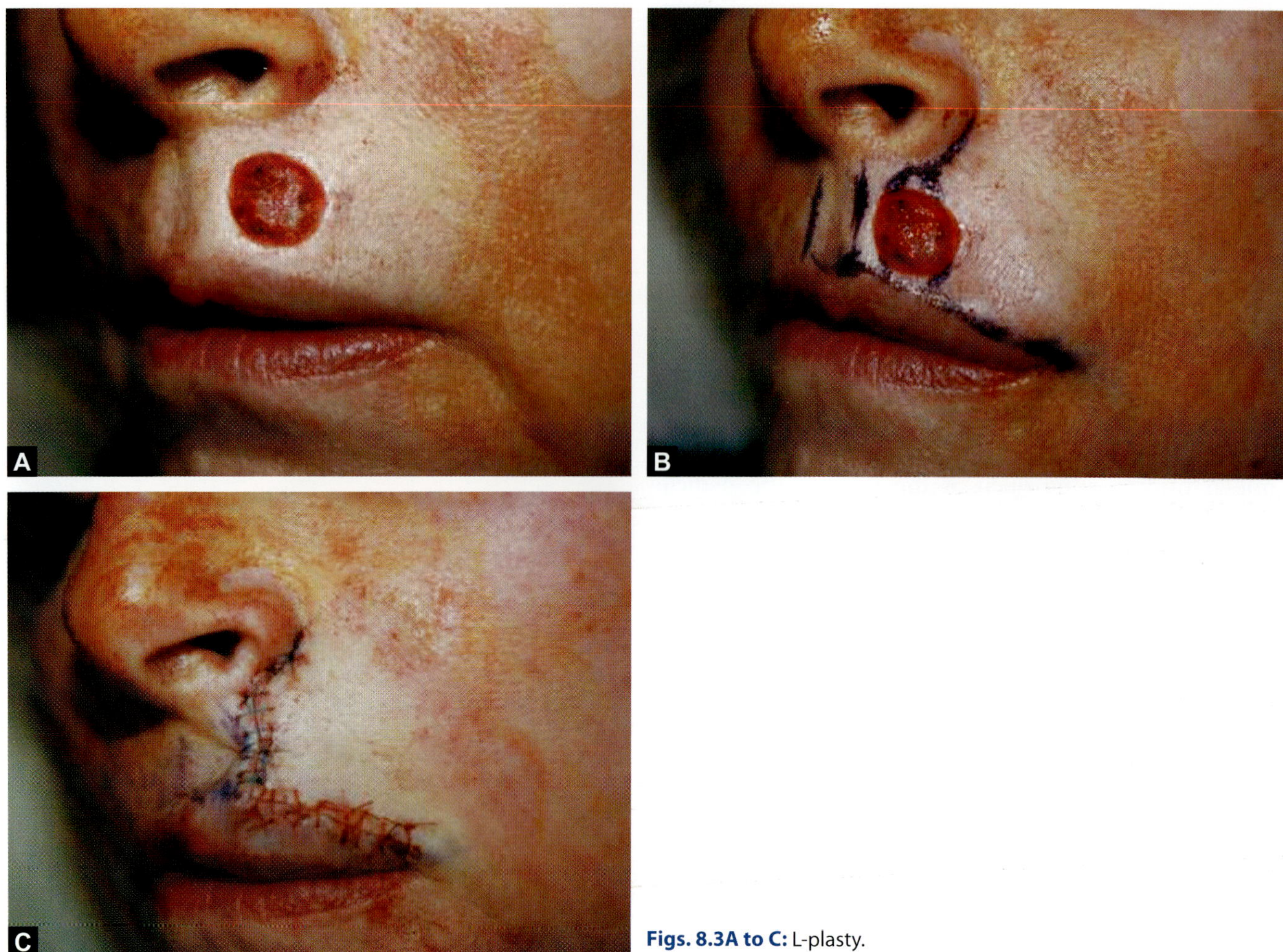

**Figs. 8.3A to C:** L-plasty.

can be cosmetically undesirable. Similar to the U-plasty, the H-plasty creates parallel lines, thus is masked in the forehead, eyebrow or glabella, central lips, and chin.[1,2]

## T- and L-Plasties

The T-plasty (or A-to-T flap) is a variation of the bilateral advancement flap in which broad opposing flaps are joined centrally to close a triangular, inverted triangular, or oval defect. The resulting standing cone is excised at the defect edge that opposes the advancing flap edges. This creates a T-shape that is ideally placed in anatomic areas with linear borders such as the central forehead, above the eyebrow, or in the temple adjacent to the hairline, or lateral lip. Redistribution of tension between the two limbs and an ample, duplicated vascular supply are advantages of this flap.[8] The vertical height should be twice as tall as the defect and the base should extend one defect diameter in each direction. A shorter vertical height can be obtained with use of an M-plasty.[9]

The key suture joins the central advancing borders of the two flaps, closing the primary defect. Standing cones should be excised after closure of the primary defect such that placement can be determined. Curvilinear or crescentic shaping of the base of the flap may be used to manage redundancy—a modification useful in naturally convex areas. If excessive vertical tension results from this modification, Burow's triangles or the rule of halves may be employed.

The unilateral variant of a T-plasty is appropriately termed an L-plasty (Figs. 8.3A to C). A single advancing limb ~2–3 times the length of the defect is designed laterally on the side that affords the most laxity. The vertical limb is excised within relaxed skin tension lines, as is the longer limb.

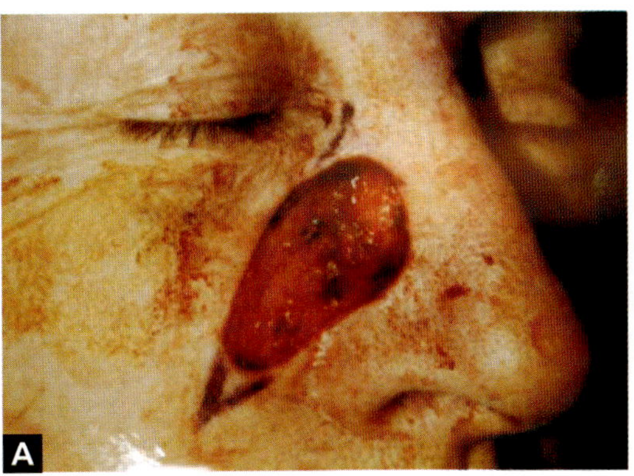

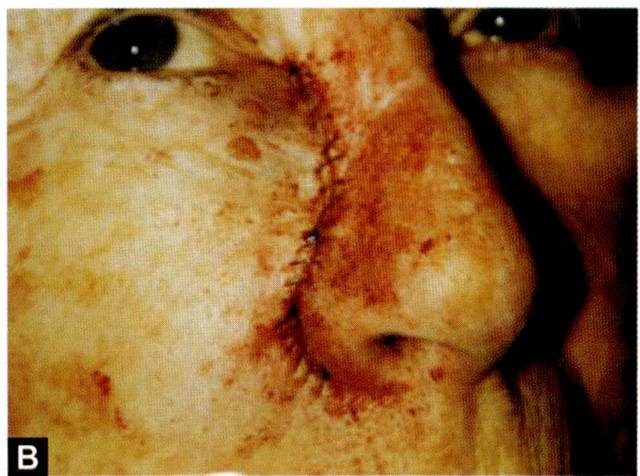

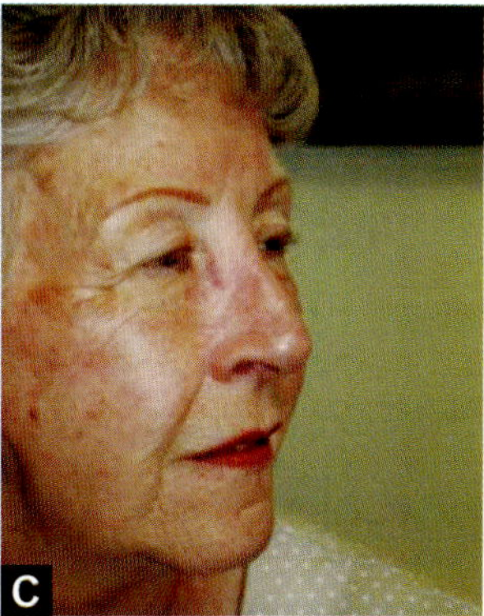


**Figs. 8.4A to C:** Cheek advancement.

## Burow's Triangle Flap

Described by Karl August von Burow in 1855, the Burow's triangle or wedge flap is an advancement flap in which two triangles are excised—one as a standing cone and another to mobilize and advance the flap. Movement is unidirectional and, as in the L-plasty, laterality is chosen based on availability of tissue laxity and ideal incision placement within cosmetic junctions or RSTLs.

This flap may also be employed for repair of two defects in close proximity. In this case, one movement closes two defects, which are housed within the two excised triangles.[10]

## Cheek Advancement

For defects of the medial cheek, nasofacial sulcus or lateral nose, the relative laxity and lateral to medial mobility of the cheek provides an ample reservoir for a unilateral advancement flap (Figs. 8.4A to C). As the cheek is a large cosmetic subunit, this flap is most useful for moderate to large sized defects. An inferior incision is made to parallel or hide within the nasolabial fold or RSTLs, and the superior incision along RSTLs or cosmetic junction units. Care must be taken with superior incisions in the infraorbital area, where downward pull of the eyelid can result in ectropion or lymphatic disruption—the latter may provoke significant and long lasting edema. Suspension, or tacking sutures placed from the dermal portion of the advancing flap edge to the periosteum can decrease excessive tension and resulting ectropion or nasofacial sulcus blunting, both relevant to cheek advancement biomechanics.[11] To avoid tying off vasculature and flap ischemia with deep tacking sutures, these should be placed parallel to the blood vessels supplying the flap.

## Helical Rim Advancement

Anatomically, the helix of the ear, with its lengthy and narrow shape, is a suitable area for a unilateral advancement flap (Fig. 8.5). The basic movement is an inferior to superior slide, with redundancies removed as an inferiorly placed standing tissue cone. First performed with a through-and-through incision, this initial version caused concern for ischemia due to interruption of blood flow when long flaps were created to cover defects of the mid-to-upper helix. Antia and Buch described an advancement in 1967, in which rather than full thickness, the depth of incision was limited to the postauricular plane, where dissection is performed above the perichondrium.[12] The flap is undermined posteriorly until the postauricular sulcus is reached. This modification allowed for improved preservation of blood supply to the helical rim, which includes connecting branches from the superior and inferior branches of the anterior auricular artery.[13]

Anatomically, this flap causes a decrease in circumference of the ear, a pliable rounded structure. Thus, cupping or shortening of the ear can occur if mobility is insufficient. To avoid this distortion, a Burow's triangle may be excised in the lobule or the curvature may be flattened with shaving of the scapha cartilage.[14] Similarly, the anatomy of the ear can cause an inward pull that may result in visible notching at the suture line if careful eversion is not performed. If eversion is insufficient, vertical mattress sutures, step cuts, and Z-plasties of the flap tips can be undertaken.[15,16]

## Crescentic Advancement Flap

In 1955, Webster published his experience with the perialar crescentic flap for upper lip repair (Fig. 8.6). This flap

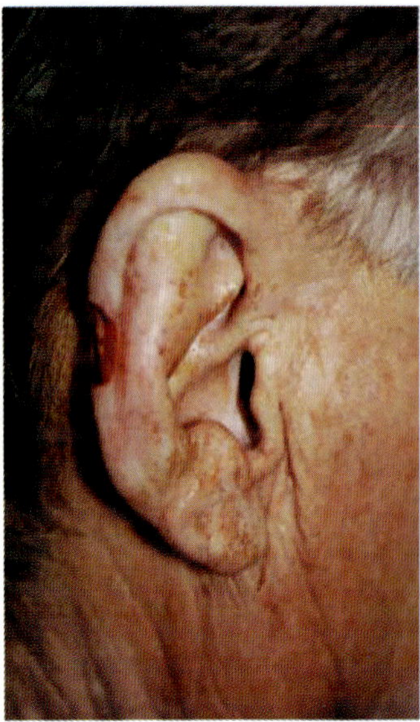
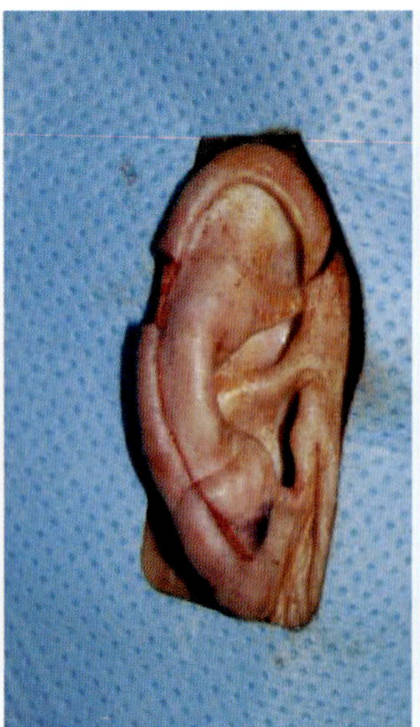
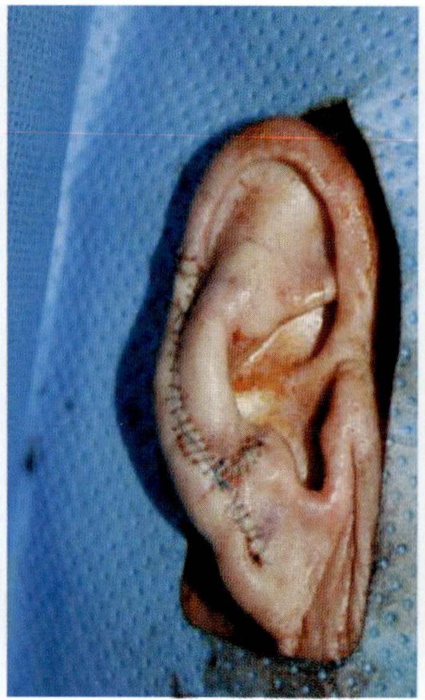
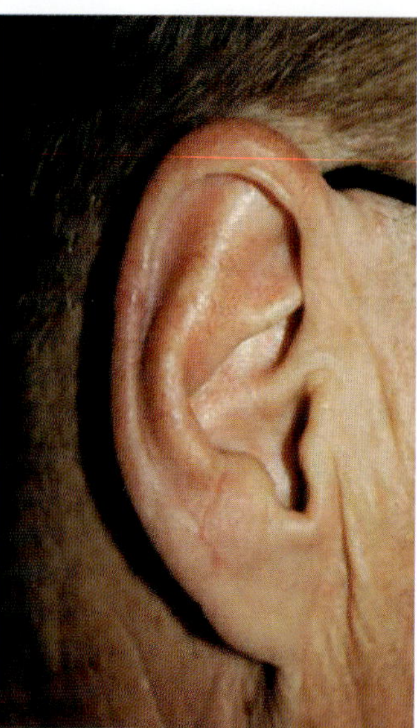

**Fig. 8.5:** Helical rim advancement.

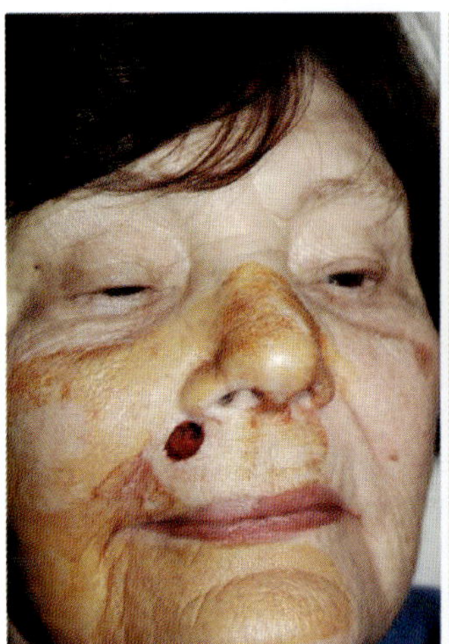
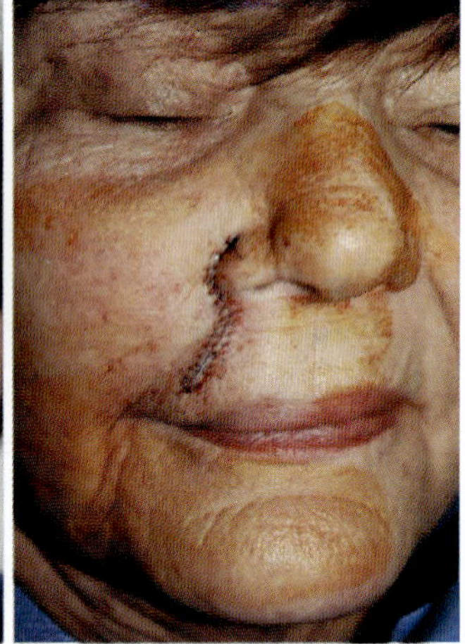

**Fig. 8.6:** Crescentic advancement.

takes advantage of both the deep curvature of the nasal ala and the nasofacial sulcus, in which incisions are easily camouflaged, and the mobility and tissue laxity of the medial cheek. By excising, in a curvilinear fashion, tissue from the perialar cheek, advancement mobility is improved and tissue redundancy is removed. The inferior incision lies along the vermillion border—along which an M-plasty may be employed to reduce incision length.

Crescentic advancements can also be used for small (under 1 cm) perialar lip and cheek defects, and has been described in the lateral nasal tip and medial ala. The latter takes advantage of the nasal crease for incision placement, and dissection is performed above the perichondrium.[17]

*Editors' note*: one potential disadvantage of this flap when used to reconstruct upper lip defects is that the isthmus of the upper lip cannot be preserved. A good alternative to maintain the isthmus intact would be designing an island pedicle flap (IPF) (V-to-Y flap) (Fig. 8.9B).

## East–West Flap

This aptly named flap is a variation based on the historical use of Burow's triangles to close surgical defects. It employs a horizontal movement that is possible after removing a superior dog-ear parallel to the long axis of the nose and an inferior dog-ear lying in the nasal tip and columella (Fig. 8.7). The two standing cones are of different heights and widths to accommodate the defect width superiorly and the columella inferiorly.[18] Ideal defects are the lateral nasal supratip and inferior or lateral sidewalls under 2 cm in diameter. Patients with thick, sebaceous skin may benefit from this laterally based closure rather than superiorly based flaps given optimal side-to-side tissue matching and low resulting tension.[18,19]

## V to Y

Flaps termed "V to Y" may refer to two distinct reconstructive options. The first is a simple advancement useful in regions that require lengthening or release from a contracted state. The second is a subcutaneous tissue pedicle flap that has been reclassified from prior denomination as an IPF.

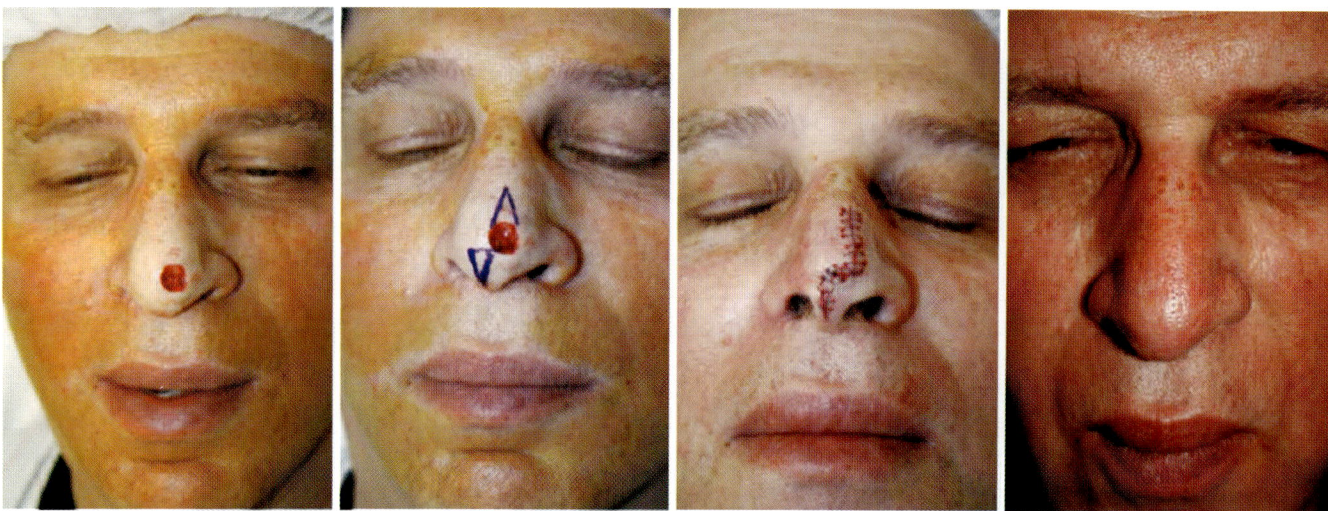

**Fig. 8.7:** East–West flap.

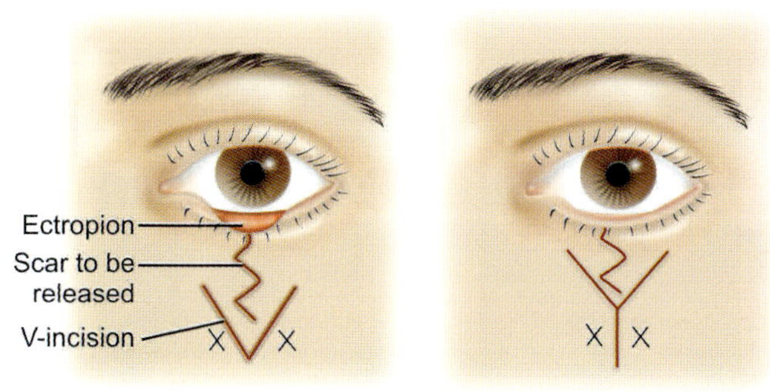


**Fig. 8.8:** Diagram of V-to-Y advancement flap for scar release.

## V-to-Y Advancement

This flap redistributes tension vectors in areas where a single linear vector is distorting, such as in the free margin of the lower eyelid. In the case of scar release, the V is incised with the tip at the scar line and advanced to alleviate adjacent tension. Subsequently, the base leg of the Y is approximated with side-to-side closure (Fig. 8.8). This is useful for areas that benefit from increased lengthening, such as burn scars, distorted free margins such as ectropion and eclabion, and lengthening of the columella to enhance nasal tip protrusion.[2]

## V-to-Y Subcutaneous Tissue Pedicle Flap

The V-to-Y subcutaneous tissue pedicle flap, also known as the subcutaneous IPF, is classified as an advancement flap due to its primary unidirectional mechanics (Figs. 8.9A and B). In the past, it was referred to as an island pedicle as it involves formation of an island of skin under which a central subcutaneous pedicle is preserved. A central vascular supply provides a distinct advantage over the classic advancement flap, which is limited by a 3:1 length-to-width ratio and risk of tension-induced ischemia.

A triangular-shaped flap is incised to the subcutis and the perimeter then undermined for a distance of 2 cm toward the fascial plane. The width of the triangle should match the widest measurement of the defect, whereas its length is measured as twice the height of the defect.

The pedicle provides blood supply to the flap and is relatively robust, consisting of subcutaneous fat, muscle, and occasionally including the superficial musculoaponeurotic system. To maintain adequate perfusion, one-third of the total flap surface should remain attached to the underlying pedicle. The reliability of its blood supply makes the IPF a wise choice for patients with increased risk of flap necrosis, such as smokers and those with prior exposure to radiation therapy. Moreover, the decreased need for extensive undermining facilitates hemostasis, and is thus beneficial in coagulopathic patients.[1]

The IPF is classically designed as an isosceles triangle, preferentially harvested from within the same cosmetic unit as the surgical wound. The length of the triangle may be up to 3–4 times the width of the surgical defect, and the angle of the apex of the triangle distal to the wound is ~30°. Local anesthesia should be infiltrated after the incisions are marked to avoid tissue distortion. The wound bed must then be made to match the shape of the advancing flap. Conversion of a circular defect into a square may

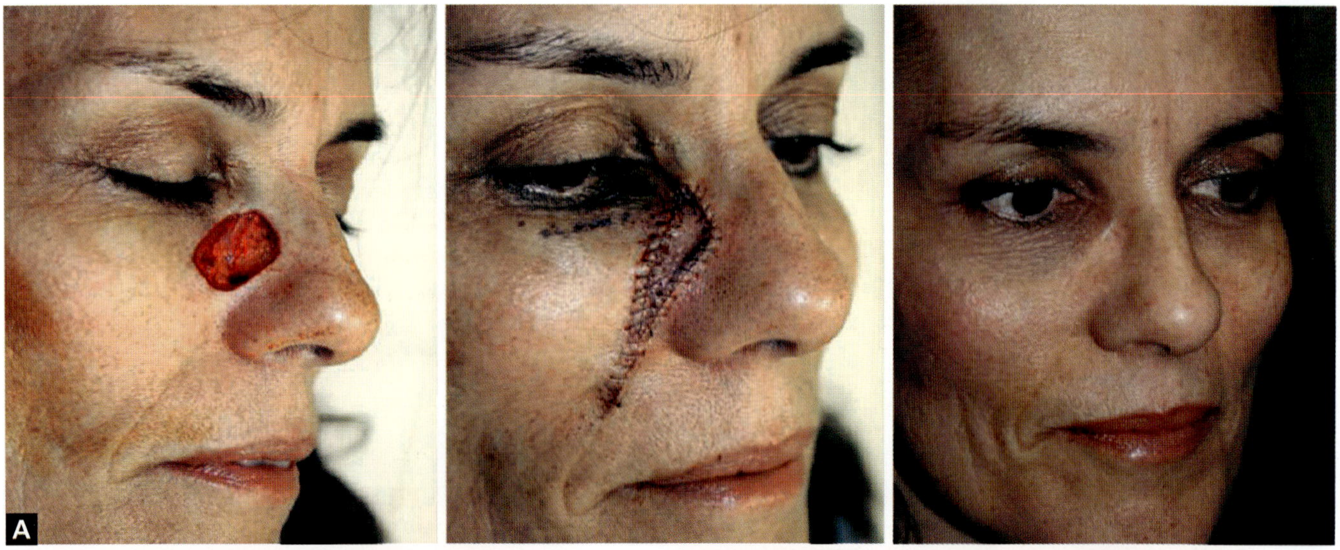

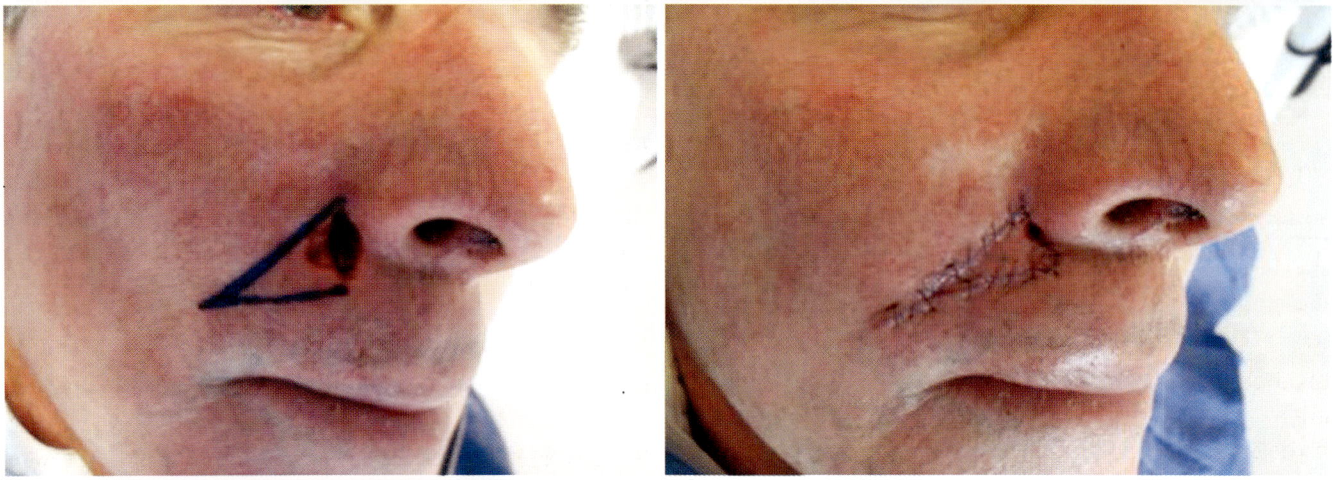

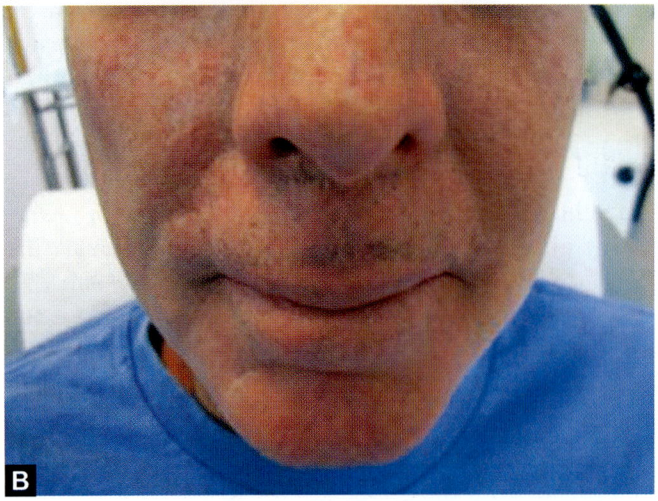

**Figs. 8.9A and B:** (A) Island pedicle flap. (B) Island pedicle flap of the upper cutaneous lip preserving the isthmus.
*Courtesy*: (Fig. 8.9B)—S Brian Jiang, MD, San Diego, California, USA.

reduce the risk of trapdooring when compared to rounding of the IPF edge.[20] The flap is sharply incised and the margins of the donor area undermined. Maintaining equal depth throughout, the margins of the original defect are similarly undermined. The central pedicle should be sized to 40–50% of the flap's area to ensure survival. Though

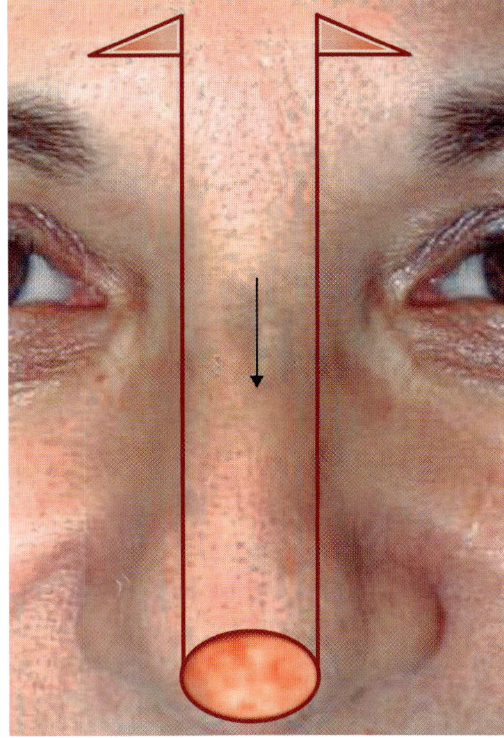

**Fig. 8.10:** Basic movement of the Rintala flap.

flap mobility cannot be achieved without undermining, this should be kept to the minimum necessary to fulfill advancement so as to maximize blood supply. The key stitch approximates the leading border of the skin island to the distal defect edge. Given the propensity of the flap to rise due to wound contraction, dermal sutures should depress the central portion of the flap by 2–3 mm. Epidermal sutures are then placed in a running cuticular or interrupted fashion.

Advantages of this flap include a lack of standing cones and decreased dead space beneath the flap, the latter reducing the incidence of hematomas and seromas. Moreover, it provides an excellent color and texture match when used within cosmetic units. A major disadvantage is the risk of a trapdoor deformity, particularly for flaps under 2 cm in size.[2] This complication appears as an elevation of the inset flap above the level of surrounding skin. Island pedicle flaps are particularly susceptible given the low peripheral tension on the freed island, which allows for undeterred inward flap contraction. Judicious undermining around the secondary defect[21] and slight undersizing can reduce the risk of pincushioning.[20,22]

The IPF is especially useful in the medial cheek below the ala and the lateral cutaneous upper lip such that the base leg of the resulting Y lies in the nasolabial fold. It is also an excellent option for the anterior or midnasal ala and brow, nasal dorsum, forehead or concha.[22-32]

Many variations of the V-to-Y advancement flap have been described. A design proposing two lateral myocutaneous pedicles may decrease potential bulkiness at the center of the flap.[33] Single myocutaneous slings may also be designed and useful for nasal reconstruction.[34,35] Buried IPFs and transposition island flaps expand its use to other anatomic sites and are discussed in other chapters.

## Rintala Flap

This is a unilateral advancement flap described by Rintala in 1969 for the reconstruction of 1.5–2.5 cm defects in the midline of the nasal dorsum. The tissue reservoir is located in the glabella, and incision lines are placed along the nasal dorsum, with bilateral Burow's triangles incised proximal to the alar grooves. Standing cones may also be placed at the corner of the eyes or above the eyebrows (Fig. 8.10). As in most flaps on the nasal dorsum, the plane of dissection should be submuscular or supraperiosteal;[36] however, care must be taken to dissect adhesions in the thinner canthal regions. Given the resulting vertical tension vector, nasal tip elevation is expected but may be desired in the appropriate patient.[37] Tip elevation may be avoided with extensive forehead undermining, releasing incisions into the galea aponeurotica and placement of a suspension suture over the nasal bone and lateral cartilage. Distal flap ischemia is a concern given the length of the pedicle and narrow pedicle. A more robust blood supply may be recruited with addition of an axial dorsal nasal flap, which employs lateral nasal vasculature.[38]

## Peng Flap

With the advantage of decreasing potential nasal tip elevation and sacrifice of healthy tissue with the Rintala flap, a "pinch" modification was described by Peng and colleagues for central nasal tip defects (Fig. 8.11).[39] A wider, shorter pedicle that curves bilaterally from the middle of the defect and extends upward along the nasofacial sulcus is then rotated and advanced, in this way "pinching" into the defect. This flap obviates the need for squaring the defect or rounding the advancing edge of the Rintala flap. Rowe and colleagues suggested a distal incision point for the flaps with the added advantage of increasing rotational movement and shortening the lateral vertical incisions.[40]

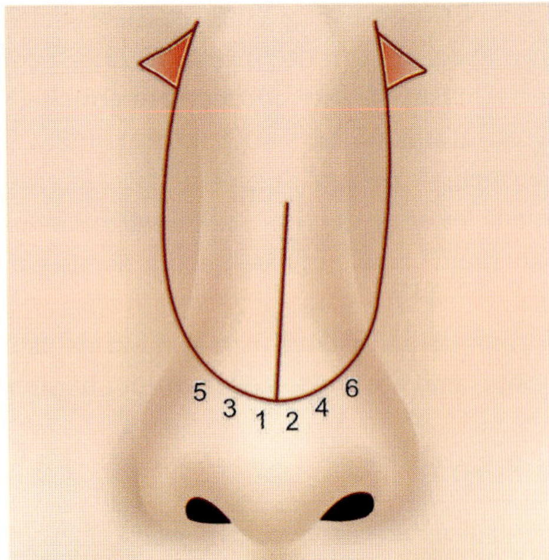


**Fig. 8.11:** Peng flap.

## APPLICATIONS

### Forehead

Defects in the lateral two-thirds of the forehead, where frontalis muscle fibers extend horizontally, are ideal sites for the horizontal incision lines created by bilateral advancement flaps. Due to the relative inelasticity of forehead skin, tension redistribution obtained with bilateral advancement is usually preferred over unilateral advancement.

Flaps should be elevated in the subcutaneous tissue plane to preserve the supraorbital and supratrochlear nerves.

### Cheek

Defects in the nasofacial sulcus that are not amenable to primary closure are good candidates for advancement flaps due to the relative mobility of cheek tissue and the aesthetic advantage of adjacent cosmetic junctions. A laterally based unilateral advancement flap for 2–4 cm defects creates scars at the infraorbital crease and nasofacial sulcus. Care should be taken to avoid blunting of the nasofacial sulcus, which can occur when advancement flaps approximate or include the nasal sidewall.

As referred to above, the V-to-Y subcutaneous tissue pedicle is ideal for medial cheek defects inferior to the nasal ala such that the length of the resulting Y lies in the nasolabial fold.

### Lip

The horizontal lines of the vermillion border, parallel to the nasal sill superiorly and the mental crease inferiorly, make defects of the upper and lower cutaneous lip amenable to bilateral advancement flaps. Also taking advantage of incision placement in the vermillion border, A–T or O–T flaps are masked well in a similar area. The V-to-Y subcutaneous advancement may also be used in the lateral upper lip, where the pedicle is based on subcutaneous cheek fat or orbicularis oris, depending on the size and location of the donor site.[38]

## REFERENCES


1. Baker SR. Local Flaps in Facial Reconstruction, 2nd edition. Elsevier; Philadelphia, PA 2007.
2. Rohrer TE, Jonathan Cook, Tri Nguyen, et al. Flaps and Grafts in Dermatologic Surgery, 1st edition. Elsevier; 2007.
3. Brodland DG. Advancement flaps. In: Roenigk RK, Roenigk HK (Eds). Roenigk & Roenigk's Dermatologic Surgery: Principles and Practice. New York: Marcel Dekker; 1996. pp. 825-34.
4. Stell PM. Letter: viability of skin flaps. Lancet. 1974;2:1385.
5. Pearl RM, Johnson D. The vascular supply to the skin: an anatomical and physiological reappraisal—part 1. Ann Plast Surg. 1983;11:99-105.
6. Kaufman AJ, Kiene KL, Moy RL, et al. Role of tissue undermining in the trapdoor effect of transposition flaps. J Dermatol Surg Oncol. 1993;19:128-32.
7. Larrabee WF, Sutton D. The biomechanics of advancement and rotation flaps. Laryngoscope. 1981;91:726-34.
8. Hirshowitz B, Mahler D. T-plasty technique for excisions in the face. Plast Reconstr Surg. 1966;37:453-8.
9. Webster RC, Davidson TM, Smith RC, et al. M-plasty techniques. J Dermatol Surg. 1976;2:393-6.
10. Boggio P, Gattoni M, Zanetta R, et al. Burow's triangle advancement flaps for excision of two closely approximated skin lesions. Dermatol Surg. 1999;25:622-5.
11. Robinson JK. Placement of the tension-bearing suture in repairing the alar facial junction. J Am Acad Dermatol. 1997;36: 440-3.
12. Antia NH, Buch VI. Chondrocutaneous advancement flap for the marginal defect of the ear. Plast Reconstr Surg. 1967;39(5): 472-7.
13. Zilinsky I, Cotofana S, Hammer N, et al. The arterial blood supply of the helical rim and the earlobe-based advancement flap (ELBAF): a new strategy for reconstructions of helical rim defects. J Plast Reconstr Aesthet Surg. 2014;68(1): 56-62.
14. Calhoun KH, Slaughter D, Kassir R, et al. Biomechanics of the helical rim advancement flap. Arch Otolaryngol Head Neck Surg. 1996;122:1119-23.
15. Ramsey ML, Marks VJ, Klingensmith MR, et al. The chondrocutaneous helical rim advancement flap of Antia and Buch. Dermatol Surg. 1995;21:970-4.
16. Butler CE. Reconstruction of marginal ear defects with modified chondrocutaneous helical rim advancement flaps. Plast Reconstr Surg. 2003;111:2009-13.
17. Eberlin KR, Nguyen B, Karia PS, et al. The Z-advancement flap for reconstruction of lateral nasal tip and medial alar defects. Dermatol Surg. 2014;40:101-9.

18. Lambert RW, Dzubow LM. A dorsal nasal advancement flap for off-midline defects. J Am Acad Dermatol. 2004;50: 380-3.
19. Geist DE, Maloney ME. The "east-west" advancement flap for nasal defects: reexamined and extended. Dermatol Surg. 2012;38:1529-34.
20. Otley CC, Roenigk RK. Surgical pearl: preparing the defect for an island pedicle flap. J Am Acad Dermatol. 1997;2:257-8.
21. Ray TL, Weinberger CH, Lee PK, et al. Closure of large surgical defects on the cutaneous upper lip using and island pedicle flap. Dermatol Surg. 2010;36:931-4.
22. Cook JL, Yildirim S, Akoz T, et al. Nasolabial V-Y advancement for closures of the midface defects. Dermatol Surg. 2001; 27:656-8. Discussion 658-60.
23. Zitelli JA, Brodland DG. A regional approach to reconstruction of the upper lip. J Dermatol Surg Oncol. 1991;17: 143-8.
24. Narsete TA. V-Y advancement flap in upper lip reconstruction. Plast Reconstr Surg. 2000;105:2464-6.
25. Kaufman AJ, Grekin RC. Repair of central upper lip (philtral) surgical defects with island pedicle flaps. Dermatol Surg. 1996; 22:1003-07.
26. Gardner ES, Goldberg LH. Eyebrow reconstruction with the subcutaneous island pedicle flap. Dermatol Surg. 2002;28: 921-5.
27. Cazualho lM, Ramos RR, Ivan DA, et al. V-Y advancement flap for the reconstruction of partial and full thickness defects of the upper lip. Scand J Plast Reconst Surg Hand Surg. 2002;36:28-33.
28. Kim KS, Huang JH, Kim DY, et al. Eyebrow island flap for reconstruction of a partial eyebrow defect. Ann Plast Surg. 2002;48:315-7.
29. Yildirim S, Aköz T, Akan M, et al. Nasolabial V-Y advancement for closures of the midface defects. Dermatol Surg. 2001;27: 656-8.
30. Guerrerosantos J. Frontalis musculocutaneous island flap for coverage of forehead of defect. Plast Reconst Surg. 2000; 105:18-22.
31. Humpreys TR, Goldberg LA, Niemer DR, et al. The postauricular (revolving door) island pedicle flap revisited. Dermatol Surg. 1996;22:148-50.
32. Fader DJ, Johnson TM. Ear reconstruction utilizing the subcutaneous island pedicle (flip flop) flap. Dermatol Surg. 1999;25:94-6.
33. Papadopoulos DJ, Trinei FA. Superiorly based nasalis myocutaneous island pedicle flap with bilevel undermining for nasal tip and supratip reconstruction. Dermatol Surg. 1999;25:530-6.
34. Willey A, Papadopoulos DJ, Swanson NA, et al. Modified single-sling myocutaneous island pedicle flap: series of 61 reconstructions. Dermatol Surg. 2008;34:1572-35.
35. Papadopoulos DJ, Pharis DB, Munavalli GS, et al. Nasalis myocutaneous island pedicle flap with bi-level undermining for repair of lateral nasal defects. Dermatol Surg. 2002;28: 190-4.
36. Ebrahimi A, Nejadsarvari N, Koushki ES, et al. Application of modified Rintala flap in nasal tip reconstruction. Am J Otolaryngol. 2012;33(6):685-8.
37. Rintala AE, Asko-Seljavaara S. Reconstruction of midline skin defects of the nose. Scand J Plast Reconstr Surg. 1969;3: 105-08.
38. Onishin K, Okada E, Hirata A, et al. The Rintala flap: a versatile procedure for nasal reconstruction. Am J Otolaryngol. 2014; 35(5):577-81.
39. Peng VT, Sturm RL, Marsh TW, et al. "Pinch modification" of the linear advancement flap. J Dermatol Surg Oncol. 1987;13: 251-3.
40. Rowe D, Warshawski L, Carruthers A. The Peng flap. The flap of choice for the convex curve of the central nasal tip. Dermatol Surg. 1995;21:149-52.

# CHAPTER 9

# Rotation Flaps

*Tushar Dabade, Bichchau Michelle Nguyen*

## INTRODUCTION

Rotation flaps utilize arciform incision and rotation of tissue to cover a wound defect. They can be used in areas of limited tissue laxity where a curved movement rather than a linear stretching of the tissue, as with advancement flaps, is preferable. Rotation flaps also redirect the final tension vectors, and by design have a large vascular supply facilitating tissue survival. Rotation flaps are often utilized over the medial cheek, chin, forehead, scalp, and occasionally nose. When performed adequately, advantages include a low flap failure and lower risk of trap door phenomenon. The challenges of these closures include masking the resulting long scar, and modifications to the standard rotation flap incision may be needed to allow for optimal functional and cosmetic restoration. The two main subtypes of rotation flaps include unilateral and bilateral, in which the donor tissue comes from adjacent tissue on one side or both sides, respectively.

## UNILATERAL ROTATION FLAPS

With a unilateral rotation flap, the incision is made from one side of the defect in a large arciform shape around the flap border. Typically, the length of the arc should be four times the diameter of the defect, with the radius of the flap being three times the diameter of the defect[1] (Fig. 9.1). This allows for enough tissue mobility, but changes depend upon the elasticity of the flap tissue and anatomical borders. If possible, the flap base should be inferior to the incision, facilitating the lymphatic drainage and decreasing flap edema.[2] Classic rotation flap locations are listed in Table 9.1.

Ideally the incision is made over a natural skin tension line or facial landmark, such as the mental crease. To a novice, the arc is often longer than expected, done purposefully to allow enough tissue laxity from the flap site to extend beyond the tissue defect for ideal closure. The majority of the undermining occurs in the area beneath the flap and around all of the borders to the incision, minimizing tension particularly at the flap's pivot point. The pivot point, or point of pivotal restraint, is the location on the flap where it rotates to cover the primary defect. Sutures are placed at the tension-bearing point (flap-tip to far side of the defect), followed by the flap border near the defect, and the area of the arc utilizing the rule of halves. Tip stitches can be placed if desired (Figs. 9.2A to C). Often near the flap's pivot point there is a resultant standing cone that can be removed, with the incision directed away from the flap base (Fig. 9.2C).

If the planned rotation flap does not adequately cover the defect, the arc can be lengthened or a "back-cut"

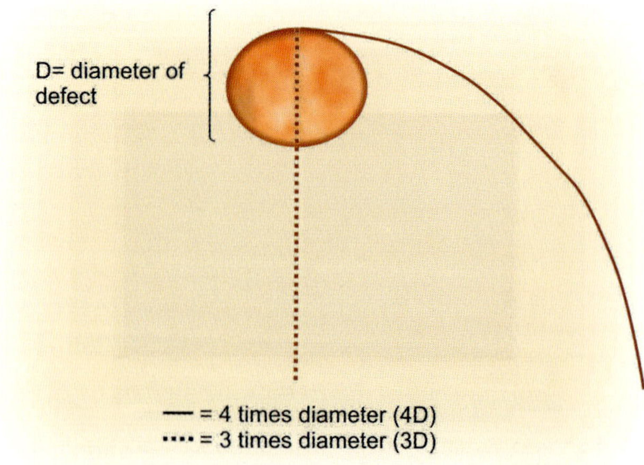


**Fig. 9.1:** Basic rotation flap design. Traditionally, the radius of the rotation flap is 2.5–3 times the defect's diameter, with the arc four times the diameter. This design may change based on anatomical site of defect.

**Table 9.1:** Common uses for rotation flap.

| *Location* | *Considerations* |
|---|---|
| Medial cheek | Utilizes large mid-cheek laxity as reservoir |
| Nose | Redirects tension and may hide incision line in natural anatomical locations |
| Chin | Utilizes mental crease as arc to cover large defects |
| Lip | Incision line may hide in nasolabial fold |
| Scalp | Classic O-to-Z location to redirect tension, useful as limited laxity due to galea aponeurotica |

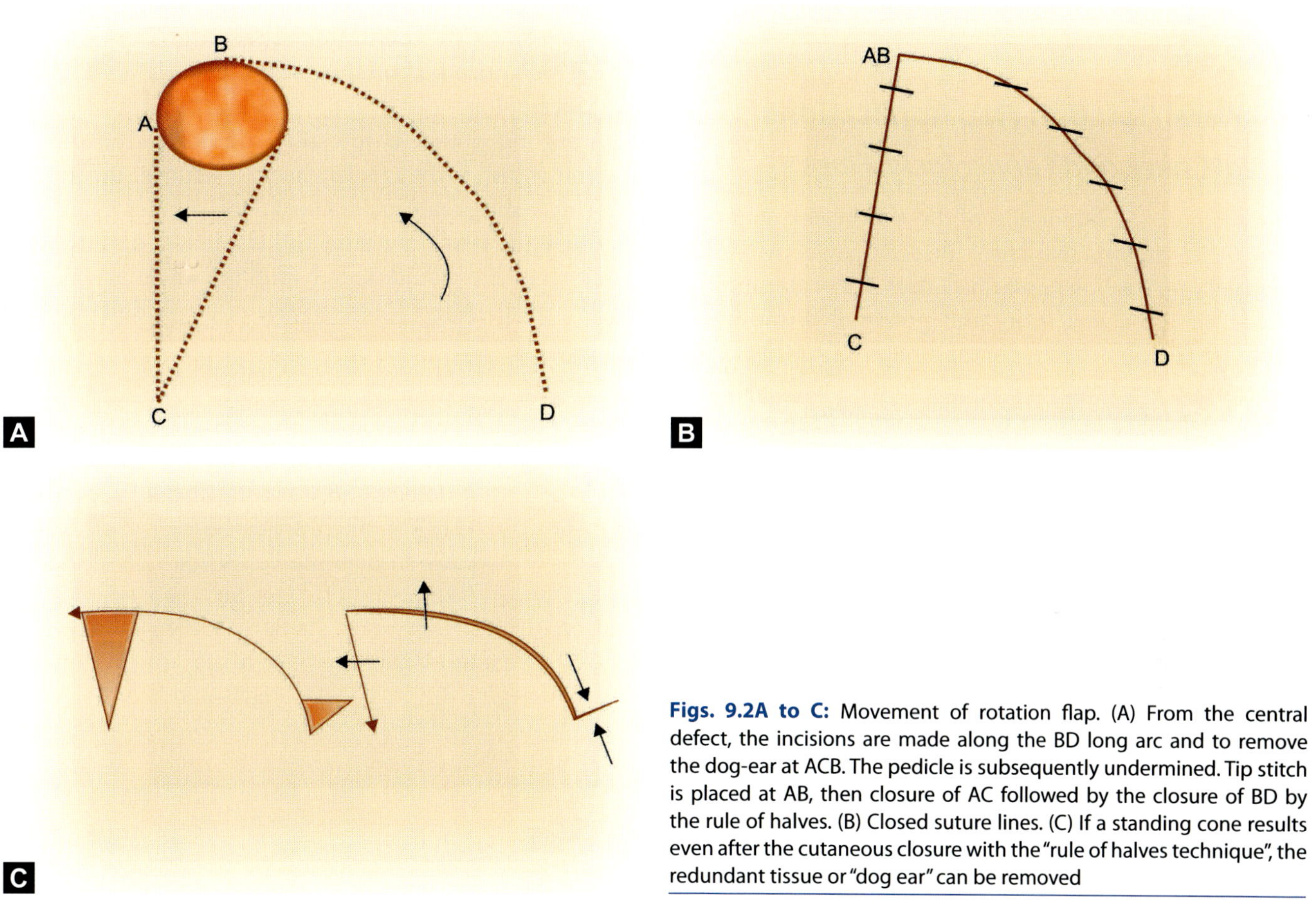

**Figs. 9.2A to C:** Movement of rotation flap. (A) From the central defect, the incisions are made along the BD long arc and to remove the dog-ear at ACB. The pedicle is subsequently undermined. Tip stitch is placed at AB, then closure of AC followed by the closure of BD by the rule of halves. (B) Closed suture lines. (C) If a standing cone results even after the cutaneous closure with the "rule of halves technique", the redundant tissue or "dog ear" can be removed

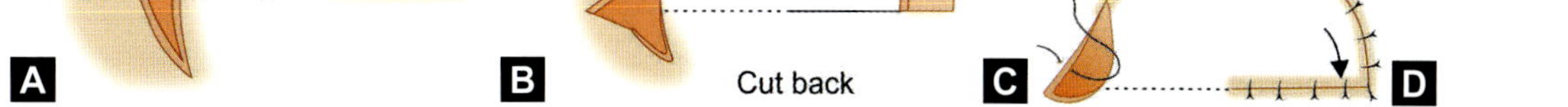

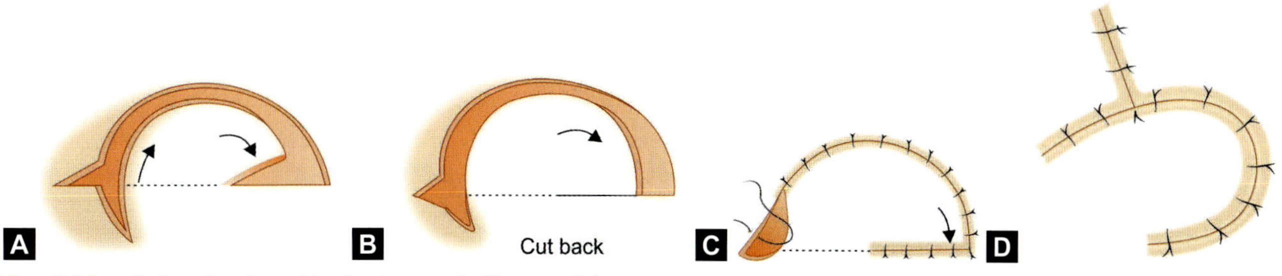

**Figs. 9.3A to D:** Rotation flap with a back-cut to facilitate pedicle rotation.

can be made to increase rotation of the pedicle (Figs. 9.3A to D). Back-cuts may decrease the vascular supply of the pedicle, with the area at highest risk of necrosis being the flap tip. With a back-cut, the scar line changes in direction and may influence overall cosmetic outcome depending upon the location.

When designing the arc shape of the traditional rotation flap, consider the direction of the tension on the flap and adjacent anatomical structures. The tension vector changes depending on the arc shape: if the curvature of the arc is accentuated further from the defect, the tension vector will be perpendicular to the defect-graft border. If the curvature is sharper, i.e. more acute angle at the start of the incision, the vector will be directed more parallel to the defect-flap border.

## Unilateral Rotation Flap Applications

### *Medial Cheek and Cervicofacial Flaps*

With a broad, lax donor site of the mid-cheek acting as the pedicle, large medial cheek defects may conveniently be closed with rotation flaps. Challenges in this area include limited medial cheek laxity and potential distortion of the adjacent inferior eyelid. As a result of these anatomical features, advancement flaps in this location are often limited by inadequate horizontal mobility of the flap, and primary closures in a horizontal orientation can cause ectropion.

For rotation flap design, one option is to curve the arc inferiorly from the defect over or parallel to the nasolabial fold, then bring the pedicle up into the defect. Undermining in the subcutaneous fatty layer allows easy rotation without difficulty. A tacking stitch stabilizing the pedicle to the periosteum over the superomedial cheek can reduce pull on the lower eyelid and thus reduce risk of ectropion.

A second option is to extend the long arc from the superior aspect of the medial cheek defect over the infraorbital rim to the preauricular cheek. This creates a horizontal to oblique tension vector, and is a useful option when primary closure would directly pull the lower eyelid inferiorly (Figs. 9.4A to C). For closure of larger defects close

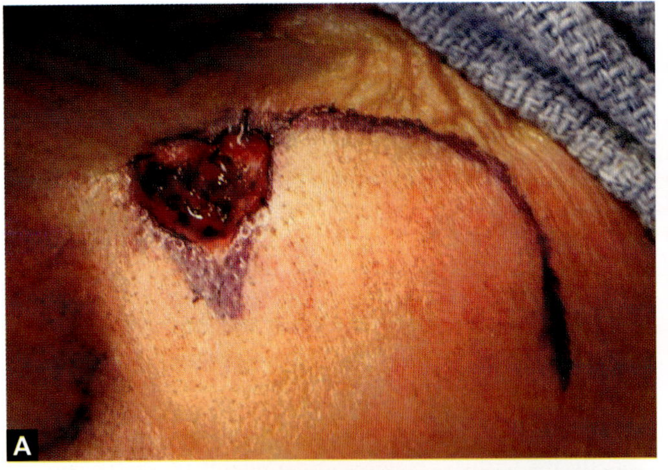


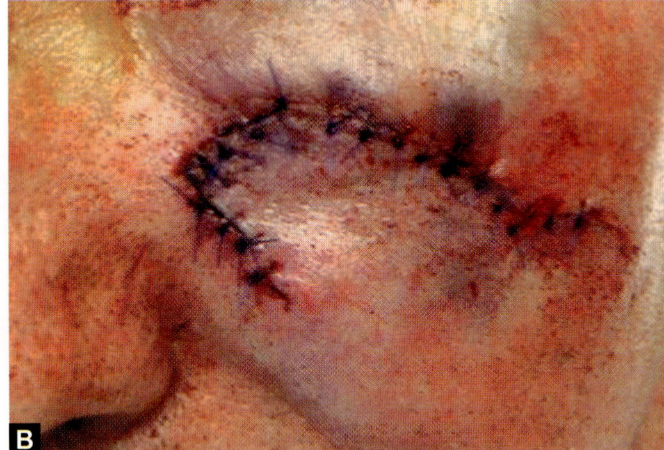


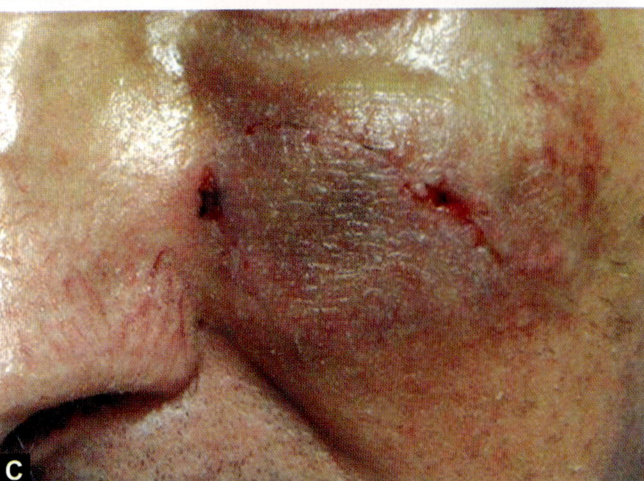


**Figs. 9.4A to C:** Medial cheek rotation flap. (A) Defect over the medial cheek with anticipated arc and dog-ear of the flap drawn. (B) Closure of the defect utilizing an arc superolaterally from the defect (C). Appearance of the flap 1-week postoperatively.
*Courtesy*: Nellie Konnikov, MD, Boston, MA, USA.

to the eyelid, extending the incision over the temple can increase tissue redundancy lateral to the orbit and decrease downward pull on the lateral eyelid. Ensuring the incisional arc does not extend into the eyelid tissue improves the consistency and appearance of the closure.

Even larger central cheek lesions may require a cervicofacial rotation flap. An arciform incision is made from the superior border of the defect laterally over the zygomatic arch then extending to the preauricular cheek and down over the neck. The resulting pedicle is sizeable, and defects up to 10 cm can be adequately closed. This hides scars within the lateral, less visible borders of the face. Some experts will place a tacking stitch over the infraorbital or zygomatic aspects to the periosteum to avoid lower eyelid ectropion. Others feel this may increase tip necrosis and may be unnecessary.[1] Undermining is often done in the subcutaneous plane, but deeper planes, i.e. submuscular and subsuperficial musculoaponeurotic, are alternatives favored by the plastic surgery literature.[3] Another variation to the neck portion of the cervicofacial rotation flap is the angle of the rotation, where the incision instead of proceeding caudally over the neck moves posteriorly after the lobule of the ear. This adds more of a horizontal movement to the pedicle and decreases visibility of the scar over the neck.[4]

## Nasal Rotation Flaps

For defects over the distal third of the nose, the dorsal nasal flap provides a useful tool to match skin quality (texture, pilosebaceous density/quality, color) with a high flap survival rate. While the nasal tip has high inherent restraint, the nasal sidewall rotates more freely, and lesions up to 2 cm can be closed in this manner.[5] The flap originally designed by Rieger and modified by Marchac and others relies on a consistent vascular supply stemming from the angular artery's position over the nasal sidewall and the perforators that extend over the dorsal nose.[6] Axial vessels stemming from the medial canthus also contribute. As such, flap failure from ischemia is low. The original design extends an incision from the defect's edge on the nasal tip along the nasofacial sulcus, extending medial to the epicanthal fold, finally with a back-cut over the glabella (Figs. 9.5A to C). Undermining occurs deep to the superficial muscular aponeurotic system (SMAS) over the perichondrium. The glabellar region may be closed primarily or using small flaps as dictated by the size of the resulting defect. Care must be taken to assess the tension on the nasal tip during the closure to ensure minimal vertical pull creating a "pig-nose" type deformity. With elderly patients this pull may be less noticeable as a natural tip ptosis occurs with age. Often a natural triangular dog-ear adjacent to the defect on the pedicle side must be removed, a maneuver that also facilitates rotation of the flap over the defect. Also, good hemostasis is important to prevent excessive edema or hematoma of the flap. The dorsal nasal flap can also be used for defects over the nasal dorsum and nasal sidewall as alternatives to bilobed transposition flaps or other closures. For smaller, more lateral defects on the nasal sidewall, a heminasal rotation flap with ipsilateral pedicle will suffice. Here, the incision extends from the medial side of the defects superiorly along the nasal sidewall toward the nasofacial sulcus, and the flap is rotated medially and inferiorly into the defect (Fig. 9.6). For larger defects, a more traditional dorsal nasal flap with contralateral pedicle extending into the glabella with or without a back-cut may be needed, and the flap rotates off-center into the defect.[5]

Medium size defect on the medial nasal ala can also be closed with a rotation flap that utilizes similar tissue within the cosmetic subunit (Figs. 9.7A and B). The defect should not exceed 50% of the alar rim to avoid functional or cosmetic distortion. The flap is created by extending the incision along the alar crease, and careful undermining and redirection of the tension vector with deep sutures to avoid distortion of the alar rim.[7]

## Lateral Upper Lip

For defects over the lateral upper cutaneous lip up to 2 cm diameter, a rotation flap can hide the arc of the incision well within the nasolabial fold[8] (Figs. 9.8A to C). The arc of the incision is made inferolaterally along the crease to free up the pedicle. A standing cone may be removed inferior to the operative defect, and extensive undermining with care to preserve superior labial artery perforators leads to better outcomes. Patients with prominent apical triangles do well with this closure.[9] An alternative closure to the rotation flap in this location is an island pedicle flap (V-to-Y advancement flap), discussed elsewhere.

## Chin

For medium-large-sized defects near the inferior border of the mental crease, rotation flaps offer the advantage of hiding the scar within this natural skin tension line and cosmetic unit border. Depending upon the location of the chin, the arc of the incision is made along the mental

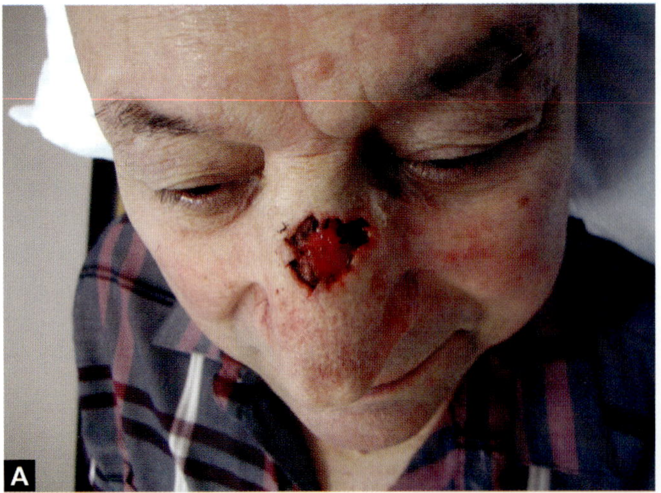


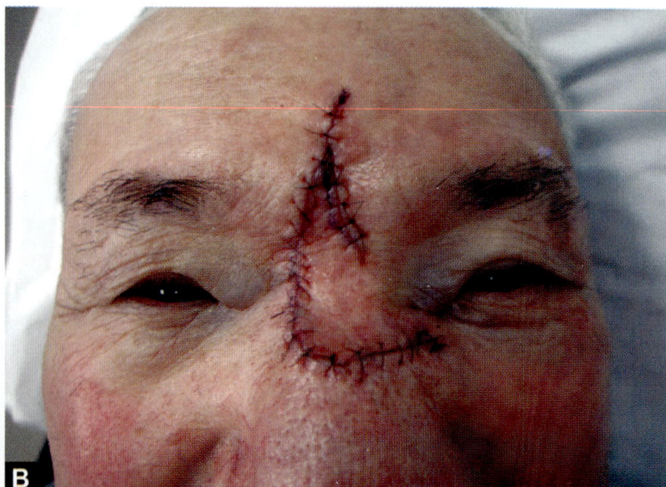


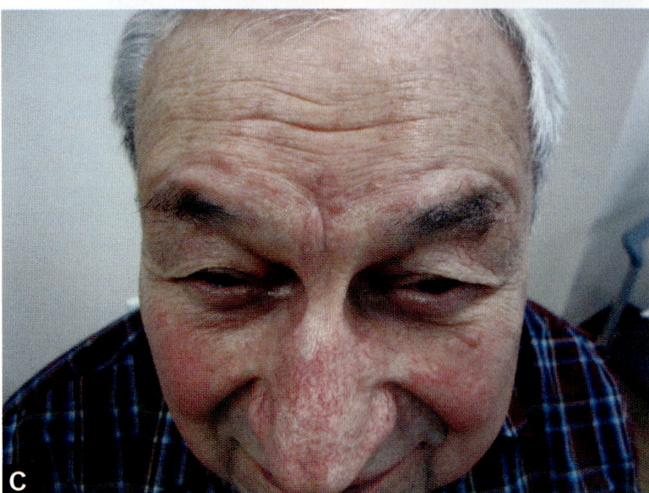


**Figs. 9.5A to C:** Design of dorsal nasal rotation flap. (A) Defect on nasal dorsum after Mohs micrographic surgery. (B) Incision extends from base of defect to the glabella. A back-cut at the glabella facilitates flap rotation downward. (C) Appearance at follow-up.
*Courtesy*: S Brian Jiang, MD, Sang Diego, California, USA.

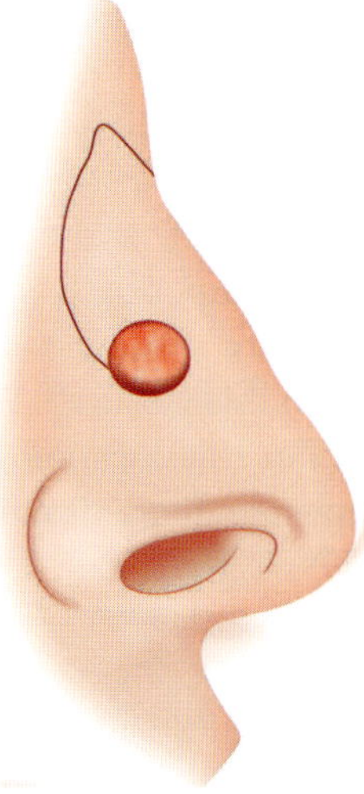

**Fig. 9.6:** Design of heminasal rotation flap for defects on nasal sidewall. Incision extends from base of defect along nasofacial sulcus to nasal root with a back-cut at the nasal root.

crease either superomedial or inferolateral to the defect. Generally, a 3:1 arc-to-defect width ratio can be adequate without the need of a back-cut.[10] Undermining is done over the mentalis muscle.

## BILATERAL ROTATION FLAPS

Bilateral rotation flaps utilize pedicles on two sides of the defect for closure. The arc of the rotation flaps may originate on the same side of the defect, as with a traditional bilateral rotation flap, or on opposite sides of the defect, as with an O-to-Z flap (Figs. 9.9A to C). These designs are useful on the scalp, forehead, and chin.

### Scalp

Unique anatomical considerations of the scalp make it ideal for rotation flaps, by simple, traditional bilateral, bilateral O-to-Z, or pinwheel design. Scalp characteristics

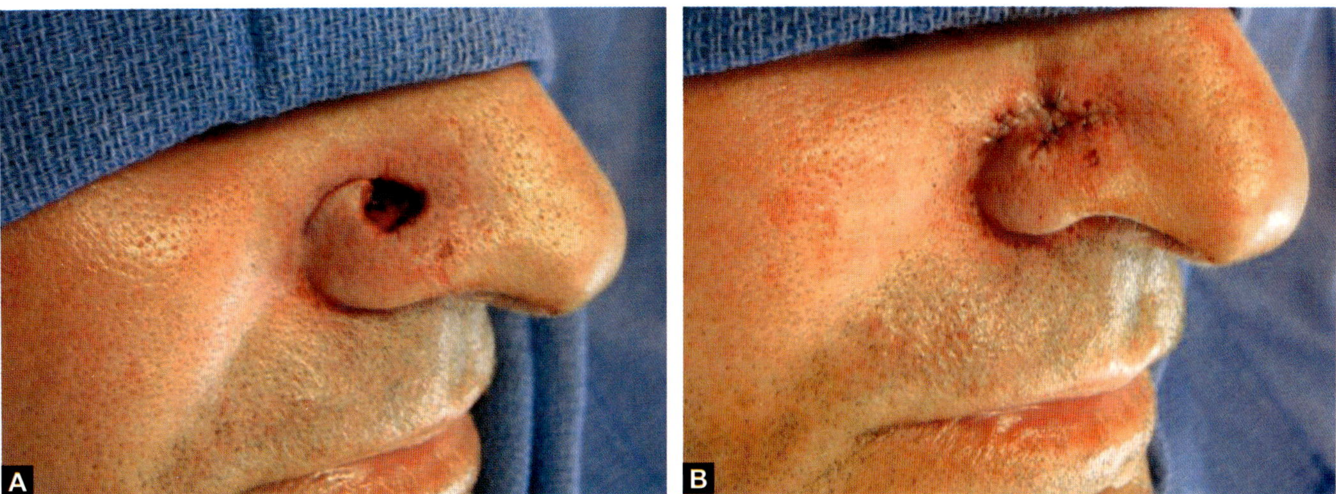

**Figs. 9.7A and B:** Nasal ala rotation flap. (A) Defect over the medial nasal ala resulting from Mohs micrographic surgery for a nodular basal cell carcinoma. (B) Rotation flap using an incision along the alar crease optimized to easily close the defect.

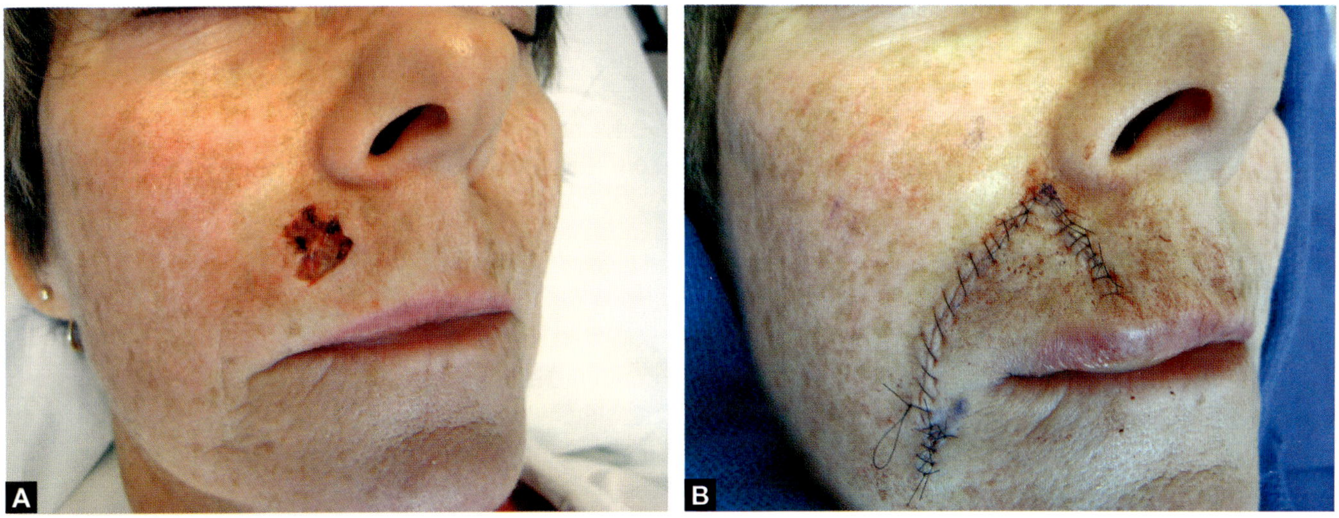

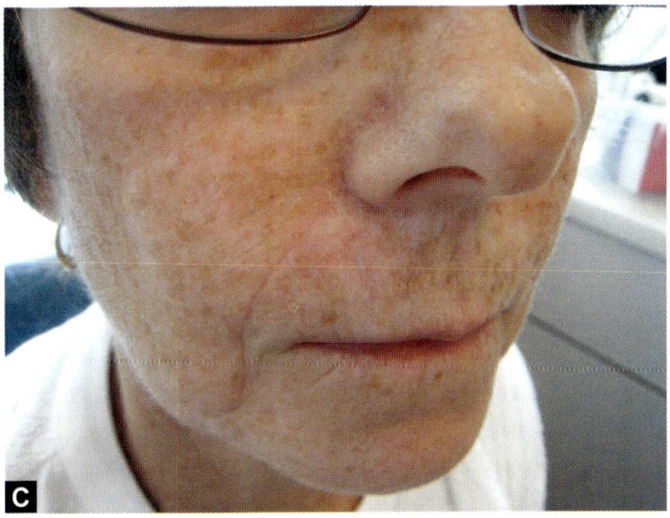

**Figs. 9.8A to C:** Right upper cutaneous lip rotation flap. (A) Mohs micrographic surgery defect on the right upper cutaneous lip. (B) Closure using a rotation flap. The arc of the incision is hidden in the nasolabial fold. (C) Appearance at follow-up.
*Courtesy*: S Brian Jiang, MD, Sang Diego, California, USA.

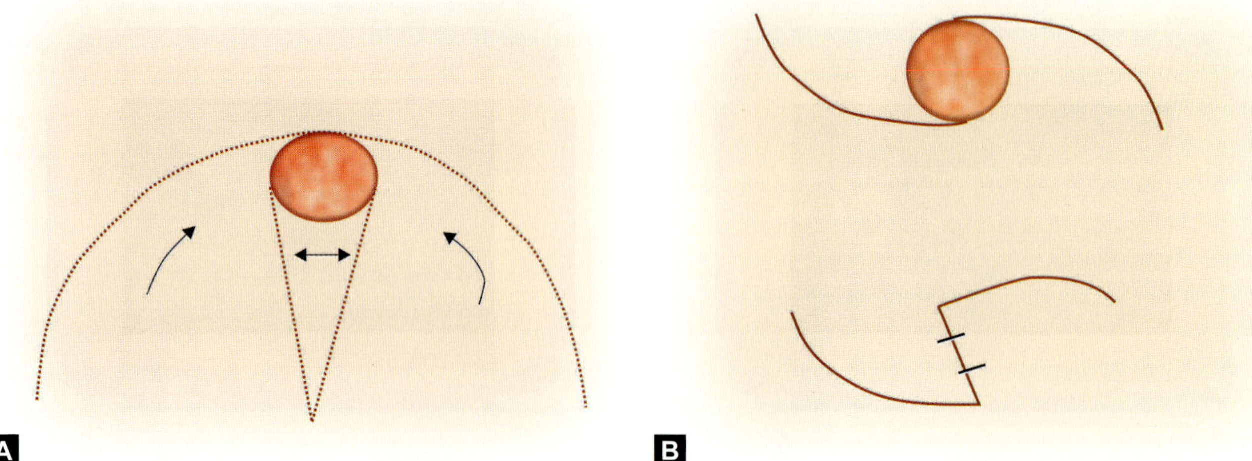


**Figs. 9.9A and B:** Bilateral rotation flaps. (A) Traditional bilateral rotation flap, with arciform incision both emanating from the same side of the defect. (B) O-to-Z rotation flap with the arcs originating on opposite sides of the defect.

include an inelastic fibrous galea aponeurotica leading to inherent restraint, a convex calvarium, and an abundance of hair follicles.[11] Traditional advancement flaps for defects are thus limited, given the taut galea and inability to stretch when covering defects. Closures under high tension lead to atrophic, noticeable scars, but can be avoided with properly designed rotation flaps.

Rotation flaps offer the advantage of a pivot motion to recruit adequate tissue when covering scalp defects. The arc of the incision should be at least the standard four times the width of the defect, again considering the galeal inelasticity. Undermining is done in the avascular subgaleal plane. If the flap does not quite close the defect comfortably, a cautious galeotomy can be done. With this maneuver, careful incisions are made in the galea perpendicular to the tension of the flap, avoiding cutting into the vascular tissue plane of the scalp.

Single rotation flaps often lead to tight closures, thus traditional bilateral, bilateral O-to-Z, or pinwheel flaps can be particularly useful. These recruit additional tissue, essentially combining rotation flaps on multiple sides of the defect. Figures 9.10A to D demonstrate a traditional bilateral rotation flap closing a large squamous cell carcinoma over the scalp. With pinwheel flaps, typically four arciform incisions are made starting 90° from each other, which converge during closure at the defect's center.[12] Lesions up to 5 cm over the scalp can be closed successfully. Fortunately, these scars are often hidden well in the hair. Also, in general on the scalp, incisions that are parallel to the direction of the follicle decrease hair follicle damage.

## Chin

Similar to the unilateral rotation flap over the chin, a bilateral rotation flap again hides the long arc of the scar in the mental crease. For larger, medial lesions over the chin, bringing tissue from both sides of the defect can offer less distortion of the cosmetic subunit and lower tension on the scar.

## SUMMARY

Rotation flaps provide unique advantages of rotational movement and recruitment of tissue from areas of limited laxity to repair medium to large size defects on the scalp, cheeks, nose, and chin. Their versatility is useful particularly in areas where often long arciform incisions can be hidden in natural junctions between cosmetic subunits. Rotation flaps are often robust with excellent vascular supply and minimal risk of trapdoor deformities. A backcut into the pedicle may be needed to facilitate flap rotation into the flap. Multiple sources of tissue laxity can be recruited using the bilateral or pinwheel variant of the rotation flaps. As with all closures, rotation flap design must take into account anatomical restrictions including free edges, e.g. eyelids, alar rim, or the vermilion lip border, to avoid distortion of key features resulting in suboptimal cosmesis. When well designed and executed, rotation flaps allow for repair of large defects with local tissue that results in better skin color and texture match yielding superior cosmetic outcomes.

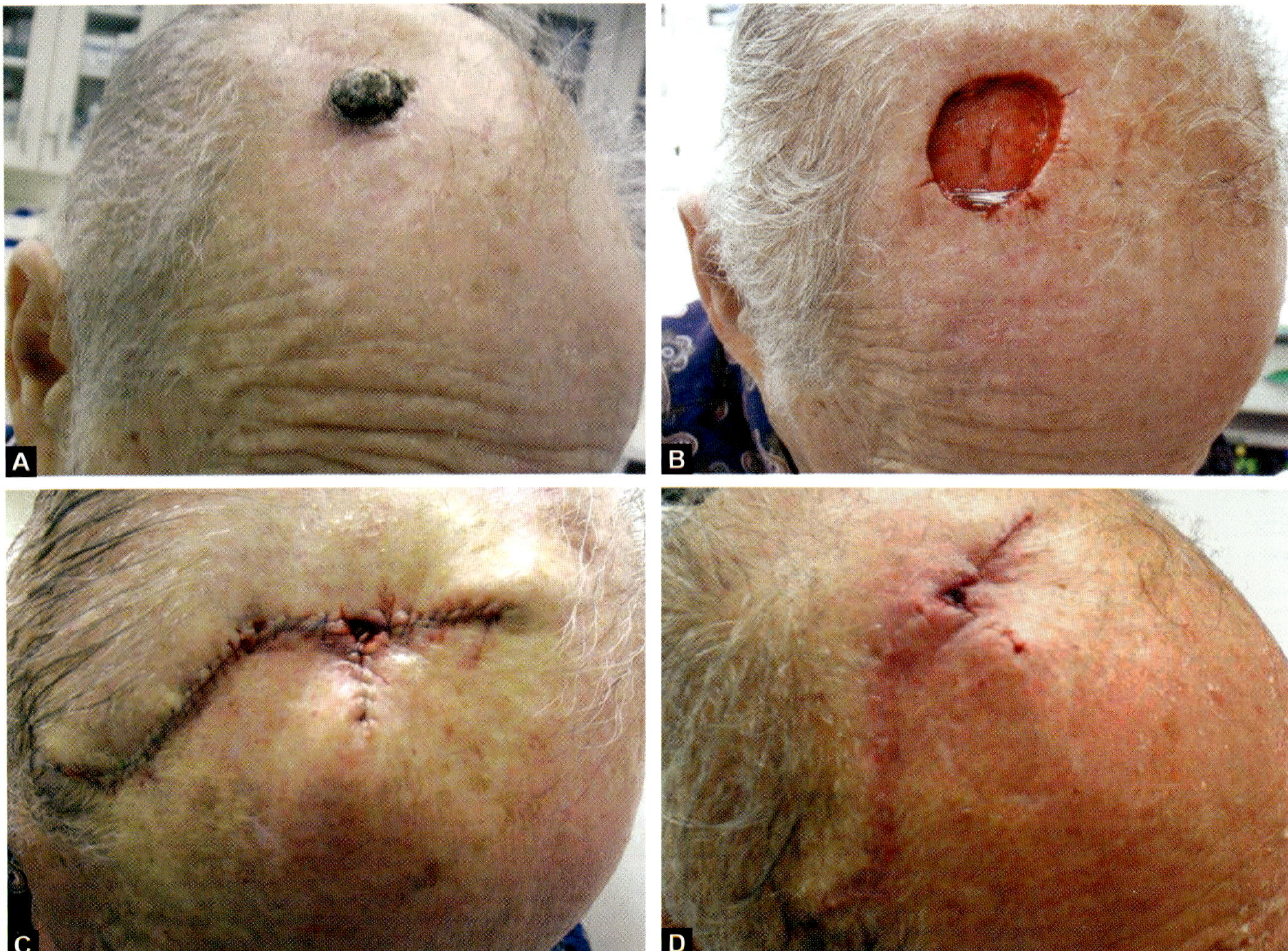


**Figs. 9.10A to D:** Right scalp bilateral rotation flap. (A) A hyperkeratotic squamous cell carcinoma over the right scalp. (B) Defect post-Mohs micrographic surgery. (C) Closure using a traditional bilateral rotation flap. A standing cone was removed at the lateral pedicle's pivot point to facilitate rotation. (D) Patient's closure 1 week postoperatively.
*Courtesy*: Chrysalyne D. Schmults MD, Boston, MA, USA.

## REFERENCES


1. Patel KG, Sykes JM. Concepts in local flap design and classification. Oper Tech Otolaryngol. 2011;22(1):13-23.
2. Dzubow LM. Dorsal nasal flap. In: Baker SR (Ed), Local Flaps in Facial Reconstruction. St Louis, MO: Mosby; 1995.
3. Austen WG Jr, Parrett BM, Taghinia A, et al. The subcutaneous cervicofacial flap revisited. Ann Plast Surg. 2009; 62(2):149-53.
4. Moore BA, Wine T, Netterville JL. Cervicofacial and cervicothoracic rotation flaps in head and neck reconstruction. Head Neck. 2005;27(12):1092-101.
5. Zavod MB, Zavod MB, Goldman GD. The dorsal nasal flap. Dermatol Clin. 2005;23(1):73-85, vi.
6. Rieger RA. A local flap for repair of the nasal tip. Plast Reconstr Surg. 1967;40(2):147-9.
7. Odobescu A, Ferland Caron G, Danino MA, et al. Alar rotation flap for full thickness medial alar defects. J Plast Reconstr Aesthet Surg. 2014;67(6):866-8.
8. Becker GD, Adams LA, Levin BC. Outcome analysis of Mohs surgery of the lip and chin: comparing secondary intention healing and surgery. Laryngoscope. 1995;105(11):1176-83.
9. Goldman GD. Rotation flaps. Dermatol Surg. 2005;31(8 Pt 2): 1006-13.
10. Colville RJ, Patel R. The mental rotation flap. J Plast Reconstr Aesthet Surg. 2011;64(3):e76-7.
11. Seline PC, Siegle RJ. Scalp reconstruction. Dermatol Clin. 2005;23(1):13-21, v.
12. Simsek T, Eroglu L. Versatility of the pinwheel flap to reconstruct circular defects in the temporal and scalp region. J Plast Surg Hand Surg. 2013;47(2):97-101.

# CHAPTER 10

# Transposition Flaps

*Jennifer Herrmann, Michelle Levender, Sarah Tuttleton Arron*

## INTRODUCTION

Transposition flaps represent an essential tool in the armamentarium of facial reconstructive surgeons. Conceptually more complex in design than advancement and rotation flaps, which move tissue across along an uninterrupted tissue plane, transposition flaps move tissue over intervening uninvolved skin. In the act of transposing over intact skin, the surgeon is able to utilize otherwise unreachable tissue reservoirs, recruiting needed tissue into areas lacking in tissue laxity. In addition, transposition flaps allow for complete redirection of tension vectors, which is particularly critical for defects near free margins including the eyelid, alar rim, and lip. These flaps also optimize cosmesis by allowing for the preservation of intact cosmetic units and essential anatomic landmarks, such as the alar-facial sulcus, which would be lost or blunted by linear repairs or other random pattern flaps. Successfully executing the geometry of these flaps requires a thorough understanding of the design of these flaps, their variations, and the tension vectors involved. This chapter discusses the most common transposition flaps, including the rhombic flap, the nasolabial transposition flap, the bilobed flap, and the Z-plasty, the variations of these flaps, and their clinical applications.

## TYPES

### Rhombic

The classic Limberg rhombic flap is constructed by conversion of a surgical defect into a four-sided rhombus with angles of 60° and 120°. The flap arms are drawn by extending a line from one of the obtuse angles that is equal in length to the short axis of the rhombus. A second line is then drawn at 60° from this first line, parallel to one of the rhombus' closest edges (Fig. 10.1).[1] Once planned, the flap is incised and elevated at a depth equal to that of the defect. The entire surrounding area is then undermined widely to fully mobilize borrowed tissue and to dissipate wound healing contractile forces. Wide undermining prevents focused wound contraction along the scar line itself, which may result in depressed wound edges or pin cushioning of the flap. A key stitch that closes the secondary defect first is placed, and the flap "transposes" into place (Fig. 10.2). The tension vector is redirected 90°, minimizing tension along the primary defect.

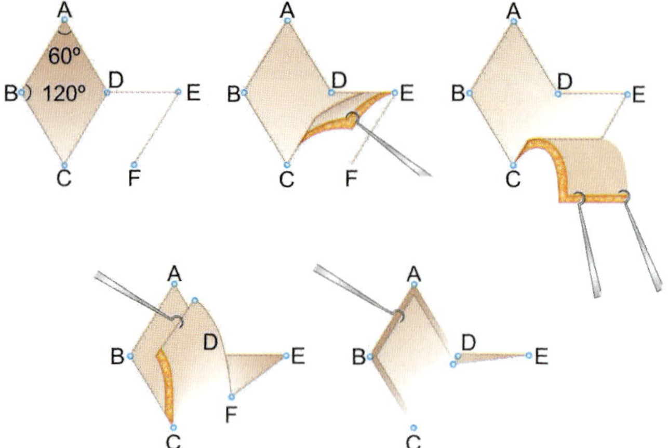


**Fig. 10.1:** Rhombic flap. Pre- and postexecution of the classic rhombic flap.

Eight distinct flaps can be created from any rhombic defect (Figs. 10.3A and B), critical analysis of adjacent skin laxity, relaxed skin tension lines, and nearby free margins should guide flap selection. Ideally, two sides of the rhombic defect are oriented perpendicular to skin tension lines, allowing the secondary operative wound to be closed

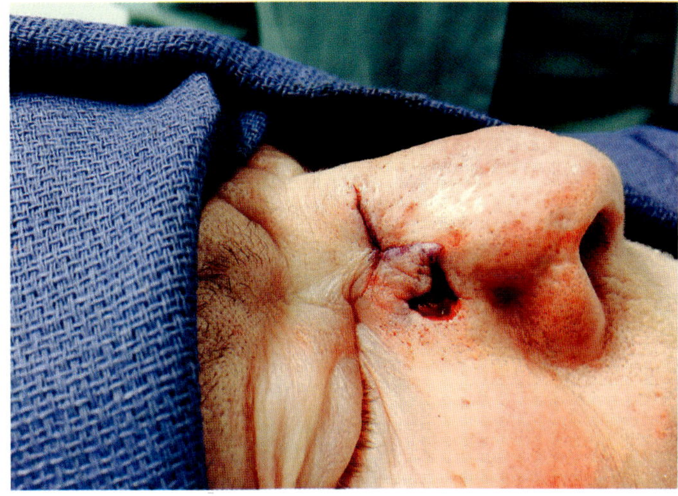

**Fig. 10.2:** Rhombic key stitch. A key stitch closes the secondary defect first, and the flap "transposes" into place.

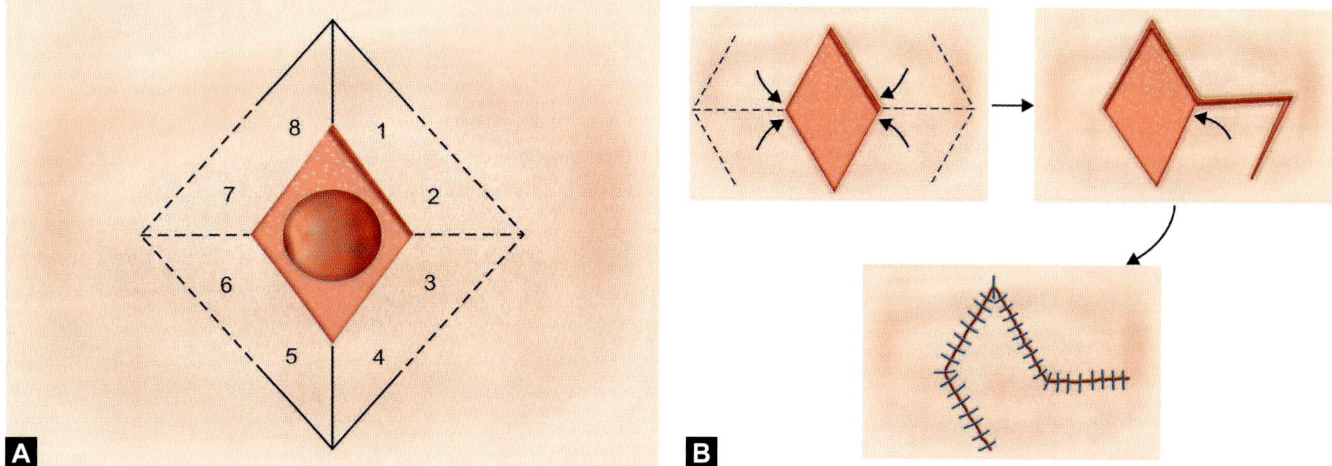


**Figs. 10.3A and B:** Rhombic flap options. (A) Eight distinct flaps can be created from any rhombic defect. (B) This schematic diagram shows four options available for rhombic flap design. The alternative four can be created with incisions from the other two points as illustrated in (A).

along them. Although a rhombic flap can be designed and executed from one of the acute angles of the rhombus, designing it off the short axis of the defect has two main advantages.[2] First, flap size is minimized, yielding shorter surgical scars, and second, the arc through which the flap rotates is kept at a minimum.[3,4]

Understanding tension forces associated with the classic rhombic design is critical to executing a successful flap. Although the Limberg flap and surgical rhombic defect are of equal size, intrinsic properties of the skin usually do not allow for a tensionless closure. Similar to rotation flaps, restraint on the flap at the pivot point of the pedicle makes the flap fall short of its destination without some movement of the recipient tissue toward the flap.[5] If this adjacent tissue is a mobile free margin, such as the eyelid, alar rim, or lip, it may be unacceptably distorted. Conversely, if the adjacent tissue is immobile, excess tension may lead to flap tip ischemia, and in severe cases necrosis. In short, although most tension is oriented perpendicularly along the line of secondary defect closure, some tension remains along the primary defect with classically executed Limberg flaps (Fig. 10.4A). Clinically, tension may be visualized as a field of hypoperfusion spanning the flap edge.

Certain modifications have been designed to overcome one or more areas of tension intrinsic to the classic rhombic design. To minimize horizontal tension, the flap may be elongated from its take-off point. This lengthening compensates for flap shortening resulting from pivotal restraint at the flap base (Fig. 10.4B). Alternatively, if the flap take-off angle is widened beyond 120°, vertical tension is reduced,

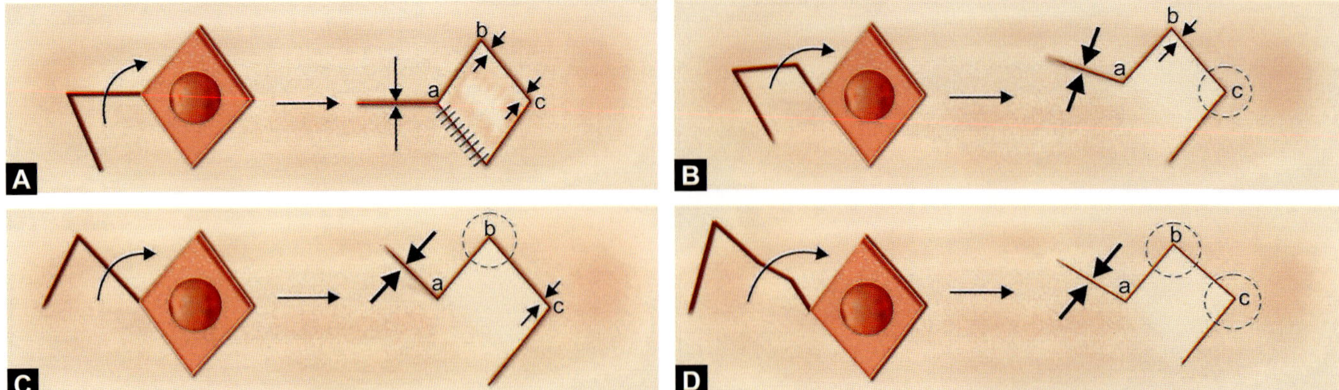


**Figs. 10.4A to D:** Methods to modify flap tension. (A) The classic rhombic flap with most tension directed along closure of the secondary defect and minor tension directed along the primary defect [points (b) and (c)]. (B) Oversizing the flap reduces tension at point (c). (C) Increasing the flap angle reduces tension at point (b). (D) Both oversizing the flap and increasing its angle reduce tension at both points (b) and (c). Dark arrows, major tension vectors; Light arrows, minor tension vectors; ... lines, tension reduced/eliminated by flap modification.

and the flap more easily reaches the most superior aspect of the defect (Fig. 10.4C). Finally, if the flap is both elongated and its angle is increased, tension will be reduced at both flap tips, leaving nearly all of the tension directed perpendicularly along the secondary defect (Fig. 10.4D). Such flap oversizing may be most useful when the surgical defect abuts a free margin, where all tension must be directed perpendicular to the primary motion of closure.

## Dufourmentel Modification

The Dufourmentel flap is a modified rhombic flap where a narrower flap tip angle and a shorter arc of rotation allow tension sharing between the primary and secondary defects.[6,7] It is designed by drawing a line from the same take-off point as a Limberg flap but at a more obtuse, 150° angle. This angle occurs at the bisection of the classic Limberg arm and a tangent drawn from the rhombic defect. A second line is then extended from the free end of line one, parallel to the long axis of the defect (Figs. 10.5A and B). This modification creates a wider flap pedicle, decreases pivotal restraint, and facilitates flap closure with less vertical tension than that in a Limberg flap. Thus, Dufourmentel flaps may be most useful when vertical tension must be eliminated to prevent pull on a free margin.

## Webster Modification

The Webster modification allows even greater tension sharing between primary and secondary defects.[8] The first arm of this flap is drawn similarly to that in a Dufourmentel modification, but the second arm is drawn at a more acute 30° angle (Fig. 10.6). This creates a thinner flap pedicle with a flap area that is only about one-half that of the recipient defect. Although this minimizes pivotal restraint and formation of a redundant tissue cone, significantly greater tension is placed in a horizontal direction upon flap closure. Excess tension may distort a free margin or result in ischemia, especially given the narrower flap pedicle. Occasionally, Webster modifications may be used in combination to close a defect where a single rhombic flap is unable to recruit adequate tissue laxity. In this case, two 30° rhombic flaps may be designed at opposite ends of a surgical defect.[9,10] Once transposed, each flap needs only to span one-half of the defect, and tension is placed along two discrete secondary defects (Fig. 10.7). Although this minimizes tension along the primary defect, the resulting complex geometric scar may limit use of this reconstructive strategy.

## Circular Defects

Postoperative defects in dermatologic surgery are typically circular or oval in shape, and the principles of rhombic reconstructions can be applied to such defects.[11-13] Because trimming a wound to create a rhombus leaves a larger defect with angles into which the flap must reach, round defects are often easier to close than traditional rhombic geometries. Location of rhombic angles around a circular defect should be determined by anatomy, adjacent tissue laxity, relaxed tension lines, and cosmetic subunit boundaries. If tension along the primary direction of closure is unacceptable, the flap can be designed slightly larger than the circular defect to account for pivotal restraint. Alternatively, if tension sharing among the defect and flap is

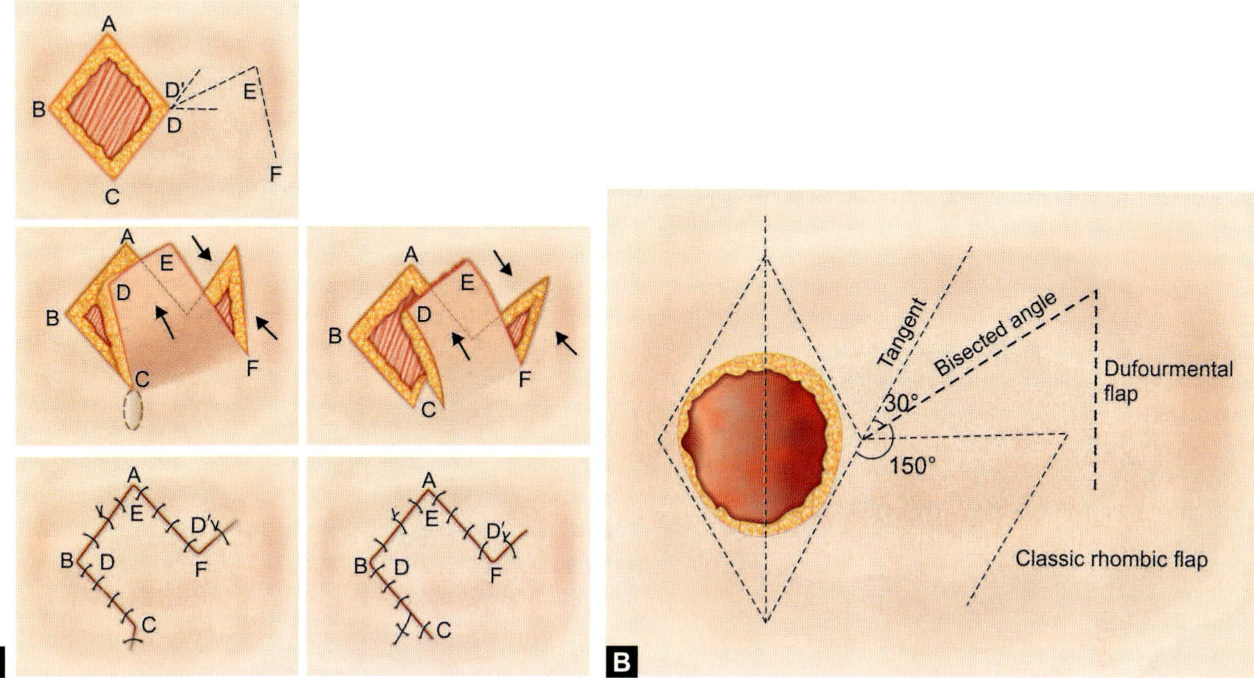


**Figs. 10.5A and B:** Dufourmentel flap. (A) A Dufourmentel flap with variation of DE flap arm arc and removal of tissue cone redundancy. (B) Drawing the Dufourmentel modification. The flap's arc of rotation is decreased compared to the classic rhombic flap.

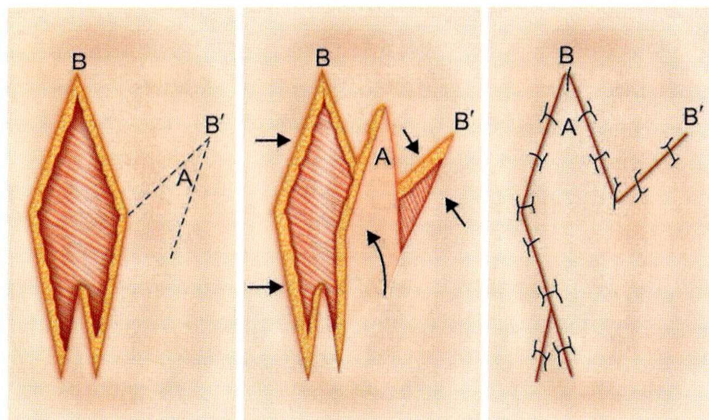


**Fig. 10.6:** Webster flap. Drawing the Webster modification. The flap's tip angle and arc of rotation are reduced compared to the classic rhombic flap.

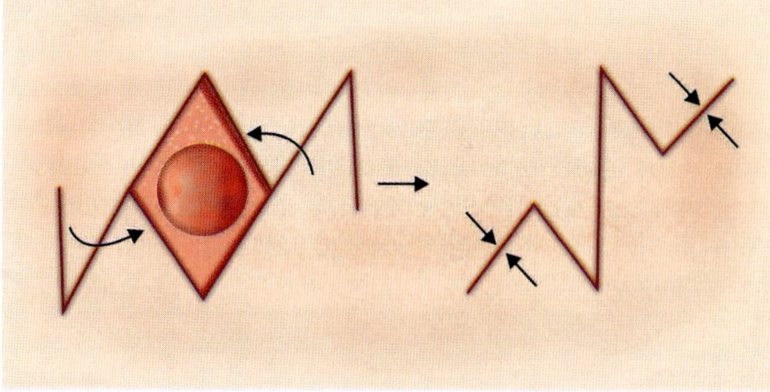

**Fig. 10.7:** Double Webster flap. Two 30° rhombic flaps may be designed at opposite ends of a surgical defect where tissue laxity is lacking. Once transposed, each flap needs only to span one-half of the defect.

permissible, the flap may be undersized to decrease scar length. Once the flap angle and size has been selected, the flap is incised, elevated, and widely undermined. A key suture closes the secondary defect first, and as the flap transposes into the round defect, either the flap tip can be trimmed or the recipient bed enlarged to accommodate the tissue. Only a cone of tissue redundancy created around the flap's pivot point must be excised as the flap is secured into place.

## Nasolabial

The single-staged nasolabial transposition flap is a modified rhombic flap where the flap is elongated, made more acute in its tip angle, and drawn at a tangent to the surgical defect (Fig. 10.8).[14] Significant skin laxity is required at the medial cheek donor site, and the flap easily transposes into its defect with nearly all tension directed along the secondary defect after a standing cone of tissue redundancy is removed. This flap is useful in repairing defects spanning the nasal ala and sidewall where transposing tissue over

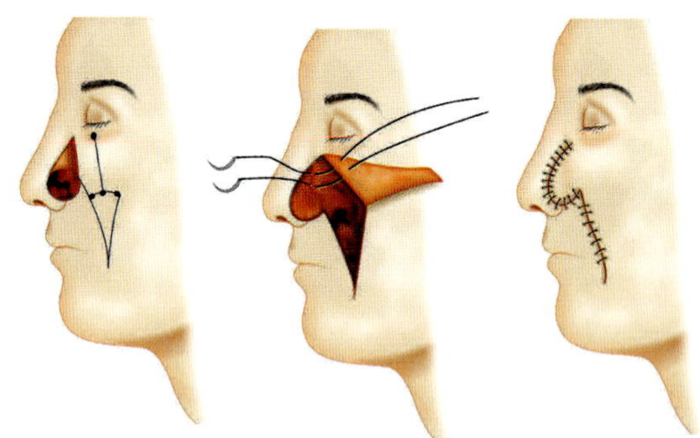

**Fig. 10.8:** Nasolabial transposition flap. Schematic of nasolabial transposition flap where medial cheek skin is recruited to cover a lateral nasal defect.

the lateral nasal crease preserves this anatomic landmark, yet blunts the more medial alar groove. If the alar groove remains intact, a two-staged melolabial interpolation flap may be more appropriate, so as not to obscure this concavity.

The flap should be designed so that the closure of the secondary defect hides in the melolabial fold but does not blunt the apical triangle. As the flap is incised and mobilized, the medial cheek is undermined widely in the superficial subcutaneous fat. Superficial undermining helps prevent flattening of the nasolabial fold when this line is closed. A key suture is then placed to close the secondary defect, directing tension away from the flap. The flap is then transposed onto the nose and judiciously thinned to match the depth of the surgical defect. Deep tacking sutures should be placed to recreate the concave alar groove and concave nasofacial sulcus. Failing to do this will result in a bulky, tented flap that creates unnatural asymmetry of the central face. Following placement of tacking sutures, the flap can be trimmed precisely. Undersized flaps may pull on the ala, while oversized flaps increase the chance of pincushioning. Because the flap loses height as it is transposed (pivotal restraint) and tacked to recreate the alar groove, it is prudent to trim after the flap is set. The excision of the superior redundant tissue cone varies depending on the operative defect. If the wound is medial, the cone is often directed toward the medial canthus. If the wound is more lateral, the cone is typically angled toward the nasal root. Care should be taken when designing and removing this tissue redundancy. Because this flap has a narrow pedicle, the excised tissue cone should be oriented so that it does not narrow the pedicle further, risking vascular compromise. Two main pitfalls of this flap are blunting of the alar crease and the tendency of this flap to pincushion. Tacking sutures can help recreate the alar groove and wide undermining around the entire flap best helps minimize the chance of pincushioning. In addition, to account for pincushioning, some surgeons either slightly undersize the flap or thin it, so that it sits slightly concave in the surgical defect. Despite these pitfalls, the single-staged nasolabial transposition flap can be a useful reconstructive solution for appropriately selected surgical defects spanning the ala and distal lateral nose.

## Bilobed

The bilobed flap is a versatile reconstructive option most often used for defects on the distal nose measuring 1.5 cm or less. It was first described by Esser in 1918[15] and refined by Zitelli in 1989.[16] Zitelli decreased the arc of rotation, which lessens buckling around the pivot point and distal distortion. The bilobed flap recruits tissue from an area of redundancy to fill an area of need more distally. Conceptually, the flap is more complex than a traditional rhombic transposition flap, given its arrangement of tandem transpositions, but like rhombic flaps, there is a significant degree of rotation incorporated into its design. The flap is planned by drawing a triangular cone laterally from the surgical defect. Next, two lines are drawn: one extending from this apex, bisecting the surgical wound; the other extending vertically at 90° from the first line. Because each lobe of the flap "transposes" along an arc, two arcs are then drawn using the triangular apex as a pivot point. The first arc extends from the center of the defect to the vertical axis, and the second extends from the lateral edge of the defect to the vertical axis. The flap lobes are then drawn, such that the primary lobe is bisected at 45° and the secondary lobe is bisected at the vertical axis. The lobes are extended back to the more inferiorly drawn arc (Fig. 10.9).

Bilobed flaps are particularly useful on the distal nose. When designing the flap in this location, the apex of the triangle drawn from the defect is typically angled toward the alar groove. Effort should also be made to align the vertical axis of the flap perpendicularly to the alar margin (Fig. 10.10A). This directs tension along the tertiary defect in a horizontal vector. Tension directed more vertically can lead to elevation of the contralateral ala by vertical tension on the secondary and tertiary closures (Fig. 10.10B).[17] Once planned, the surgical defect should be deepened to the perichondrium and the flap sharply incised. Critical to the flap's perfusion is inclusion of the nasalis muscle in the

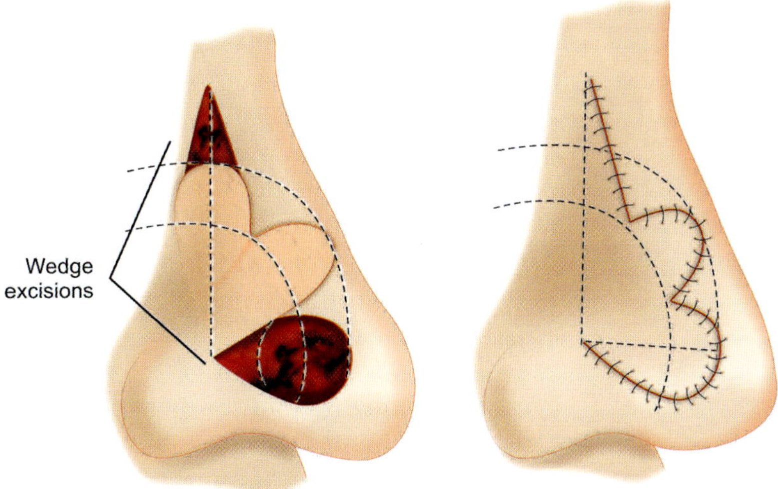


**Fig. 10.9:** Bilobed flap. Schematic of the classic bilobed flap as described by Zitelli.

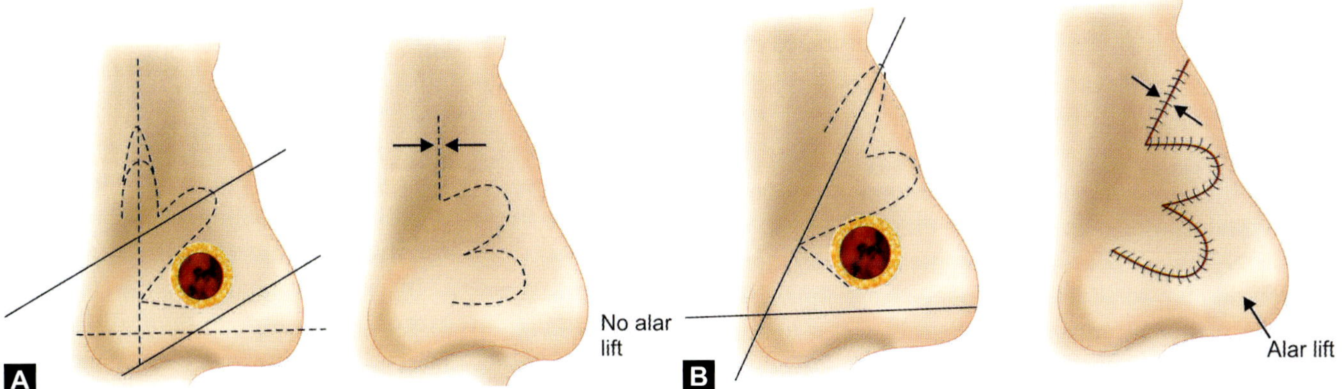


**Figs. 10.10A and B:** Bilobed flap angle planning. (A) Effort should be made to orient the secondary lobe perpendicular to the alar rim to prevent alar lift. (B) A secondary lobe that is not aligned perpendicularly to the alar rim can lead to contralateral alar lift/distortion.

flap. The flap should be elevated below this muscle and widely undermined above the perichondrium and periosteum. To increase flap mobility, undermining may be extended around the flap's pivot point and to the naso facial sulcus. A key suture is placed to close the tertiary defect first, which pushes the primary and secondary lobes into place. The primary lobe should be thinned extensively and inset level or slightly concave in the defect to account for anticipated pincushioning. The secondary lobe is then similarly trimmed and sutured into place. Depending on the stiffness and availability of nasal skin, the flap lobe sizes, their points of origin, and their angles of rotation can be modified to create best outcomes.[17] Several principles can help guide the surgeon in choosing modifications of this technique:

- For thinner, more mobile skin, the primary and secondary lobes may be slightly undersized to decrease the arc of rotation, minimizing tension associated with pivotal restraint.
- For thicker immobile skin, the primary flap is best designed the same size as the primary defect. Undersizing the lobe will create tension with closure that may unacceptably raise the ipsilateral alar rim. Conversely, oversizing may bulldoze the lobe, depressing the ala.
- For immobile skin, adjusting the flap's pivot point more superiorly decreases the necessary arc of rotation, relieving pivotal restraint. The flap can be designed as depicted in Figure 10.11.

Bilobed repairs can be elegant reconstructive solutions to distal nasal defects. Analysis of nasal skin quality and

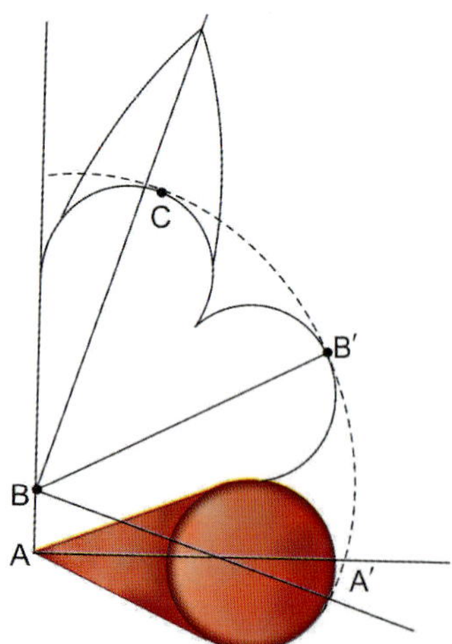


**Fig. 10.11:** Bilobed fulcrum modification. Adjusting the bilobed flap's pivot point more superiorly decreases the necessary arc of rotation, relieving pivotal restraint, which allows the flap to more easily transpose into place.

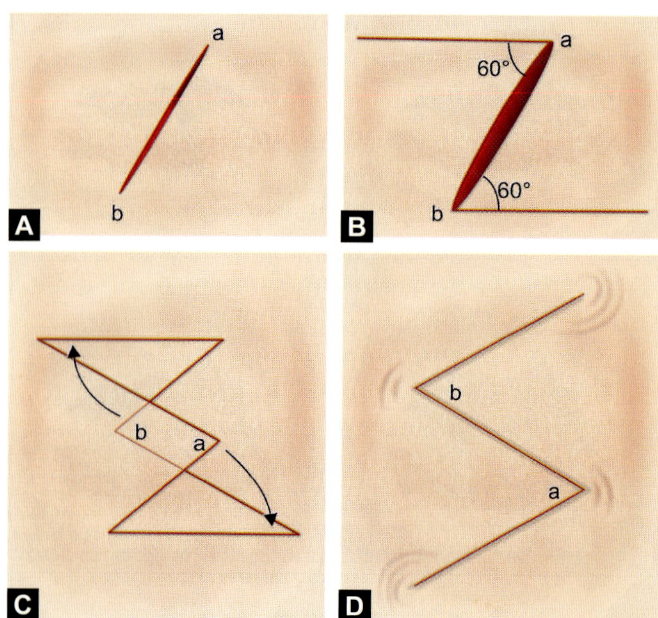


**Figs. 10.12A to D:** Classic Z-plasty. (A) Orientation of scar from (a) to (b). (B) Scar excised and two additional limbs are cut equal in length to the scar and parallel to the relaxed skin tension lines. (C) The flaps are transposed over one another. (D) The resultant scar is reoriented by 90° and lengthened by 75%.

laxity, careful planning, and precise execution are critical for excellent results.

## Z-plasty

Z-plasty transposition flaps are those where two triangular flaps are transposed over one another into a Z-shape. These flaps thus achieve scar lengthening and reorientation of relaxed skin tension lines. The angle size and length of the common diagonal (common limb) may be varied to achieve added closure length and reorientation. In a traditional Z-plasty (Fig. 10.12A), two flap arms of equal length are drawn at 60° around the common limb (Fig. 10.12B).[18,19] The flap is incised, widely undermined in the subcutaneous fat, and each limb is transposed into the defect created by the other arm (Fig. 10.12C). This creates a tissue length gain of 75% and scar reorientation by 90° (Fig. 10.12D). An angle of 30° lengthens a scar by 25%, an angle of 45° by 50%, an angle of 75° by 100%, and an angle of 90° by 125%. Angles less than 60° are easier to transpose, but yield less scar lengthening and reorientation. Although angles >60° maximize scar lengthening and realignment, they are more difficult to transpose, given increased pivotal restraint.

# APPLICATIONS

## Rhombic

The rhombic flap is particularly useful for defects involving the upper two-thirds of the nose, the medial and lateral canthus, the lateral forehead and the temple.[20] For defects of the nasal root, upper nasal sidewall and medial canthus linear repair may result in webbing in the canthus. The rhombic flap works well to maintain the normal anatomic concavity in this area. Moreover, the geometric lines of the flap are well camouflaged within the naturally occurring glabellar creases and "bunny lines" (Figs. 10.13A and B). Essential to repair of defects of the lateral forehead, temple, and lateral canthus is to avoid any pull on the free margin of the eyelid (Figs. 10.14A and B). The rhombic flap achieves this by allowing for the redirection of tension vectors and the sharp lines and acute angles of the flap hide well in the crow's feet. The editors also find transposition flaps very useful to repair defects on the anterior ear since these flaps are able to mobilize the tissue reservoir of the preauricular area and maintain distinct cosmetic units (Figs. 10.15A to C).

The applications of this flap extend beyond the single rhombic flap. Defects of the nasal dorsum and supratip/tip may be closed with an extended vertically oriented linear repair. However, when the defect is too large, a bilateral rhombic flap can be employed (Figs. 10.16A and B).[21] The two rhombi are designed lateral to the defect, as mirror images of one another; with each rhombic designed to repair half the defect. They can be based superiorly or inferiorly and they share a medial Burow's triangle.

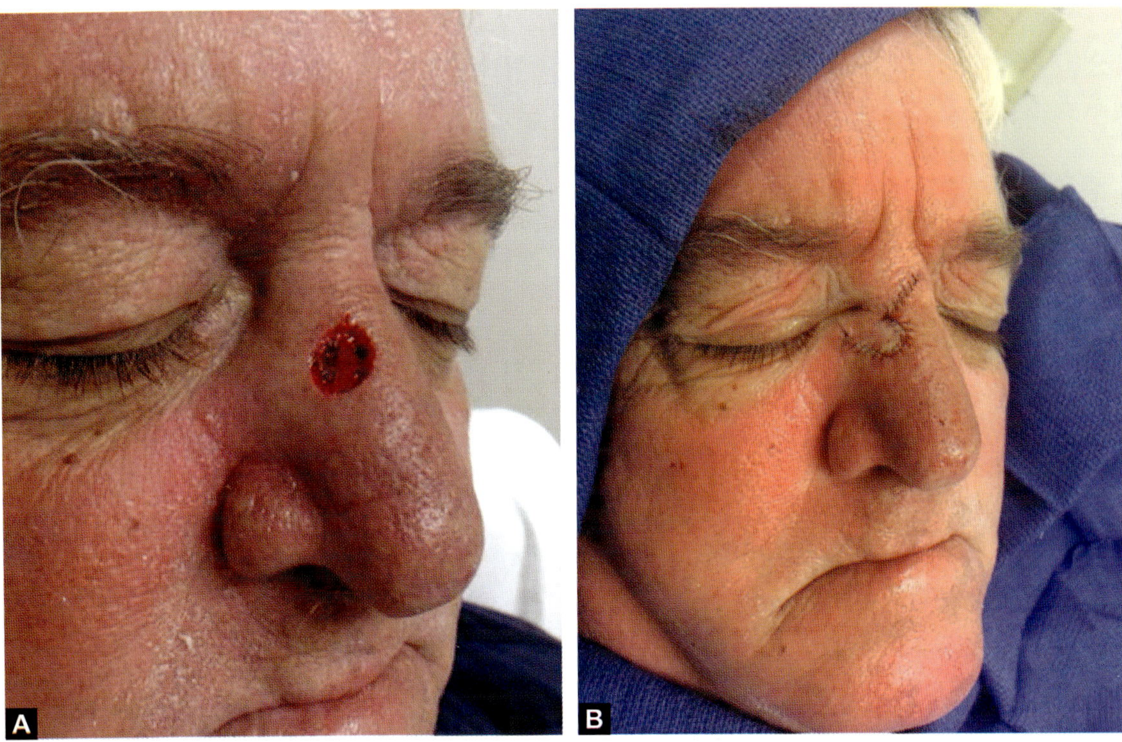


**Figs. 10.13A and B:** Utilization of rhombic flap in the upper nasal sidewall. (A) Surgical defect. (B) The geometric lines of the rhombic flap are readily camouflaged in the "bunny lines" of the upper nose.

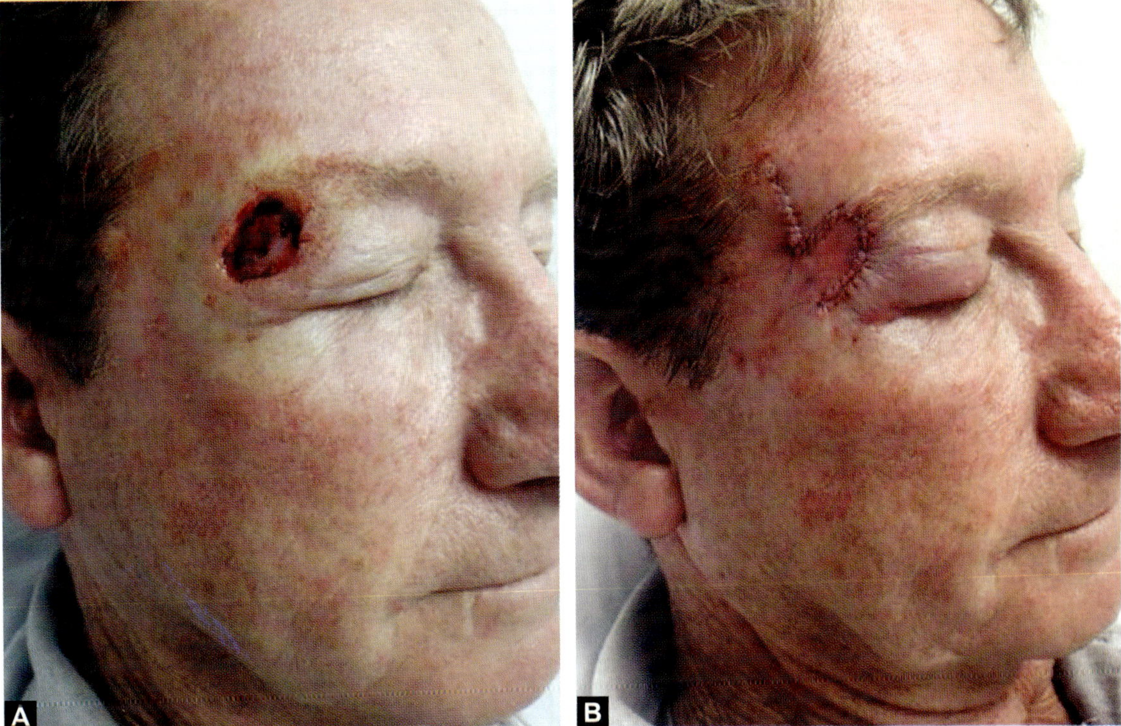


**Figs. 10.14A and B:** Utilization of the rhombic flap in the eyelid. (A) Surgical defect. (B) The rhombic flap effectively closes the eyelid defect while preventing any distortion of the free margin of the eyelid.

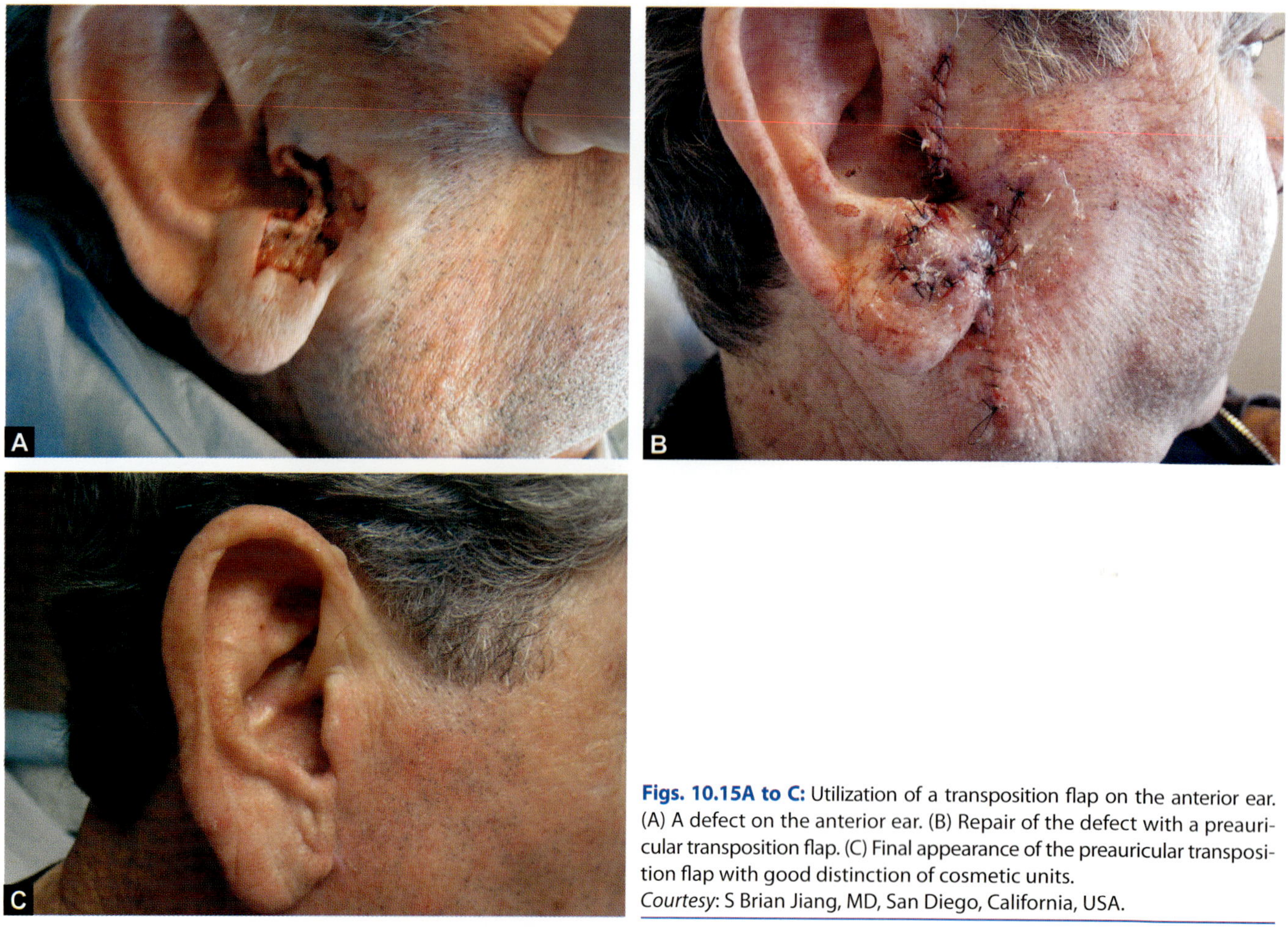

**Figs. 10.15A to C:** Utilization of a transposition flap on the anterior ear. (A) A defect on the anterior ear. (B) Repair of the defect with a preauricular transposition flap. (C) Final appearance of the preauricular transposition flap with good distinction of cosmetic units.
*Courtesy*: S Brian Jiang, MD, San Diego, California, USA.

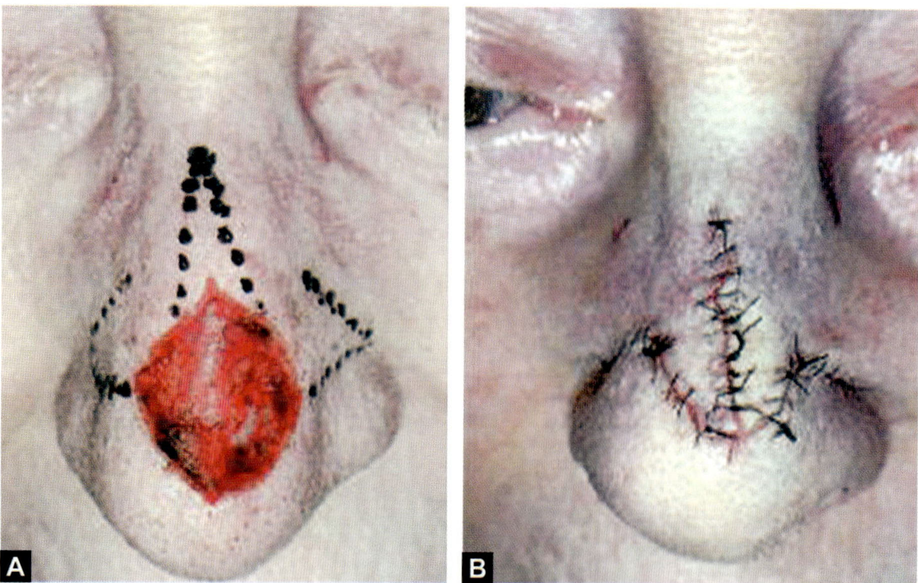


**Figs. 10.16A and B:** Bilateral rhombic flap. (A) Two rhombic flaps designed as mirror images of one another designed to repair a large defect of the nasal tip and supratip, executed with a shared central Burow's triangle.

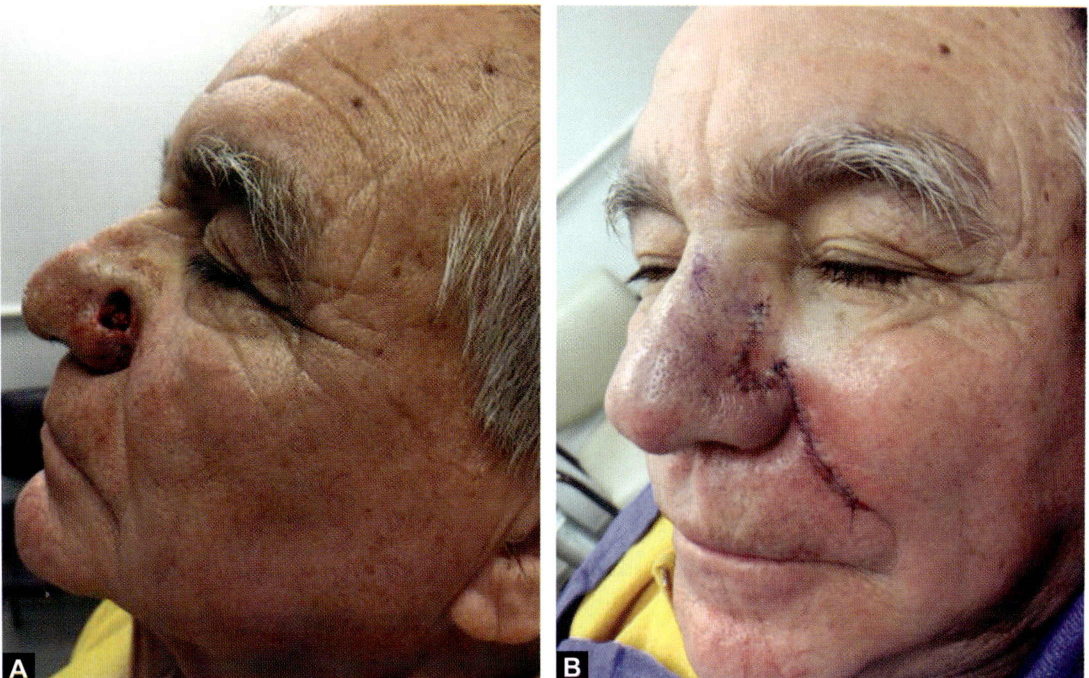


**Figs. 10.17A and B:** Classic nasolabial transposition flap. (A) A defect spanning the nasal ala and the superior alar crease. (B) Nasolabial transposition flap used to repair the defect with sutures hidden in the nasolabial fold and along the nasal sidewall.

## Nasolabial

The nasolabial or melolabial flap is a banner flap that takes advantage of the generous tissue reservoir of the relatively sebaceous skin of the medial cheek. This flap is used to close large defects of the nasal sidewall and nasal ala. It lends itself well to oblong defects that lay perpendicular to the donor site. Inherent in the design of this flap is the aesthetically optimal placement of the secondary defect along the nasolabial fold. Unlike the similarly named interpolation flap, this nasolabial transposition flap has the advantage of requiring only a single stage. It does however run the risk of blunting the nasofacial sulcus and alar crease and as such is best reserved for defects in which the superior alar crease is already compromised (Figs. 10.17A and B).

The nasolabial transposition flap is classically a laterally based flap used to repair defects of the lateral nose. However, a medially based single-stage nasolabial flap has recently been described to repair moderate to large defects of the nasal tip (Figs. 10.18A and B).[22] Traditionally repair options for this location include dorsal nasal rotation flaps, staged interpolated forehead flaps, and skin grafts. A nasolabial flap that transposes over uninvolved alar and nasal sidewall skin may be a useful reconstruction alternative, eliminating a large forehead scar or graft harvest site scar.

## Bilobed

As previously detailed the bilobed flap is primarily used for defects of the lower third of the nose (Figs. 10.19A and B).[23] It is particularly well suited for defects in this location because of its ability, via the two lobes, to mobilize the adjacent thick sebaceous tissue that can otherwise be quite difficult to match.[24] The flap is ideally laterally based, however it can work as a medially based flap as well.[25]

In addition to its value in nasal reconstruction, the bilobed flap is versatile and a variety of extranasal applications have been described.[26] In virtually any location the flap can be used to take advantage of remote tissue reservoirs and, off the nose, there is more flexibility in the design of the lobes. The bilobed flap has been successfully used to repair defects of the hand, cheek, chin, ear, and lip, among others, and should be kept in mind when approaching challenging defects in any location (Figs. 10.20A and B).

The trilobed flap is a useful modification of the bilobed flap that expands its use to larger defects of the nasal tip and nasal ala (Figs. 10.21A to D).[27] In the trilobed design, a third lobe is added that recruits tissue from a more distant reservoir and minimizes pivotal restraint. The lobes of the trilobed flap are designed with a small 45°–50° angle of rotation, but the addition of the third lobe allows for a broader arc of

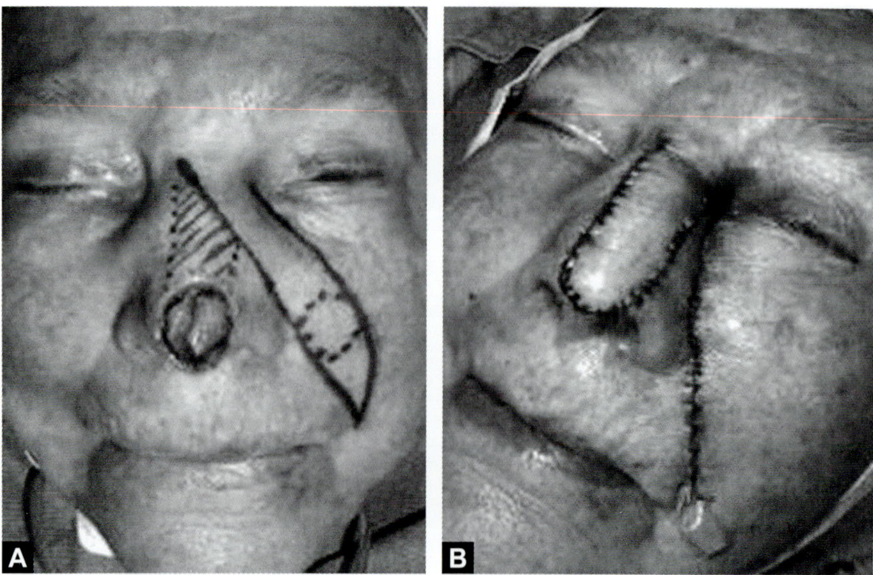


**Figs. 10.18A and B:** Novel variation and use of the nasolabial transposition flap. (A) For this large defect of the nasal tip, a medially based nasolabial transposition flap is designed to utilize the melolabial tissue reservoir. (B) The defect is closed in a single stage.

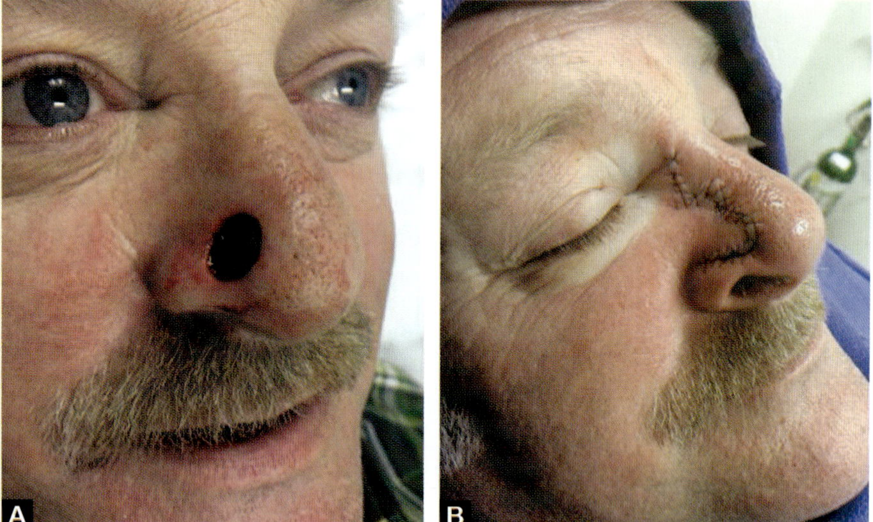


**Figs. 10.19A and B:** Bilobed flap. (A) Surgical defect. (B) Classic use of bilobed flap to repair defect of the lower third of the nose.

rotation, with a superiorly oriented dog ear and a vertically oriented tertiary lobe.

## Z-plasty

The Z-plasty is most widely used as a technique for scar revision. By transposing two equally-sized triangle flaps on either side of the scar, the scar is reoriented and lengthened. Reorientation of a scar may be desired to move a scar that crosses multiple anatomic units or borders into a natural line or shadow of the face, for example, the melolabial fold.[28] This technique is also useful for correcting a scar that distorts a free margin, including ectropion or an elevated oral commissure. Webbing in the medial canthus or nasal ala can also be addressed with a Z-plasty. In these repairs, the common arm of the flap is drawn along the web and the flap arms reorient skin tension after transposition (Figs. 10.22A to F).

Z-plasties can also be used to lengthen contracted scars that restrict mobility, lift structures that may have been depressed by other surgical repairs, break up geometric

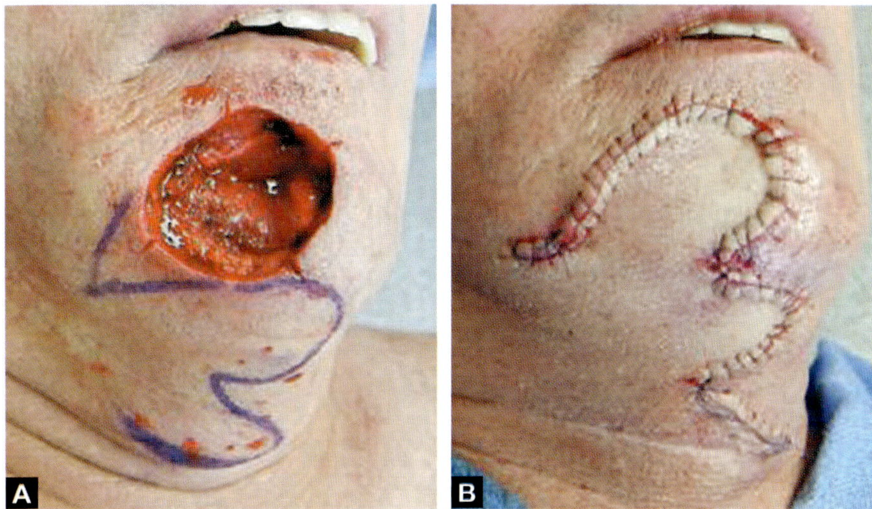


**Figs. 10.20A and B:** Extranasal uses of the bilobed flap. (A) The bilobed flap designed to take advantage of tissue reservoir in the anterior neck to repair a large defect of the chin. (B) Closure of a large defect on the chin with a bilobed flap.

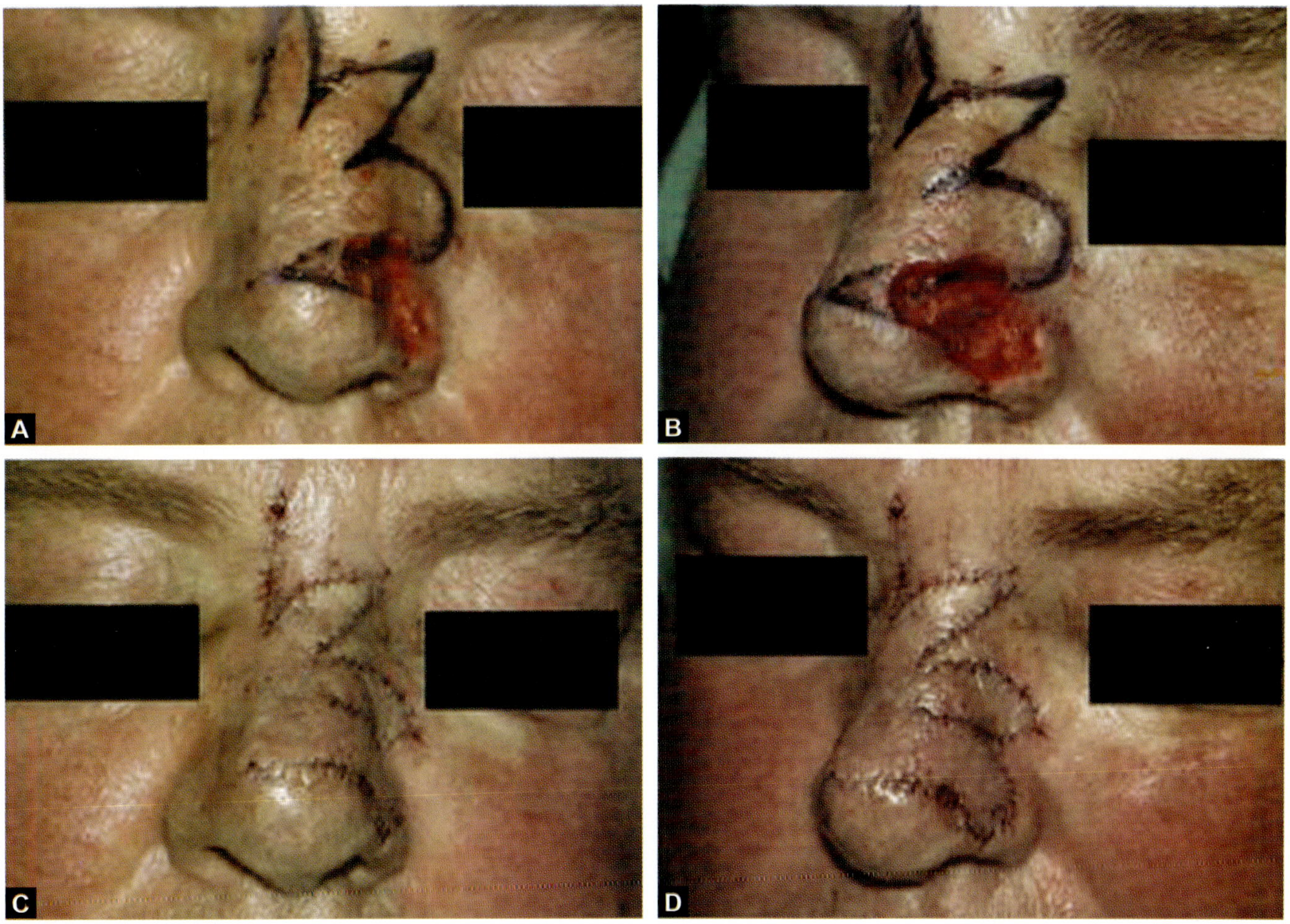

**Figs. 10.21A to D:** Trilobed flap. (A) A modification of the bilobed flap with three lobes rather than two (frontal view). (B) Lateral view. (C) Closure of the alar defect with a trilobed flap (frontal view). (D) Lateral view.

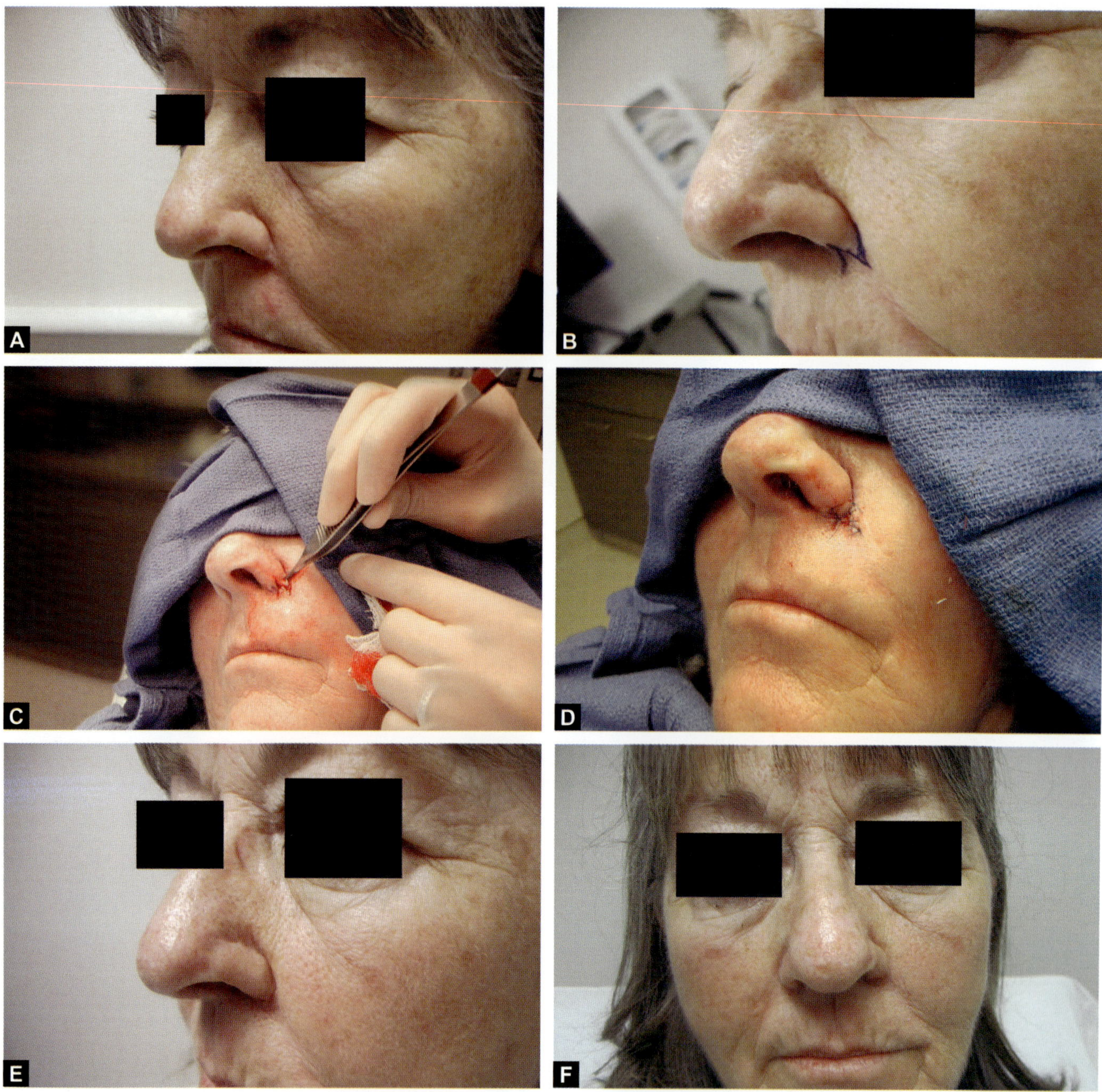

**Figs. 10.22A to F:** Utilization of a Z-plasty to correct webbing of the alar crease. (A) Preoperative alar web. (B) Z-plasty design with the common limb drawn along the web. (C) Flap incised and Z-plasty arms transposed into place. (D) Immediate postoperative Z-plasty repair. (E) Oblique view. (F) frontal view of corrected web 8 weeks postrepair.

scars, or recreate creases. In addition to being invaluable in the correction of cosmetically unfavorable scars, the Z-plasty can be incorporated into primary repair design to optimize cosmetic outcomes. Long straight lines on the face can attract the eye, even when the scar is very fine. One or multiple Z-plasties can be incorporated into the design of the repair to break up the linearity, as well as camouflage some of the lines within the horizontal creases resulting in a shorter much less noticeable scar (Figs. 10.23A to C).[29]

A Z-plasty can also be used in combination with other flaps at the time of primary closure. A double Z-plasty can be added to a traditional rhombic flap to increase tissue

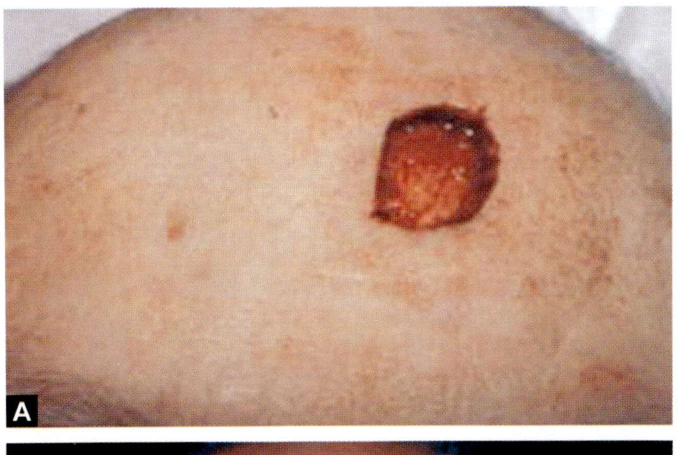

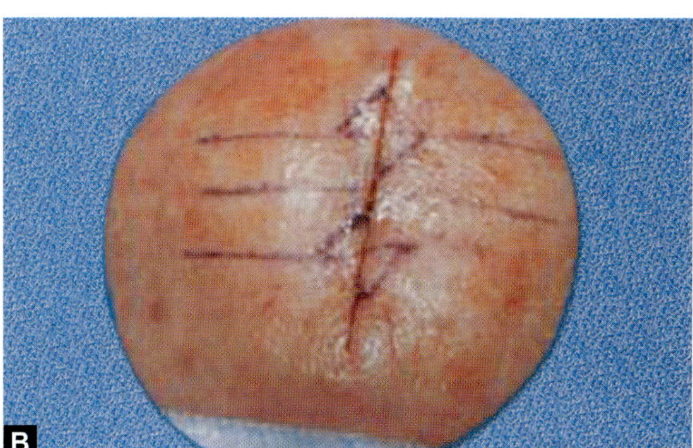

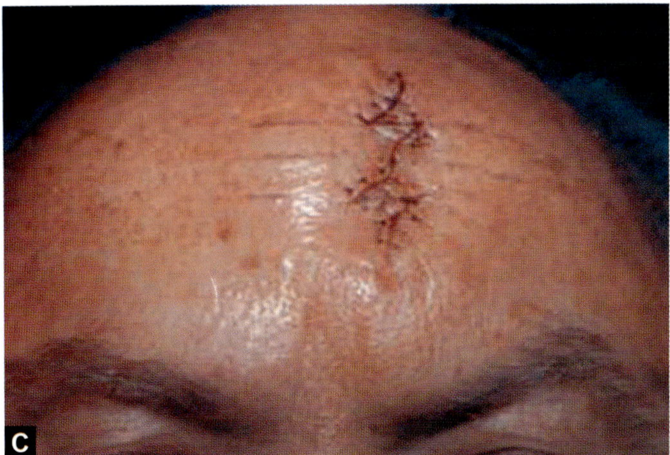

**Figs. 10.23A to C:** Utilization of Z-plasty to camouflage linear repair. (A) A large defect on the forehead. (B) Z-plasty employed at time of primary repair to break up a lengthy vertical linear repair. (C) The scar is partially hidden within the horizontal rhytids of the forehead.

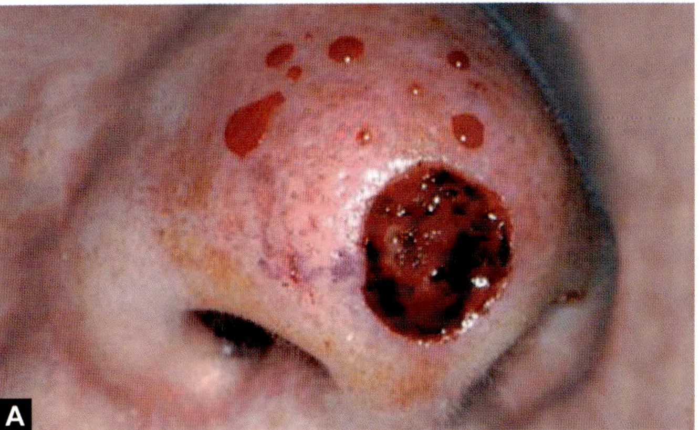

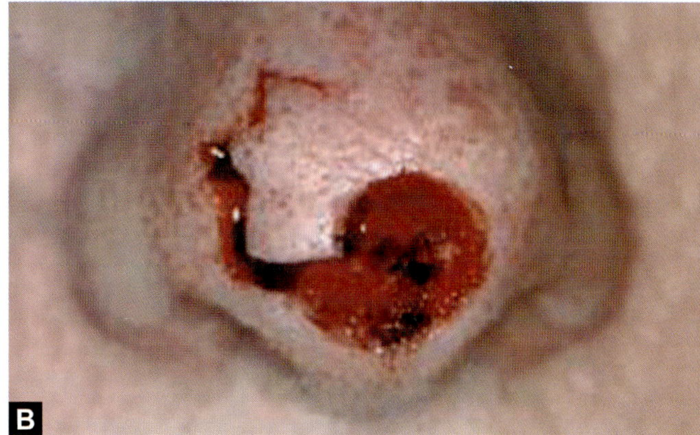

**Figs. 10.24A and B:** Combination double Z-plasty with rhombic flap. (A) Nasal tip defect. (B) Addition of a double Z-plasty to a rhombic flap to increase tissue mobility in the relatively immobile sebaceous skin of a nasal tip defect.

mobility while minimizing distortion of surrounding tissue.[30,31] The first Z-plasty triangle is designed at a 90°–105° angle from the rhombic and a 60° angle in the triangle tip and the second Z-plasty triangle is at 90° from the first, again with a 60° angle in the tip (*See* Figs. 10.24A and B).

## SUMMARY

Transposition flaps are invaluable tools for the reconstructive surgeon. A thorough understanding of the geometry at the foundation of the design of these complex flaps is essential to their successful execution. Once mastered, these techniques offer unparalleled opportunity for precise tissue matching, utilization of distant tissue reservoirs, and protection of free margins and preservation of cosmetic units. The classic transposition flaps discussed here, the rhombic, the nasolabial, the bilobed, and the Z-plasty, can be utilized to repair a wide array of cutaneous defects. With a little imagination these classic flaps can be adapted with a variety of modifications to significantly expand their application and to precisely address the unique characteristics and challenges presented with each new defect.

## REFERENCES


1. Limberg AA. Design of local flaps. In: Gibson T (Ed). Modern Trends of Plastic Surgery. London: Butterworth-Heinemann; 1966. pp. 38-61.
2. Borges AF. Choosing the correct Limberg flap. Plast Reconstr Surg. 1978;62:542-5.
3. Brobyn TJ, Cramer LM, Hulnick SJ. Facial resurfacing with the Limberg flap. Clin Plast Surg. 1976;3:481-90.
4. Fee WE Jr, Gunter JP, Carder HM. Rhomboid flap principles and common variations. Laryngoscope 1976;86:1706-11.
5. Dzubow LM. The dynamics of flap movement: effect of pivotal restraint on flap rotation and transposition. J Dermatol Surg Oncol. 1987;13:1348-53.
6. Lister GD, Gibson T. Closure of rhomboid skin defects: the flaps of Limberg and Dufourmental. Br J Plast Surg. 1972; 25: 300-14.
7. Dufourmental C. Le fermeture des pertes de substance cutanee limitees "Le lambeau de rotation en L pour losange" det "LLL." Ann Chir Plast. 1962;7:61-6.
8. Webster RC, Davidson TM, Smith RC. The thirty degree transposition flap. Laryngoscope. 1978;88(1 Pt 1):85-94.
9. Becker H. The rhomboid-to-W technique for excision of some skin lesions and closure. Plast Reconstr Surg. 1979;64:444-7.
10. Katoh H, Nakajima T, Yoshimura Y. The double-Z-rhomboid plasty: an improvement in design. Plast Reconstr Surg. 1984;74:817-24.
11. Dzubow LM. Mohs surgery report: design of an appropriate rhombic flap for a circular defect created by Mohs microscopically controlled surgery. J Dematol Surg. 1988; 14:124-6.
12. Quaba AA, Sommerland BC. "A square peg into a round hole": a modified rhomboid flap and its clinical application. Br J Plast Surg. 1987;40:163-70.
13. Webster RC, Benjamin BJ, Smith RC. Closure of circular defects. Laryngoscope. 1987;88:534-8.
14. Zitelli JA. The nasolabial flap as a single-stage procedure. Atch Dermtol. 1990;126:1445-8.
15. Esser JFS. Gestielte locale Nasenplanstik mit Zwizipfligem lappen Deckung des Sekundaren Detektes vom ersten Zipfel durch den Zweiten. Stsch Z Chirurgie. 1918;143:385-90.
16. Zitelli JA. The bilobed flap for nasal reconstruction. Arch Dermatol. 1989;125:957-9.
17. Cook JL. A review of the bilobed flap's design with particular emphasis on the minimization of alar displacement. Dermatol Surg. 2000;26:354-62.
18. Lee KK, Mehrany K, Swanson NA. Surgical revision. Dermatol Clin. 2005;23:141-50.
19. Salam GA, Amin JP. The basic Z-plasty. Am Fam Physician. 2003;67:2329-32.
20. Rohrer TE, Bhatia A. Transposition flaps in cutaneous surgery. Dermatol Surg. 2005;31(8 Pt 2):1014-23.
21. Desciak EB, Eliezri YD. Bilateral rhombic flaps for defects on the nasal dorsum and supra-tip. Dermatol Surg. 2003;29 (11):1163-5.
22. Beustes-Stefanelli M, O'Toole G, Schertenleib P. The midline-based nasolabial transposition flap: a new single-stage technique for nasal tip reconstruction. Ann Plast Surg. 2015;74(4):426-31.
23. Zitelli JA. The bilobed flap for nasal reconstruction. Arch Dermatol. 1989;125(7):957-9.
24. Cook JL. Reconstructive utility of the bilobed flap: lessons from flap successes and failures. Dermatol Surg. 2005;31 (8 Pt 2):1024-33.
25. Skaria AM. The medial based bi- or trilobed flap for repair of distal alar defects. Dermatology. 2013;227(2):165-70.
26. Ricks M, Cook J. Extranasal applications of the bilobed flap. Dermatol Surg. 2005;31(8 Pt 1):941-8.
27. Albertini JG, Hansen JP. Trilobed flap reconstruction for distal nasal skin defects. Dermatol Surg. 2010;36(11): 1726-35.
28. Fader DJ, Wang TS, Johnson TM. The Z-plasty transposition flap for reconstruction of the middle cheek. J Am Acad Dermatol. 2002;46(5):738-42.
29. Pomaranski MR, Krull EA, Balle MR. Use of the Z-plasty technique for forehead defects. Dermatol Surg. 2005;31(12): 1720-3.
30. Becker H. Double Z-plasty for rhombic defects. Plast Reconstr Surg. 1983;72(6):917.
31. Johnson SC, Bennett RG. Double Z-plasty to enhance rhombic flap mobility. J Dermatol Surg Oncol. 1994;20(2): 128-32.

# CHAPTER 11

# Staged Flaps

*Jesse M Lewin, John A Carucci*

## INTRODUCTION

The staged interpolation flap is a workhorse for dermatologic surgeons reconstructing complex defects following tumor extirpation that cannot be repaired adequately with local adjacent tissue transfers or grafts. The principle underlying the staged interpolation flap is to elevate tissue with a strong arterial supply from one location and transpose it over uninvolved skin in order to cover and nourish the recipient site with well-matched donor tissue. The pedicle with a rich blood supply is then divided after a defined period of time after neovascularization has occurred.[1]

The first interpolation flaps were "median forehead flaps" performed by Sushruta Samhita, in approximately 600 BC.[2] The operation was performed by members of a caste of potters known as the Koomas and grew out of the Indian practice of amputating the tip of the nose as punishment for a variety of crimes, ranging from robbery to adultery. Centuries later the classic "Indian rhinoplasty" was propagated in the United States by Kazanjian in 1946, who published on the "vertical flap" from the midline of the forehead.[3] Later the vertical axis of the "median" forehead flap was shifted to the paramedian position which allows for greater ease of rotation and length and is currently favored.[4,5] At present dermatologic surgeons perform staged interpolation flaps to reconstruct complex defects primarily of the nose, ear, and lip. While many other surgical subspecialties perform multiple staged flaps with intravenous sedation or general anesthesia, staged interpolation flaps have been demonstrated to be safe and with low complication rates in the hands of dermatologic surgeons using local anesthesia.[6] In addition, a large series that examined patients treated with Mohs micrographic surgery followed by reconstruction by dermatologic surgeons revealed similar rates of major complications in office versus hospital-based settings.[7] Patients undergoing Mohs micrographic surgery also value the fact that the surgery is done on an outpatient basis and that it does not require general anesthesia.[8]

The key principles for any interpolated pedicle flap include a rich blood supply from the stalk, no tension or torsion of the pedicle, and appropriate defect and patient selection. Since interpolated pedicle flaps require at least two procedures, the inset and takedown, and patients will have an undivided pedicle for several weeks, it is crucial that they understand their operative course, have reasonable expectations, and are involved in the decision to undergo this type of reconstruction. Furthermore, the authors suggest that prior to reconstruction, patients be offered the option of viewing pictures of patients who have undergone these procedures prior to division of the pedicle in order to have a full understanding of the procedure. Patients should also be assessed for functional status and any comorbidities that may impair their ability to tolerate the procedure or perform necessary aftercare. This chapter covers the applications and proper execution of the melolabial interpolation flap, mastoid pedicle flap, paramedian forehead flap, and Abbe "lip switch" flap.

### Melolabial Interpolation Flap

#### *Applications*

The cheek-to-nose interpolation flap or melolabial interpolation flap is useful for defects of the caudal nose including nasal tip, ala, and alar rim where a local flap may obscure a cosmetic subunit junction such as the alar crease or alar facial sulcus. The donor portion of this flap is harvested from cheek, leaving a secondary defect which can be closed in the melolabial fold allowing excellent scar

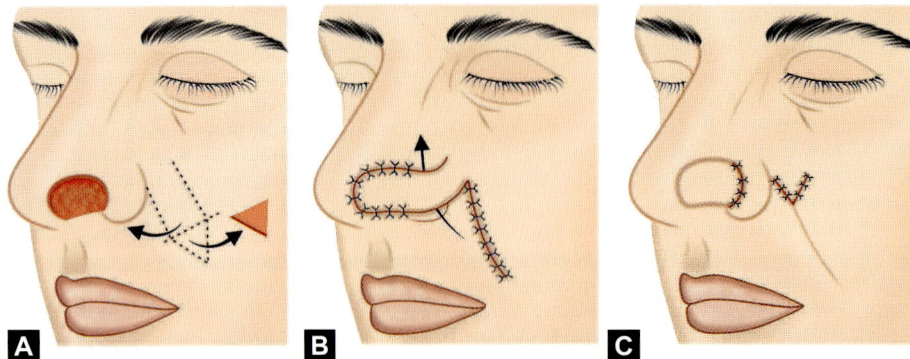


**Figs. 11.1A to C:** Schematic of melolabial interpolation flap. (A) Defect of nasal ala and alar rim with pedicle marked lateral to melolabial crease. (B) Flap elevated, inset, and sutured into nasal defect. (C) Pedicle is divided and secondary cheek defect is closed.

camouflage (Figs. 11.1A to C). The melolabial fold is created by the insertion of the superficial muscular aponeurotic system into the skin at the junction of the cutaneous lips and the cheek. The melolabial interpolation flap is considered a random-pattern flap, rather than a purely axial flap as it is supplied by perforating vessels from the angular artery which penetrate the levator labii muscle in the region of the alar facial sulcus.[9] When approaching reconstruction of defects on the caudal third of the nose, factors such as the size and depth of the defect, involvement of cartilage or mucosa, patient comorbidities, and potential for functional impairment all play into the choice of repair.

Options include full-thickness skin grafts or composite grafts, secondary intention healing for small defects of the dorsum, tip or sidewall, local flaps such as bilobe or trilobe transposition flaps, nasolabial transposition flaps, and paramedian forehead flaps for larger defects. The melolabial interpolation flap is advantageous over the one-stage nasolabial transposition flap in that it does not deform the alar facial sulcus or alar groove. It is imperative that whenever possible flaps should be designed as to not cross borders that separate aesthetic subunits, in particular a concave border such as the alar facial sulcus.[10] When the sulcus is effaced by a nasolabial transposition flap as in the repair of a caudal nasal defect it is difficult to restore the contour between the ala and cheek. Another consideration when approaching a caudal nasal defect involving the ala is to assess the need for structural support with a cartilage strut to replace lower lateral alar cartilage or fibrofatty subdermal tissue. Adequate structural support with cartilage is imperative to maintain nasal valve patency as well as to resist the forces of contraction and preserve nasal architecture. The authors favor the use of auricular donor cartilage from the helix or antihelix as a strut for this location. Lastly, if a "through-and through" defect is present resulting in loss of nasal mucosa, it is important to consider a mucosal flap, since adequate function of the nose requires a thin internal layer best supplied by vascularized mucosa.[11]

## *Planning and Execution*

Prior to the administration of additional local anesthesia into the nose or cheek which tumesces and distorts the anatomy, the surgeon should carefully mark the melolabial fold and the intended pedicle which frequently originates lateral to the fold (Fig. 11.2A). The defect or recipient site should be prepared by removing any remaining dermal and subcutaneous tissue in order to allow meticulous inset of the full-thickness pedicle. However, it is not necessary to expand the defect if the surrounding portion of the alar subunit is intact and structurally sound. A template of the defect is then traced and cut using foil or a telfa pad and then used to design and size the pedicle.

Once appropriately drawn and planned, the melolabial pedicle flap is incised to the level of subcutaneous fat and elevated. The flap is designed and elevated such that it will pivot 90° clockwise when harvested from the left cheek, or counterclockwise when harvested from the right cheek. It is crucial to ensure adequate pedicle width and depth in order to maintain a robust and thick pedicle at the superomedial portion of the flap in order to nourish the flap. Flap mobility is attained by careful and judicious dissection of subcutaneous fat with sharp undermining scissors at the lateral borders of the pedicle while visualizing the pedicle base and with awareness of the extent of "reach" necessary to inset the flap. Hemostasis with electrocautery can be performed at this time around the pedicle if necessary, however, care should be taken not to compromise or devitalize adjacent dermis.

After the pedicle is elevated, skin hooks are used to ensure that it will sit in the recipient site without tension and with minimal torsion. Much of the fat on the portion of the pedicle that will be inset is carefully thinned until only the subdermal plexus remains. At this point the flap can be sewn into the recipient defect with a tacking stitch to ensure that it sits at the appropriate level insofar as it is even with the surrounding tissue and is not under tension. Once the surgeon is satisfied with placement of the pedicle in the recipient bed, deep absorbable sutures and then superficial nonabsorbable sutures are placed to inset the medial, superior, and inferior portions of the flap into the defect (Fig. 11.2B). At times vertical mattress sutures can be used for the top layer of the nasal portion of the inset flap to ensure adequate eversion and strength. The secondary cheek defect is then closed in two layers. Meticulous hemostasis intraoperatively and an appropriate dressing is applied in order to minimize the risk of postoperative bleeding. Some surgeons use a bolster dressing over the nasal portion of the flap to increase apposition of the flap to the wound bed. In our practice, the patient is seen on postoperative day 1 for the first dressing change in order to check the flap and reinforce appropriate wound care.

In 1 week the patient returns for removal of sutures from the secondary defect closed in the melolabial fold and at the recipient site. In 2–3 weeks, the pedicle can be divided and the final inset is done after "freshening" the edges of the lateral portion of the nasal defect (Figs. 11.2C and D). If further thinning of the flap is necessary it can be done at this point; however, while "pincushioning" should be avoided, conversely, the surgeon does wish to ensure that the curve of the ala is maintained with adequate convexity. After division and inset of the flap, the portion of the cheek, which supplied the pedicle base, is closed in two layers with removal of a superior standing cone if necessary. In our practice, patients are typically seen in 2 months to ensure adequate cosmesis and function (Fig. 11.2E). While much attention has been paid in the literature to the first stage of the melolabial interpolation flap, the takedown and final inset is crucial to ultimate function and cosmesis and the importance of this step should not be understated. In our hands staged melolabial interpolation flaps are reliable and produce reproducibly good cosmetic and functional results for defects of the nasal ala, tip, and rim (Figs. 11.3 to 11.6).

### *Complications and Pitfalls*

The most feared complication of the staged melolabial interpolation flap is necrosis or flap failure that can be a result of excess pedicle tension or torsion at the base of the flap, in addition to several other factors. One large series of 256 interpolation flaps done by a single Mohs surgeon revealed no major complications, with the most common minor complication being bleeding in 7% of patients, followed by infection in 4.3% of patients, most of whom had not received postoperative antibiotics prophylactically.[6] There was one case of total flap necrosis and two cases of partial flap necrosis which were attributed to tobacco smoking and poor flap design for a large defect. A more common pitfall of staged melolabial interpolation flaps is "trapdoor" or "pincushion" deformity of the ala. The risk of pincushioning can be lessened by meticulous thinning of the flap, and when it occurs it often softens and flattens over time, but can be surgically revised in 6 months if deemed necessary by the surgeon and patient. Intralesional kenalog has also been used to hasten resolution of "pincushioning."

## Mastoid/Retroauricular Pedicle Flap

### *Applications*

The two-staged mastoid pedicle flap is advantageous for large defects (>2–2.5 cm) of the outer auricle involving the middle or upper pinna (Fig. 11.7). These extensive defects typically involve exposed cartilage or loss of perichondrium and are thus not well suited for coverage with a full-thickness skin graft which may not survive or for local flaps which may distort the complex surface anatomy of the ear. The mastoid scalp has been shown to be an excellent tissue reservoir due to its blood supply and textural match for ear reconstruction.[12,13] However, it should be noted that some mastoid scalps that have dense hair are not good tissue matches for ear reconstruction. Unlike most interpolation flaps, with the mastoid interpolation flap there is no pivotal movement, but rather the flap is advanced over the intervening postauricular sulcus into its recipient bed. This random-pattern flap derives its blood supply from the robust blood supply of the retroauricular scalp. Other reconstructive options that can be considered for upper and central helical defects include chondrocutaneous advancement and rotation flaps. As discussed above for the melolabial interpolation flap, it is crucial to assess the need for structural support with cartilage prior to repair with a mastoid interpolation flap. For defects of the scaphoid

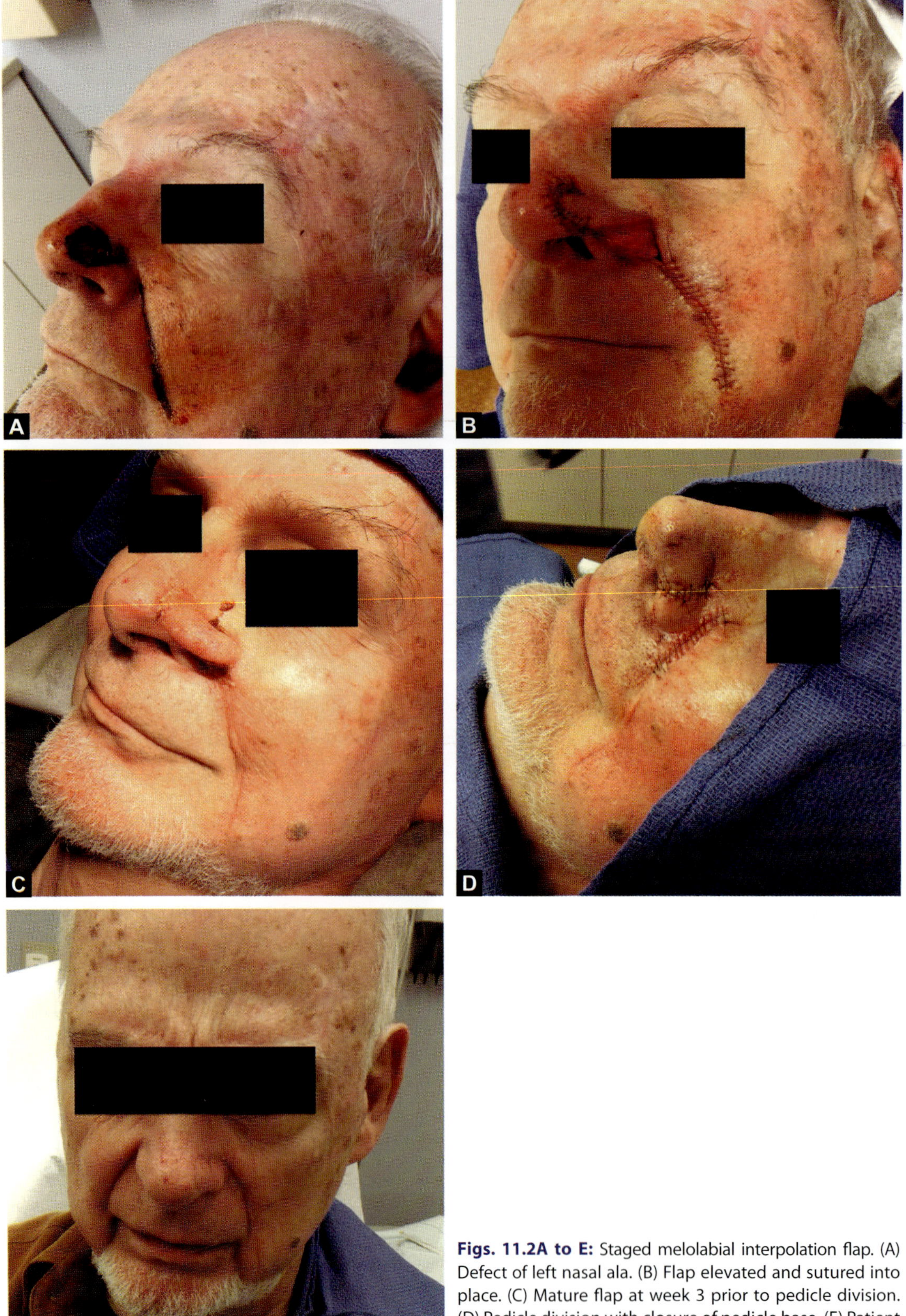


**Figs. 11.2A to E:** Staged melolabial interpolation flap. (A) Defect of left nasal ala. (B) Flap elevated and sutured into place. (C) Mature flap at week 3 prior to pedicle division. (D) Pedicle division with closure of pedicle base. (E) Patient at 2-month follow-up without revision or resurfacing.

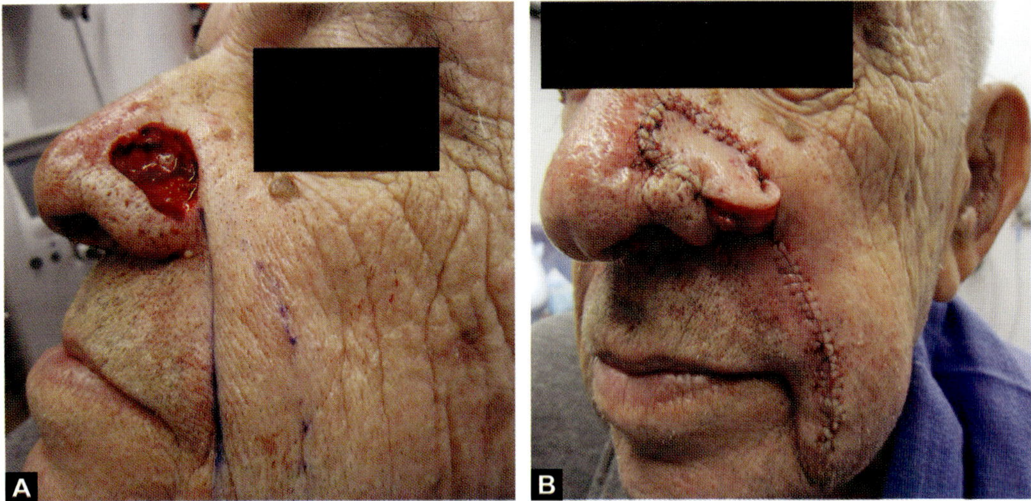


**Figs. 11.3A and B:** Staged melolabial interpolation flap. (A) Defect of left nasal ala, supra-ala, and sidewall. (B) Flap elevated and sutured into place.

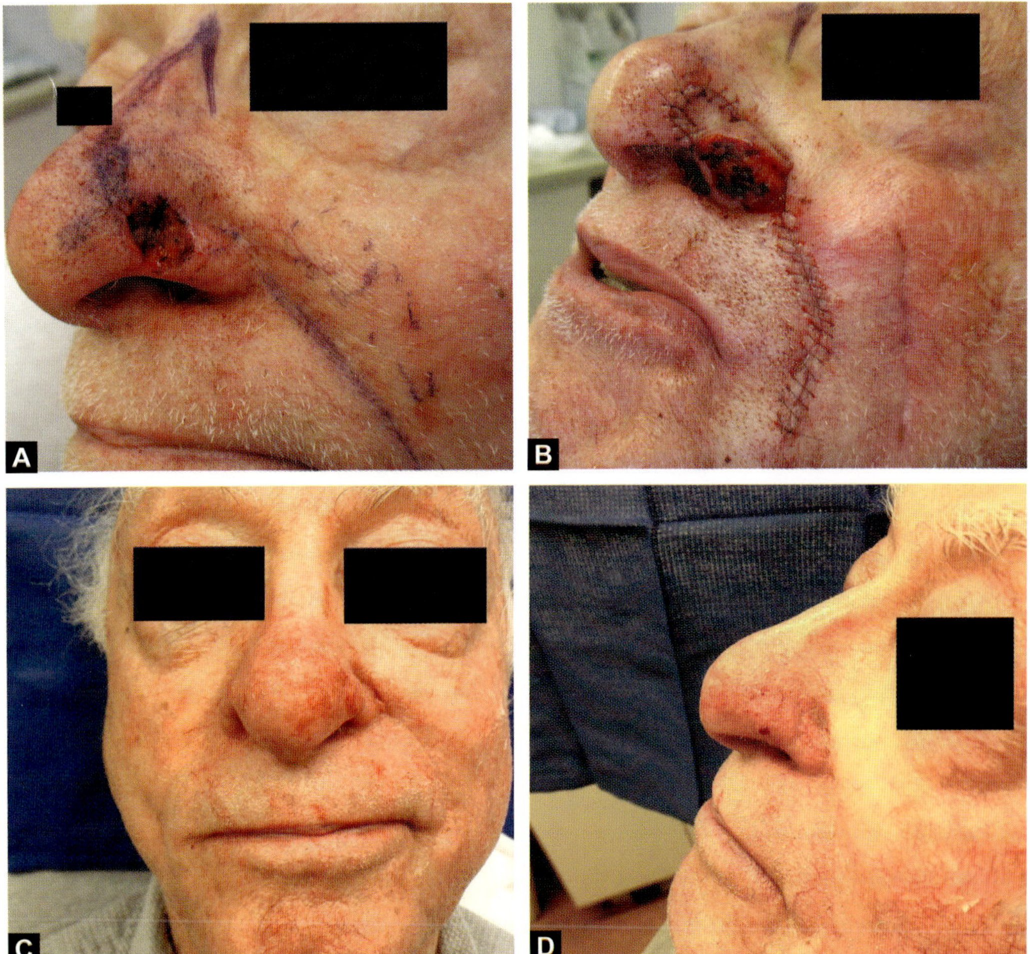


**Figs. 11.4A to D:** Staged melolabial interpolation flap. (A) Defect of the left nasal ala encroaching upon alar rim. (B) Flap elevated and sutured into place. (C) Frontal view at 2-month follow-up. (D) Final result lateral view.

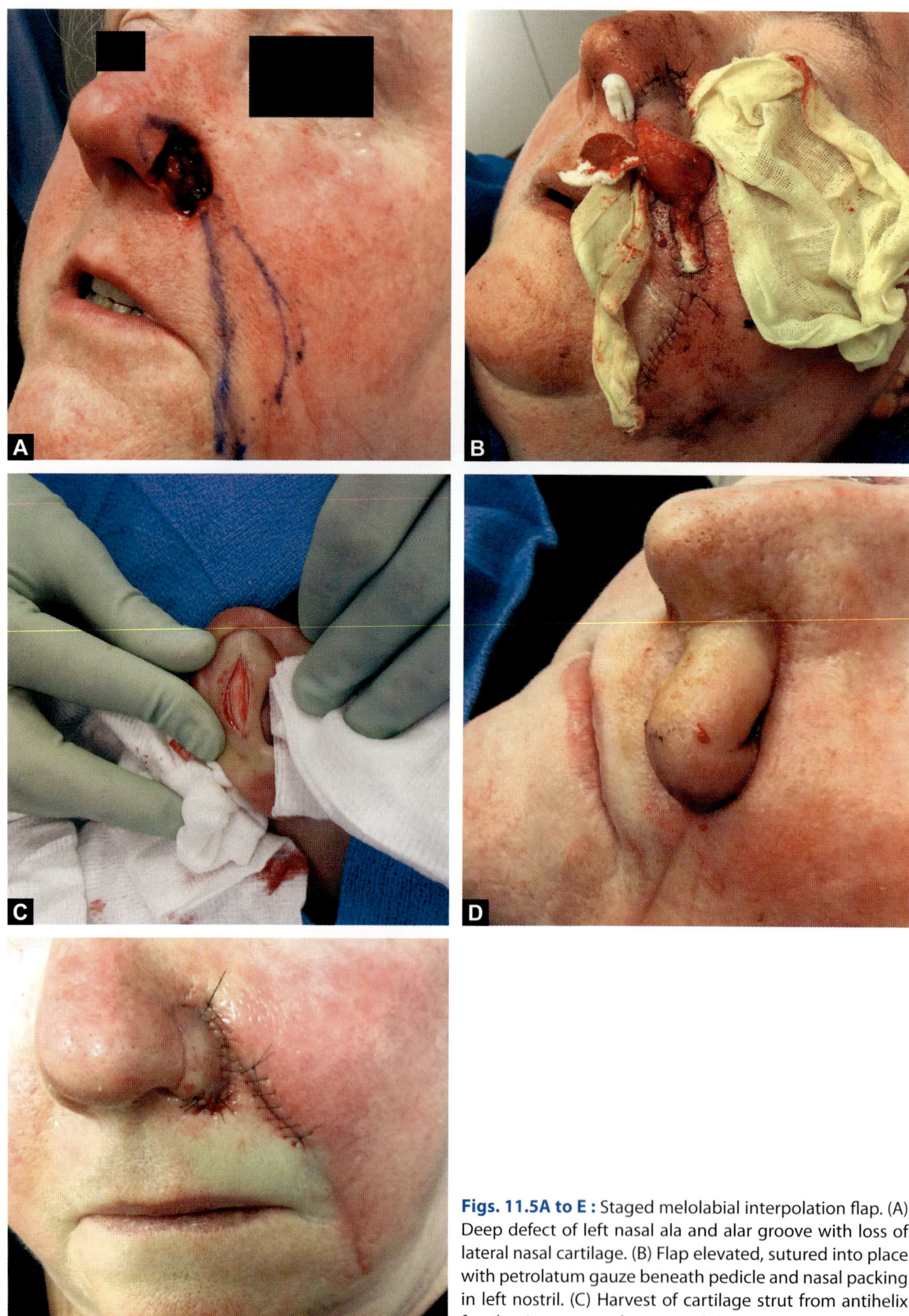


**Figs. 11.5A to E :** Staged melolabial interpolation flap. (A) Deep defect of left nasal ala and alar groove with loss of lateral nasal cartilage. (B) Flap elevated, sutured into place with petrolatum gauze beneath pedicle and nasal packing in left nostril. (C) Harvest of cartilage strut from antihelix for alar rim structural support. (D) Mature pedicle prior to division at week 3. (E) Following division of pedicle.
*Courtesy*: (C) S Brian Jiang, MD, San Diego, California, USA.

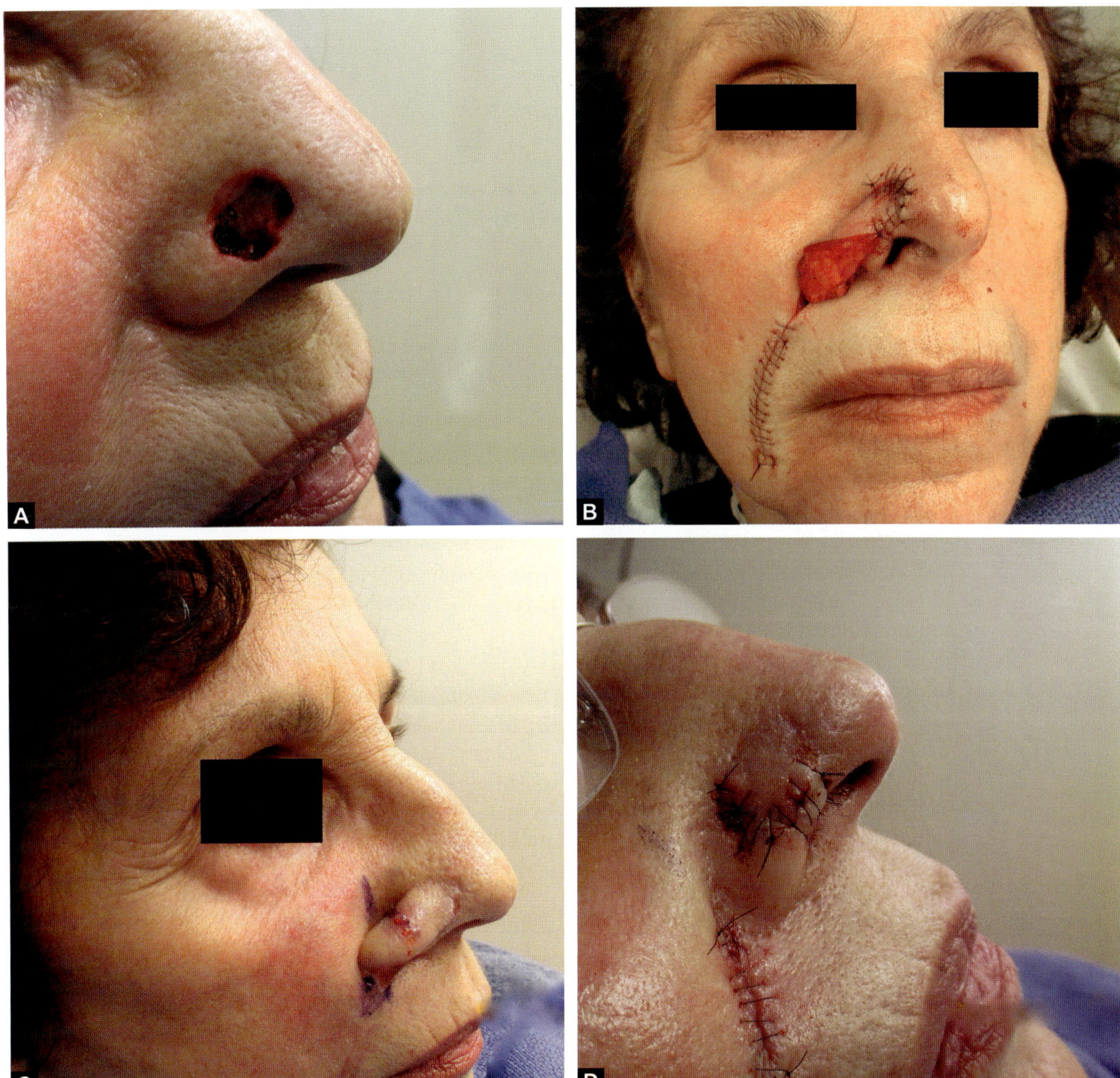


**Figs. 11.6A to D:** Staged melolabial interpolation flap. (A) Defect of right nasal ala. (B) Flap elevated and sutured into place. (C) Mature pedicle prior to division at week 3. (D) Following division of pedicle.

and triangular fossa, a staged pull-through interpolation flap can also be employed (Figs. 11.8 and 11.9).

## *Planning and Execution*

When approaching a mastoid interpolation flap the surgeon must first fashion a template based upon the auricular defect to be repaired and then place this on the postauricular scalp for appropriate sizing of the flap. Prior to incision of the flap the surgeon must take great care to ensure adequate length and width of the flap to be advanced over the helix. The flap is then incised from the postauricular sulcus back to the hairline to the level of subcutaneous fat and elevated above mastoid fascia (Fig. 11.10B). It is then

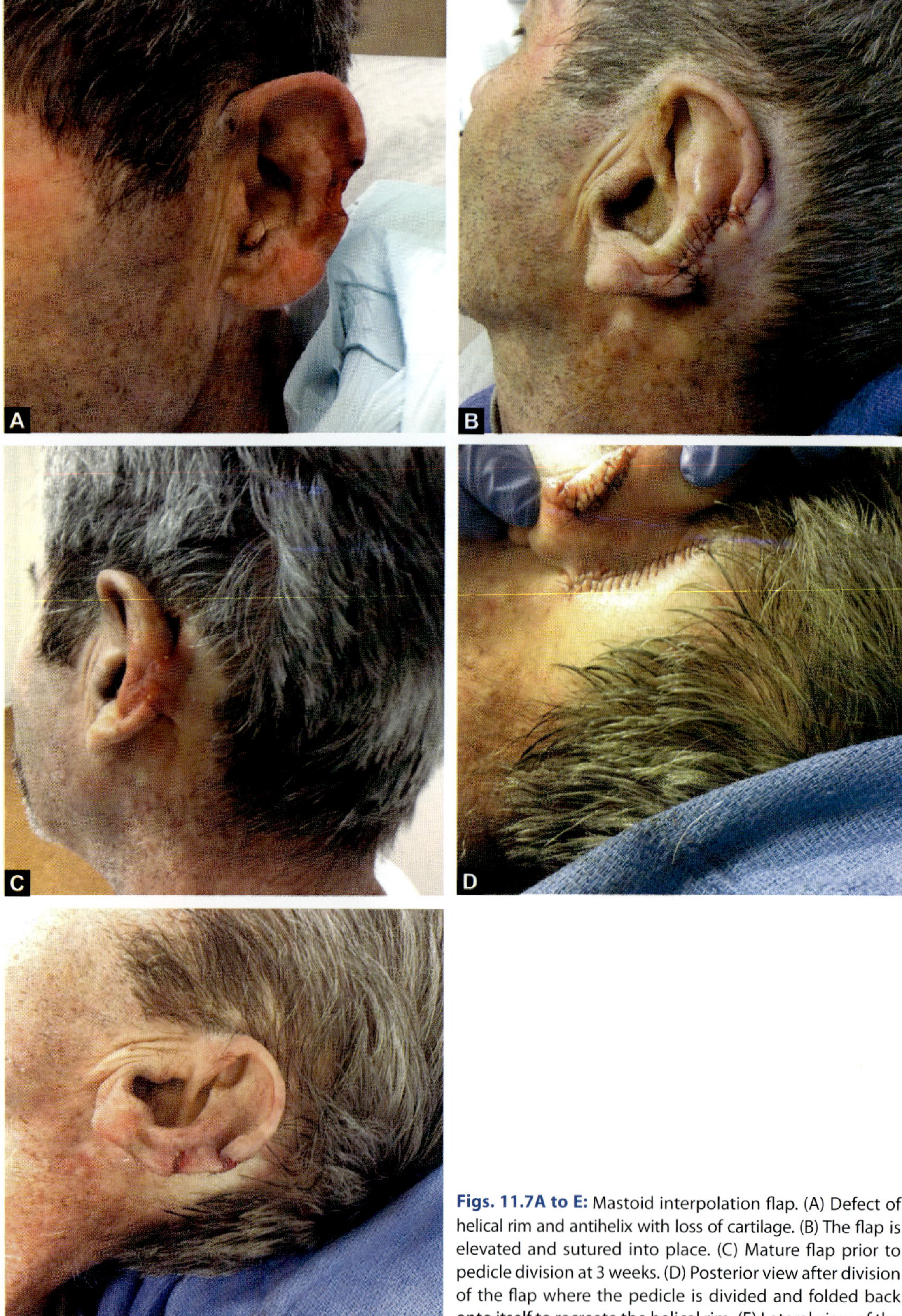

**Figs. 11.7A to E:** Mastoid interpolation flap. (A) Defect of helical rim and antihelix with loss of cartilage. (B) The flap is elevated and sutured into place. (C) Mature flap prior to pedicle division at 3 weeks. (D) Posterior view after division of the flap where the pedicle is divided and folded back onto itself to recreate the helical rim. (E) Lateral view of the ear following division.

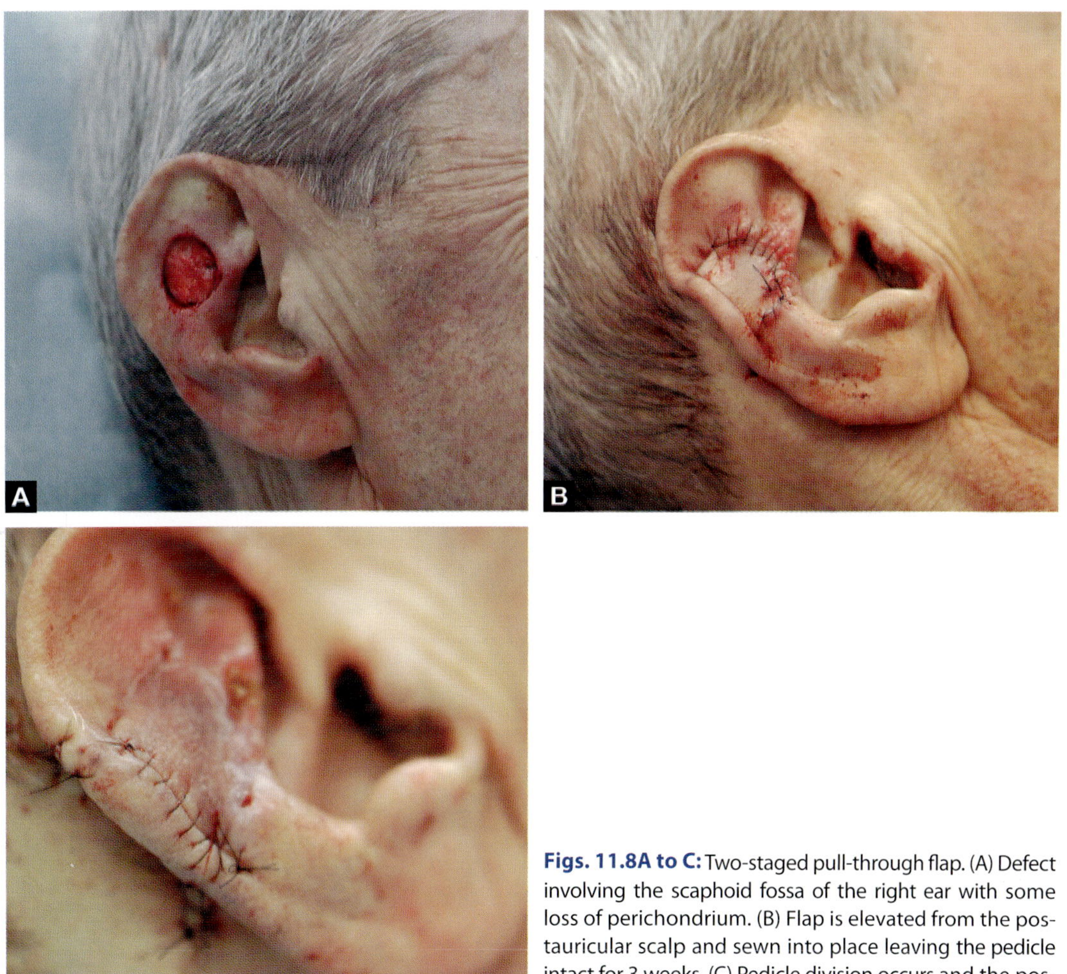


**Figs. 11.8A to C:** Two-staged pull-through flap. (A) Defect involving the scaphoid fossa of the right ear with some loss of perichondrium. (B) Flap is elevated from the postauricular scalp and sewn into place leaving the pedicle intact for 3 weeks. (C) Pedicle division occurs and the posterior portion of the flap is sutured to the helical rim.

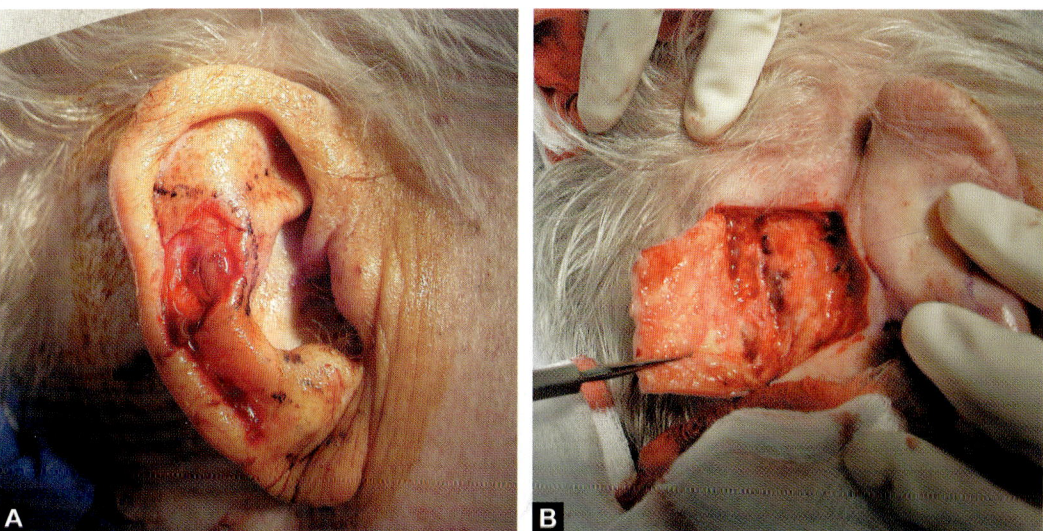


**Figs. 11.9A and B:** Two-staged pull-through flap. (A) Defect involving the scaphoid fossa, helical rim, and antihelix of the right ear with loss of cartilage. (B) Flap is elevated from the postauricular scalp above the level of the fascia and reflected back with a skin hook.

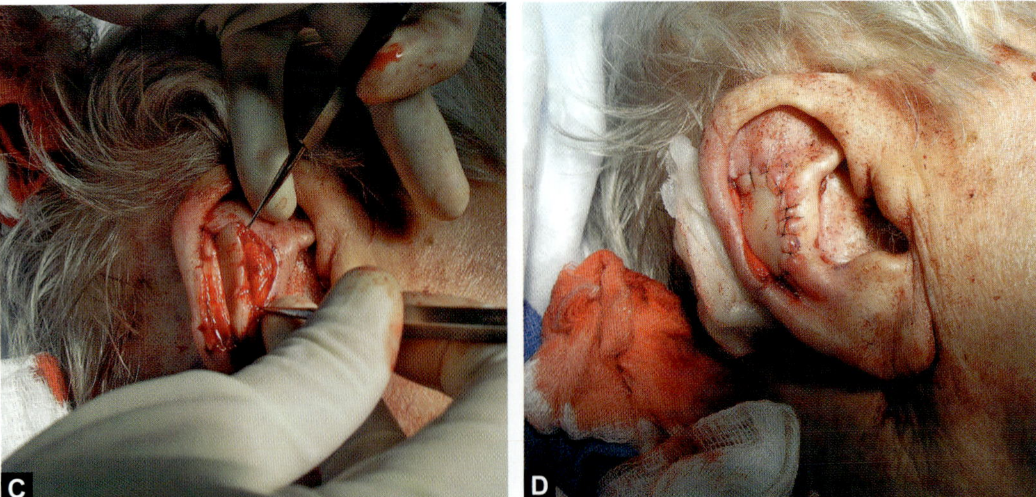

**Figs. 11.9C and D:** (C) The remainder of the anterior and posterior surface of the defect is incised to allow for a window to pull the pedicle through from posterior to anterior. (D) The flap is sewn into place to the anterior portion of the remaining antihelix.

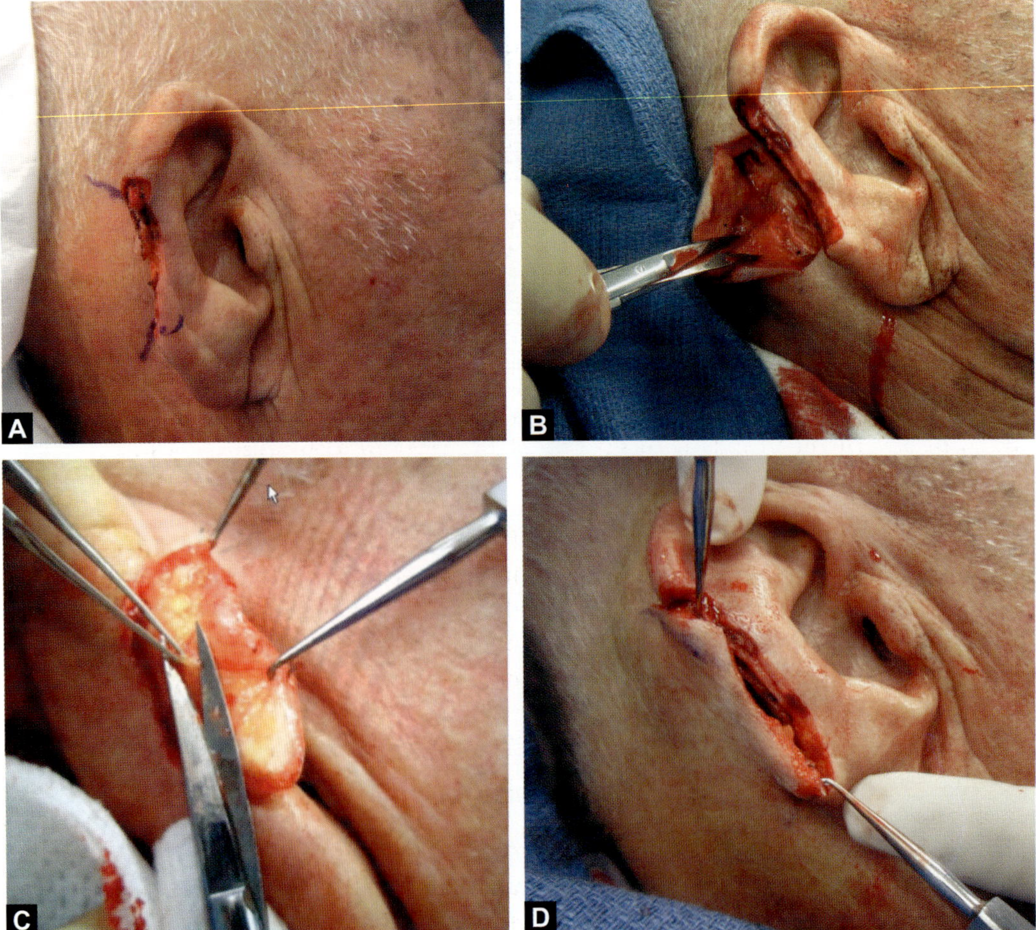

**Figs. 11.10A to D:** Mastoid interpolation flap. (A) Defect of helical rim with exposed cartilage. (B) The flap is incised and elevated from the post-auricular scalp above the level of the fascia and reflected back. The flap is elevated and dissected above the level of fascia. (C) The pedicle can then be meticulously thinned as necessary. (D) Skin hooks are used to ensure adequate reach of the flap to the recipient site.

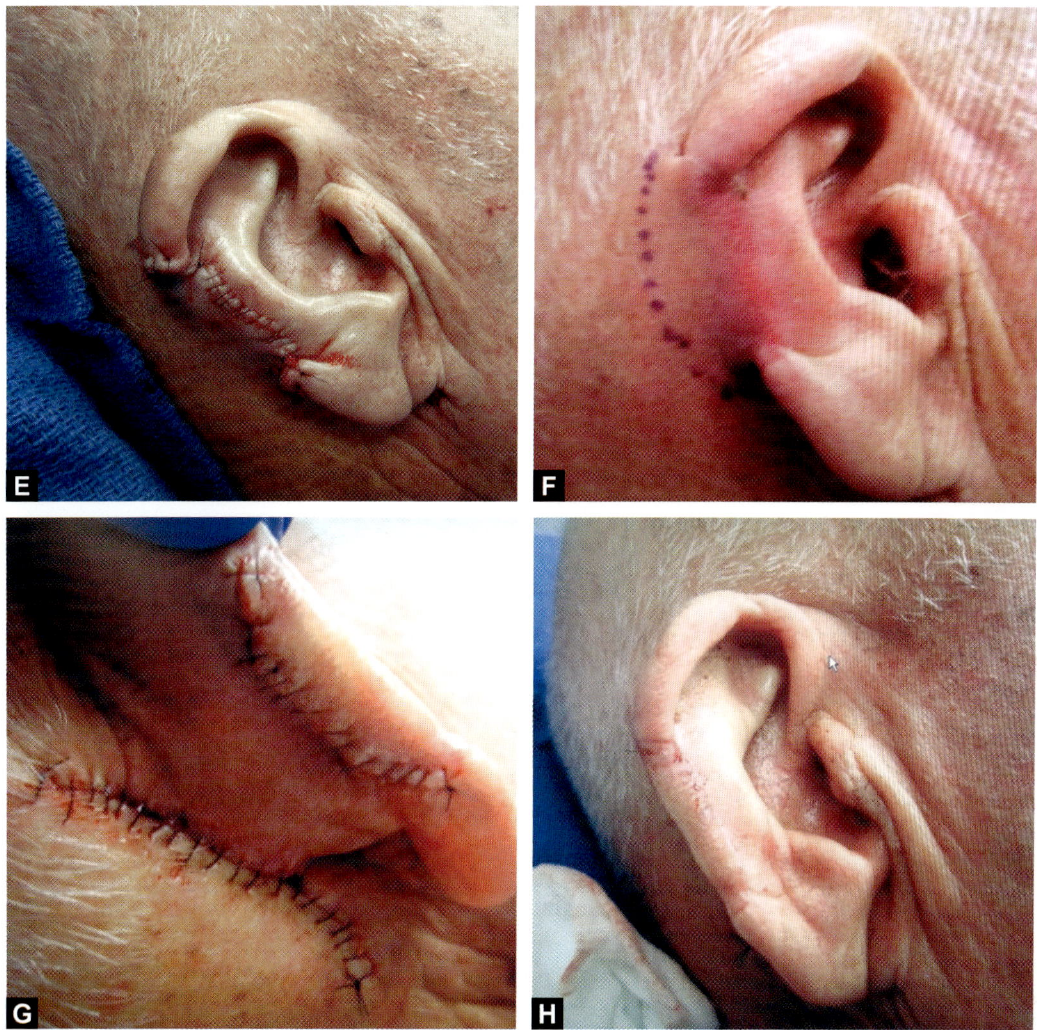


**Figs. 11.10E to H:** (E) The flap is sewn into place. (F) At 3 weeks the mature flap prior to division. (G) The pedicle is divided and the flap is sewn into place on the posterior surface of the helix and the donor site is closed. (H) Lateral view following pedicle division.

thinned prior to inset into the recipient defect. After elevation of the flap, skin hooks are used to gently advance the flap over the ear to ensure coverage without tension that could compromise its viability and survival (Fig. 11.10D).

Once it is determined that the flap has adequate reach without tension in horizontal and vertical planes to cover the defect, adequate hemostasis of the posterior bed of the flap should be ensured to avoid postoperative bleeding. In addition, some surgeons favor the use of hemostatic agents or dressings followed by packing of the posterior surface of the flap, which remain in place for variable periods of time. The flap can then be sewn into the recipient defect with either one or two layers of sutures depending on tension and surgeon preference. In 3 weeks, the pedicle can be divided near the scalp and the remaining portion of the flap will be curved over the helix and posterior ear where it recreates the helical rim (Figs. 11.10 to 11.13). At times through-and-through sutures are used for the helical portion of the flap in order to secure the healed anterior portion of the flap to the newly inset posterior portion. The portion of the mastoid scalp that served as the donor or base of the flap can be left to heal by secondary intention, closed primarily, or covered with a full-thickness skin graft.

Similarly, a two-staged interpolated banner style pedicle flap can be performed for deep defects of the anterior auricle using preauricular skin between the tragus and sideburn as the donor.[14] Alternatively, postauricular skin can be used (Figs. 11.14A to H). The pedicle can be based superiorly or inferiorly based depending on whether it is used to cover a defect on the upper or lower anterior ear. This is done as

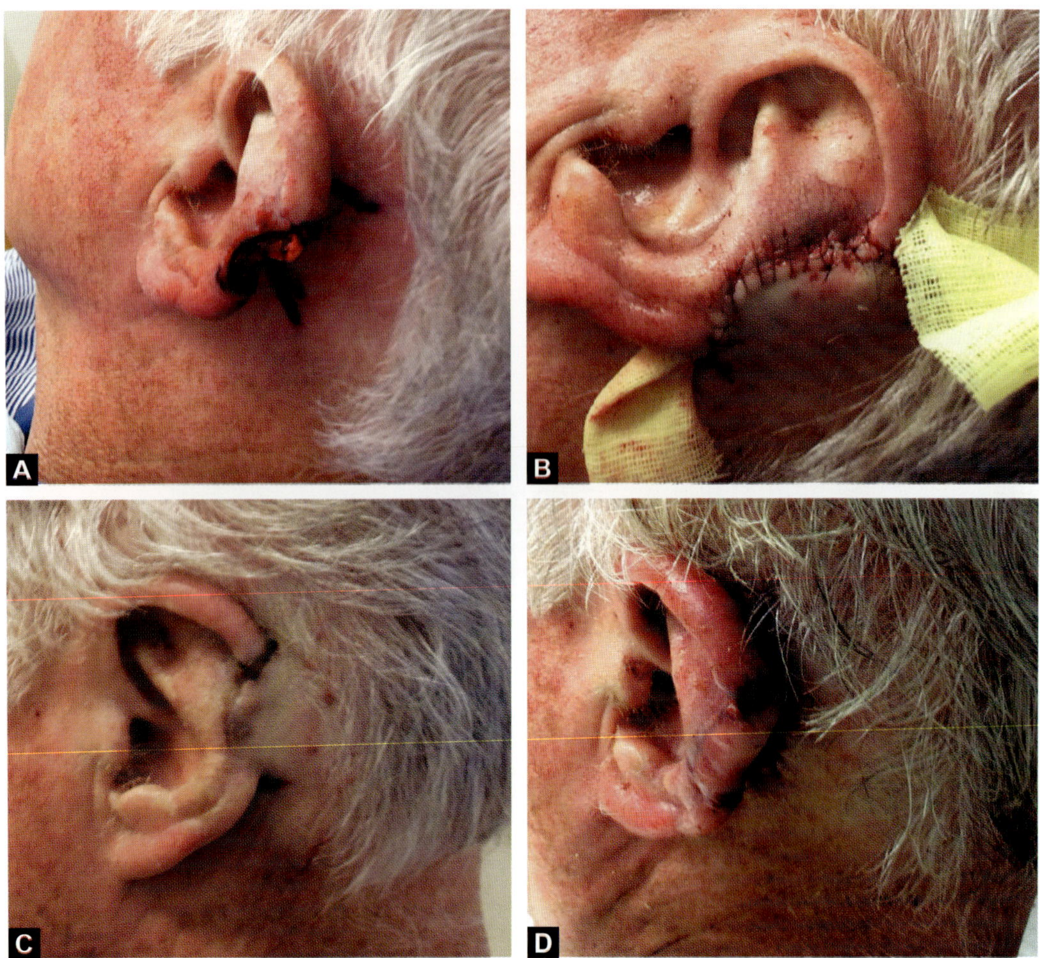


**Figs. 11.11A to D:** Mastoid interpolation flap. (A) Defect of mid-helical rim with exposed cartilage. (B) The flap is elevated and sutured into place with petrolatum gauze placed beneath the pedicle. (C) Mature flap prior to pedicle division at 3 weeks. (D) Posterior view after division of the flap with primary closure of the donor site.

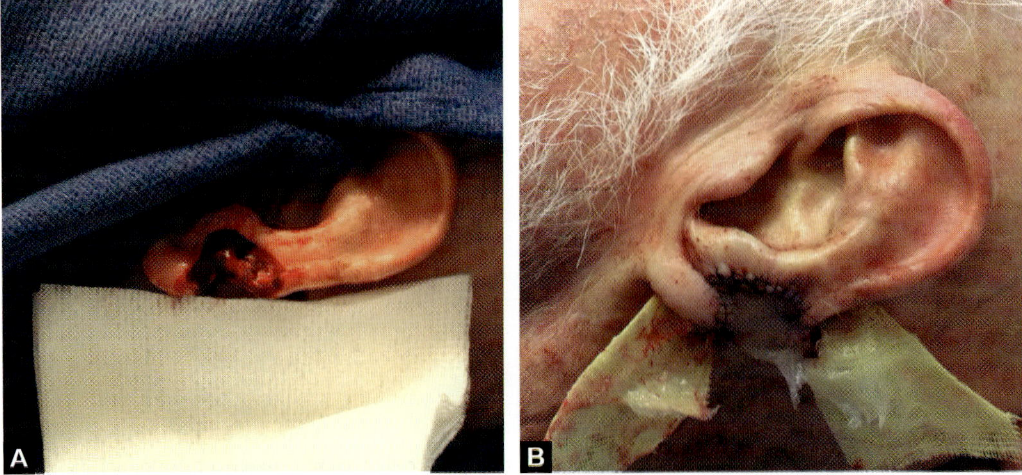


**Figs. 11.12A and B:** Mastoid interpolation flap. (A) Defect encompassing the lower helical rim and encroaching upon the lobule and posterior portion of the tragus with exposed cartilage. (B) The flap is elevated and sutured into place.

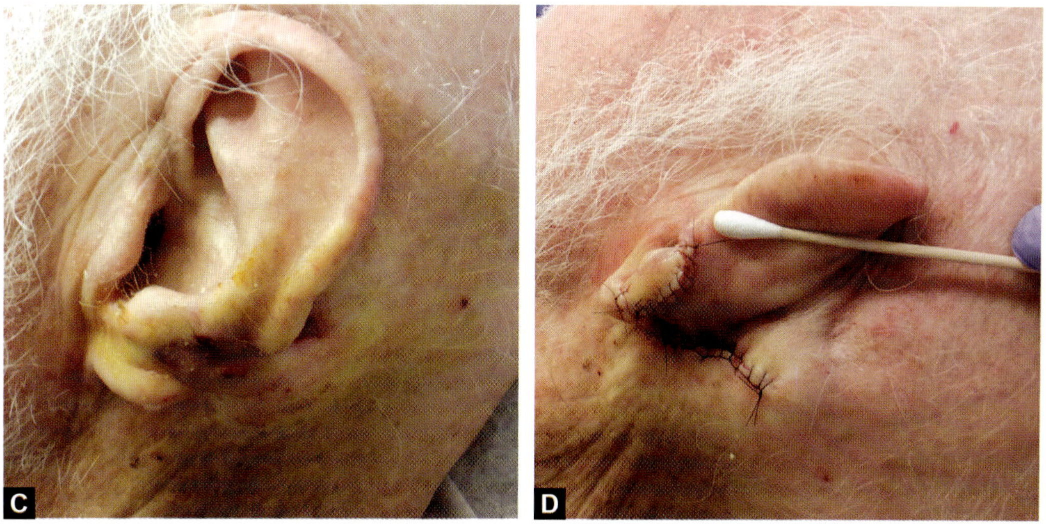

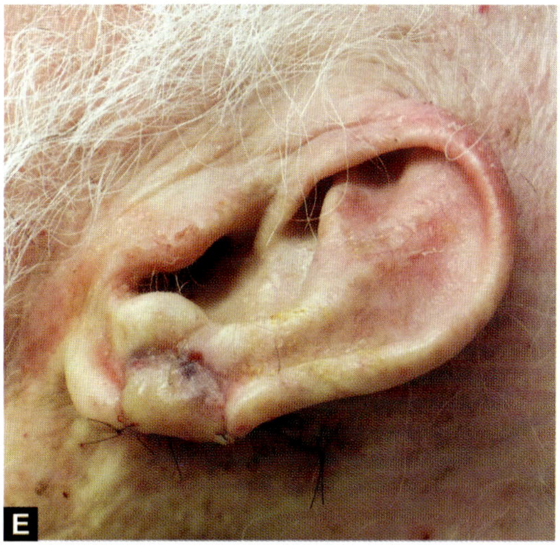

**Figs. 11.12C to E:** (C) Mature flap prior to pedicle division at 3 weeks. (D) Posterior view after division of the flap. (E) Lateral view of the ear following division.

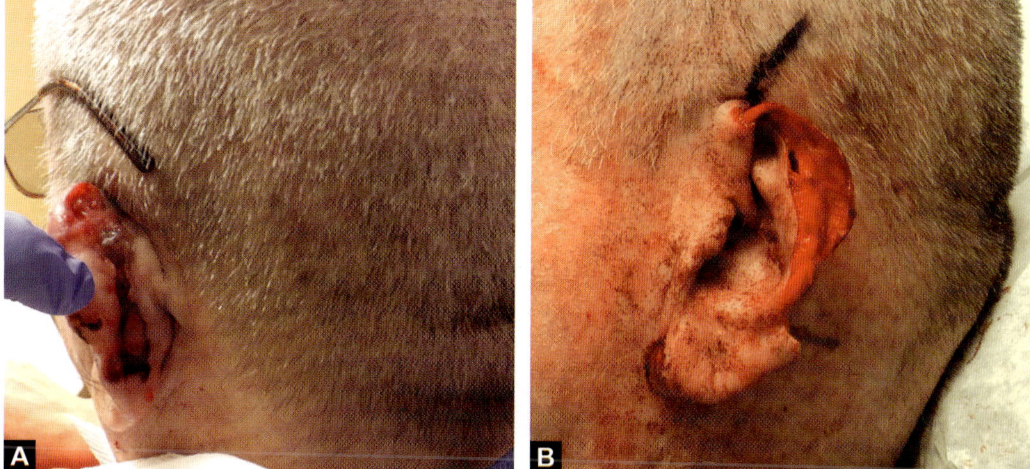

**Figs. 11.13A and B:** Mastoid interpolation flap. (A) A neglected infiltrative basal cell carcinoma of the posterior auricle prior to Mohs micrographic surgery. (B) Complete loss of the upper two-third of the helical rim, antihelix, and scaphoid fossa with a thin layer of cartilage remaining following Mohs extirpation (lateral view).

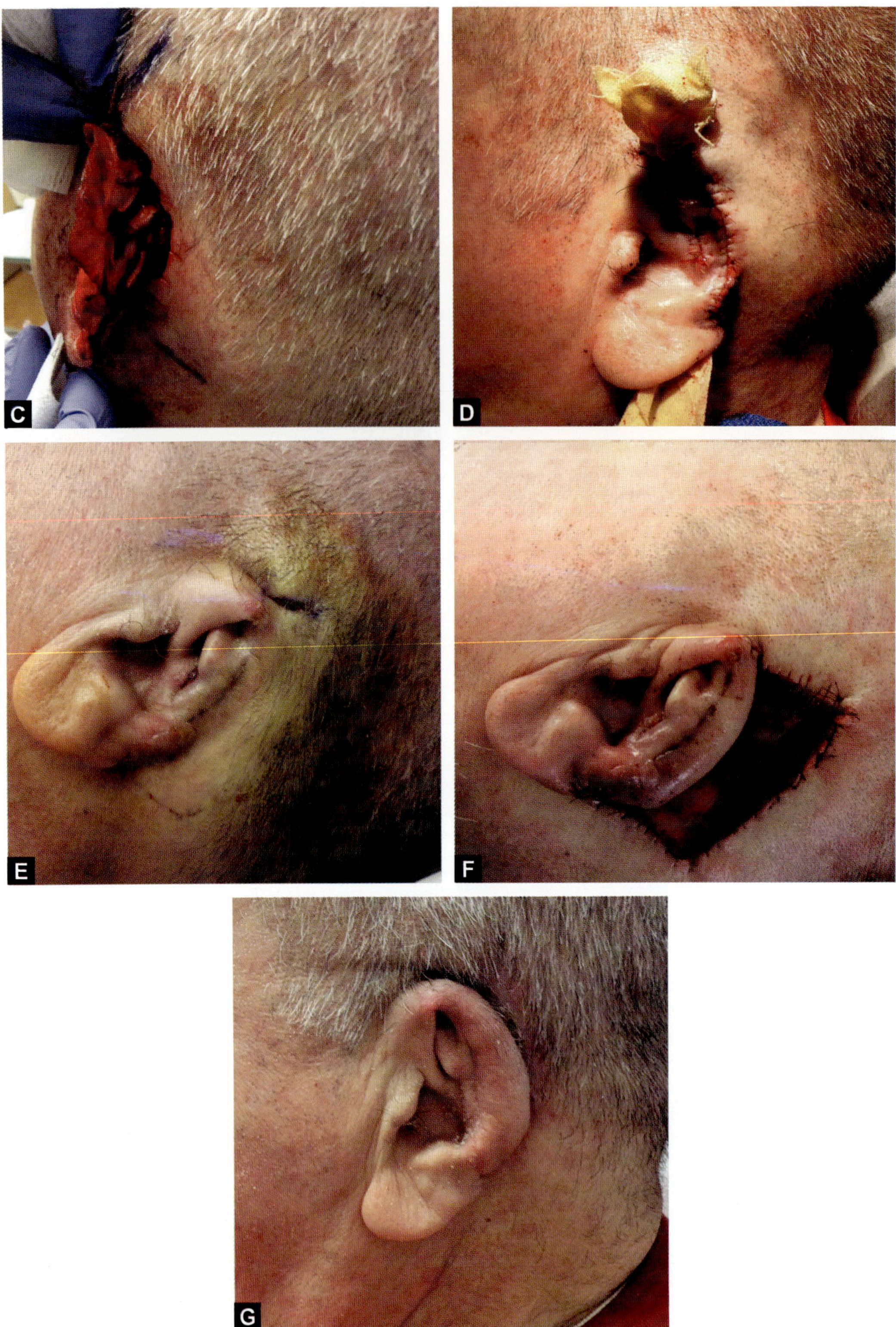


**Figs. 11.13C to G:** (C) Near total loss of the posterior auricle following Mohs extirpation of the tumor (posterior view). (D) The flap is elevated and sewn into place; petrolatum gauze separates the pedicle from the postauricular scalp. (E) Mature flap prior to pedicle division at 3 weeks. (F) Following division of the pedicle, the flap is sewn to the posterior surface of the auricle and the donor scalp is covered with a xenograft sewn into place with fast absorbing gut. (G) Two months follow-up.

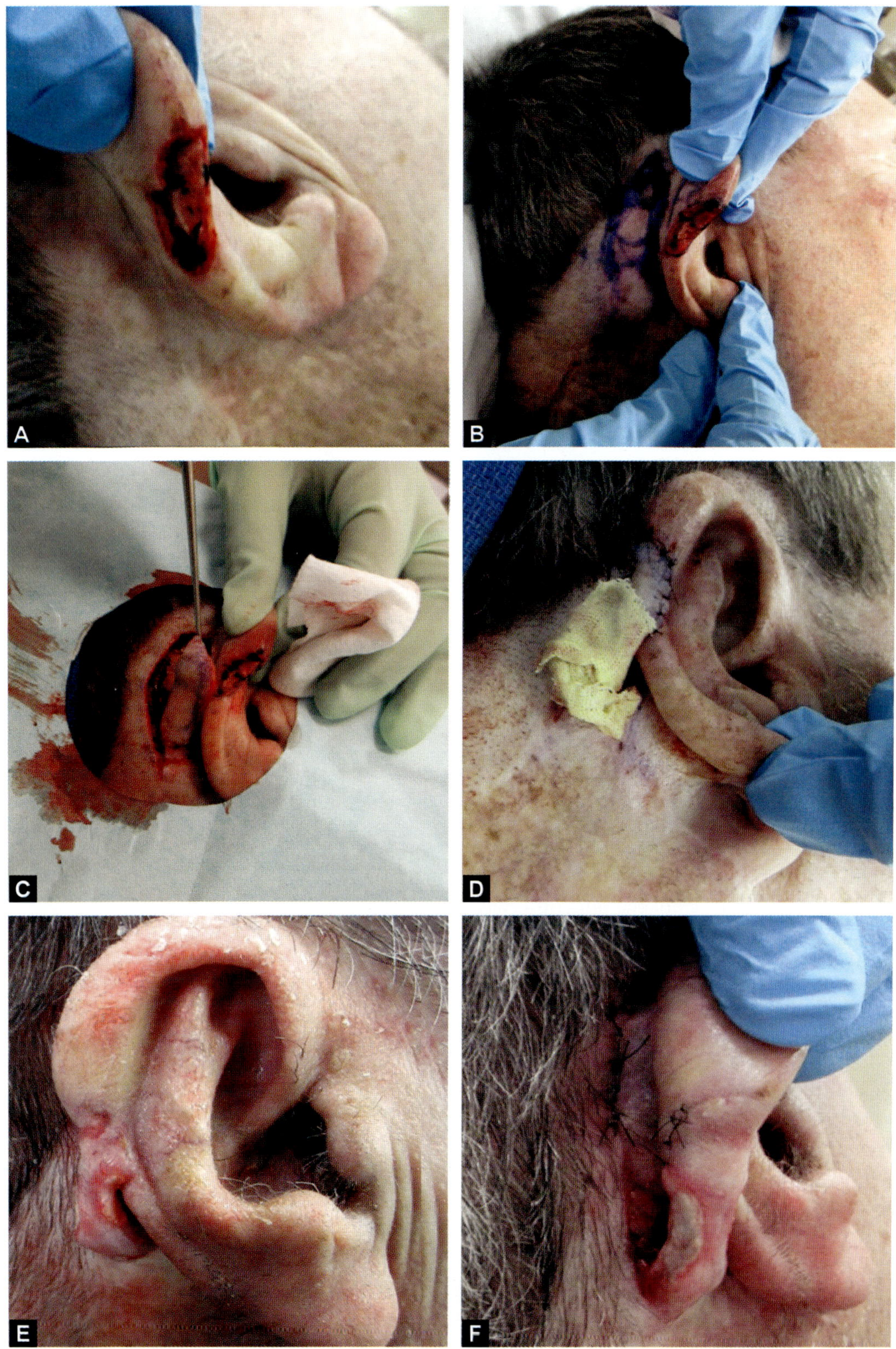


**Figs. 11.14A to F:** Postauricular staged banner flap for defect of the helix. (A) Defect following Mohs extirpation of tumor. (B) Design of flap on the postauricular scalp. (C) The flap is then cut and elevated with a skin hook. (D) The flap is sewn into place and wrapped with petrolatum gauze around the pedicle. (E) Mature flap prior to pedicle division at 2 weeks. (F) Posterior view of donor site prior to pedicle division at 2 weeks.

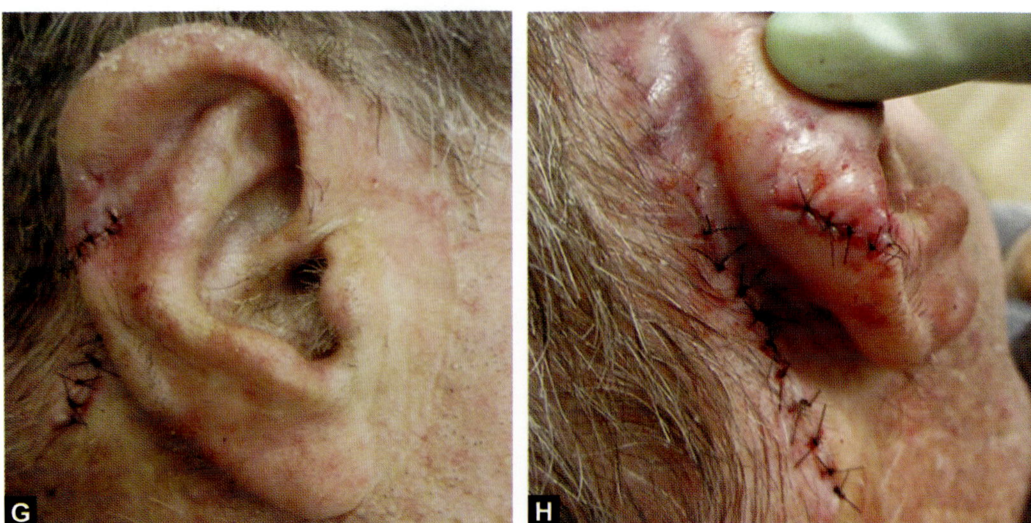

**Figs. 11.14G and H:** (G) Following division of the pedicle, the flap is sewn into place. (H) Posterior view showing the repaired donor site. *Courtesy*: S Brian Jiang, MD, San Diego, California, USA.

an alternative to the single-staged banner style transposition flap which is also employed for similar defects.[15]

### *Complications and Pitfalls*

In a review of 58 interpolated retroauricular flaps, there were no major complications, and the overall rate of minor complications was low; the most common complication was bleeding occurring in 18 patients with only 1 patient requiring electrocoagulation for hemostasis.[6] The authors reported 1 case of partial-thickness necrosis of a retroauricular interpolation flap in a smoker, but otherwise observed no cases of flap necrosis. Given the involvement of auricular cartilage in this flap, chondritis is occasionally observed and can be treated effectively with nonsteroidal anti-inflammatories until resolution. In terms of technical pitfalls, surgeons may at times underestimate the distance necessary to reach from the mastoid scalp to the anteromedial portion of the auricular defect. This can be avoided by precise measurement prior to incision of the flap, and correction when necessary via extension toward the hairline of the base of the pedicle flap if undersized.

## Paramedian Forehead Flap

### *Applications*

Paramedian forehead flaps are invaluable for repairing medium to large defects of the nose and periocular region. It is considered to be the preferred method for covering nasal defects too large to repair with full-thickness skin grafts, local nasal transposition, rotation or advancement flaps, composite auricular grafts, or melolabial interpolation flaps. The rich blood supply of the paramedian forehead flap and the sebaceous quality of the donor forehead makes them excellent choices for reconstruction of large and deep nasal defects (Figs. 11.15A to F). The paramedian forehead flap is an axial flap that is supplied by the supratrochlear artery which is consistently located 1.7–2.2 cm from the glabella.[16] The supratrochlear artery exits the orbit by piercing the orbital septum, passing under the orbicularis oculi and over the corrugator supercilii before passing through the orbicularis and frontalis muscles and into superficial subcutaneous tissue.[16] Some surgeons employ Doppler to confirm the location of the supratrochlear artery prior to harvesting the flap. While the supratrochlear artery is considered to be the main nourishment for this flap, studies have suggested that the secondary supply is significant and that the flap could likely survive even when the ipsilateral supratrochlear artery was occluded.[17,18] The pedicle of the paramedian forehead flap contains skin, subcutaneous tissue, muscle, and the supratrochlear artery.

### *Planning and Execution*

When approaching a nasal defect located primarily on one side of the nose, the contralateral paramedian location should be used as the pedicle base. This minimizes pedicle rotation and thus torsion on the flap and its vascular supply.

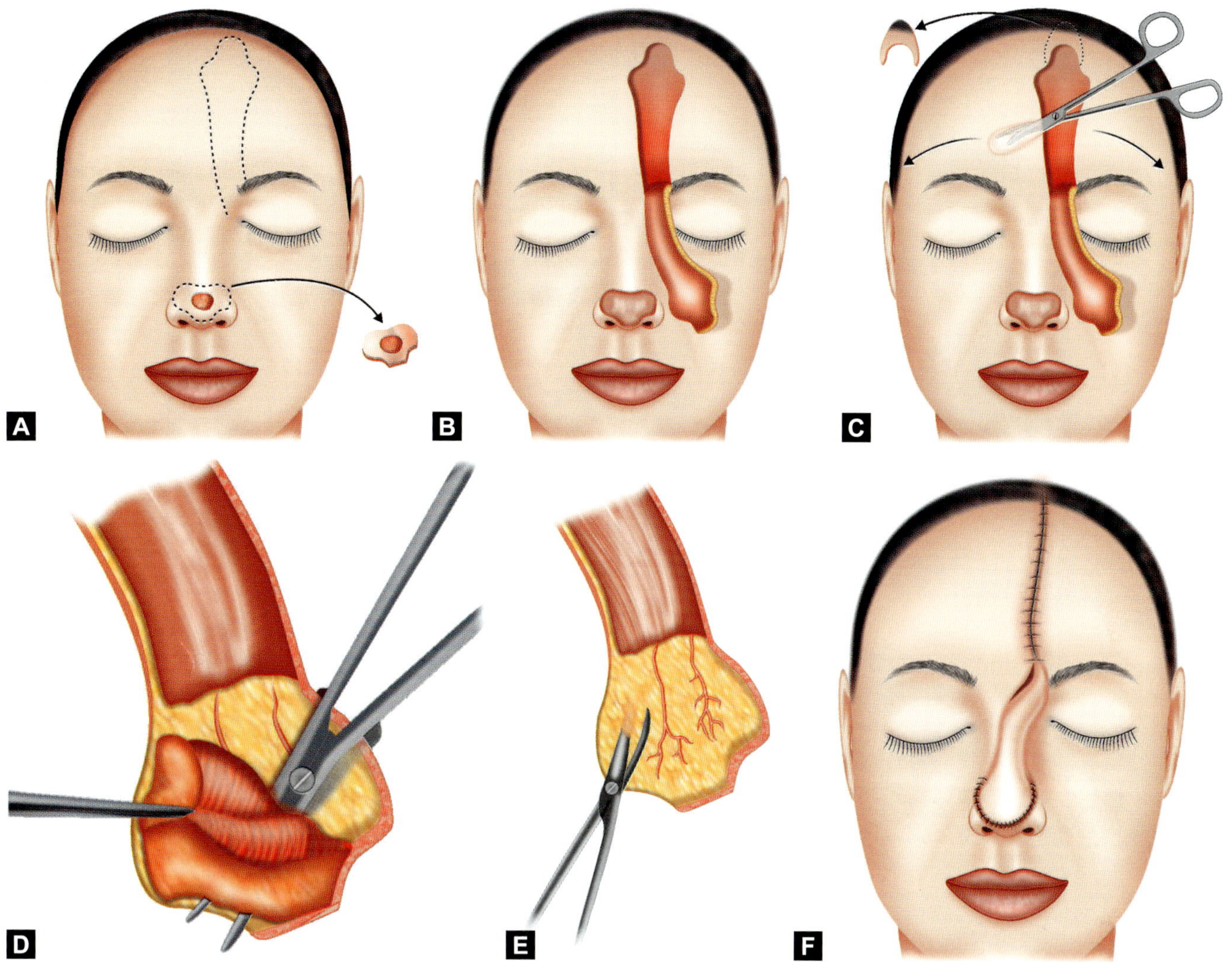


**Figs. 11.15A to F:** Paramedian forehead flap schematic. (A) A nasal tip defect with the base of a paramedian forehead flap drawn over the medial eyebrow with the pedicle 2 cm from midline and a vertical axis. (B) The flap is elevated. (C) Undermining of the subfascial plane and removal of the standing cutaneous deformity allows for closure of the donor site. (D) The galea and frontalis muscle is removed from the distal flap. (E) The subcutaneous fat is thinned from the distal tip. (F) The flap is sutured in place at the recipient site and the donor site is closed.

The defect to be repaired should first be dissected down to perichondrium or periosteum in order to provide a uniformly deep and wide recipient site for the flap to be inset (Figs. 11.16 to 11.19). The nasal defect should be squared off to create an angular defect rather than curvilinear since round defects are more likely to undergo concentric scar contraction and result in a trapdoor deformity.[19] A template of the recipient defect should be made with foil or a telfa pad and then be inverted and rotated and placed on the forehead at the superior portion of the future pedicle. It is important to ensure adequate length of the pedicle in order to avoid tension once it is rotated down into position over the defect (Fig. 11.20F). The preferred pedicle width for the paramedian forehead flap is generally 1.5 cm; however, pedicles as narrow as 1.0–1.2 cm have been reported.[4,5]

After the forehead is anesthetized with either supraorbital and supratrochlear nerve blocks, or local regional anesthesia, the flap is incised and elevated. Of note the authors favor using tumescent anesthesia on the forehead with 1.5 cc of 1% lidocaine with 1:100,000 epinephrine mixed with 10 cc normal saline and 0.5 cc sodium bicarbonate. The superior portion of the flap adjacent to the hairline is incised to the level of frontalis muscle, whereas the inferior portion of the flap is incised to the subfascial plane just above periosteum. Blunt dissection around the

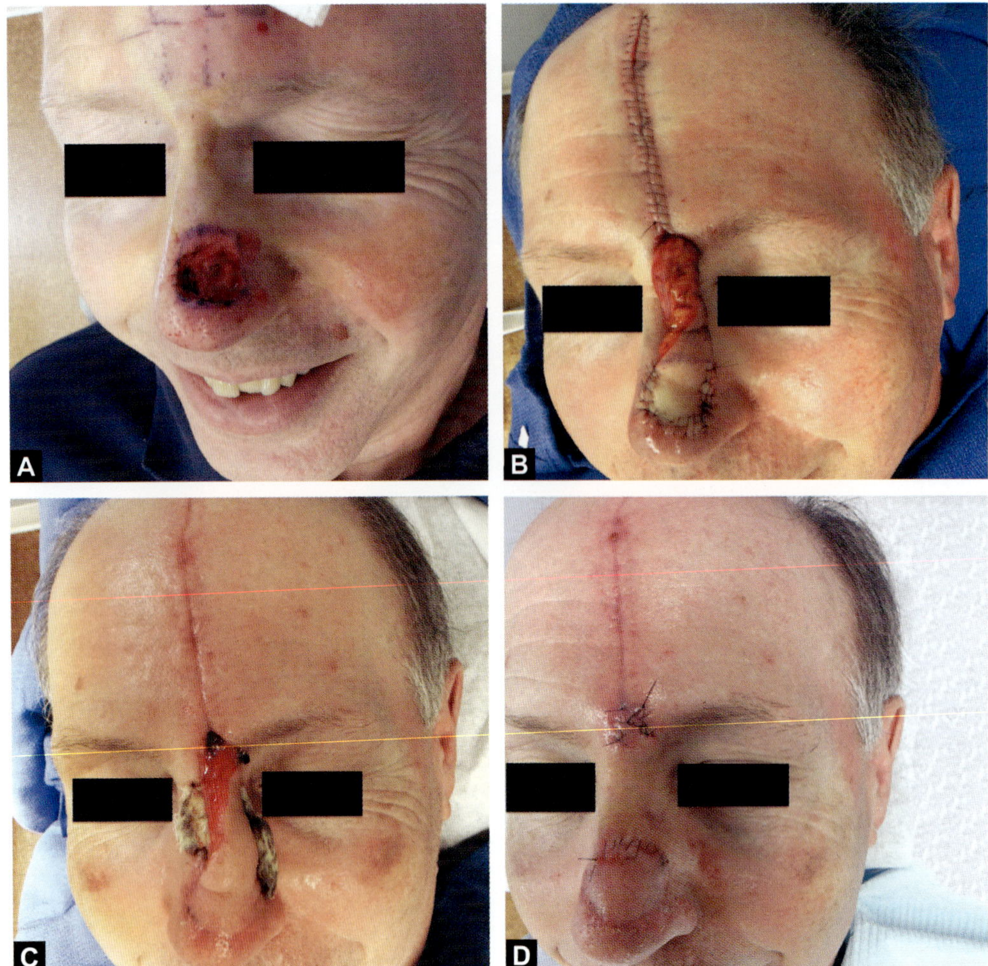

**Figs. 11.16A to D:** Paramedian forehead flap for a defect of the nasal tip. (A) Defect following Mohs extirpation of tumor and prior to skeletonization of the operative wound. (B) Flap at immediate closure with pedicle in place under little tension and entire forehead donor site closed. (C) Prior to pedicle division at 3 weeks. (D) Immediately following pedicle division, thinning of the flap and inset with closure of the forehead.

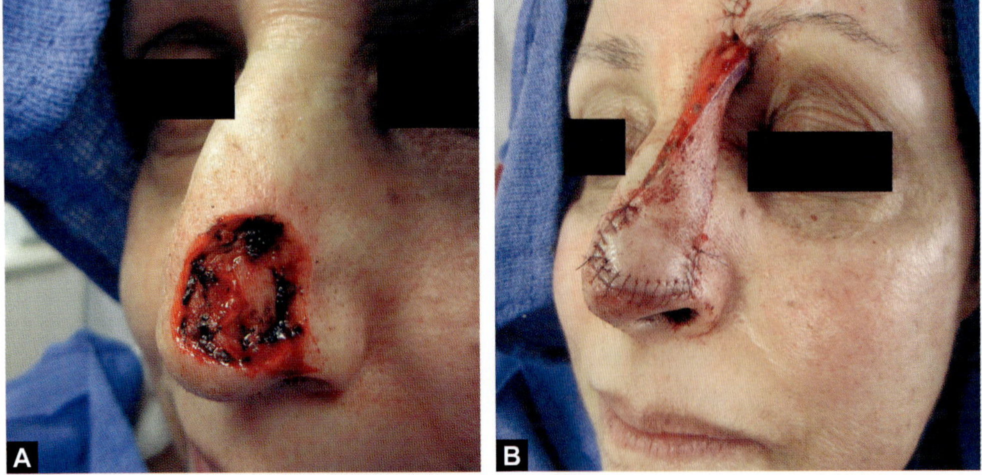

**Figs. 11.17A and B:** Paramedian forehead flap for a defect of the nasal tip, supratip, and medial ala. (A) Defect following Mohs extirpation of tumor and prior to skeletonization of the operative wound. (B) Flap at immediate closure with pedicle sewn in place under little tension.

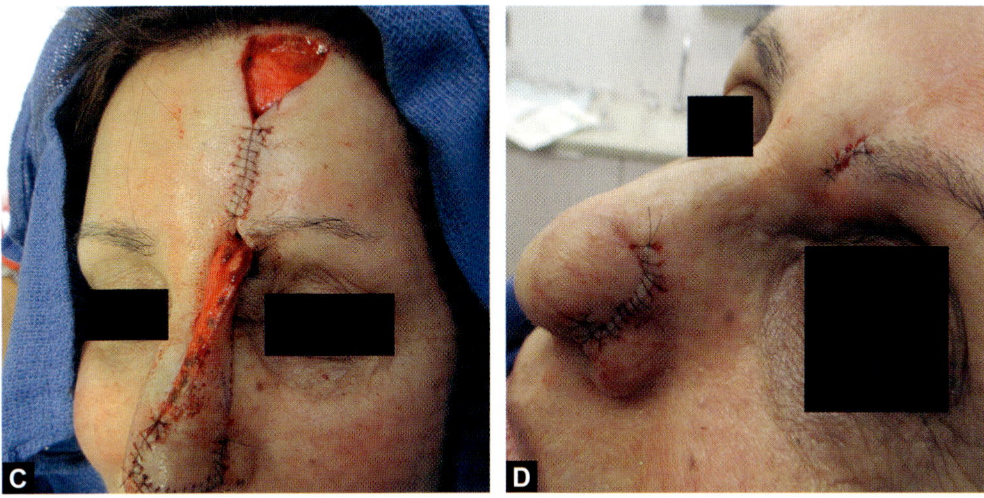


**Figs. 11.17C and D:** (C) In this case, the upper portion of the forehead donor site was left to heal by secondary intention. (D) Immediately following pedicle division, thinning of the flap, and inset.

pedicle is done to allow for mobility down toward the root of the nose with care not to disrupt the neurovascular bundle in the area of the corrugators. The flap is inset into the nasal recipient defect prior to undermining the forehead in the subfascial plane and performing a bilayered closure. At times the superior portion of the forehead donor site may not be closed completely due to excessive tension and can be left to heal by secondary intention with good cosmetic result (Fig. 11.17C).

The donor portion of the flap should be thinned of most of its subcutaneous fat in order to sit neatly in the recipient bed while retaining its subdermal vascular plexus. The flap is then pivoted in an arc and sutured into the recipient site with either one or two layers of sutures depending on surgeon preference, and at times tacking sutures to the base of the defect to ensure stability and tissue apposition. Hemostasis should be achieved on the stalk of the pedicle to prevent postoperative bleeding after the vasoconstrictive effects of the epinephrine in the local anesthetic have worn off. Some surgeons will use a hemostatic dressing for the exposed portion of the flap pedicle. The patient may return the following day to ensure that the flap is well vascularized and a dressing change can be done if necessary. The patient will return in 1 week for removal of top layer stitches from the forehead and nasal sites.

The pedicle is typically divided in 3 weeks. The division is often done at the superior margin of the defect thus releasing the superior portion of the pedicle. The nasal portion of the flap can then be trimmed and thinned so the superior portion can be sutured into the recipient site, typically with superficial sutures only as there is no wound tension. The glabellar portion of the pedicle or stump is then excised, the edges freshened, and the defect closed linearly if feasible. If granulation tissue is present at either the recipient site or the glabella, it can be excised or debrided allowing for precise closure of these areas. A bolster dressing can be placed over the nasal portion of the repair as with full-thickness skin grafts depending on surgeon preference, however, it is imperative that these dressings are not attached tightly as to impair circulation to the distal flap. At times forehead flaps can be combined with advancement or rotation flaps when the defect encompasses multiple anatomic subunits or entire subunits can be removed when multiple defects are present (Figs. 11.20 and 11.21).

## Complications and Pitfalls

The paramedian forehead flap is a well-vascularized interpolation flap and thus is rarely subject to flap necrosis. Out of 290 paramedian forehead flaps performed by one Mohs surgeon the most common complication was postoperative bleeding in 33 patients, all occurring within 24 hours of the procedure, and none requiring hospitalization.[6] The authors also reported two cases of total full-thickness necrosis, two cases of partial full-thickness necrosis, one case of full-thickness necrosis of the donor site, and six cases of partial thickness necrosis of the flap, noting that 8 of these 11 patients were tobacco users, and 4 of

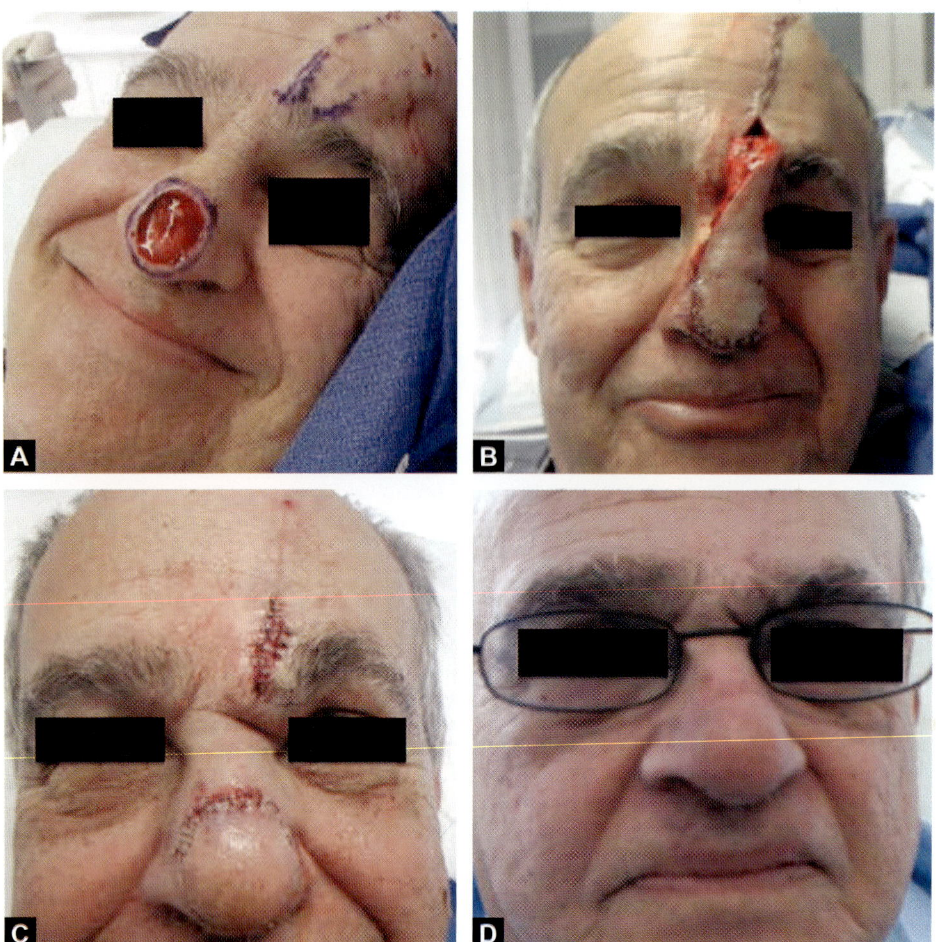

**Figs. 11.18A to D:** Paramedian forehead flap for a defect of the nasal tip. (A) Defect following Mohs extirpation of tumor and prior to skeletonization of the operative wound. (B) Flap at immediate closure with pedicle in place. (C) After pedicle division, thinning of the flap and inset with closure of the forehead. (D) Final result.

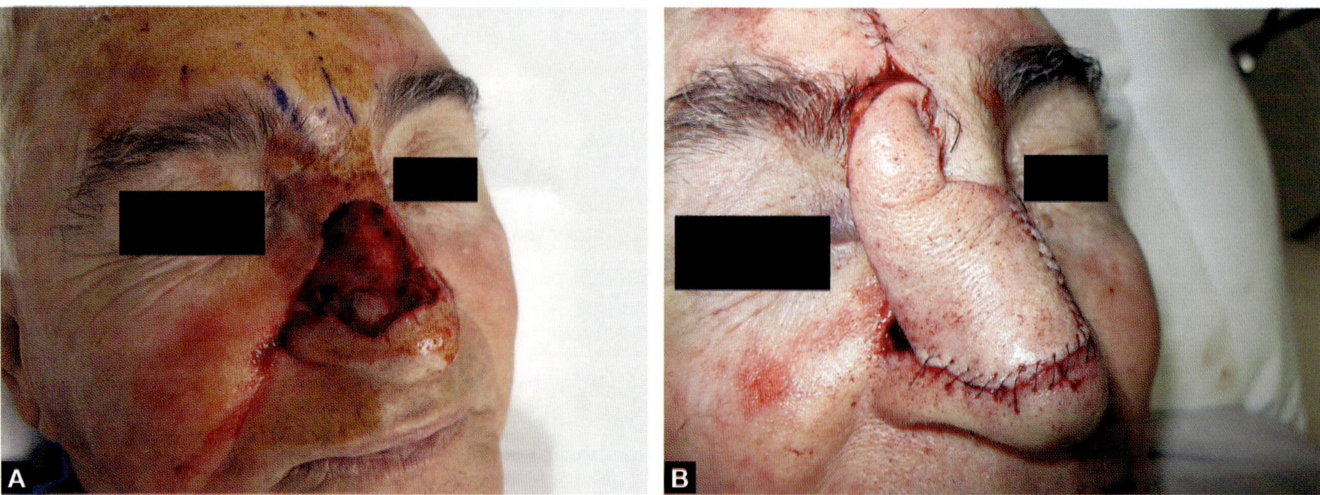

**Figs. 11.19A and B:** Paramedian forehead flap for a defect of the right nasal dorsum and tip. (A) Defect following Mohs extirpation of tumor with exposed lateral nasal cartilage. (B) Flap at immediate closure with pedicle in place.

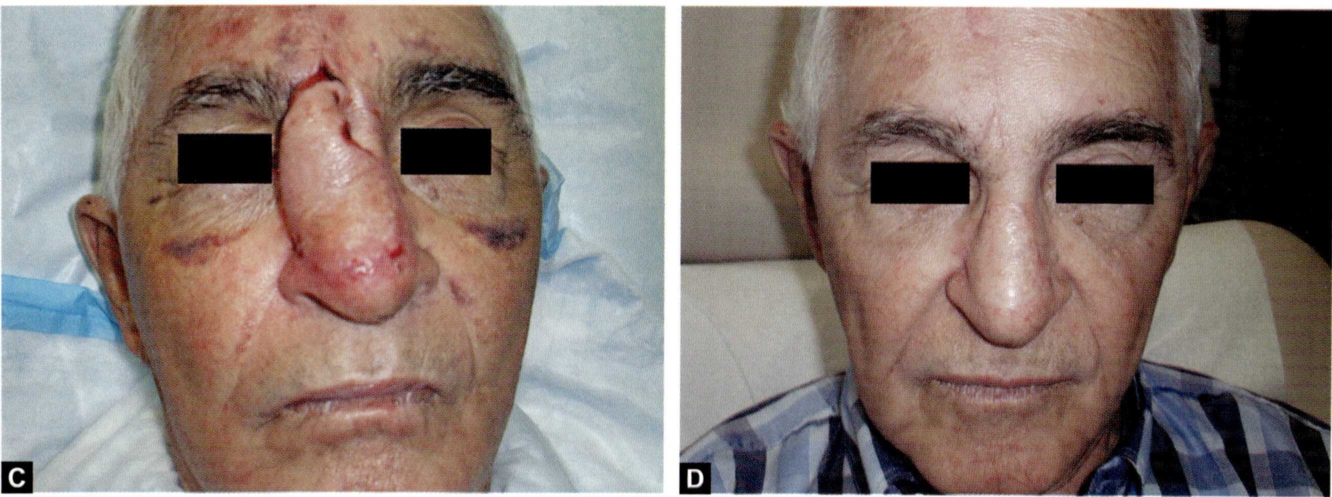


**Figs. 11.19C and D:** (C) Mature flap at week 3 prior to pedicle division. (D) Result 2 months postoperatively.

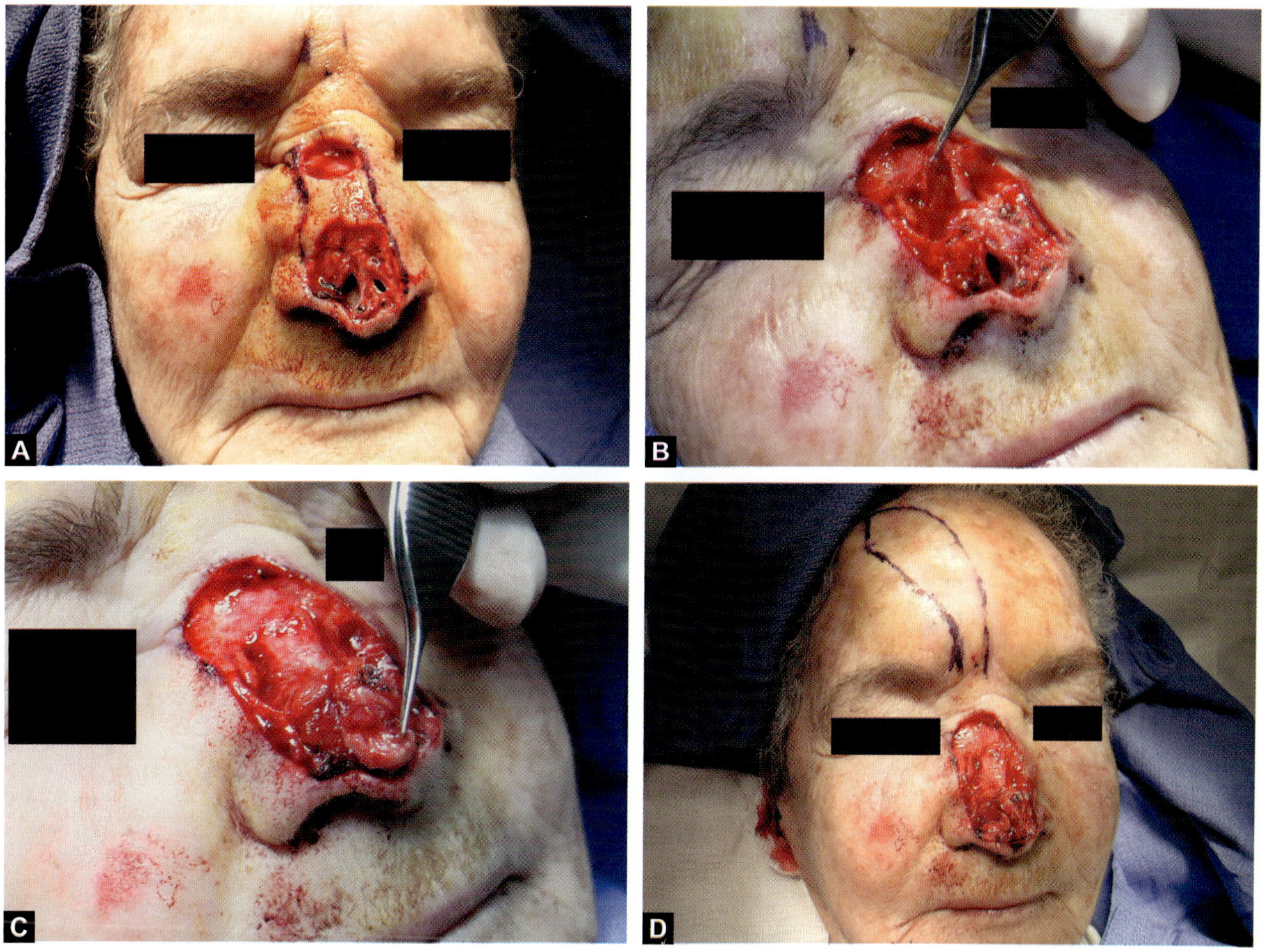

**Figs. 11.20A to D:** Paramedian forehead flap for 2 complex defects of the nasal dorsum and tip repaired en bloc. (A) Adjacent defects following Mohs surgery of the nasal dorsum and a through and through defect of the nasal tip. (B) Following excision of the subunit creating one larger defect with exposed mucosa and cartilage. (C) Mucosal hinge flap lifted and moved into place. (D) Mucosal lining and cartilage in place and forehead flap drawn prior to incision and elevation.

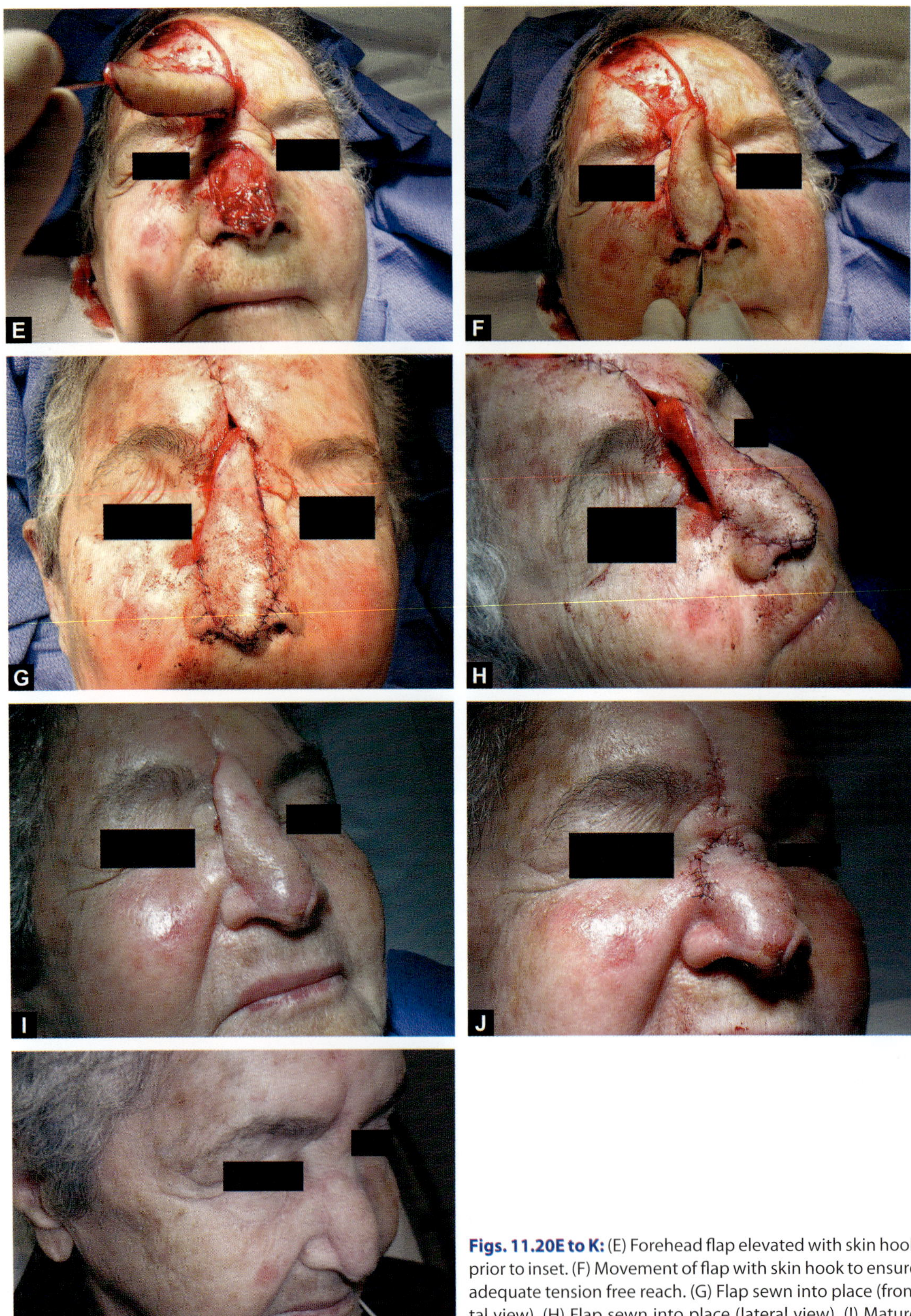


**Figs. 11.20E to K:** (E) Forehead flap elevated with skin hook prior to inset. (F) Movement of flap with skin hook to ensure adequate tension free reach. (G) Flap sewn into place (frontal view). (H) Flap sewn into place (lateral view). (I) Mature flap at 3 weeks prior to division. (J) Immediately following division of pedicle with closure of glabella. (K) Final result.

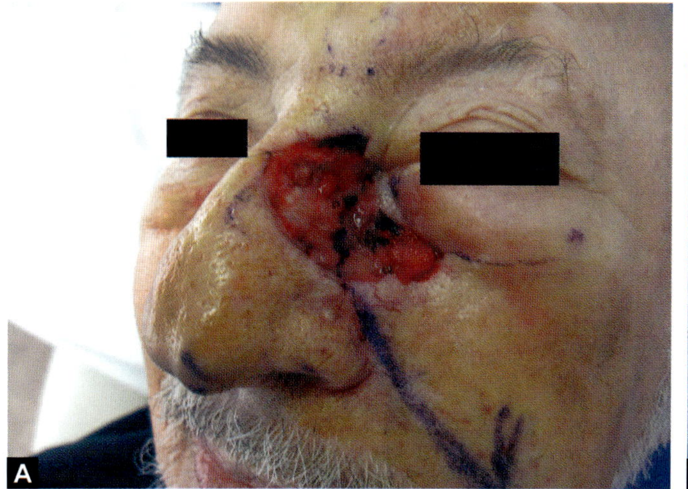

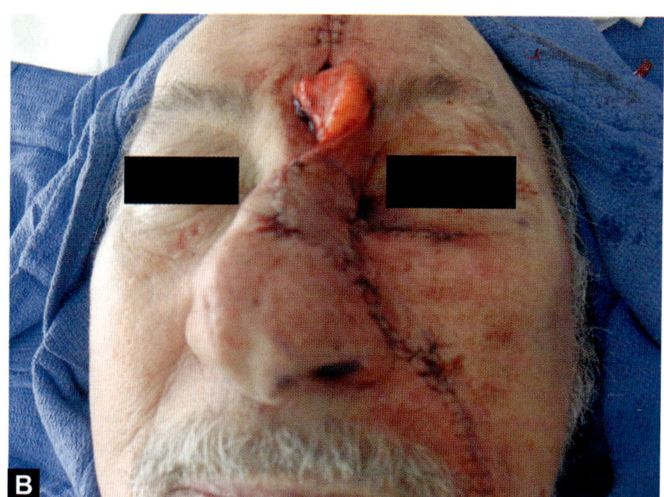

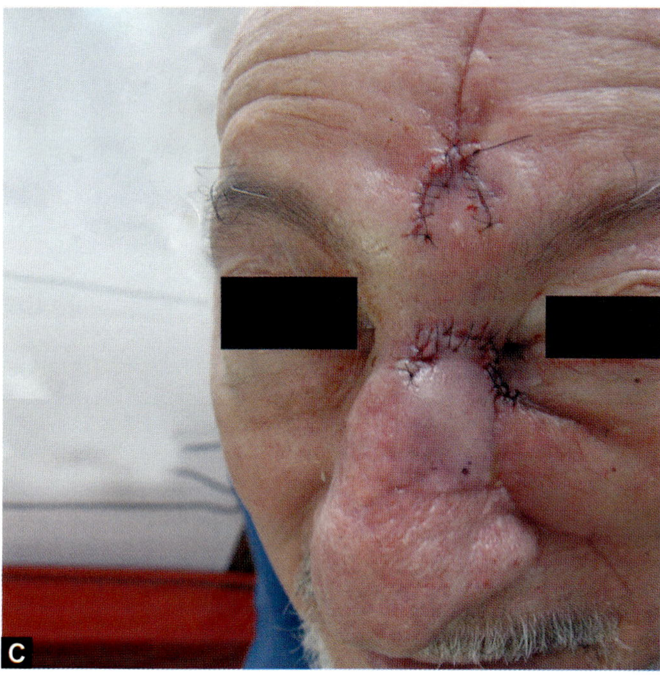

**Figs. 11.21A to C:** Paramedian forehead flap and inferomedially based rotation flap for a complex defect of the nasal sidewall, superior medial cheek, and lower eyelid. (A) Defect following Mohs extirpation of tumor spanning nasal sidewall, superior medial cheek, and lower eyelid. (B) Paramedian forehead flap plus inferomedially based rotation flap. (C) Following division of paramedian pedicle at 3 weeks.

the 11 had experienced significant postoperative bleeding requiring intervention.[6]

Most patients undergoing paramedian forehead flaps by dermatologic surgeons will go home on the day of surgery. However, postoperative pain, headache, and reflex nausea lasting 24–36 hours are not uncommon and the patient should be provided with adequate oral analgesic and antiemetic medications and a backup plan if these measures fail to control their symptoms.[20] In the authors' experience, there are rare instances in which patients who are elderly or debilitated may benefit from an overnight admission to the hospital on the day of the procedure for observation and pain control.

As with melolabial interpolation flaps, there is potential for "trapdooring" or "pincushioning" of the nasal recipient site if the flap is not adequately thinned or the defect skeletonized. In such cases the surgeon can revise the flap by debulking this area after adequate healing time is allowed (Figs. 11.22A and B).

Lastly, while great care is taken to ensure cosmesis, the function of the nasal valve is crucial and should be prioritized. Prior to covering a defect with a paramedian forehead flap it is important to recreate the nasal valve if it has been compromised during tumor extirpation otherwise the patient will have long-term difficulty with nasal patency and breathing (Figs. 11.23A to D). In addition,

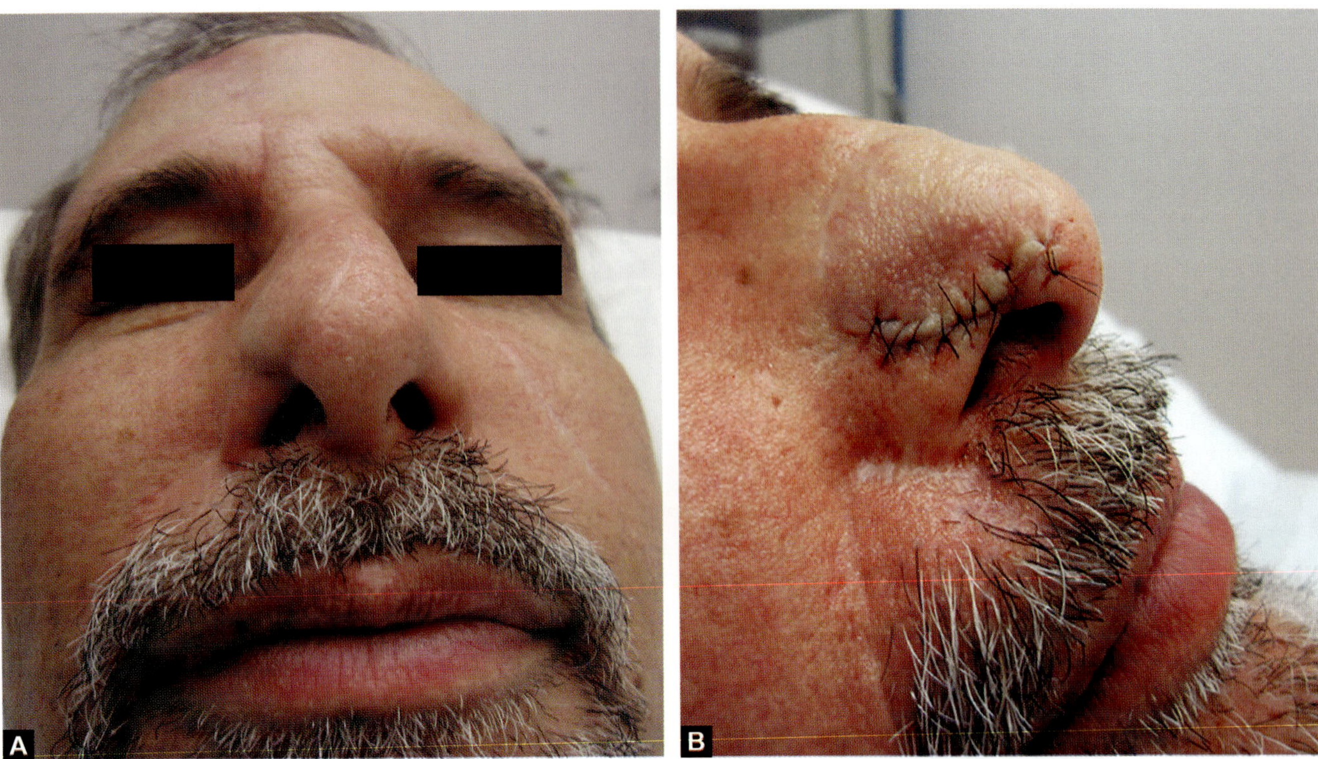

**Figs. 11.22A and B:** Revision of trapdoor deformity following paramedian forehead flap. (A) Trapdoor deformity following paramedian forehead flap. (B) Debulking and thinning of trapdoor deformity.

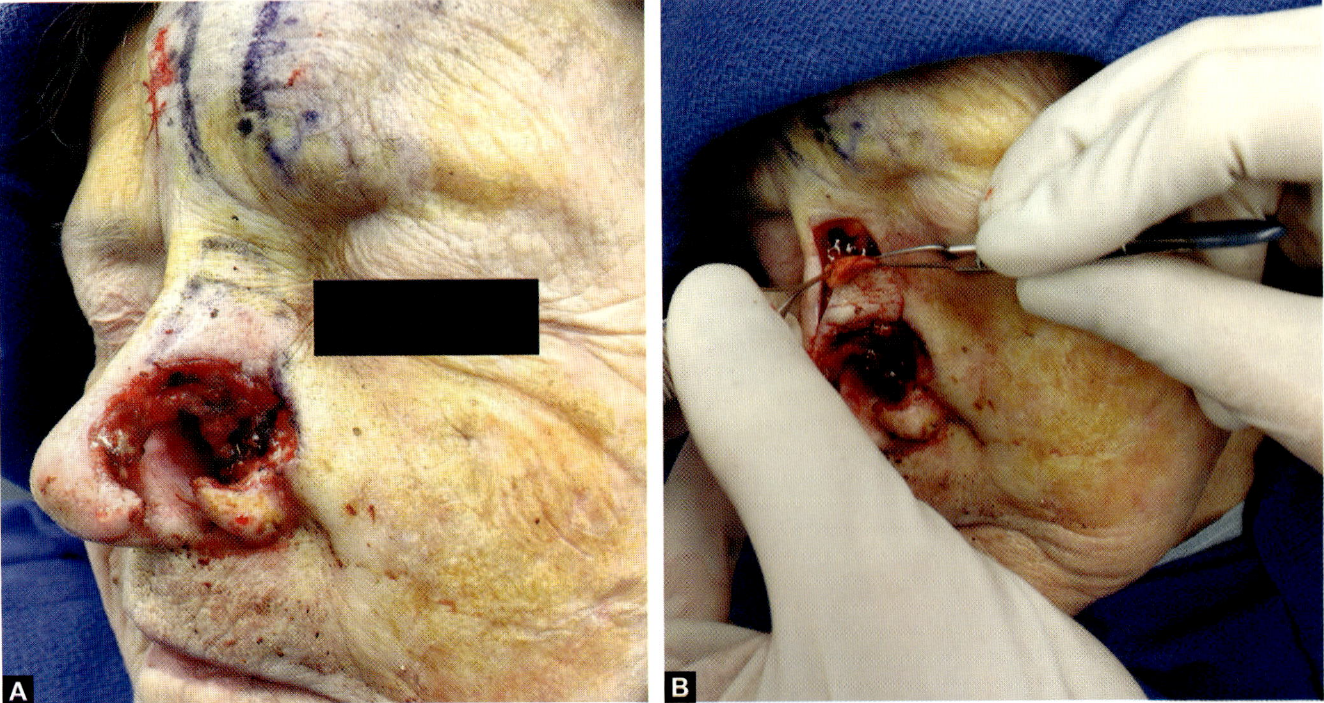

**Figs. 11.23A and B:** Repair of full-thickness defect of the nose. (A) Defect after removal of deeply invasive squamous cell carcinoma on the nose. (B) Development of lining flap.

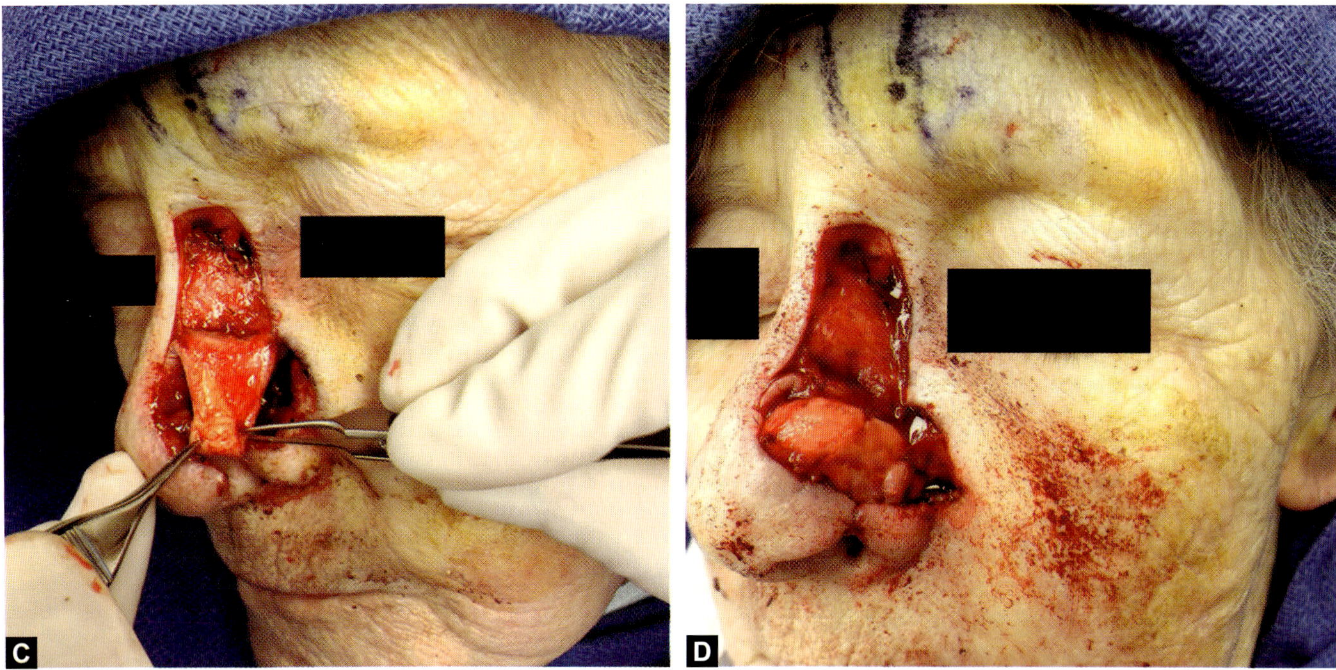


**Figs. 11.23C and D:** (C) Lining flap turned over in "page of book" fashion. (D) Cartilage graft on the ala.

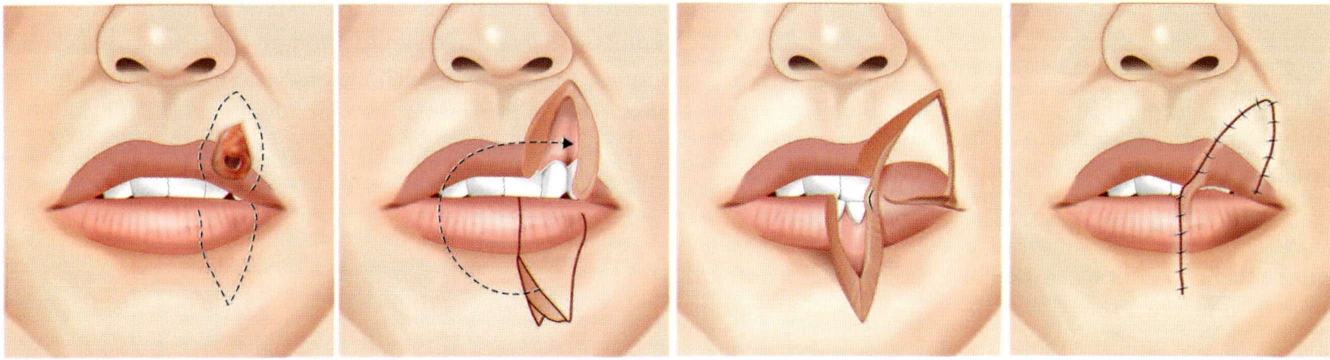

**Fig. 11.24:** Schematic of Abbe flap.

while much attention is given to the nasal or recipient portion of the reconstruction, it is also important to elegantly repair the forehead for cosmesis. Patients should be made aware of potential sensory deficits or neuralgia of the forehead due to interference with the supratrochlear neurovascular bundle and be counseled that these deficits are usually temporary.

## Abbe Flap

### *Applications*

In 1836, Sabattini first described "cross-lip transfer" of full-thickness lip tissue, which was later modified in 1898 by Abbe who published on the transfer of a triangular-shaped full-thickness segment of lip tissue from the lower lip to a full-thickness upper lip defect.[21-23] The Abbe lip switch flap is useful for defects where a wedge repair or local tissue transfer flap will not lead to symmetry of the upper and lower lip or adequate function.[24] Specifically, Abbe flaps are useful for full-thickness wounds of the upper cutaneous and vermillion lip that encompass >1/3 of the length of the lip (Fig. 11.24). This axial pedicle flap derives its blood supply from the inferior labial artery as well as perforating branches from the orbicularis muscle. The inferior labial artery is located 1 cm below the free margin of the lower lip most frequently between mucosa and orbicularis and less frequently within the orbicularis oris.[25] The full-thickness nature of Abbe flaps allows for restoration of the orbicularis oris sphincter which is crucial for function of the mouth and in most cases full motor and sensory function after healing.

### Planning and Execution

Prior to any reconstruction it is crucial to mark aesthetic subunit boundaries, in particular the vermillion border should be marked prior to infiltration of anesthesia as misalignment leads to obvious deformity. Anesthesia of the upper and lower lip can be achieved with infraorbital and mental nerve blocks and/or local anesthesia. A template should be made using foil or a telfa pad of the upper lip defect to approximate the height and width of donor tissue necessary; however, often the lower lip donor portion of the flap is undersized in order to avoid a bulky pedicle. The pedicle is based medially or laterally depending on the location of the recipient defect on the upper lip. The donor lower lip should be marked similarly to a wedge resection and incised through skin, subcutis, and muscle, leaving the inferior labial artery and a small amount of mucosa and submucosa intact (Figs. 11.25A to F).

Once the full thickness of the pedicle is incised the surgeon must ensure axial movement allowing rotation into the recipient upper lip defect without tension. This can be done with skin hooks to avoid crushing tissue. Next the donor site is closed beginning with mucosa using absorbable sutures, followed by approximation of orbicularis muscle, dermis, and epidermis. The flap can then be inset and sewn into the upper lip defect as a layered closure in the aforementioned order. For the vermillion lip the authors advocate using silk suture for patient comfort. The patient returns in 1 week for epidermal suture removal and in 3 weeks for pedicle division. Division of the flap pedicle at 3 weeks is achieved via incision of the stalk between the upper and lower lip. The flap takedown is relatively uncomplicated and the most crucial step is careful realignment of the upper vermillion lip. The base of the pedicle can be repaired linearly or with an advancement flap if necessary.

### Complications and Pitfalls

One of the main complications of the Abbe flap is trapdoor deformity of the recipient site and the tendency of the recipient site to appear bulky while the patient is at rest. However, some of this edema results from lymphatic and venous congestion and will resolve with time. In other cases, true trapdoor deformity is the result of oversizing the donor flap and results in lip protrusion. Some authors note that if orbicularis muscle is not carefully approximated there may be greater wound contraction resulting in a depressed scar around the borders of the flap thus highlighting the appearance of a trapdoor deformity.[20]

It has been reported that patients undergoing Abbe flaps sustain at least temporary loss of sensation with return of pain sensation detected 2 months following flap transfer, followed by tactile sensation at 3 months, cold sensation at 6 months, and warmth at 9 months.[26] It is crucial that patients undergoing Abbe flaps are prepared for the appearance and functional deficits that they will encounter for the 3 weeks prior to pedicle division. In the postoperative period, it is important to balance pain control with the potential for opiate-induced nausea and vomiting which would compromise the flap. The authors recommend avoiding opiate based analgesia or premedicating with antiemetics if a codeine-based medication is to be administered. Prior to pedicle division, a diet limited to liquids and soft foods that require minimal biting and chewing is advised as to not disrupt the flap. Patients must also be counseled extensively on the lengthy recovery period and impairment with speech and function following the first stage of the procedure. In a small series of eight patients who underwent Abbe flaps by a single Mohs surgeon there were no minor or major complications reported.[6]

## SUMMARY

Reconstruction of complex defects of the nose, ear, and lip following surgical extirpation of cutaneous malignancies is both challenging and rewarding. Following tumor clearance the surgeon must achieve satisfactory function, followed by optimal cosmesis. Many defects encountered by dermatologic surgeons are easily repaired with linear repairs, local adjacent tissue transfers, or skin grafts. In cases where defects are not amenable to these options, staged interpolation flaps become useful and necessary. However, the number of staged interpolation flaps performed by dermatologic surgeons after Mohs micrographic surgery is only 0.3%.[27] This suggests that some dermatologic surgeons are not comfortable with multiple staged repairs and are likely to refer these cases to other surgical specialties. It is the authors' hope that this chapter provides clear and concise guidance regarding the appropriate application and execution of melolabial interpolation flaps, mastoid interpolation flaps, paramedian forehead

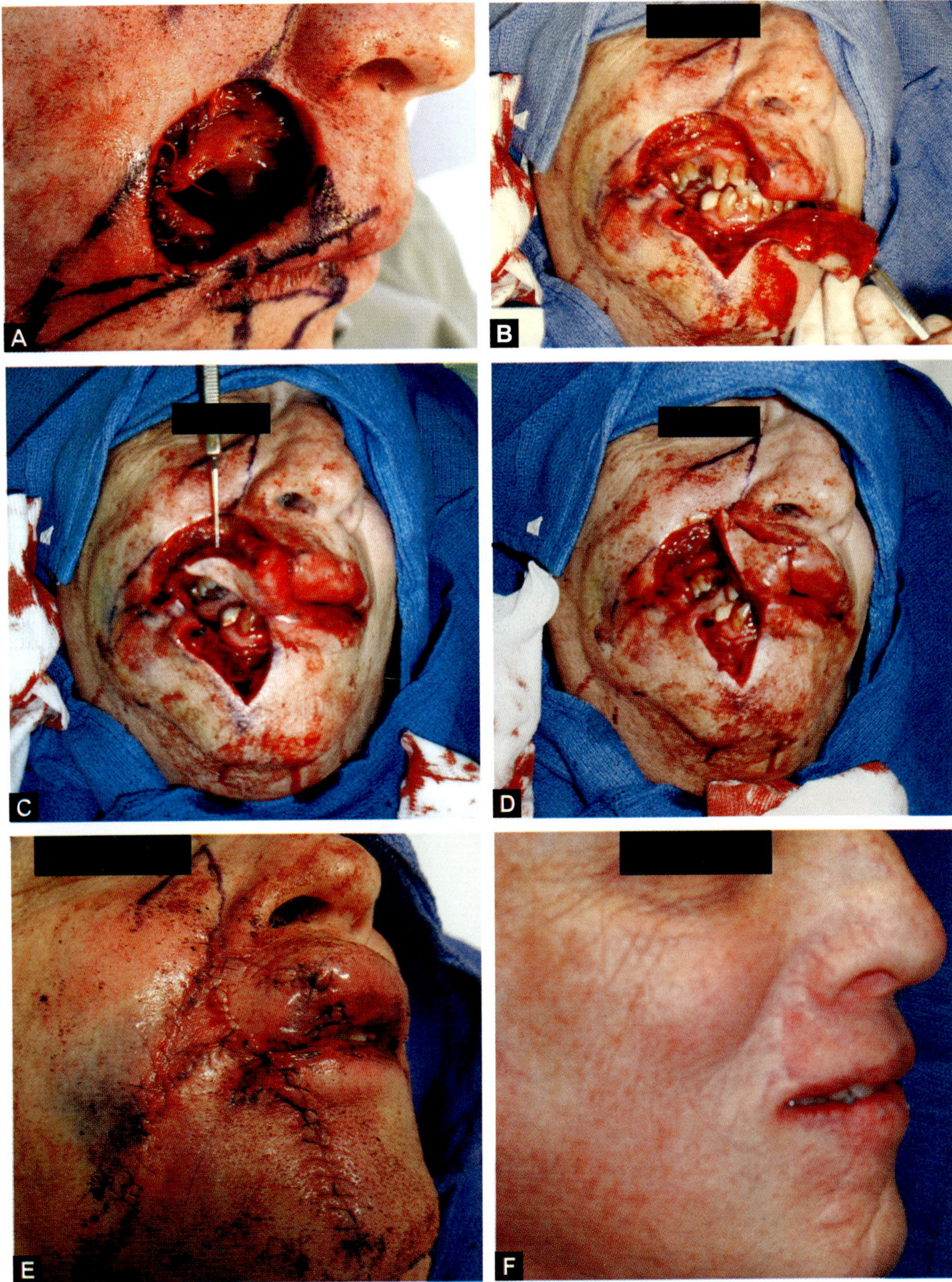


**Figs. 11.25A to F:** Complex full-thickness defect of the cutaneous and mucosal lip repaired with an advancement flap and Abbe flap. (A) Defect following Mohs micrographic surgery tumor extirpation resulting in full thickness through and through defect of the cutaneous upper lip and extending onto the mucosal upper lip. (B) Excision of remaining upper mucosal and cutaneous lip and wedge resection of lower lip. (C) Lower lip with orbicularis muscle elevated with a skin hook to ensure reach to primary defect on upper lip. (D) A tacking stitch is placed to align the donor lower mucosal lip with the upper vermillion lip as well as the tip of the lower cutaneous lip to the superior portion of the upper cutaneous lip. (E) A laterally based V-to-Y advancement flap is harvested and used to close a portion of the lateral cutaneous lip and the lip switch is sewn into place. (F) Final result at follow-up with complete preservation of function. Note excellent placement of the oral commissure and vermillion border.

flaps, and Abbe flaps. Regardless of the type of flap selected, with a strong foundation of surgical skills and knowledge of facial skin thickness, contour, and function, dermatologic surgeons should be confident in their ability to use staged interpolation flaps to reconstruct complex defects.

## REFERENCES

1. Friduss M, Dagum P, Mandych A, et al. Forehead flap in nasal reconstruction. Otolaryngol Head Neck Surg. 1995:113 (6):740-7.
2. Bhishagratna KKL, ed. Sushruta Samhita. Calcutta, India: Bose; 1907-1916..
3. Kazanjian V. Reconstruction of the ala using septal flap. Trans Am Acad Ophthalmol Otolaryngol. 1937;42:338.
4. Menick FJ. Aesthetic refinements in use of forehead for nasal reconstruction: the paramedian forehead flap. Clin Plast Surg. 1990;17(4):607-22.
5. Baker SR, Naficy S. Principles of Nasal Reconstruction. St Louis, MO: Mosby; 2002.
6. Newlove T, Cook J. Safety of staged interpolation flaps after Mohs micrographic surgery in an outpatient setting: a single-center experience. Dermatol Surg. 2013;39(11):1671-82.
7. Kimyai-Asadi A, Goldberg LH, Peterson SR, et al. The incidence of major complications from Mohs micrographic surgery performed in office-based and hospital-based settings. J Am Acad Dermatol. 2005;53(4):628-34.
8. Chuang GS, Leach BC, Wheless L, et al. Preoperative expectations and values of patients undergoing Mohs micrographic surgery. Dermatol Surg. 2011;37(3):311-9.
9. Herbert DC. A subcutaneous pedicled cheek flap for reconstruction of alar defects. Br J Plast Surg. 1978;31(2):79-92.
10. Baker SR, Johnson TM, Nelson BR. The importance of maintaining the alar-facial sulcus in nasal reconstruction. Arch Otolaryngol Head Neck Surg. 1995;121(6):617-22.
11. Burget GC, Menick FJ. Nasal support and lining—the marriage of beauty and blood-supply. Plast Reconstr Surg. 1989;84 (2):189-203.
12. Renard A. Postauricular flap based on a dermal pedicle for ear reconstruction. Plast Reconstr Surg. 1981;68(2):159-65.
13. Johnson TM, Fader DJ. The staged retroauricular to auricular direct pedicle (interpolation) flap for helical ear reconstruction. J Am Acad Dermatol. 1997;37(6):975-8.
14. Field LM. The preauricular tubed pedicle flap. J Dermatol Surg Oncol. 1989;15(6):614-8.
15. Mellette JR Jr. Ear reconstruction with local flaps. J Dermatol Surg Oncol. 1991;17(2):176-82.
16. Shumrick KA, Smith TL. The anatomic basis for the design of forehead flaps in nasal reconstruction. Arch Otolaryngol Head Neck Surg. 1992;118(4):373-9.
17. McCarthy JG, Lorenc ZP, Cutting C, et al. The median forehead flap revisited: the blood supply. Plast Reconstr Surg. 1985;76(6):866-9.
18. Mellette J. The paramedian forehead flap for nasal reconstruction. Facial Plast Surg Clin North Am. 1998;6(3):365-78.
19. Jewett BS. Interpolated forehead and melolabial flaps. Facial Plast Surg Clin North Am. 2009;17(3):361-77.
20. Baker SR. Local Flaps in Facial Reconstruction, 3rd edition. St Louis, MO: Mosby; 2014.
21. Mazzola RF, Lupo G. Evolving concepts in lip reconstruction. Clin Plast Surg. 1984;11(4):583-617.
22. Sabattini P. Cenno Storico dell'Origine e Progressi della Rinoplastica e Cheiloplastica. Bologna: Belle Arti; 1838.
23. Abbe R. New plastic operation for relief of deformity due to double hairlip. Med Rec. 1898;53:477.
24. Burget GC, Menick FJ. Aesthetic restoration of one-half the upper lip. Plast Reconstr Surg. 1986;78(5):583-93.
25. Schulte DL, Sherris DA, Kasperbauer JL. The anatomical basis of the Abbe flap. Laryngoscope. 2001;111(3):382-6.
26. Smith JW. The anatomical and physiologic acclimatization of tissue transplanted by the lip switch technique. Plast Reconstr Surg Transplant Bull. 1960;26:40-56.
27. Donaldson MR, Coldiron BM. Mohs micrographic surgery utilization in the Medicare population, 2009. Dermatol Surg. 2012;38(9):1427-34.

CHAPTER

# 12

# Skin, Cartilage, and Composite Grafts

*Syril Keena T Que, Omar A Ibrahimi*

## INTRODUCTION

Skin and cartilage grafting is a useful reconstructive modality for the dermatologic surgeon. Sites in dermatologic surgery where grafts are most commonly used include the nasal tip and ala, ears, medial canthus, digits, and extremities. Generally, grafts are considered in areas where it is not possible to do a primary closure without significant distortion, where healing by secondary intention is likely to lead to poor cosmesis, when a patient cannot tolerate a larger reconstructive procedure, or for defects where the use of a flap is likely to violate aesthetic units and result in pincushioning or when a sufficient tissue reservoir does not exist.

Grafts can be classified according to the source of the donor tissue. An autograft is taken from a donor site on an individual and placed at a recipient site on the same individual. A homograft is obtained from an individual and transplanted to another individual of the same species. A xenograft is a graft transplanted between species (i.e. from a pig to a human). The nomenclature of grafts also depends on the thickness of skin and subcutaneous tissue involved. These graft types include full-thickness, split-thickness, cartilage, and composite grafts.

A full-thickness skin graft includes the epidermis, dermis, and adnexal structures, while a split-thickness skin graft contains epidermis and varying amounts of dermis. The advantage of using a full-thickness skin graft over a split-thickness graft is the more complete filling of surgical defects, the improved color and texture match, and the lower risk of contracture. The benefits of using a split-thickness graft are the lower rate of graft failure and the ability to fill in larger defects, including defects >5 cm. Some argue that split-thickness skin grafts allow for better monitoring for tumor recurrence as well.

Cartilage grafts are useful when significant amounts of supporting tissue and/or cartilage are removed during an excision, resulting in potential structural and functional deficits. Replacement of cartilage can be achieved by grafting cartilage separately and subsequently covering it with a cutaneous graft or flap or by grafting a composite graft, which consists of both cartilage and overlying skin. A composite graft has a higher rate of graft failure than a cartilage graft alone.

Generally, a graft undergoes several stages after it is attached to the wound bed: (i) imbibition, where fibrin and granulation tissue are deposited to underlying tissues and the graft absorbs nutrients passively through the wound bed,[1] (ii) inosculation, which involves the formation of anastomoses between graft vessels and existing vessels,[2] and (iii) neovascularization, defined as the formation of new vessels. Graft survival is dependent on these three stages. Graft necrosis may result when a hematoma or seroma forms because any fluid accumulation between the graft and wound bed impairs the processes of imbibition and inosculation.

## GRAFT TYPES

### Full-Thickness Skin Grafts

#### *Indications and Contraindications*

Indications for using a full-thickness skin graft (Figs. 12.1A to C) include the following: when primary closure could cause significant distortion, when secondary intention healing is likely to lead to poor cosmesis, when patients cannot tolerate larger flaps, or when the use of a flap may not give a superior cosmetic result, i.e. wide, superficial defects on the ear or bald scalp. Full-thickness skin grafts are also considered when margin control is difficult or

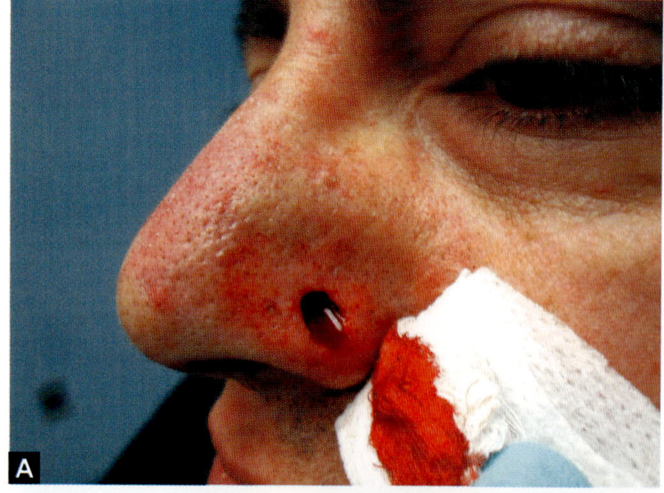


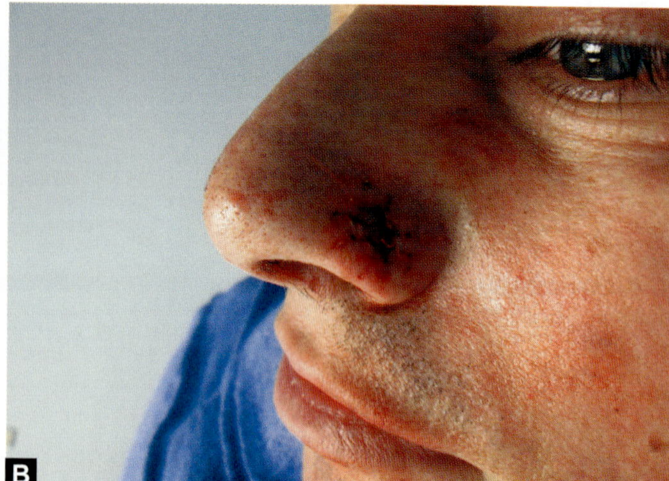


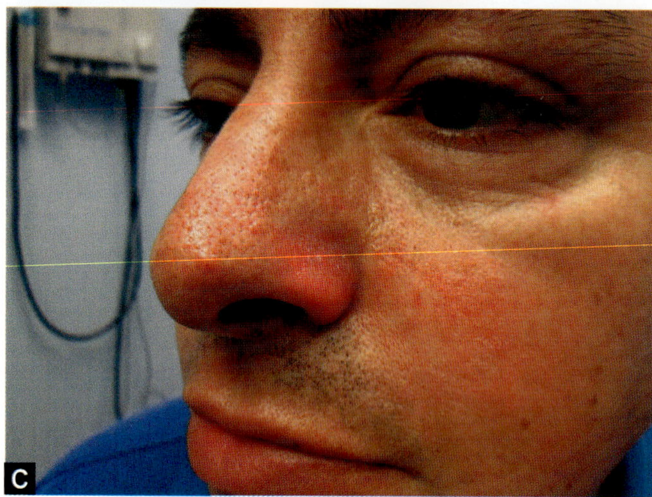


**Figs. 12.1A to C:** Full-thickness skin graft. (A) Appearance of defect on left nasal ala following basal cell carcinoma tumor extirpation with Mohs surgery. (B) Full-thickness graft from left conchal bowl immediately postreconstruction. (C) Appearance of surgical site 3 months post-Mohs and reconstructive surgery.

when dealing with aggressive cancers, as grafts make it easier to monitor for skin cancer recurrence.

The major contraindication for using full-thickness skin grafts is the presence of avascular tissue, i.e. areas of exposed bone or cartilage with no periosteum or perichondrium. Additional preparation (i.e. fenestrating cartilage on the ear) or other reconstructive modalities should be considered because these sites will not support full-thickness skin grafts.

## *Preoperative History and Donor Site Considerations*

Preoperative evaluation before the placement of a full-thickness skin graft should include assessment of bleeding tendencies, use of anticoagulants, history of hypertension, diabetes mellitus, smoking history, and other factors that may decrease the likelihood of graft survival. Smoking is one factor that plays a significant role in graft loss. Nicotine impairs healing through vasoconstriction.

The method for harvesting full-thickness skin grafts begins with the selection of an appropriate donor site. Selection of a donor site should take into consideration the color, texture, thickness, sun exposure, and sebaceous qualities of the skin around the surgical defect. For a defect on the nasal ala (Figs. 12.1A to C) and tip, where skin is thick, the conchal bowl, forehead, or preauricular skin (Figs. 12.2A to E) are ideal donor sites.[3] Postauricular skin, which is thinner and less exposed to the sun, might be considered as a donor site for defects of the nasal sidewall.

## *Description of Technique*

Harvesting and placing a full-thickness skin graft over a surgical defect begins by making a template of the defect on gauze, Telfa (Covidien, Mansfield, MA, USA) or

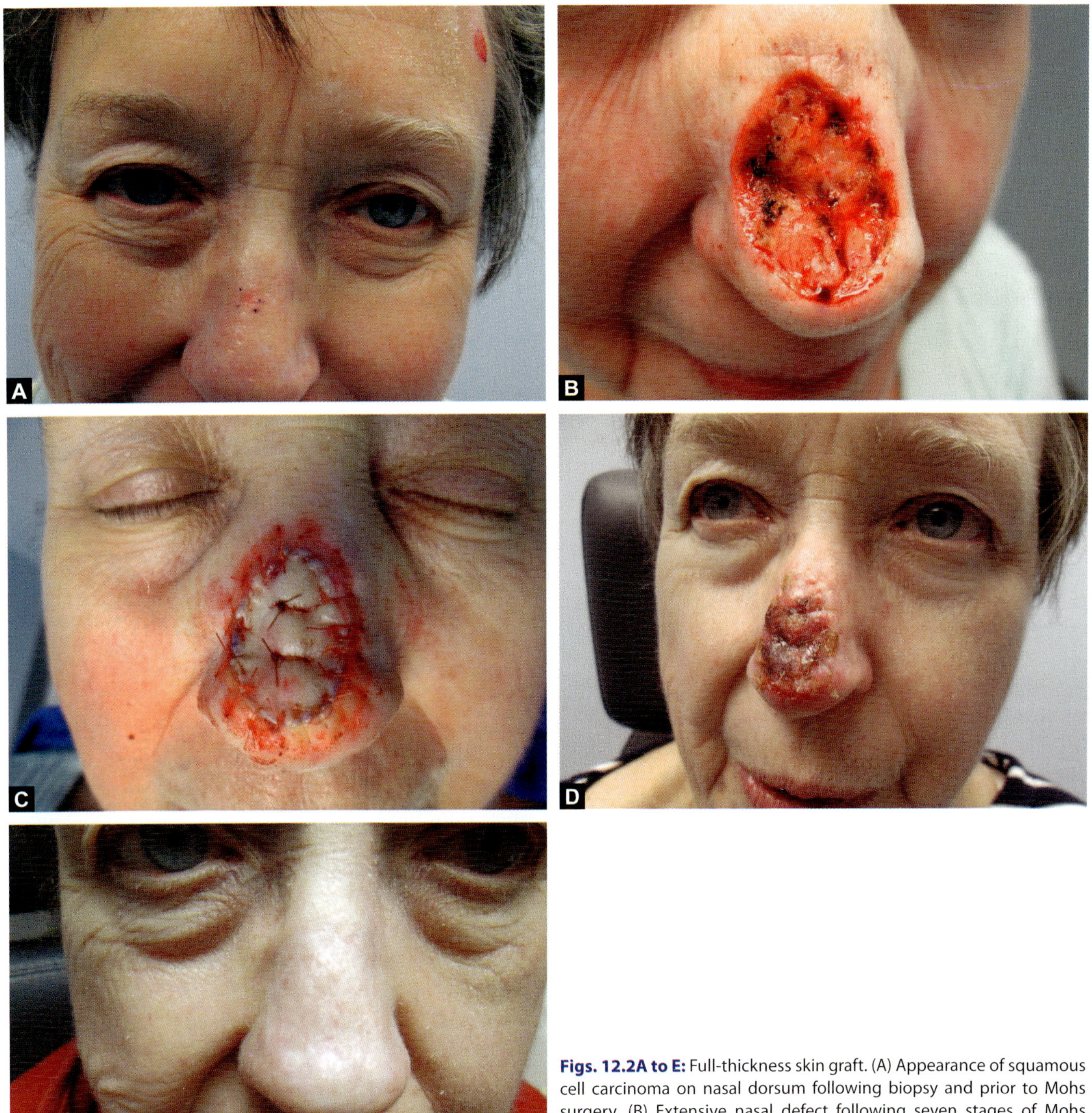


**Figs. 12.2A to E:** Full-thickness skin graft. (A) Appearance of squamous cell carcinoma on nasal dorsum following biopsy and prior to Mohs surgery. (B) Extensive nasal defect following seven stages of Mohs surgery to remove tumor. (C) Full-thickness graft from left preauricular cheek immediately postreconstruction. (D) Appearance of graft 1 week postreconstructive surgery. (E) Appearance of graft 2 years following reconstructive surgery.

aluminum foil. This template is applied to the donor site and is used to outline the area that will be removed. The graft should be 3–5% larger in size than the template to allow for natural contraction of the graft after it has been harvested. Local anesthesia is injected into the donor and recipient sites, and the sites are prepped with chlorhexidine and draped in a sterile manner. The donor tissue is excised and immediately placed in a Petri dish containing normal saline, where excess adipose tissue is trimmed using curved Iris or Supercut scissors. Trimming excess adipose tissue enhances nutrient and oxygen delivery during the processes of imbibition and inosculation. Removal of any cartilage not needed for structural support also increases the chances of graft survival, although meticulous surgical technique should allow for harvesting a full thickness skin graft without any underlying cartilage.[4]

At this stage, the graft is ready to be attached to the defect. A series of simple interrupted sutures or a running suture technique can be used to anchor the graft in place. Basting sutures that anchor the graft to the wound bed are not necessary but are generally recommended if grafts are large or placed over convex surfaces.[5] Any basting sutures should be placed while at least half of the graft is still free so that hemostasis can be achieved before the entire perimeter of the graft has been adhered to the wound bed.[6] After all perimeter sutures are placed, a petrolatum ointment is applied, and a bolster dressing can be applied to protect and immobilize the graft. A bolster dressing typically consists of a nonadherent layer such as Xeroform (Johnson & Johnson Medical, Arlington, TX, USA) or Adaptic (Johnson & Johnson Medical, Arlington, TX, USA) followed by gauze, foam, or cotton balls as a top layer. Three to four sutures at opposite ends can be tied over the dressing or a strong, elastic, adhesive tape such as Hypafix (Smith & Nephew, London, UK) can be used to secure the bandage. The bolster dressing serves to provide constant pressure, which ensures complete adherence between the graft and wound bed and increases the chance of graft survival. The bolster dressing is especially useful for grafts on the extremities or areas more likely to get traumatized. Bolster dressings and any non-absorbable sutures should be removed after 1 week.

Grafts may also be attached using cyanoacrylate tissue adhesives, such as 2-octyl cyanoacrylate.[7] Some advantages of tissue adhesives over suturing is faster closure time and ability of the tissue adhesive to act as a water and antimicrobial barrier. The cyanoacrylate tissue adhesive also enhances graft survival by helping to maintain close contact between the graft and the wound bed.

## Postoperative Care and Complications

The most common short-term complications for full-thickness skin grafts include graft hypertrophy, partial graft failure, and graft contraction, which occurred in ~11% of full-thickness grafts according to the Australian Mohs database, which records all patients treated with Mohs surgery in Australia and monitored by the Skin and Cancer Foundation between 1993 and 2002.[8]

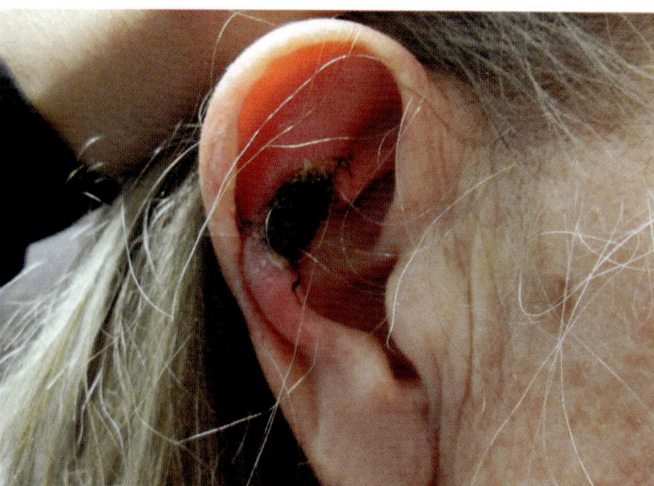

**Fig. 12.3:** Necrosis of full-thickness skin graft. Black appearance of graft 1 week postprocedure indicates graft failure.

### *Transient Graft Hypertrophy Following a Full-thickness Skin Graft*

Grafts have been reported to undergo hypertrophy weeks after surgery, even in the absence of hematoma or fluid accumulation. Treatment modalities to correct for graft hypertrophy include silicone gel sheets, topical and intralesional corticosteroids, dermabrasion, and $CO_2$ laser resurfacing. Spot dermabrasion can be used as early as 6 weeks, but it is advisable to wait until the graft has significantly matured for 3–4 months, in case the hypertrophy is temporary. In one case report, a patient who developed hypertrophy of her full-thickness skin graft experienced spontaneous resolution of the graft thickness with gentle manual massage alone.[9]

### *Graft Necrosis*

A full-thickness skin graft is ideally expected to be light pink in color when the bolster dressing is removed 1 week after the surgery. A white graft indicates the lack of revascularization and signals that the graft will fail. A black graft signifies necrosis (Fig. 12.3). There can be a range of normal color changes to the graft, ranging from pink or red to darker blue or purple. Skin graft necrosis is more likely to occur in men than in women.[10] This may be because men have a greater sebaceous gland density in the nose, which affects the process of skin graft vascularization, either by promoting a larger number of microorganisms that affect wound healing or by affecting wound edge apposition.

*Indications for Postoperative Antibiotics*

Some indications for postoperative antibiotics include delayed grafts, a lengthy surgery >6 hours, and surgical sites close to mouth or nostrils. Full-thickness skin grafts on the nose more often become necrotic than grafts on other parts of the face, possibly because bacteria in the nose causes a subclinical wound infection or compromises circulation. A higher rate of graft survival has been reported in patients receiving antibiotics after having a full-thickness skin graft placed on the nose—86% of graft survival was reported with a 3-day course of azithromycin at day 10 versus 36% survival without antibiotics ($p$ = 0.002).[11] Aside from the indications mentioned above, infection of skin grafts is rare and the routine use of prophylactic antibiotics is not recommended. However, many surgeons still prefer to use postoperative antibiotics when performing a full-thickness skin graft (FTSG) includes the epidermis, dermis in locations with high risk for surgical site infection. There is a more in depth discussion of antibiotic use for cutaneous surgery in our preoperative considerations chapter.

*Hematoma and Seroma*

The development of hematomas or seromas can affect graft survival and are prevented with the use of meticulous hemostasis, in addition to basting sutures and/or a bolster dressing, both of which maintain contact between the wound bed and the graft. Additionally, patients are advised to avoid strenuous activity for at least 2 weeks postoperatively, as this may raise their blood pressure. Medications that increase the risk of bleeding that are not medically necessary can also be avoided prior to surgery. For all medically necessary antithrombotic therapy, the evidence in the literature suggests the continuation of these medications when undergoing cutaneous surgery. For patients on warfarin, screening the international normalized ratio to maintain the therapeutic range of 2–3.5 one week prior to surgery is recommended.[12-14] There is a more detailed discussion of antithrombotic use during cutaneous surgery in our preoperative considerations chapter.

*Cosmetic Concerns*

To optimize the cosmetic results of a graft, dermabrasion or laser resurfacing may be considered 6 weeks to 6 months postoperatively.[15] Any evidence of graft hyperpigmentation can be treated with topical hydroquinone and/or tretinoin.

*Variations of the Technique Delayed*

*Full-thickness skin grafts*

Delay of skin graft placement by more than one day was correlated with subsequent skin graft success ($p$ = 0.015).[10] Delayed skin grafting is an option for patients undergoing Mohs surgery who are not candidates for an immediate full-thickness skin graft (i.e. the graft bed is a large avascular surface or the defect is too deep to be covered by a full-thickness graft).[16] It is also useful for patients who lack an appropriate donor site. Delaying placement of a full-thickness skin graft to 12–14 days after Mohs micrographic surgery gives the surgeon time to determine which patients can instead be allowed to heal by secondary intention. Delaying skin graft placement also allows for the formation of granulation tissue in the wound base, which helps to fill in some of the defect and guarantees adequate vascularity.[17] It additionally prevents the incidence of hematoma and seroma formation, which could complicate graft survival. Studies have shown that there is no difference in texture irregularity, hypopigmentation, hyperpigmentation, or erythema when the placement of skin grafts is delayed rather than immediate.[18]

Prior to placement of a delayed full-thickness skin graft, the surgical defect can be cleansed daily with dilute acetic acid at a ratio of 3 tablespoons of vinegar to 1 quart of clean tap water. It is otherwise covered for 1–3 weeks and allowed to granulate. Since the delay between tumor excision and reconstruction can slightly increase the risk of infection, it may be beneficial to start the patient on preoperative and/or postoperative antibiotics, specifically antibiotics that cover *Staphylococcus aureus* and *Streptococcus pyogenes*. There is limited evidence for the use of prophylactic antibiotics in delayed full-thickness skin grafts, but many surgeons prefer to use antibiotics postoperatively for procedures on certain anatomic sites, i.e. locations with high risk for surgical infection. On the day of surgery, the wound is scrubbed with chlorhexidine, peripheral margins are cleaned, and any eschar is removed. The full-thickness skin graft is then placed as mentioned above.

*Cartilage, Dermal Grafts, Subcutaneous Hinge Flap, Myocutaneous Hinge Flap, and Porcine Xenografts*

If immediate reconstruction is preferred for a deep defect, cartilage or dermal grafts can be used as tissue filler prior to the placement of a full-thickness skin graft.[19-22] Another option is to use a subcutaneous or myocutaneous hinge flap to occupy the base of the defect with well-vascularized tissue, with the remaining defect covered by a full-thickness skin graft.[23,24] For defects involving the nasal dorsum, sidewall, supratip, or ala, a myocutaneous hinge flap can be performed by outlining and excising a standing cone immediately superior to the defect. After the skin is removed, underlying muscle is incised, elevated above the periosteum, and turned downward into the defect in a "hinge" motion, thereby providing a rich vascular bed for the graft. The previously excised standing cone is then used to fill in the defect. The subcutaneous hinge flap is created in a similar manner and is useful for nasal defects extending to the cheek. This flap is performed by transposing subcutaneous tissue from the cheek in a "hinge" motion toward the defect, followed by a cheek advancement flap. Any remaining defect can be covered using a full-thickness skin graft.

Porcine xenografts and other synthetic grafts are also options for promoting granulation and enhancing autograft survival. They are sometimes used temporarily in situations where delayed repairs are being considered and help to protect and preserve vital structures such as bone, cartilage, tendons, and nerves prior to the placement of the autograft.[25] Synthetic grafts are usually replaced every 7–10 days until an autograft is placed.[26,27] Porcine grafts are obtained from domestic swine and harvested with a dermatome as split-thickness skin grafts of 0.01 inch thickness. The porcine xenograft is usually replaced every 7–14 days until an autograft is ready to be placed.

*Purse-string Sutures*

The purse-string suture is a subcuticular stitch placed around the periphery of a circular or oval defect to advance the skin from the entire periphery and to reduce the size of the defect.[28] The remaining defect can then be covered with a full-thickness skin graft. This technique can help minimize large defects so that they can be covered with relatively smaller full-thickness grafts.

*Burow's Graft*

A Burow's graft uses the skin adjacent to a defect as the donor site and therefore provides a superior tissue and color match compared to grafts from other locations. To obtain a Burow's graft, tissue removed from the dog-ear repair of a partial primary closure is defatted, trimmed, and sutured into the residual defect. For large defects on the nasal sidewall, ala, or cheek, one option is to use a cheek advancement flap in combination with a melolabial Burow's graft.[29] This technique is very useful and can be utilized in many anatomical locations with limited tissue mobility. The editors frequently use Burow's grafts on the nose, scalp, hands, and feet.

*Hair-bearing Grafts*

Hair-bearing grafts can be performed on locations like the eyebrows, with some important considerations.[30] When performing a hair-bearing graft, hair density and orientation of hair follicles must match that of the recipient site. In contrast to full-thickness skin grafts on nonhair bearing skin, hair-bearing grafts should be defatted minimally, with only the fat between hair bulbs removed, if possible. Care must be taken to preserve the hair follicles.

## Split-Thickness Skin Grafts

### *Indications and Contraindications*

Much of the literature for split-thickness skin grafts comes from burn patients or from patients with chronic ulcers. Split-thickness skin grafts tend to be used less often by Mohs surgeons due to the less than ideal cosmesis resulting from split-thickness skin grafts. The main advantages of split-thickness skin grafts are the ability to cover larger surface areas and the higher likelihood of graft survival. Because they are semitransparent, they are also useful for excised tumors that are aggressive and have a possibility of recurring. One of the main disadvantages is poor cosmesis, as the color and texture may not necessarily match that of the recipient site. A split thickness skin graft is more likely to experience contraction and may also result in a depressed appearance because of its inability to completely fill a deep defect. These types of grafts should be used with caution near free margins, including the eyes, oral commissure, and nasal alae. Split-thickness skin grafts are most commonly used in Mohs repair for large defects on the scalp or legs.[31,32]

### *Donor Site Considerations*

The most common donor sites for split-thickness skin grafts are the upper thighs, lateral hips, inner aspect of upper arms, low back, and abdomen.[5] These are all locations where a large area of skin can be removed but where the area can remain hidden beneath clothing.

### *Description of Technique*

The donor site is prepped with chlorhexidine and local anesthesia and draped in a sterile fashion. After a template is made to ensure a graft of the correct size, the split-thickness skin graft is obtained by one of several methods: (i) by pinch graft, which involves using forceps, a skin hook, needle tip or suction to elevate the skin and a scalpel or scissors to shave off the skin,[33] (ii) by using a Weck blade, which can be placed flat on taut skin and advanced to harvest a split-thickness skin graft of uniform size, or (iii) by using a powered dermatome to cut grafts of a fixed diameter and thickness. Once obtained, the graft is transferred to a sterile saline-containing Petri dish or directly to the recipient site. The donor site is temporarily covered with gauze soaked in 1% lidocaine with 1:100,000 epinephrine. At this point, a mechanical meshing device can be used to create fenestrations within the graft, if desired. The presence of fenestrations prevents blood and serum from accumulating under the graft, therefore increasing the likelihood of graft survival. Fenestrations additionally help to expand the surface area of split-thickness skin grafts by 24–35% and are useful for defects >8 cm in diameter.[5]

After harvesting and preparing the split-thickness skin graft, it can be attached to the recipient site using a combination of basting sutures centrally and running or interrupted sutures 5–6 mm apart peripherally. The edges do not require careful approximation because graft skin that does not make direct contact with the wound bed will naturally slough off. After sutures are placed, a bolster or pressure dressing may be applied to maintain adequate contact between the graft and the wound bed.

Additionally, the donor site is treated as an abrasion and covered with petrolatum gauze or another moist occlusive dressing. To help reduce pain at the donor site, one might consider using a dressing soaked in lidocaine or other anesthetic.[34] A pressure dressing over the donor site, in particular a dressing containing calcium alginate,[35] can be used to reduce the amount of serum exudate since there typically is a significant amount of drainage over the donor site for the first 48 hours.

### Postoperative Care and Complications

*Graft Failure*

Graft failure can result from the development of hematoma or seroma. Bolster dressings help prevent this complication. The other option is to create fenestrations within the graft that allow the blood and other fluid to leak out instead of accumulating under the graft.

*Cosmetic Concerns*

Color and texture mismatch is a predictable complication of a split-thickness skin graft. Split-thickness skin grafts often remain erythematous and become hyper- or hypopigmented compared to surrounding skin. Patients should be advised to minimize sun exposure and to use sunscreens. Additionally, the absence of adnexal structures often predisposes the graft site to xerosis and scaling. Contraction of the graft is another major concern, and contraction of facial grafts can result in alar retraction, ectropion, helical rim distortion, and other facial deformities.[36] It is best to avoid split-thickness skin grafts in these regions.

### Variations of Technique

*Intermediate-thickness Graft*

To overcome the disadvantages of either full-thickness or split-thickness skin graft, some surgeons advocate the use of an intermediate-thickness graft (Figs. 12.4A to D), which is obtained by using a No. 15 or No. 10 blade to score the edges of skin elevated by tumescent anesthesia, with a resultant depth <1 mm.[37] In comparison, full-thickness skin grafts tend to be 1–4 mm deep and split-thickness skin grafts tend to be 0.5–1 mm deep.

*Combined Flap and Graft Technique for Large Defects on the Scalp*

For large defects on the scalp with exposed bone, it is difficult to use a split-thickness graft alone because of the low rate of graft survival. In this case, it may be possible to combine a rotation flap with a split-thickness skin graft to achieve better results. For this technique, a flap is created adjacent to the primary defect, with a width equal to that of the primary defect. The flap is incised to the deep dermis, leaving the galea and periosteum intact, and rotated into the primary defect. The flap is closed in a layered manner and the donor site is closed with a split-thickness skin graft.[38]

## Cartilage Grafts

### Indications, Contraindications and Donor Site Considerations

Cartilage grafts are used for deep defects of the nasal alae (Figs. 12.5A to C) or sidewall, where there is loss of alar shape, loss of nasal valve function, or the risk of rim retraction.[39] The nasal sidewall and dorsum are sections of the nose less likely to require cartilage grafting.[40]

Free cartilage that is used to repair a defect on the nose, ear, or lower eyelid can be obtained from the nasal septum, ear, or rib. Cartilage obtained from the ear, which is classified as elastic cartilage, has excellent pliability

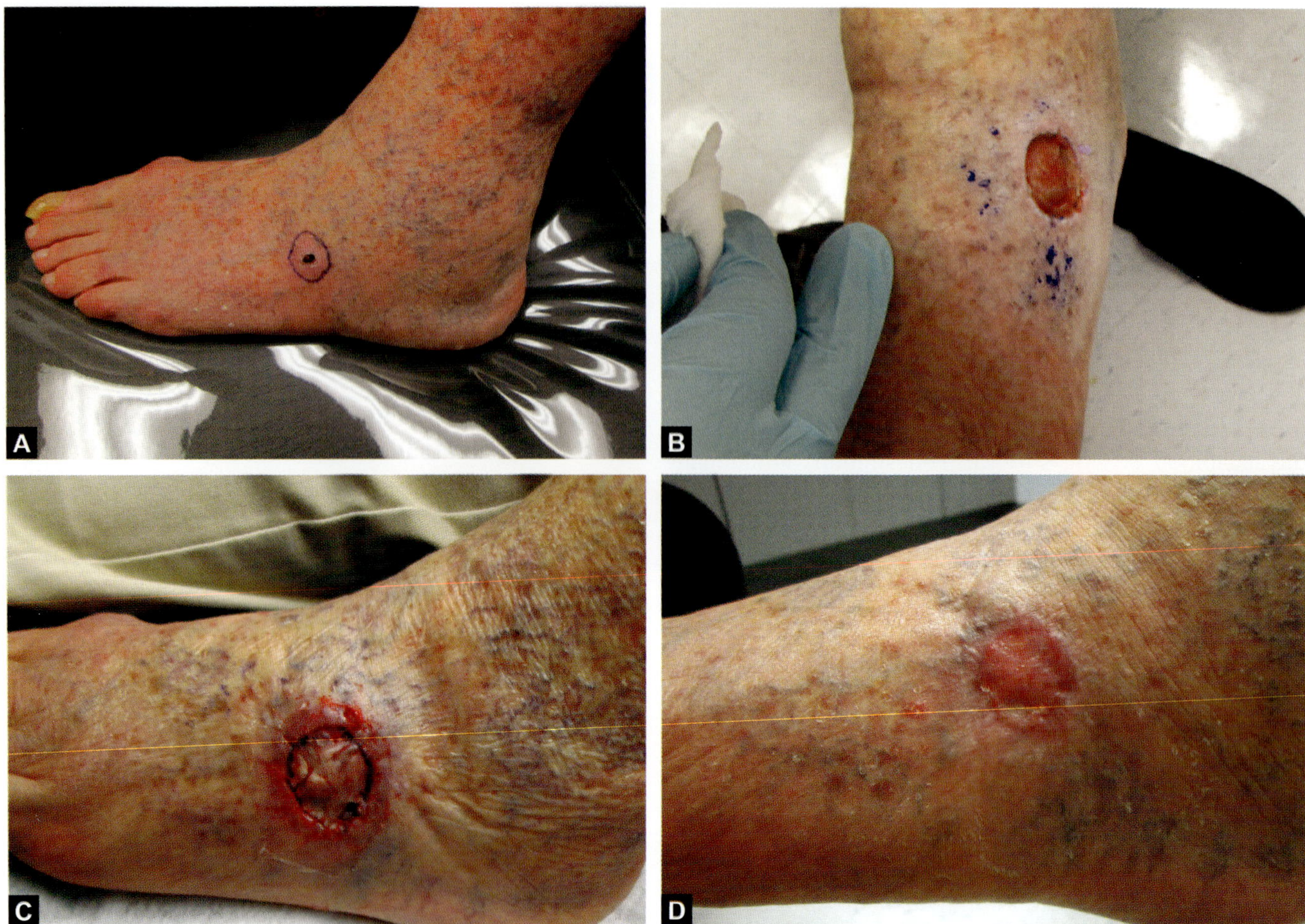

**Figs. 12.4A to D:** Intermediate-thickness skin graft. (A) Appearance of biopsy-proven squamous cell carcinoma on the left dorsal foot prior to Mohs surgery. (B) Defect following tumor extirpation with Mohs surgery. (C) Appearance following placement of intermediate-thickness skin graft. (D) Appearance of graft site 3 months following procedure.

compared to the other types of cartilage and is the most frequently used donor site for free cartilage in dermatologic surgery.[41,42] The antihelix is a donor site that is readily accessible and easily repaired. Other reasons to choose this site over the concha or the helix include the fact that the cartilage in this area is more pliable, has greater memory than other types of cartilage, and is less brittle. Nasal septum and costal cartilage is less flexible but has greater rigidity and strength. Taking cartilage from a rib is performed infrequently in Mohs surgery, however, as it may result in complications that include iatrogenic pneumothorax, chest wall scarring, and postoperative pain.[43] Cartilage that is actively inflamed due to infection, trauma, or other disorders (collagen vascular diseases, rheumatic disease, immunologic disorders) should not be harvested.[44]

## Description of Technique

### *Nasal alae*

A cartilage graft, which is 4–6 mm longer than the surgical defect, is obtained, typically from the ear. After injecting local anesthesia and prepping the donor site on the ear with chlorhexidine, the auricular skin is incised and skin flaps are raised to expose the underlying cartilage. Blunt dissection is used to free the inferior portion of the cartilage from underlying soft tissue and hemostasis is obtained from the donor site as soon as the cartilage is removed. Subdermal pockets are created on the anterior and lateral aspects of the defect, and the cartilage graft is inserted into these pockets to prevent migration of the cartilage. The cartilage graft can then be secured with tie-over sutures, which are first inserted at the base of the defect

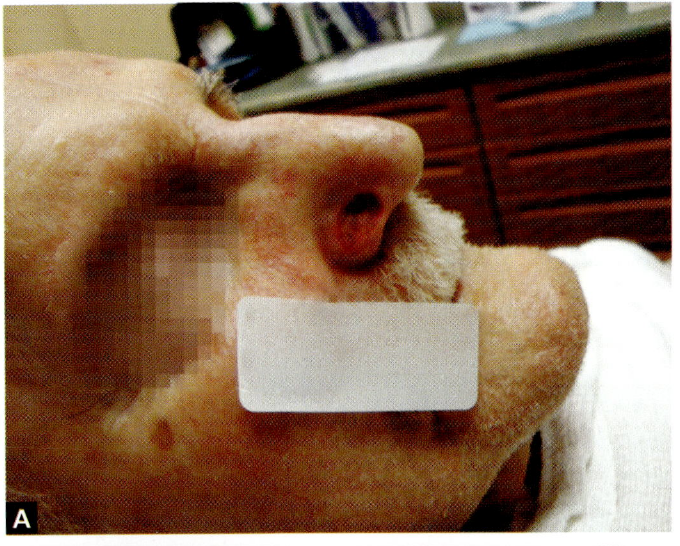
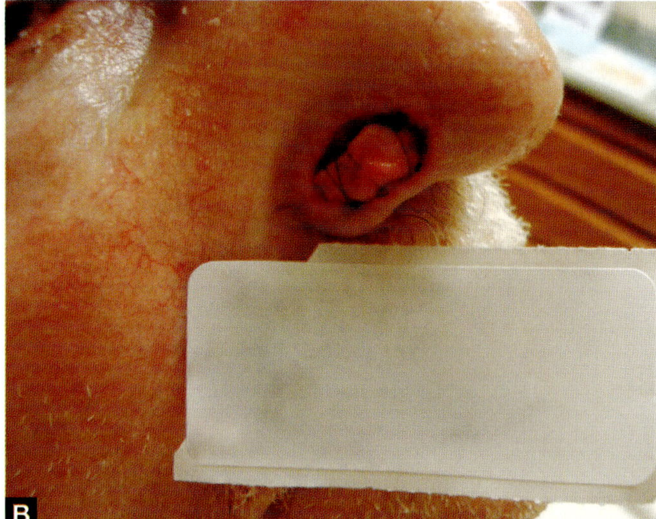
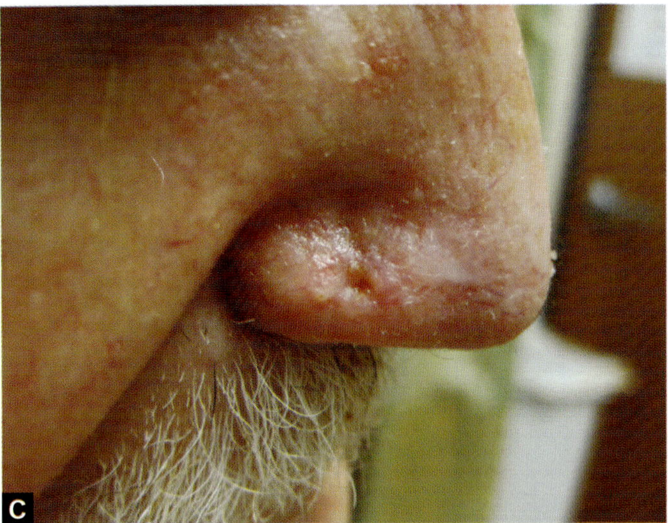

**Figs. 12.5A to C:** Free cartilage grafting to repair a deep nasal ala defect. (A) Appearance of defect on right nasal ala near free margin following tumor extirpation with Mohs surgery. (B) Placement of cartilage graft to wound bed. (C) Appearance of graft site at 12 weeks post-Mohs and reconstructive surgery.
*Courtesy*: Daniel Eisen MD, Sacramento, CA, USA.

and tied over the top of the cartilage without ever penetrating the cartilage.

Cartilage grafts can be combined with flaps or full-thickness skin grafts.[21] Another option for preventing alar collapse is to use a cartilage graft followed by second intention healing.[22] A dressing composed of nonstick products such as Adaptic (Johnson & Johnson Medical, Arlington, TX, USA) or Xeroform (Johnson & Johnson Medical, Arlington, TX, USA) can be used to cover the area.

*Nasal Tip*

Nasal tip revision can be achieved with the use of a "tripod" graft.[45] The nasal tip is marked, ear cartilage grafts are harvested from the concha, and the grafts are sculpted and molded to have lateral and medial crura as well as a shield graft in the center. The whole graft is then inserted via endonasal or external approach and inserted into pockets made in the nose. The graft is then sutured into the lower lateral cartilage of the nose and the anterior skin with 5-0 polyglactin sutures. The conchal bowl donor site can be closed or allowed to heal by secondary intention.[46] Another option for reconstructing the nasal tip is to use a septal extension graft, using autologous septal cartilage as the donor material for the graft.[47]

*Ear*

Partial defects of the helix can be repaired in a single stage using a postauricular advancement flap combined with an ipsilateral conchal cartilage graft.[48] Alternatively, the defect can also be repaired with a staged interpolation flap from the neck/scalp combined with antihelical or conchal cartilage graft.

### Postoperative Care and Complications

Ice packs can be applied to the grafted area postoperatively to minimize graft edema. Oral antibiotics are often used for surgery around the nose and ear because of the high bacterial colonization in this area. The ear is prone to infection with *Pseudomonas*, which can be prevented with the use of gentamicin ointment or oral fluoroquinolones.

Aside from infection, other complications associated with cartilage grafts include necrosis, contraction, and textural changes. Contraction and textural changes can be addressed by using dermabrasion or laser resurfacing 6 weeks to 6 months postoperatively.

## Composite Grafts

### Indications, Contraindications, and Donor Site Considerations

A composite graft is a modified full-thickness skin graft with more than one tissue component, with cartilage for the most part being the additional component. Composite grafts from the ear have been used for full-thickness defects of the lower 1/3 of the nose—to reconstruct the nasal tip and to repair alar retraction as well as septal perforation. The ear helix is most often used as a donor site for alar reconstruction because its curved contour is similar to the curvature of the alar rim. The concha of the ear is useful as a donor site for even deeper nasal defects because of the increased bulk of the concha. Composite grafts not only provide structural support but additionally replace missing skin.

A major limitation to the use of composite grafts is the lower rate of graft survival. Cartilage itself is avascular and relies on passive diffusion of oxygen and nutrients from adjacent tissue. Composite grafts should be limited to a diameter of 1–2 cm to keep all points of the graft within proximity of a vascular source.[49] Grafts larger than this are at risk for central necrosis. To reduce the risk of necrosis, perforations can be created through a large piece of cartilage to allow granulation tissue to penetrate and provide nutrition to the cartilage.

### Description of Technique

After donor and recipient sites are anesthetized with local anesthesia and cleaned with chlorhexidine, the defect is measured and a template made. A tongue-in-groove technique is usually implemented to increase the stability of the graft and its chance for survival. To carry out this technique, two cartilaginous wings are marked out and removed from the donor site. These wings are inserted into pockets created on both sides of the defect. This technique ensures that the graft stays within the defect. The skin overlying the graft is then sutured using two layers, often using an absorbable suture for the deeper layer followed by a nonabsorbable suture. The cartilage itself does not need to be sutured.

The donor site may be closed by primary repair or with the aid of an advancement, transposition, or rotation flap if the donor is the helical crus or rim. The concha, if used as the donor site, is often allowed to heal by second intention.

### Postoperative Care and Possible Complications

Ice packs can be applied to the grafted area postoperatively to minimize graft edema. Oral antibiotics are often used because of the high bacterial colonization around the nose.

*Ways to Improve Outcomes of Composite Graft*

One of the deterrents to using composite grafts is the low rate of graft survival. Corticosteroids,[50] hyperbaric oxygen therapy,[51,52] and postoperative cooling[53] are methods that have been documented to increase the survival of composite grafts. In one study involving an auricular composite graft, preoperative steroids were administered 1 hour before surgery and postoperatively for 3 days. With this regimen, graft survival increased from 23% to 71%. The hypothesized mechanism for increased survival with corticosteroids involves cell membrane stabilization, inhibition of phospholipase and inflammatory mediators, stimulation of gluconeogenesis, and reduction of lactic acid levels.[54]

## SUMMARY

Skin and cartilage grafting is a safe and effective closure technique for dermatologic surgery. Essential to success of grafts is an understanding of the indications, techniques, appropriate donor sites, and possible complications. Grafts can be used alone or in combination with flaps and other reconstructive techniques to improve cosmesis and functional outcome. Attention to hemostasis and the use of bolster dressings can help to prevent graft failure by decreasing the development of hematoma and seroma formation. Prophylactic antibiotics can be considered for sites more likely to get infected and for cases when there is a 1–3 week delay between tumor excision and surgical reconstruction. With careful planning and attention to detail, surgical reconstruction with cutaneous and cartilage grafts can have a successful outcome.

## REFERENCES


1. Maeda M, Nakamura T, Fukui A, et al. The role of serum imbibition for skin grafts. Plast Reconstr Surg. 1999;104 (7):2100-7.
2. Converse JM, Smahel J, Ballantyne DL Jr, et al. Inosculation of vessels of skin graft and host bed: a fortuitous encounter. Br J Plast Surg. 1975;28(4):274-82.
3. Tan E, Mortimer N, Salmon P. Full-thickness skin grafts for surgical defects of the nasal ala—a comprehensive review, approach and outcomes of 186 cases over 9 years. Br J Dermatol. 2014;170(5):1106-13.
4. Mellette JR Jr, Swinehart JM. Cartilage removal prior to skin grafting in the triangular fossa, antihelix, and concha of the ear. J Dermatol Surg Oncol. 1990;16(12):1102-5.
5. Acosta AE, Aasi SZ, MacNeal RJ, et al. Skin grafting. In: Surgery of the Skin: Procedural Dermatology, 2nd edition. Edinburgh: Mosby Elsevier; 2010. pp. 309-27.
6. Adnot J, Salasche SJ. Visualized basting sutures in the application of full-thickness skin grafts. J Dermatol Surg Oncol. 1987;13(11):1236-9.
7. Ranario JS, Shimizu IB. Full-thickness skin grafts secured using 2-octylcyanoacrylate and adhesive strips. Dermatol Surg. 2014;40(2):203-5.
8. Leibovitch I, Huilgol SC, Richards S, et al. The Australian Mohs database: short-term recipient-site complications in full-thickness skin grafts. Dermatol Surg. 2006;32(11):1364-8.
9. Rajpara S, Affleck A, Varma S. Transient graft hypertrophy following full-thickness skin graft. Br J Dermatol. 2010;163 (3):658-9.
10. Thibault MJ, Bennett RG. Success of delayed full-thickness skin grafts after Mohs micrographic surgery. J Am Acad Dermatol. 1995;32(6):1004-9.
11. Kuijpers DI, Smeets NW, Lapière K, et al. Do systemic antibiotics increase the survival of a full thickness graft on the nose? J Eur Acad Dermatol Venereol. 2006;20(10): 1296-301.
12. Henley J, Brewer JD. Newer hemostatic agents used in the practice of dermatologic surgery. Dermatol Res Pract. 2013;2013:279289.
13. Blasdale C, Lawrence CM. Perioperative international normalized ratio level is a poor predictor of postoperative bleeding complications in dermatological surgery patients taking warfarin. Br J Dermatol. 2008;158(3):522-6.
14. Stables G, Lawrence CM. Management of patients taking anticoagulant, aspirin, non-steroidal anti-inflammatory and other anti-platelet drugs undergoing dermatological surgery. Clin Exp Dermatol. 2002;27(6):432-5.
15. Nehal KS, Levine VJ, Ross B, et al. Comparison of high-energy pulsed carbon dioxide laser resurfacing and dermabrasion in the revision of surgical scars. Dermatol Surg. 1998;24(6):647-50.
16. Adams DC, Ramsey ML. Grafts in dermatologic surgery: review and update on full- and split-thickness skin grafts, free cartilage grafts, and composite grafts. Dermatol Surg. 2005;31(8 Pt 2):1055-67.
17. Robinson JK, Dillig G. The advantages of delayed nasal full-thickness skin grafting after Mohs micrographic surgery. Dermatol Surg. 2002;28(9):845-51.
18. Lewis R, Lang PG Jr. Delayed full-thickness skin grafts revisited. Dermatol Surg. 2003;29(11):1113-7.
19. Meyers S, Rohrer T, Grande D. Use of dermal grafts in reconstructing deep nasal defects and shaping the ala nasi. Dermatol Surg. 2001;27(3):300-5.
20. Otley CC. Alar batten cartilage grafting. Dermatol Surg. 2000;26(10):969-72.
21. Zopf DA, Iams W, Kim JC, et al. Full-thickness skin graft overlying a separately harvested auricular cartilage graft for nasal alar reconstruction. JAMA Facial Plast Surg. 2013; 15(2):131-4.
22. Ibrahimi OA, Campbell T, Youker S, et al. Nonanatomic free cartilage batten grafting with second intention healing for defects on the distal nose. J Drugs Dermatol. 2012;11(1): 46-50.
23. Fader DJ, Wang TS, Johnson TM. Nasal reconstruction utilizing a muscle hinge flap with overlying full-thickness skin graft. J Am Acad Dermatol. 2000;43(5 Pt 1):837-40.
24. Johnson TM, Baker S, Brown MD, et al. Utility of the subcutaneous hinge flap in nasal reconstruction. J Am Acad Dermatol. 1994;30(3):459-66.
25. Davis DA, Arpey CJ. Porcine heterografts in dermatologic surgery and reconstruction. Dermatol Surg. 2000;26(1): 76-80.
26. Gladsjo JA, Kim SS, Jiang SI. Review of the use of a semi-synthetic bilaminar skin substitute in dermatology and a case series report of its utility in Mohs surgery. J Drugs Dermatol. 2014 May;13(5):537-41.
27. Müller CS, Schiekofer C, Körner R, et al. Improved patient-centered care with effective use of Integra® in dermatologic reconstructive surgery. J Dtsch Dermatol Ges. 2013;11 (6):537-48.
28. Brady JG, Grande DJ, Katz AE. The purse-string suture in facial reconstruction. J Dermatol Surg Oncol. 1992;18(9): 812-6.
29. Kim KH, Gross VL, Jaffe AT, et al. The use of the melolabial Burow's graft in the reconstruction of combination nasal sidewall-cheek defects. Dermatol Surg. 2004;30(2 Pt 1): 205-7.
30. Fritz TM, Burg G, Hafner J. Eyebrow reconstruction with free skin and hair-bearing composite graft. J Am Acad Dermatol. 1999;41(6):1008-10.
31. Ibrahim AM, Rabie AN, Borud L, et al. Common patterns of reconstruction for Mohs defects in the head and neck. J Craniofac Surg. 2014;25(1):87-92.

32. Shareef M, Hussain W. "Skimming the surface": a review of split-thickness skin grafting practices and preferences among U.K. dermatological surgeons. Br J Dermatol. 2013; 169(4):943-4.
33. Wheeland RG. The technique and current status of pinch grafting. J Dermatol Surg Oncol. 1987;13(8):873-80.
34. Raza MS, Nazim T, Khan FA. Comparison of bupivacaine moistened dressing and conventional dressing for pain relief on skin graft donor sites. J Coll Physicians Surg Pak. 2014;24(6):416-9.
35. Läuchli S, Hafner J, Ostheeren S, et al. Management of split-thickness skin graft donor sites: a randomized controlled trial of calcium alginate versus polyurethane film dressing. Dermatology. 2013;227(4):361-6.
36. Adams DC, Ramsey ML. Grafts in dermatologic surgery: review and update on full- and split-thickness skin grafts, free cartilage grafts, and composite grafts. Dermatol Surg. 2005;31(8 Pt 2):1055-67.
37. Sage RJ, Moy RL, Kampp J, et al. Intermediate-thickness skin grafting for repair of cutaneous defects after Mohs micrographic surgery. Dermatol Surg. 2010;36(8):1305-8.
38. Aldabagh B, Cook JL. Reconstruction of scalp wounds with exposed calvarium using a local flap and a split-thickness skin graft: case series of 20 patients. Dermatol Surg. 2014;40(3):257-65.
39. Campbell T, Eisen DB. Free cartilage grafts for alar defects coupled with secondary-intention healing. Dermatol Surg. 2011;37(4):510-3.
40. Woodard CR, Park SS. Reconstruction of nasal defects 1.5 cm or smaller. Arch Facial Plast Surg. 2011;13(2):97-102.
41. Ratner D, Skouge JW. Surgical pearl: the use of free cartilage grafts in nasal alar reconstruction. J Am Acad Dermatol. 1997;36(4):622-4.
42. Sage RJ, Leach BC, Cook J. Antihelical cartilage grafts for reconstruction of mohs micrographic surgery defects. Dermatol Surg. 2012;38(12):1930-7.
43. Immerman S, White WM, Constantinides M. Cartilage grafting in nasal reconstruction. Facial Plast Surg Clin North Am. 2011;19(1):175-82.
44. Son SB, Han WH, Park JH, et al. Aggravation of relapsing polychondritis due to the infection and its manifestation on a nasal tip graft. Clin Exp Otorhinolaryngol. 2014;7(1): 63-5.
45. Pedroza F, Pedroza LF, Achiques MT, et al. The tripod graft: nasal tip cartilage reconstruction during revision rhinoplasty. JAMA Facial Plast Surg. 2014;16(2):93-101.
46. Rohrer TE, Dzubow LM. Conchal bowl skin grafting in nasal tip reconstruction: clinical and histologic evaluation. J Am Acad Dermatol. 1995;33(3):476-81.
47. Lin J, Chen X, Wang X, Gao X, et al. A modified septal extension graft for the Asian nasal tip. JAMA Facial Plast Surg. 2013;15(5):362-8.
48. Hu J, Zhang Q, Zhang Y, et al. Partial helix defect repair by use of postauricular advancement flap combined with ipsilateral conchal cartilage graft. J Plast Reconstr Aesthet Surg. 2014;67(8):1045-9.
49. Maves MD, Yessenow RS. The use of composite auricular grafts in nasal reconstruction. J Dermatol Surg Oncol. 1988;14(9):994-9.
50. Aden KK, Biel MA. The evaluation of pharmacologic agents on composite graft survival. Arch Otolaryngol Head Neck Surg. 1992;118(2):175-8.
51. Renner G, McClane SD, Early E, et al. Enhancement of auricular composite graft survival with hyperbaric oxygen therapy. Arch Facial Plast Surg. 2002;4(2):102-4.
52. Lewis D, Goldztein H, Deschler D. Use of hyperbaric oxygen to enhance auricular composite graft survival in the rabbit model. Arch Facial Plast Surg. 2006;8(5):310-3.
53. Hirasé Y. Postoperative cooling enhances composite graft survival in nasal-alar and fingertip reconstruction. Br J Plast Surg. 1993;46(8):707-11.
54. Harbison JM, Kriet JD, Humphrey CD. Improving outcomes for composite grafts in nasal reconstruction. Curr Opin Otolaryngol Head Neck Surg. 2012;20(4):267-73.

# CHAPTER 13

# Combination Repairs

Sailesh Konda, Swati Kannan, Suneel Chilukuri

## INTRODUCTION

The previous chapters have introduced the fundamentals of reconstruction with a wide array of versatile flaps and grafts. These workhorses of reconstruction are the foundation of every dermatologic surgeon's toolkit and have the ability to close a majority of surgical defects while preserving the cardinal rules of reconstruction: form, function, and free margins. However, during the course of one's practice, situations may arise when closure of a surgical defect with the use of a single flap or graft is not ideal either due to its large size, involvement of multiple cosmetic subunits, or the inability to adhere to the cardinal rules of reconstruction. Ideally, large defects involving more than one cosmetic subunit should be repaired as separate single-unit defects with each repair completed within its own cosmetic subunit. When these situations arise, the dermatologic surgeon may resort to individualized solutions utilizing a combination of repair options to close a surgical defect and allow for optimal cosmetic outcomes.

Over a decade ago, Robinson prospectively evaluated 500 facial surgical defects during a 10-year period with a diameter of 1.5–4.0 cm secondary to Mohs micrographic surgery for nonmelanoma skin cancers. She performed repairs of surgical defects confined to one cosmetic subunit with a primary closure or single local flap when feasible. When surgical defects bridged cosmetic subunits, segmental reconstruction was performed with combinations of local flaps and grafts to minimize scarring and deformity by placing the scar at the junction of cosmetic subunits. Most often, segmental repair was utilized in the following locations: eyebrow, lip, chin, nasal alar–cheek junction, and the nasal sidewall–cheek junction.[1]

Herein, we will describe a variety of combination repair options categorized by anatomic locations. Many of these combination repairs take advantage of reservoirs of lax skin while respecting cosmetic subunit boundaries. Figure 13.1 depicts the cosmetic subunits of the face. When possible, the reconstructive scar should be hidden within these cosmetic boundaries. As we will utilize combinations of reconstructive techniques previously described, please refer to earlier chapters in this book for in-depth details on flap or skin graft mechanics. These combination repairs are not meant to be an exhaustive list but rather a foundation to assist the dermatologic surgeon with conceptualizing the versatility that combination repairs provide during reconstruction of challenging surgical defects.

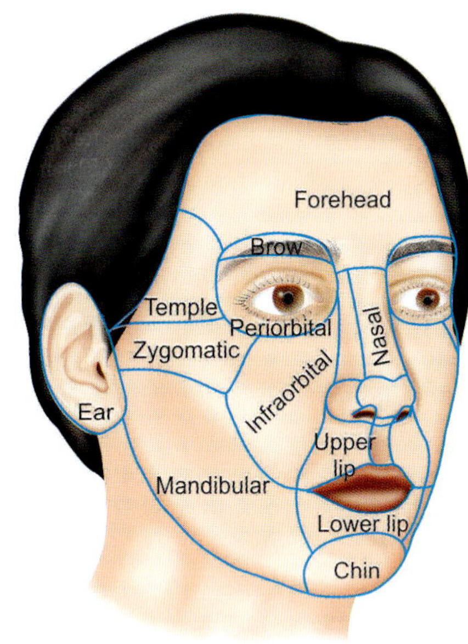


**Fig. 13.1:** Cosmetic subunits of face.

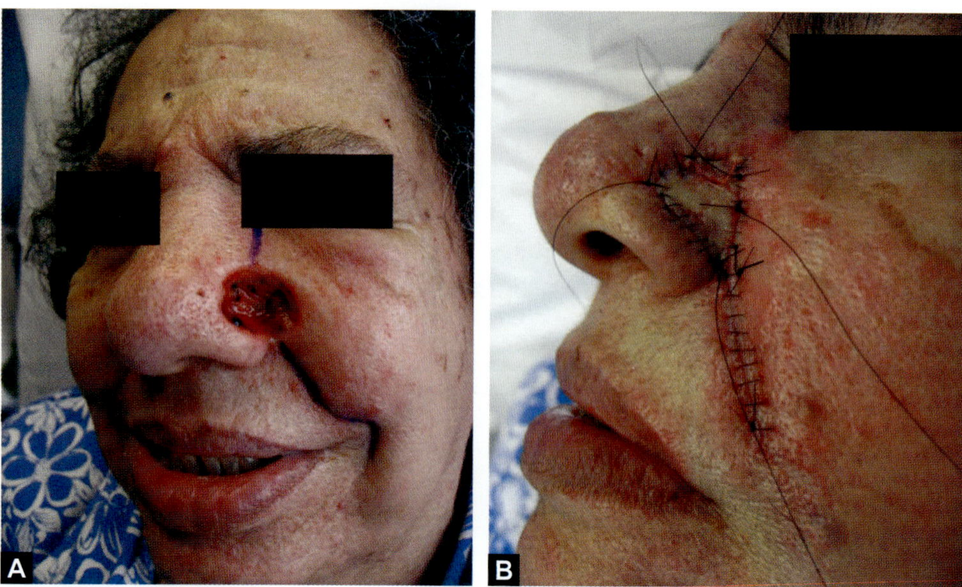


**Figs. 13.2A and B:** (A) Mohs surgical defect of the lateral nasal sidewall and medial cheek; surgical marker depicting planned cheek advancement flap, which will be combined with a V-Y advancement flap from the nasolabial fold. (B) Cheek advancement flap in combination with a V-Y advancement flap from the nasolabial fold.

## NASOFACIAL SULCUS

The nasofacial sulcus is an important cosmetic subunit boundary that separates the nasal sidewall, medial cheek, and the upper cutaneous lip. This cosmetic subunit boundary has a complex interaction of contours and preservation of these landmarks is paramount during reconstruction. Ideally, the reconstruction should be divided into two parts with the cheek undertaken first to recreate the nasofacial sulcus prior to reconstructing the nasal sidewall. The contralateral nasofacial sulcus may be used as a template to achieve facial symmetry during the reconstruction. Many of these combined repair options prove useful as the surgical scars can be hidden in the nasofacial sulcus and/or nasolabial crease while avoiding blunting of the sulcus.

For surgical defects involving the nasal sidewall and medial cheek, a cheek advancement flap combined with a full-thickness nasolabial Burow's graft can provide excellent cosmetic results.[2,3] As the medial cheek is advanced to the nasofacial sulcus and nasolabial fold, superior and inferior Burow's triangles are removed to facilitate advancement and avoid standing cone deformities. Once removed, either Burow's triangle skin can be defatted, shaped to fill the remaining defect on the nasal sidewall, and secured as a full-thickness skin graft (FTSG). Similarly, a cheek advancement flap can be combined with a V-Y advancement flap from the nasolabial fold (Figs. 13.2A and B). For larger defects involving the nasal alar or perialar areas, a V-Y advancement flap and Burow's graft combination may be considered.[4] The V-Y advancement flap is advanced from the nasolabial sulcus up to the nasofacial sulcus to cover the cheek defect. A full-thickness Burow's graft is then taken from the distal third portion of the flap to reconstruct the remainder of the nasal alar defect. This combination repair preserves the nasofacial sulcus angle while hiding the final scar (Figs. 13.3A to D).

When the dermatologic surgeon encounters larger surgical defects at the nasofacial sulcus that extend laterally toward the central cheek and medially toward the nasal dorsum and/or nasal tip, a cheek advancement flap may not provide enough tissue recruitment to recreate the nasofacial sulcus. Instead, a V-Y advancement flap with its medial border along the nasolabial fold can be used to recreate the nasofacial sulcus followed by a paramedian forehead flap, if needed, to reconstruct the nasal dorsum and/or tip. Meticulous care should be taken to preserve the alar groove and apical triangle of the lip. If the surgical defect on the nose involves >50–70% of the cosmetic subunit, the defect can be enlarged to the borders of the involved cosmetic subunit prior to repair to allow the final scars to hide within cosmetic subunit boundaries. Depending on the size of the wound, a FTSG may be added to repair the nasal portion of the defect.

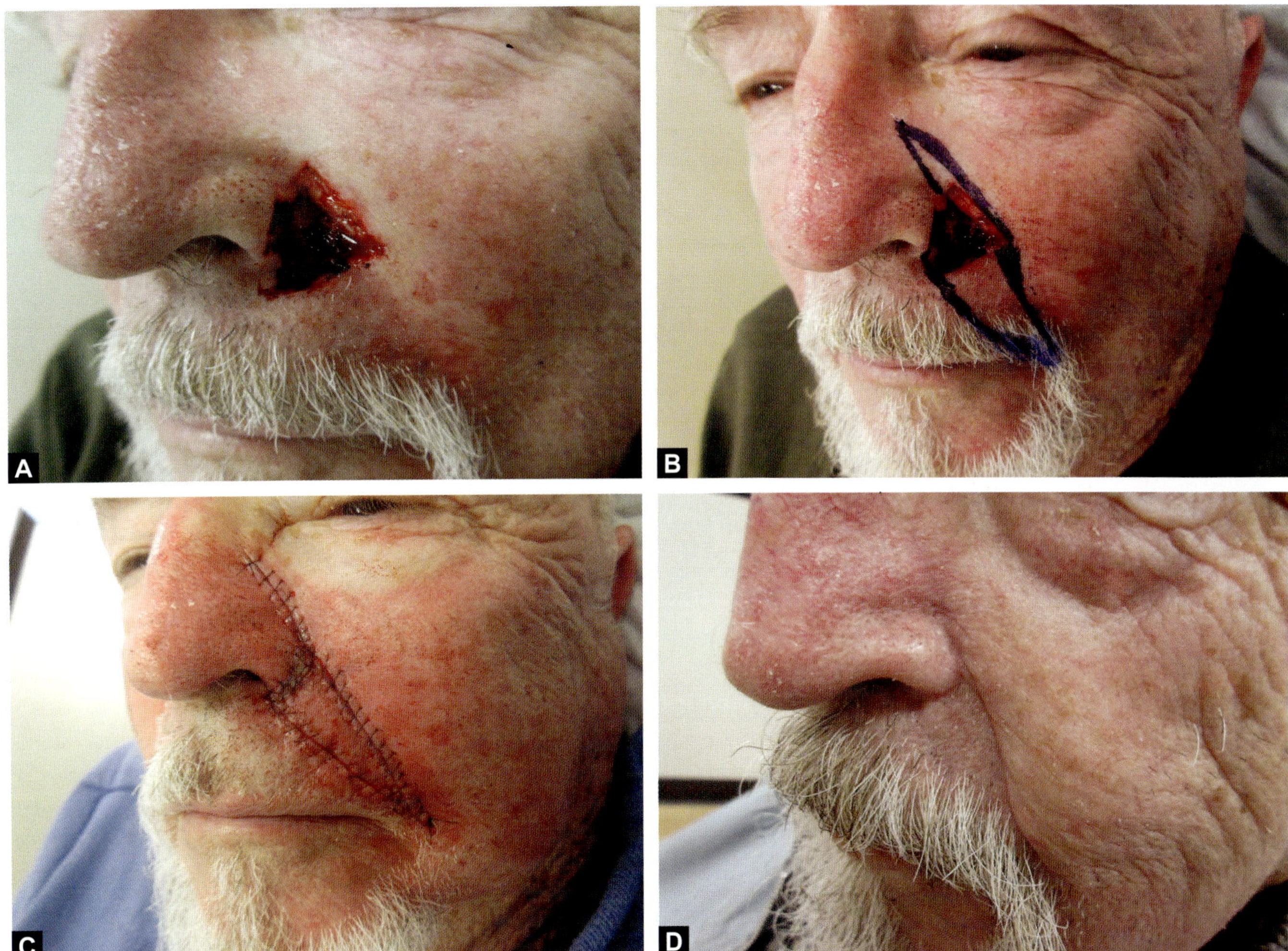

**Figs. 13.3A to D:** (A) Mohs surgical defect involving the nasal ala, upper cutaneous lip, and cheek. (B) Surgical markings depicting planned cheek advancement flap combined with a V-Y advancement flap to address the lip defect. (C) Repair showing combination of a V-Y advancement flap of the upper cutaneous lip, a Burow's graft of the nasal ala, and a cheek advancement flap. (D) Appearance at 4-month follow-up.
*Courtesy*: S Brian Jiang, MD, Sang Diego, California, USA.

## CHEEK

The cheek is the largest cosmetic subunit of the face and has an adequate tissue reservoir to repair most surgical defects utilizing primary closure or a local flap. Occasionally, very large surgical defects may need to be repaired with the use of a combination repair to avoid distorting free margins. Additionally, if a defect crosses a cosmetic subunit boundary of the cheek, consider repairing the defect with two separate closures. Davis and colleagues have used a double purse-string closure to maximize circumferential tissue recruitment for a large surgical defect of the cheek.[5] The first purse-string was placed in the plane between the subcutis and the superficial musculoaponeurotic system and the second purse-string was placed within the superficial dermis. This combined approach reduced the surgical defect to 8% of the original size. Ciatti and Greenbaum have also used the purse-string suture in combination with bilateral advancement to repair large preauricular cheek, cheek/zygomatic arch, and temple surgical defects. Complete closure was achieved in one case and the other two cases had partial closure followed by healing by secondary intention. Excellent cosmetic results were achieved in all cases.[6] Similarly, a purse-string closure can be combined with a rhombic transposition flap or a FTSG.

Another option for large cheek defects is to recruit the inferior tissue reservoir of the mandibular cheek with a large bilobed flap. If the defect cannot be completely

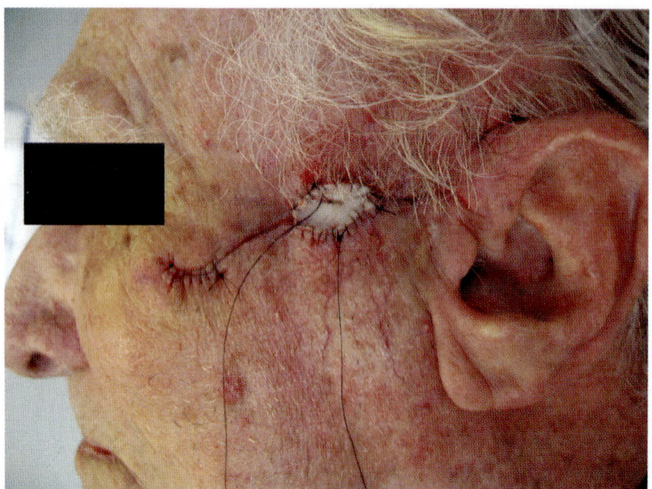

**Fig. 13.4:** Repair of a Mohs surgical defect of the zygomatic cheek with a primary closure in combination with a full-thickness skin graft from a preauricular donor site.

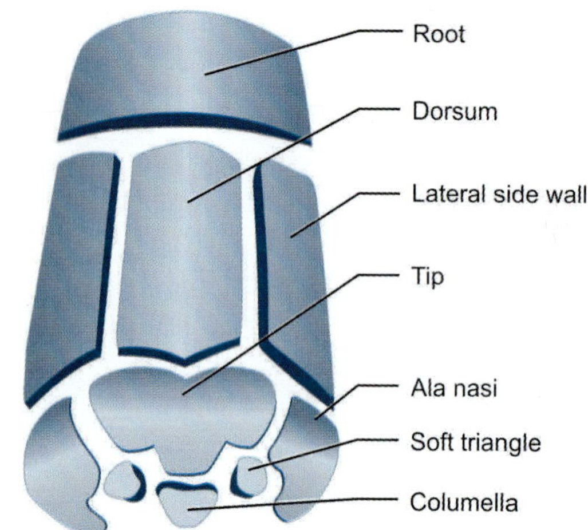


**Fig. 13.5:** Cosmetic subunits of the nose.

closed with the bilobed flap, the standing cone removed adjacent to the surgical defect can be utilized as a FTSG to close the remainder of the defect. Similarly, standing cones from bilateral advancement flaps can also be used as Burow's FTSGs. An example of a large surgical defects of the zygomatic cheek repaired with primary closure combined with a FTSG is depicted in Figure 13.4. Alternatively, primary closure can be combined with secondary intention healing in lieu of a FTSG. Another option to consider in the repair of large cheek surgical defects involves the use of a rhombic transposition flap to repair a portion of the defect combined with an advancement flap to repair the remainder of the defect. Placing these incision lines within cosmetic subunit boundaries and relaxed skin tension lines will optimize the final cosmetic result.

## NOSE

The nose is a complex three-dimensional pyramidal structure supported by a framework of bone and cartilage. It can be subdivided into the following cosmetic subunits: root, dorsum, lateral side walls, tip/supratip, alae nasi (alae lobules), soft triangles, and columella; there may be slight variations of this cosmetic unit breakdown depending on the referenced text. Skin cancers commonly infiltrate two or more subunits of the nose. Figure 13.5 depicts the cosmetic subunits of the nose and, when possible, repair scars should be hidden within these cosmetic boundaries. Each individual's nose has unique peaks and valleys that cast a complex interplay of light and shadows. The dermatologic surgeon should take this into account along with the nasal cosmetic subunits when planning where to create surgical incisions allowing for an optimal cosmetic outcome.

### Nasal Sidewall/Ala

When faced with a defect involving both the nasal sidewall and ala, the reconstructive surgeon must carefully restore the appropriate contour of the nose. First, consider repair of the nasal sidewall. Common reconstructive options for the sidewall include a primary closure, an advancement flap, bilobed flaps, and a rhombic flap. With any of these options, there is typically redundant skin that can be utilized as a FTSG for the alar defect. Consider enlarging the defect to involve an entire cosmetic subunit of the nose before sizing the skin graft, as this will allow suture lines to hide within cosmetic subunit boundaries.

### Nasal Dorsum/Tip

The purse-string closure is a versatile reconstructive option; however, its use in combination closures of surgical defects on the nasal dorsum or tip has rarely been reported. Lackey and colleagues described three patients with surgical defects localized to either the nasal dorsum or nasal supratip, which were reconstructed with a purse-string closure followed by a full-thickness preauricular skin graft to repair the remainder of the reduced defect.[7] They suggest using absorbable poliglecaprone 25 over a nonabsorbable suture to allow gradual loss of strength over 2–3 weeks to minimize the risk of pincushioning of the graft, commonly seen in sebaceous areas such as the nose. To minimize the quilt-like appearance of a FTSG scar, we utilize dermabrasion or fractionated nonablative or ablative lasers to the repaired area 4–6 weeks following placement of the FTSG. The patient may require a series of dermabrasion or laser to minimize the final surgical scar.

If a FTSG is not an option, Redondo describes a one-stage reconstruction with a combination of dorsal nasal flap and a superiorly based nasolabial flap for large defects on the nasal tip. Using this type of closure, the incision lines are placed along the alar crease, nasolabial sulcus, nasofacial junction, and glabellar frown lines. The superior portion of the flap arising from the glabella and nasolabial fold should be undermined in the subcutaneous plane, whereas the remaining portion is lifted beneath the musculature. The rotation flap covers the nasal dorsum, and the transposition nasolabial flap covers the alar defect, columella, and the tip.[8]

## Nasal Dorsum/Sidewall/Supratip

When faced with small-to-medium-sized deep soft tissue defects of the nasal dorsum, side wall, supratip, and alae nasi, any significant loss of soft tissue must be restored prior to cutaneous reconstruction. A nasalis muscular hinge flap can immediately fill the soft tissue defect while providing a rich vascular bed to support further cutaneous reconstruction.[9] This technique takes advantage of skin laxity superior to the surgical defect to allow for primary closure of the secondary donor site. The muscular hinge flap is outlined superiorly to the surgical defect with an anticipated standing cone. After the overlying donor skin is removed, it is saved for later use as a FTSG. The underlying muscle is incised, elevated above the periosteum, and turned into the surgical defect as an inferior-based hinge flap. Once the donor site is closed, the FTSG is then placed over the muscular hinge flap to close the primary defect.[9] This versatile muscular hinge flap can be utilized as a component of varied combination repairs. For example, if a deep surgical defect extends to involve the alar rim/crease, a muscular hinge flap can be used in conjunction with a cartilage graft to buttress the alar rim. The overlying skin can then be closed with a FTSG or ipsilateral nasolabial interpolation flap. The editors often utilize a subcutaneous/muscular hinge flap in combination with a FTSG for reconstruction of deep nasal alar defects that also involve the medial cheek (Figs. 13.6A to F).

## Full-thickness Nasal Surgical Defects

Nasal defects extending full-thickness to the nasal mucosa are challenging, as repair of the nasal mucosa is imperative to achieve optimal functional and cosmetic outcomes. If the nasal mucosa is left to heal by secondary intention, the overlying flap may contract significantly leading to nasal distortion and airway obstruction. Possible repair options for the nasal mucosa include an intranasal mucosal advancement flap from the vestibule, middle vault, or septum; labial buccal, or hard palate mucosal grafts; a septal hinge flap consisting of mucosa and cartilage for support; a nasolabial transposition skin flap rotated 180° on its own axis; or a cutaneous hinge flap from the lateral nasal sidewall.[10] After repairing the nasal mucosa, a skin flap is required for reconstruction of the cutaneous defect.

Plotner and Gloster have described a combination hinge and nasolabial transposition flap for repair of full-thickness nasal alar defects.[10] The hinge flap is taken from the lateral nasal sidewall superior to the alar full-thickness defect and rotated on its base using a hinge maneuver. After the hinge flap is sutured into place, the apex is trimmed to match the size of the primary nasal mucosal defect. Thus, epidermis now replaces the excised nasal mucosa, thereby creating a recipient vascular bed for cutaneous reconstruction. A nasolabial interpolation flap from the cheek is then utilized to repair the remaining cutaneous defect, hiding the final scar in the nasolabial sulcus. Bickle and Bennett have also described successful use of combination hinge flap with an FTSG for a through-and-through nasal defect near the right alar rim.[11] A cartilage graft harvested from the conchal bowl to buttress the alar rim is combined with a nasolabial interpolation flap from the cheek. The distal aspect of the flap can be folded onto itself encasing the cartilage graft for inner mucosa coverage (Figs. 13.7A to C).

Qian and colleagues describe a combination repair for full-thickness alar defects utilizing an auricular skin-cartilage composite graft and a nasolabial flap.[12] The use of skin-cartilage composite grafts is limited to smaller defects ranging from 1.0 to 1.5 cm due to inadequate vascular supply; however, the addition of the robust nasolabial flap allows for repairs of slightly larger defects while restoring the alar rim. The skin-cartilage composite graft, with the same measurement as the alar defect, is obtained from superior helix. The concave side of the graft forms the nasal vestibule and the convex side is bare cartilage. The skin at the margin

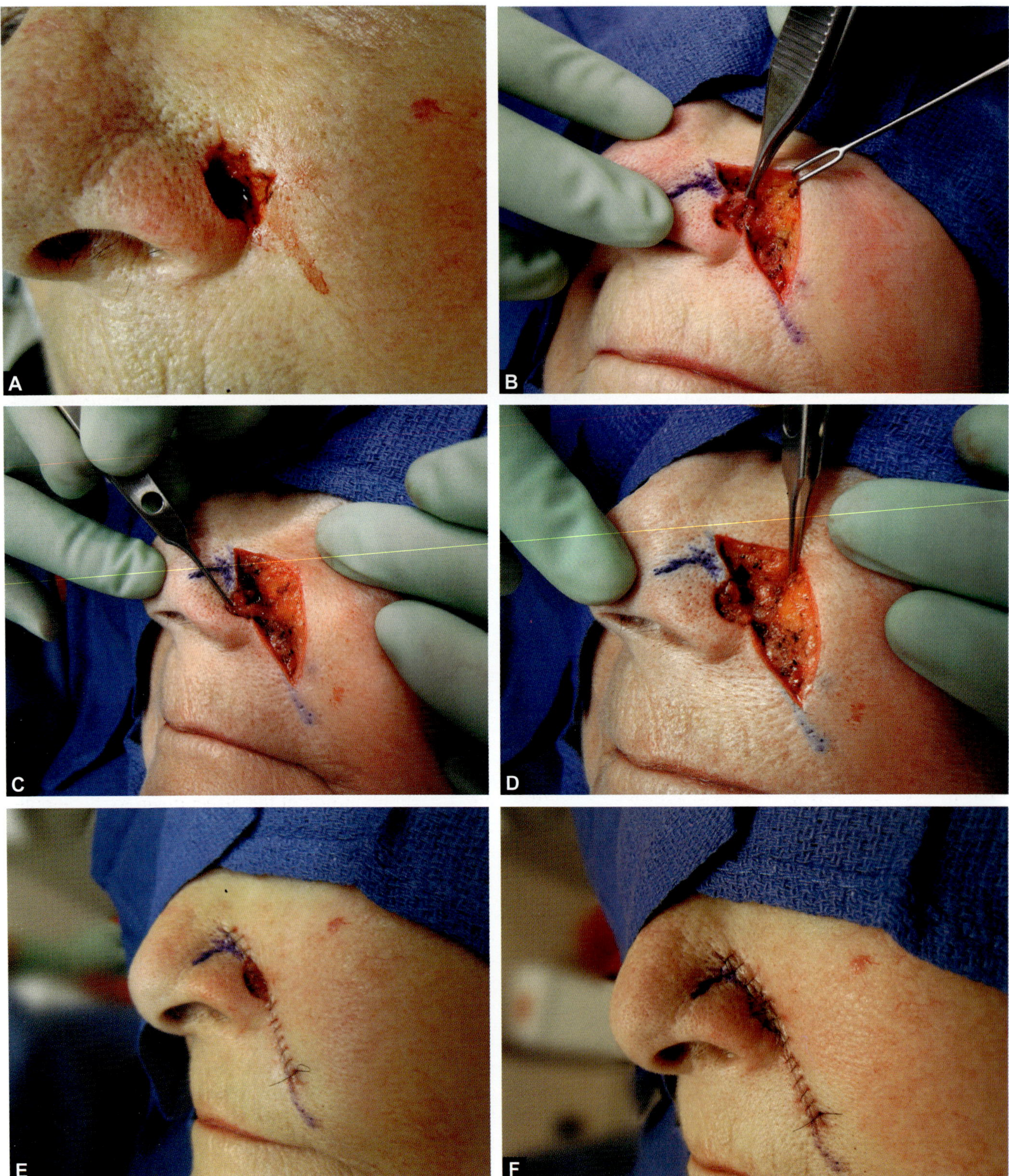


**Figs. 13.6A to F:** (A) Deep Mohs surgical defect involving the lateral nasal ala and medial cheek. (B) Subcutaneous muscular hinge elevated. (C) Muscular hinge moved into place. (D) Hinge secured into defect. (E) Donor site sutured. (F) Skin graft in place.
*Courtesy*: S Brian Jiang, MD, Sang Diego, California, USA.

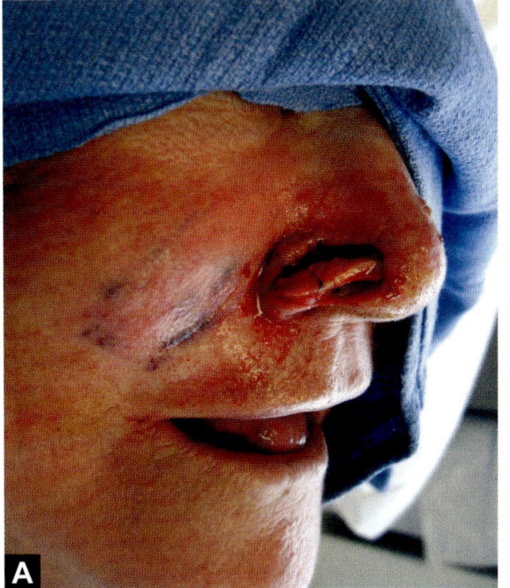

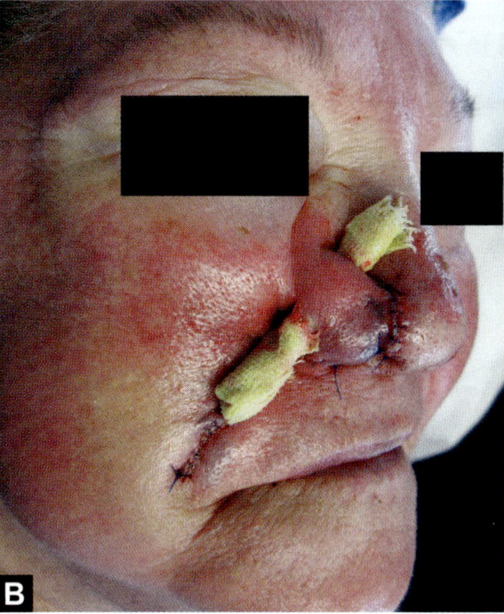

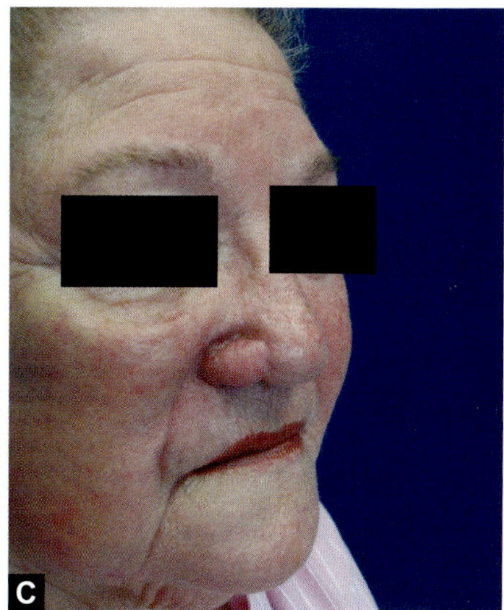


**Figs. 13.7A to C:** (A) Full-thickness Mohs surgical defect of the alar rim; cartilage graft harvested from conchal bowl secured in place to buttress alar rim; faint surgical marker depicting planned nasolabial interpolation flap. (B) Nasolabial interpolation flap sutured over the defect with the distal aspect of the flap folded onto itself around the cartilage graft for inner mucosa coverage. (C) Three-month postoperative results after pedicle takedown.

of the nostril is left smaller than the cartilage to allow the nasolabial flap to be sutured along the inner side of the nostril. Then, the nasolabial interpolation flap is rotated and sutured in place to cover the defect along the nasal ala and the cartilage.

### Nasal Sidewall/Dorsum/Ala

Large central defects involving multiple nasal subunits pose a reconstructive challenge. Kaufman described a combination repair for a large defect involving the right paranasal cheek, right nasal sidewall, dorsum and ala.[13] The paranasal portion of the defect was closed with a cheek advancement to the nasolabial sulcus. A standing cone from the advancement flap was used as a FTSG to repair a small portion of the defect involving the nasal ala and the alar crease. Lastly, a larger FTSG from supraclavicular skin was used to repair the remainder of the nasal sidewall and dorsum. As seen here, there is no limitation to the creativity or number of combined options.

## FOREHEAD

Smaller surgical defects on the forehead can usually be closed primarily or with O-L, O-T, A-T, O-Z, or H-plasty advancement flaps along relaxed skin tension lines. Larger surgical defects involving the paramedian and lateral forehead may need a combination repair with a median forehead rotation flap and an advancement lateral U-shaped flap as described by Redondo.[14] The median forehead rotation flap should not exceed 3–3.5 cm in width so that the donor defect can be closed primarily. The flap receives its blood supply from the ipsilateral or both supratrochlear arteries and is rotated into the medial defect on a pivot point. The U-shaped advancement flap should not exceed a 4:1 length-to-width ratio and is a combined rotation and advancement flap with a curvilinear incision from the inferior lateral portion of the defect down to the temple. Burow's triangles are taken as needed to assist with tissue movement.

Forehead surgical defects may also cross over cosmetic subunits with involvement of the glabella. When both the forehead and glabella are involved, a repair option should be selected that avoids any superior or medial movement of the eyebrows. This can be accomplished with a superolaterally based rhombic transposition flap and an inferolateral primary repair described by Desai and Donnelly.[15] Alternatively, large surgical defects of the forehead and glabella can also be closed with an inferiorly based rhombic transposition flap and superiorly based O-T advancement flaps as described by Blake and Maher.[16]

### Temple

Larger surgical defects on the temple may be difficult to close with a single repair. Judicious care should be taken

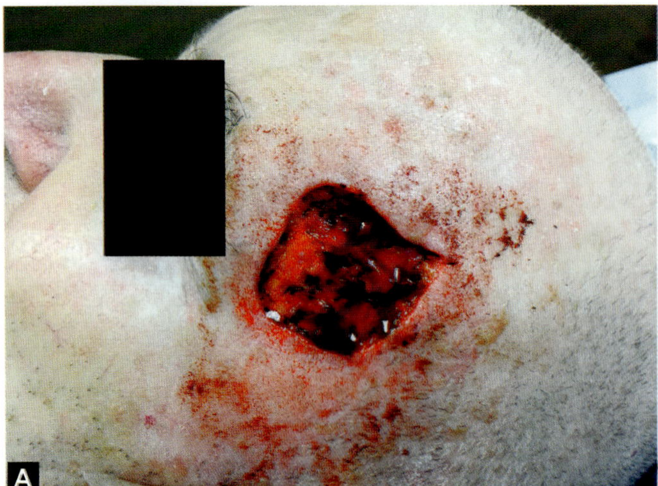


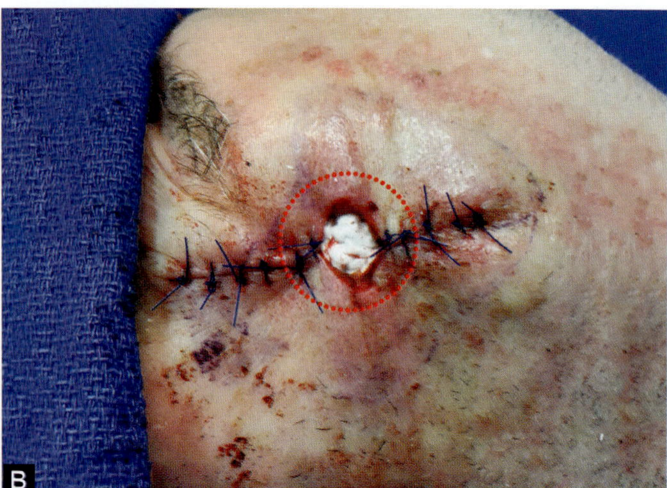


**Figs. 13.8A and B:** (A) Mohs surgical defect of the temple. (B) Primary repair used to close lateral edges of defect followed by a centrally placed double purse-string suture. Red-dotted circle depicts where purse-string sutures were placed. The remainder of the defect was allowed to heal by secondary intention.

to avoid damaging the temporal branch of the facial nerve. A primary repair can be used to close the lateral edges of the defect followed by a purse-string suture to reduce the size of the central portion of the defect. The remainder of the wound can then heal by secondary intention. Figures 13.8A and B depict a large wound of the temple that was repaired with a primary repair and a centrally placed double purse-string repair with the remainder of the defect allowed to heal by secondary intention. Surgical defects in this area can also be closed with a combination of a rhombic transposition flap and a primary repair. Alternatively, given the concave surface of the temple, a rhombic transposition flap can be combined with secondary intention healing if the remainder of the surgical defect is difficult to close with a primary repair or an additional flap.

## Temple/Lower Eyelid

When surgical defects involve the lateral lower eyelid and canthus with extension toward the temple (Fig. 13.9A), the dermatologic surgeon is faced with the challenge of reconstructing the lower eyelid with a horizontal tension vector when there is a paucity of lateral tissue. One reconstructive option that has been regaining popularity in recent years is the temporoparietal fascia flap, which has been used in combination repairs for the lip, ear, eyelid, and even oral cavity.[17] The scalp overlying the temporal fossa is comprised of six layers: skin, temporoparietal fascia, loose areolar tissue, temporalis fascia, temporalis muscle, and pericranium. The temporoparietal fascia is a pliable 2–4-mm thick layer of richly vascularized connective tissue, usually perfused by the superficial temporal artery, and can be recruited for advanced reconstructive options. Blunt undermining at the temple just deep to the hair follicles will reveal the temporoparietal fascia. Figures 13.9B and C show a 3–4 mm width temporoparietal fascia flap that has been hinged over and sutured in place to the remaining lateral lower lid margin, which effectively recreates the contour and tension vectors of the lower eyelid while minimizing risk of ectropion. The inset of the flap was followed by primary closure of the lateral portion of the defect on the temple and a Burow's skin graft on the medial portion of the defect on the lateral lower eyelid. Another option would be to repair the lateral portion of the defect on the temple with a rhombic transposition flap.

## Scalp

Reconstruction of the scalp is challenging due to its limited elasticity and relatively poor vascularity. Further complications occur when large surgical defects extend to or involve bone since deep defects limit the use of primary closures or skin grafts as viable options. These surgical defects may be left to heal by secondary intention or reconstructed with advancement, rotation, or transposition flaps, full- or split-thickness delayed skin grafts, or skin grafting after bone burring to stimulate fine bleeding. Halpern and colleagues have described a combination repair for reconstruction of scalp defects extending to bone using a galeal hinge flap to create a suitable vascular bed

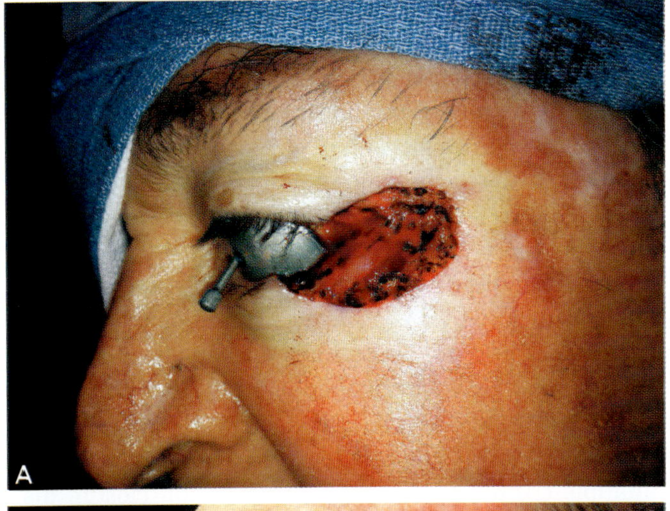


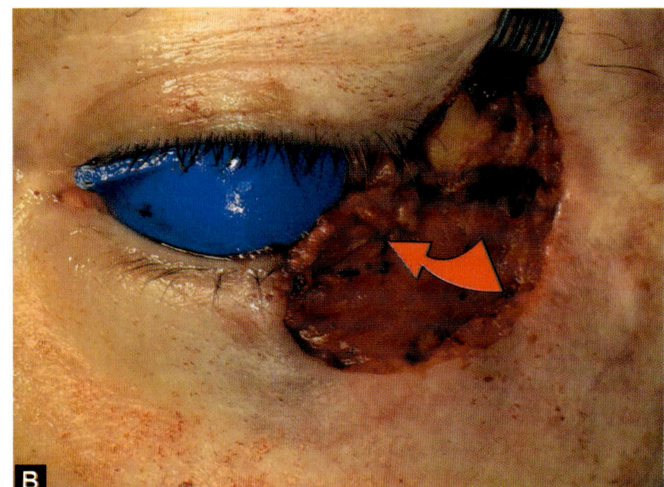


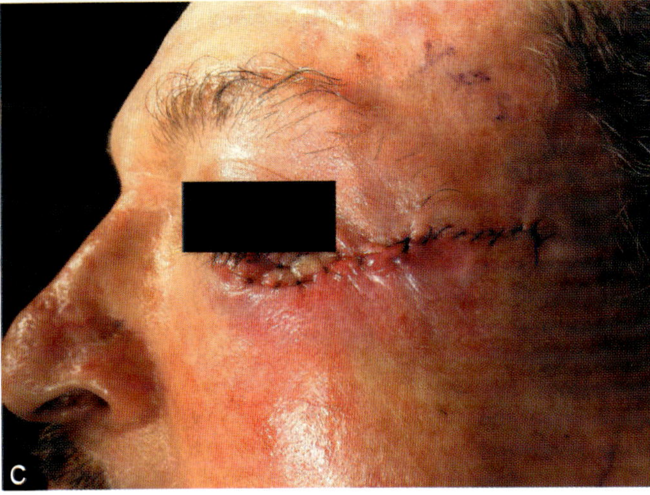


**Figs. 13.9A to C:** (A) Mohs surgical defect of the lateral lower eyelid and canthus with extension toward the temple. (B) Three to four millimeter width temporoparietal fascia flap (red arrow) has been hinged over and sutured in place to remaining lateral lid margin. (C) Immediately after reconstruction; primary closure of the lateral portion of the surgical defect on the temple and a Burow's skin graft on the medial portion of the surgical defect on the lateral lower eyelid.

followed immediately by a full- or split-thickness skin graft.[18] To create the galeal hinge flap, a distal area of the galea aponeurotica is bisected, and a partial-thickness layer of galea is dissected from its base and transposed into position to cover the exposed periosteum of the adjacent surgical defect. A purse-string suture may also be placed before galeal hinge flap placement to reduce the size of the surgical defect. After recreating a vascular bed, the overlying skin can be closed with a full- or split-thickness skin graft or any number of the aforementioned traditional reconstructive options. Lam and colleagues describe a variation of this flap named the reverse galeal hinge flap.[19] After undermining in the subgaleal plane, the galea is bisected toward the surgical defect from below the elevated scalp tissue.

Another reconstructive option is to recruit a banner type flap from adjacent scalp tissue to cover the exposed bone of the surgical defect followed by a split-thickness skin graft harvested from the thigh to repair the secondary defect created by flap recruitment. Aldabagh and Cook successfully performed this combination flap and graft technique for 20 scalp defects ranging in size from 6.25 to 37.6 cm$^2$ resulting in good aesthetic outcomes. The only reported complications were 20% skin graft necrosis in one patient and a methicillin-resistant *Staphylococcus aureus* wound infection in another patient that resolved with antibiotic treatment.[20]

## Infraorbital Cheek/Lower Eyelid

Smaller surgical defects on the cheek can usually be closed primarily along relaxed skin tension lines or with advancement (i.e. nasolabial, V-Y advancement), rotation, or rhombic transposition flaps. Larger surgical defects involving the infraorbital cheek and/or lower eyelid may need a combination repair to preserve cosmetic subunit boundaries and minimize the risk of ectropion. Kaufman described reconstruction of an infraorbital cheek and lower eyelid defect with a combination of a primary closure and a Burow's graft.[21] The inferior portion of the surgical defect on the cheek was closed with primary closure and the resulting adjacent standing cone was excised and used as a Burow's graft to close the superior portion of the surgical defect on the lower eyelid. Using a Burow's graft from adjacent skin to reconstruct the lower eyelid allows for a similar color, texture, and thickness match as opposed to a distant donor site. Care should be taken to not undersize the Burow's graft as postoperative graft contraction can result in ectropion.

If a primary closure is not ideal, a V-Y advancement flap with its medial border along the nasofacial and nasolabial sulci can be advanced superiorly to close the inferior portion of the surgical defect on the cheek followed by a FTSG to repair the superior portion of the surgical defect on the lower eyelid. Several iterations exist for this combination repair.

Another combination repair that preserves cosmetic subunit boundaries and can be useful in this area is a rhombic transposition flap along with a Tripier flap, a single-lobe transposition flap from the upper eyelid.[22] The inferior portion of the surgical defect on the cheek is closed with a rhombic transposition flap with a double Z-plasty followed by a Tripier flap from the upper eyelid, which is transposed into the superior portion of the defect on the lower eyelid. Herman and Bennett include a double Z-plasty at the inferior base of the rhombic transposition flap to allow for greater extension and movement.[22]

An advancement cheek flap and a subcutaneous pedicle propeller flap may also be combined to repair large defects involving the infraorbital cheek.[23] Rozas-Muñoz and colleagues described a vertical cheek advancement flap covering nearly 70% of the inferior portion of the surgical defect on the cheek. A lateral subcutaneous flipped island pedicle flap from the right temple was then used to repair the superior portion of the surgical defect on the lower eyelid. The width of the pedicle should match the width of the remaining superior surgical defect to minimize risk of ectropion. The risks of the subcutaneous pedicle propeller flap include trapdoor formation and necrosis secondary to pedicle torsion.

## Medial Canthus

The medial canthus is a challenging location for reconstruction, as it is the convergence point for four distinct cosmetic subunits: upper eyelid, nasal root, nasal sidewall, and lower eyelid. Additional challenges include the recruitment of tissue reservoirs in a relatively small surgical work field, recreation of the natural concave contour, prevention of ectropion, prevention of postoperative lymphedema, and the match of appropriate color, texture, and thickness. Useful repairs for smaller defects of the medial canthus include primary closures, transnasal flaps, V-Y advancement flaps, transposition flaps, and skin grafts. Secondary intention may also be useful; however, if a defect juxtaposes or also involves the eyelids, secondary intention should be avoided as this may increase the risk of developing ectropion.

When a large surgical defect of the eyelid involves multiple cosmetic subunits, a combination closure may once again prove useful. Yildirim and colleagues describe the use of combined nasolabial V-Y advancement and glabellar V-Y advancement flaps for the closure of 23 large surgical defects of the medial canthus.[24] The glabellar V-Y and nasolabial V-Y advancement flaps were incised down to the galea aponeurotica and subcutaneous tissue, respectively, with preservation of intact pedicles. These V-Y advancement flaps were then advanced until they approximated each other in the center of the medial canthal surgical defect. At 6 months, no complications were reported.[24]

## Vermillion Lip—Mucosal/Cutaneous Lip Junction

The lip is a multilayered structure composed of skin, muscle, and mucosa and plays a prominent aesthetic and functional role within the lower face. A prominent component of the lip is the vermilion and its border; this border signifies a noticeable anatomic boundary between the mucosa and the cutaneous lip and can be easily distorted during reconstruction. Smaller and partial-thickness defects along the vermilion can be repaired via primary repair, local flaps, or even secondary intention. However, secondary intention near the vermilion border sometimes results in lip free-margin distortion. Full-thickness grafts from labial or buccal mucosa are substandard options of reconstruction as these often develop trapdoor deformity and mismatch of color, texture, and thickness. Larger defects require more complex reconstructive methods, often utilizing a combination of various repairs, to preserve oral competency and to prevent distortion, displacement of the vermilion border, and eclabium.

One option for repairing a partial-thickness defect involving the vermilion border utilizes a combination of FTSG and partial mucosal advancement.[25] A graft from the perialar, nasolabial, or preauricular skin is placed on the anterior portion of the defect, followed by advancement of the mucosa to repair the posterior mucosal defect. Prior to graft placement, the vermilion border should be marked to maintain alignment of the border. Benefits of this combined closure include decreased risk of dysesthesia, scar size, and healing time compared to an exclusively mucosal advancement.

Mucosal advancement flaps are the preferred method of repair for large defects localized to the lower vermilion; however, this flap can frequently result in scar contraction, increased redness of the lip, hypoesthesia, and upward movement of beard hairs in men. Kaufman reported a bilateral vermilion rotation flap to repair central defects of up to 40% of the width of the lower vermilion lip; this flap rotates adjacent vermilion skin to the central defect. This technique maintains dimensions of the lip and decreases the aforementioned risks.[26-28]

A combination of Karapandzic and Abbe flaps can be used for large defects of the lower lip. An Abbe flap is performed laterally while the Karapandzic flap is raised on the contralateral portion of the defect. This combination results in an even distribution of the donor sites between the upper and lower lips but inevitably reduces the size of the oral aperture.[29] For larger defects involving greater than two-thirds of the lower lip, Salgarelli and colleagues report a combination of the staircase technique and Sabattini–Abbe flap for reconstruction in nine patients. After full-thickness resection, an Abbe flap is used to repair the central third of the defect by rotating the median upper lip flap with its underlying pedicle onto the central lower lip defect. The second stage utilizes a bilateral symmetric staircase advancement flap for the remainder of lower lip reconstruction.[30]

If a defect involves both the upper cutaneous and vermilion lip and the philtrum, reconstruction utilizing a V-Y island pedicle advancement and mucosal advancement can be performed (Figs. 13.10A to E). Goldberg and colleagues illustrate such a combination repair to reconstruct a large full-thickness defect on the right lip involving the vermilion.[31] A V-Y island pedicle advancement taken from the superior edge repairs the right upper lip skin and muscle, while the mucosal defect is reconstructed using a mucosal transposition flap from the inferior portion of the adjacent left upper lip.[28,32] Bilateral rhombic transposition flaps present another novel repair option for reconstruction of philtral defects. A rhombic flap can be transposed into the center from either side of the philtral crest.[28,33] If there is blunting of the philtral column, injectable hyaluronic acid fillers may be used to recreate the philtrum.

Larger surgical defects of the philtrum and Cupid's bow can be repaired with bilateral vermillion rotation flaps completed by incision along the vermillion border laterally to the oral commissures. These rotation flaps are then recruited medially to reconstruct the surgical defect followed by a W-plasty on the central upper cutaneous lip to recreate the contour of the philtrum and Cupid's bow.

In cases of smaller defects involving the partial-thickness of muscle and mucosa of the lateral upper cutaneous and/or vermilion lip, a combination of partial wedge repair and advancement flap can be performed. A partial wedge repair closes the subcutaneous tissue and muscle, whereas a laterally recruited advancement flap repairs the cutaneous defect.[34]

## EAR

Similar to the nose, the ear is a complex three-dimensional structure, supported by a framework of cartilage that is easily deformed with wound tension or scar contracture. The skin on the anterior surface of the ear is thin and adherent to the underlying cartilage, while the skin on the posterior surface of the ear is thicker with greater mobility. The dermatologic surgeon must be cognizant of cosmetic subunits and tension vectors when selecting a repair option. Larger partial thickness defects of the conchal bowl may be allowed to heal by secondary intention or may be repaired with a combination of FTSGs, rotation flaps, and/or secondary intention. If a deep conchal bowl defect with loss of cartilage extends to involve the antihelix or antitragus, other creative combination repairs can be utilized. The conchal bowl portion can be repaired with a revolving door, postauricular artery island, or postauricular transposition flap followed by a FTSG to repair the antihelix or antitragus portion. Larger defects of the helical rim can be repaired with single or bilateral helical rim advancement flap(s) or with a postauricular interpolation flap followed by a wedge excision or FTSG to repair the remainder of the defect.

The posterior surface of the ear has greater mobility and allows the dermatologic surgeon greater flexibility when tackling surgical defects with combination repairs. Larger defects of the posterior central ear can be repaired with an advancement flap recruited from laterally based

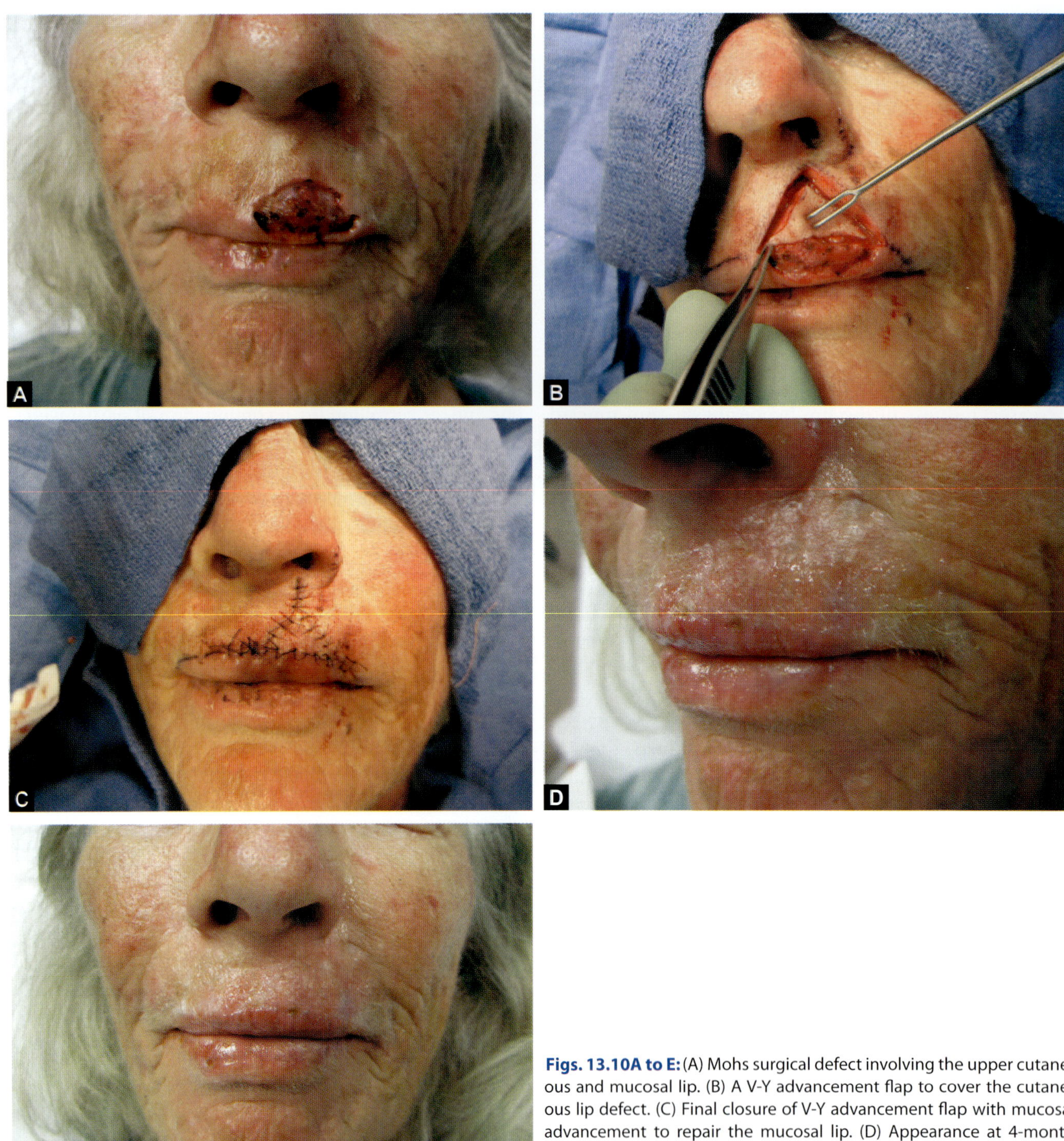


**Figs. 13.10A to E:** (A) Mohs surgical defect involving the upper cutaneous and mucosal lip. (B) A V-Y advancement flap to cover the cutaneous lip defect. (C) Final closure of V-Y advancement flap with mucosal advancement to repair the mucosal lip. (D) Appearance at 4-month follow-up (lateral view). (E) Appearance at 4-month follow-up (frontal view).
*Courtesy*: S Brian Jiang, MD, Sang Diego, California, USA.

postauricular skin followed by a rhombic transposition flap recruited from skin either superior or inferior to the defect. Defects of the superior or inferior aspect of the posterior ear can be repaired with a transposition flap from postauricular skin and, if needed, a FTSG can be used to repair the remainder of the defect (Figs. 13.11A to F).

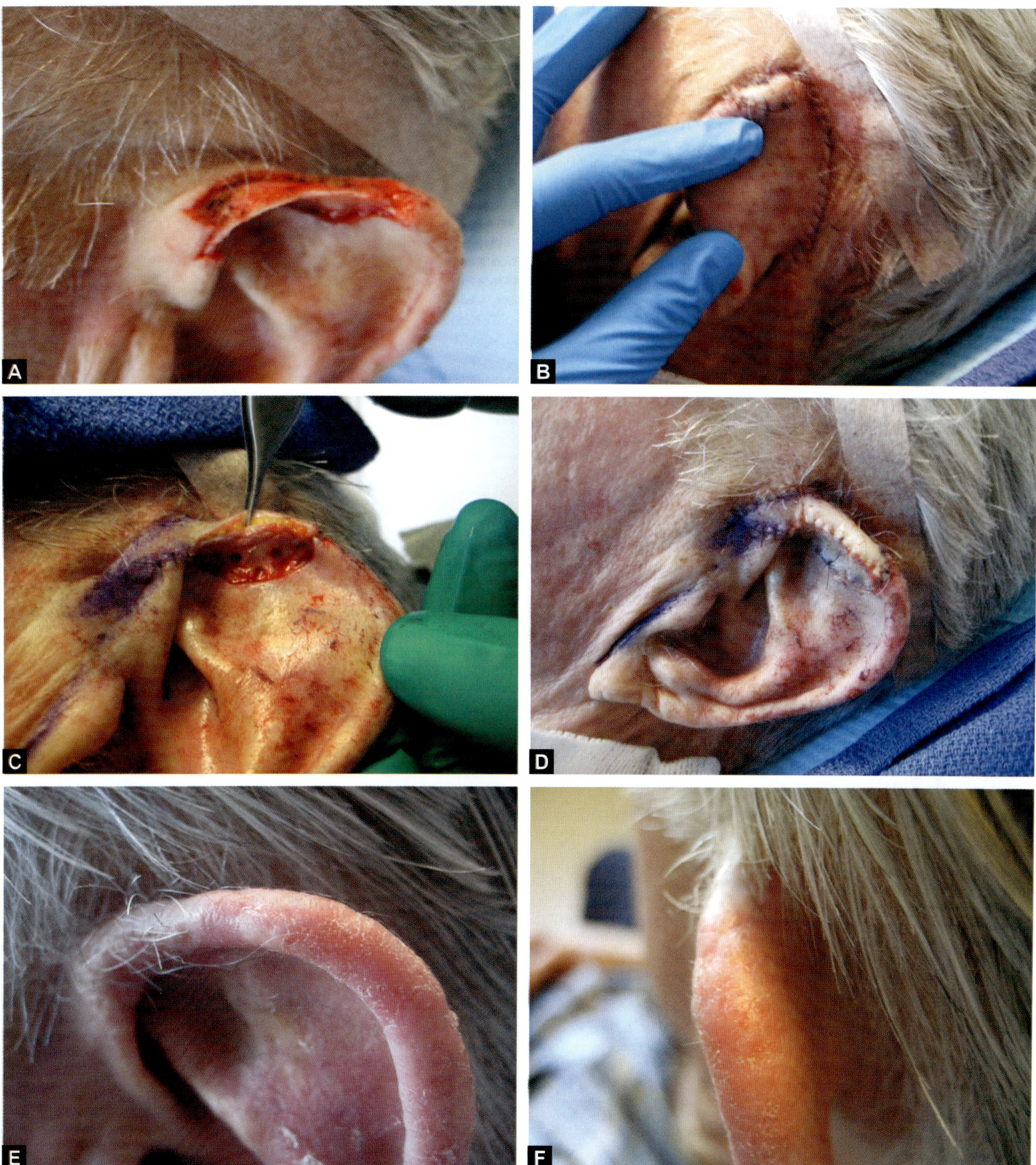


**Figs. 13.11A to F:** (A) Mohs surgical defect involving the superior anterior and posterior helix and scaphoid fossa. (B) Transposition flap placed to repair the superior posterior helical defect. (C) The transposition flap extends to repair the superior anterior portion of the helix. Note the 2 mm punch defects created within the exposed cartilage to assist with perfusion. (D) A full-thickness skin graft covers the defect in the scaphoid fossa. (E) 4-month follow-up (anterior view). (F) Four-month follow-up (posterior view).
*Courtesy*: S Brian Jiang, MD, Sang Diego, California, USA.

Hollmig and Leach described a combination repair for a large full-thickness surgical defect involving the concha, antitragus, and postauricular sulcus with extension to the retroauricular and mastoid region.[35] A large inferiorly based rotation flap was used to close the postauricular sulcus, retroauricular, and mastoid portions of the defect and a Burow's triangle was saved from this repair. A transposition flap was then raised from within the center of the rotation flap and turned over like a page in a book to repair the posterior portion of the ear. The Burow's triangle was then used as a FTSG to repair the anterior portion of the ear. The FTSG received vascular support from the underlying transposition flap from the posterior side of the ear.[35]

## CHIN

The chin is delineated by the labiomental crease superiorly and the mandible inferiorly. This cosmetic unit contains areas of convexity and concavity. While many reconstructive modalities exist, poorly planned reconstruction can lead to contour deformities and functional disability of the lower lip. Useful repair options along the labiomental crease include O-T, A-T, and V-Y advancement flaps along with rotation and bilobed flaps. Bilateral V-Y advancement and rotation flaps may be effective in symmetrically recruiting laterally based tissue reservoirs from both sides of the defect. If a defect crosses the labiomental crease, a combination repair can be performed to preserve the labiomental crease. The portions of the defect superior to and inferior to the labiomental crease may be repaired with two distinct flaps. Secondary intention may also be useful in areas of concavity around the labiomental crease. If a defect is laterally based along the labiomental crease, a V-Y advancement flap with tissue borrowed from the concavity of the chin may be utilized and the secondary defect can be left to heal by secondary intention. Defects that cross the mental protuberance to involve the upper neck should also undergo separate cosmetic subunit repair.

## CONCLUSION

Defects involving multiple cosmetic subunits require judicious planning to attain optimal cosmetic and functional outcomes. Functional goals of reconstructive surgery include preservation of symmetry and distinct boundaries between cosmetic subunits, sensation and motor function, and overall form of the particular cosmetic subunit. Thus, a surgeon may need to consider a combination of repairs such as primary and secondary intention, flaps, and grafts to close a particular defect. While future studies may be considered to evaluate and standardize which combination repairs provide the best cosmetic outcomes at the junction of two distinct cosmetic subunits, these combination repairs are unique to each patient. In addition, difficulty lies in obtaining sample sizes with adequate power. The dermatologic surgeon's discretion is paramount in deciding which repair option a patient is best suited for given the surgical defect, location, and any comorbidities. By understanding the adaptability and mechanics of innovative closure techniques, the dermatologic surgeon can individualize a particular combination repair to reconstruct a challenging defect. We hope that this chapter has provided a foundation of combination repairs to help stimulate thinking outside of the box for creative surgical reconstructive solutions.

## REFERENCES


1. Robinson JK. Segmental reconstruction of the face. Dermatol Surg. 2004;30:67-74.
2. Kim KH, Gross VL, Jaffe AT, et al. The use of the melolabial Burow's graft in the reconstruction of combination nasal sidewall-cheek defects. Dermatol Surg. 2004;30:205-7.
3. Maher IA, Lavigne K. Use of the standing cone allows for subunit repair of a large composite cheek and nose defect. Dermatol Surg. 2014;40:1255-8.
4. Yi SM, Lee KG, Kim JH, et al. Single-stage reconstruction of nasal ala and perialar defect with island pedicle flap and Burow's graft. Dermatol Surg. 2011;37:851-4.
5. Davis JC, Baillis B, Love WE. Novel stacked double purse-string closure. Dermatol Surg. 2014;40:1409-12.
6. Ciatti S, Greenbaum SS. Modified purse-string closure for reconstruction of moderate/large surgical defects of the face. Dermatol Surg. 1999;25:215-9; discussion 219-20.
7. Lackey J, Mendese G, Grande D. Using an absorbable purse-string suture to reduce surgical defects of the nose before placement of full-thickness skin grafts. Dermatol Surg. 2015;41:657-60.
8. Redondo P. Elongated dorsal nasal flap with superiorly based nasolabial flap for large nasal tip defects: 1-stage reconstruction. Dermatol Surg. 2014;40:912-5.
9. Fader DJ, Wang TS, Johnson TM. Nasal reconstruction utilizing a muscle hinge flap with overlying full-thickness skin graft. J Am Acad Dermatol. 2000;43:837-40.
10. Plotner AN, Gloster HM Jr. Combined hinge and nasolabial transposition flap for repair of a full-thickness nasal alar defect. Dermatol Surg. 2011;37:371-4.
11. Bickle K, Bennett RG. Combined hinge flap full-thickness skin graft for a through-and-through nasal defect. Dermatol Surg. 2008;34:389-92.
12. Qian C, Yaodong X, Xiaoming H, et al. Repair of full-thickness alar defects. Dermatol Surg. 2012;38:1639-44.

13. Kaufman AJ. Repair of nasal defect following Mohs surgery. Dermatol Surg. 2001;27:995-7.
14. Redondo P. Repair of large defects in the forehead using a median forehead rotation flap and advancement lateral U-shaped flap. Dermatol Surg. 2006;32:843-6.
15. Desai RS, Donnelly HB. Repair of a glabellar and inferior forehead defect. Dermatol Surg. 2006;32:112-4.
16. Blake B, Maher I. Reconstruction of a large defect of the glabella and forehead. Dermatol Surg. 2015;41:280-2.
17. Mavropoulos JC, Bordeaux JS. The temporoparietal fascia flap: a versatile tool for the dermatologic surgeon. Dermatol Surg. 2014;40(Suppl 9):S113-9.
18. Halpern M, Adams C, Ratner D. Galeal hinge flaps: a useful technique for immediate repair of scalp defects extending to periosteum. Dermatol Surg. 2009;35:127-30.
19. Lam T, Miletta N, Bingham JL. The reverse galeal hinge flap: another valuable technique in the repair of scalp defects extending to the calvarium. Dermatol Surg. 2015;41:533-6.
20. Aldabagh B, Cook JL. Reconstruction of scalp wounds with exposed calvarium using a local flap and a split-thickness skin graft: case series of 20 patients. Dermatol Surg. 2014; 40:257-65.
21. Kaufman AJ. Reconstruction of a large surgical defect involving the lower eyelid and infraorbital cheek. Dermatol Surg. 2003;29:284-6; discussion 286-7.
22. Herman AR, Bennet RG. Reconstruction of a large surgical defect on the lower eyelid and infraorbital cheek. Dermatol Surg. 2005;31:689-91.
23. Rozas-Munoz E, Pujol RM, Toll A. Reconstruction of defects of the infraorbital malar cheek. Dermatol Surg. 2011;37: 1675-8.
24. Yildirim S, Akoz T, Akan M, et al. The use of combined nasolabial V-Y advancement and glabellar flaps for large medial canthal defects. Dermatol Surg. 2001;27:215-8.
25. Seavolt MB, McCall MW. Repair of partial-thickness Mohs defects of the vermilion lip with a combination of full-thickness graft and mucosal advancement. Dermatol Surg. 2005;31:1333-5.
26. Sand M, Altmeyer P, Bechara FG. Mucosal advancement flap versus primary closure after vermilionectomy of the lower lip. Dermatol Surg. 2010;36:1987-92.
27. Litani C, Maize JC, Cook J. An interesting observation in lip reconstruction. Dermatol Surg. 2010;36:704-12.
28. Kaufman AJ, Rohrer TE. Novel flaps for lip reconstruction. Skin Therapy Lett. 2006;11:4-9.
29. Ilankovan V, Ethunandan M, Ee Seah T. Part II: reconstruction of specific defects- lips/chin. In: Local Flaps in Facial Reconstruction—A Defect Based Approach. Switzerland: Springer; 2015. pp. 247-315.
30. Salgarelli AC, Bellini P, Magnoni C, et al. Synergistic use of local flaps for total lower lip reconstruction. Dermatol Surg. 2011;37:1666-70.
31. Goldberg LH, Peterson SR, Silapunt S. Reconstruction of a large surgical defect involving the upper lip. Dermatol Surg. 2005;31:206-9.
32. Ray TL, Chow S, Lee PK. Myocutaneous island pedicle "sling" flap for correction of central upper cutaneous (philtral) lip defects. Dermatol Surg. 2010;36:671-4.
33. Jacono AA, Bassiri M, Talei B. Bilateral transposition lip flaps: a novel single-stage reconstruction of central upper lip defects involving Cupid's bow. JAMA Facial Plast Surg. 2015;17:219-23.
34. Spinowitz AL, Stegman SJ. Partial-thickness wedge and advancement flap for upper lip repair. J Dermatol Surg Oncol. 1991;17:581-6.
35. Hollmig ST, Leach BC. Reconstruction of a complex auricular defect. Dermatol Surg. 2015;41:1175-8.

# CHAPTER 14

# Reconstruction of the Nose

***Bassel H Mahmoud, Suzanne M Olbricht***

## INTRODUCTION

The nose is the central feature that defines a person's face and allows for normal respiration. Its unique anatomy combined with its aesthetic and functional importance makes reconstruction a challenging process. The goals of reconstruction are to maintain airway patency and to restore a normal appearance. The patient should experiment preoperatively with nasal respiration (breathing from both nostrils, then with one nostril occluded and then the other) in order to define the normal state for the patient. Postoperatively, the patient will be more sensitive to feelings of stuffiness in the nostril which may be the result of surgery but may also have been present prior to surgery. In addition, the natural and normal appearance of a nose usually includes some asymmetry. It is often useful to point out to the patient in a mirror how naturally asymmetric their nose is prior to instilling local anesthesia.

The nose is a three-layered structure covered by skin, supported by cartilage and bone, and lined by perichondrium and mucous membrane.[1] A detailed knowledge of the anatomy of the nose (discussed in Chapter 3) is essential in designing the reconstructive plan.

An important concept in nasal reconstruction is the recognition of cosmetic subunits. These subunits remain consistent across all patient populations despite varying ethnic characteristics. The nose is divided into the following subunits (Fig. 14.1):

1. The dorsal subunit of the nose, which extends from the root to the supratip depression. The lateral ridges of the dorsum meet the nasal sidewalls. This skin has a thin epidermis with few sebaceous units, and a thin dermis intertwined with the musculature of the nose. The upper half is supported and shaped by the nasal bone and the lower half by the septal and lateral nasal cartilage.

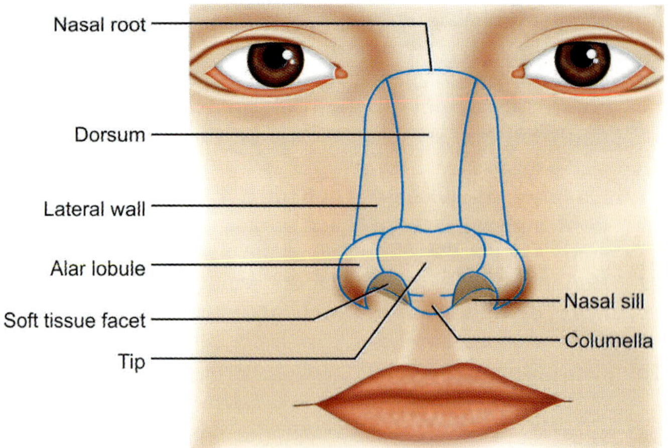


**Fig. 14.1:** Cosmetic subunits of the nose.

2. The nasal sidewall, which extends from the medial canthus to the lateral ridge of the dorsum superiorly. The posterior border of the sidewall is defined by its junction with the soft slope of the cheek skin. The inferior border is its confluence with the alar lobule and nasal tip. The epidermis is similar to the dorsum of the nose but the dermis is thicker and there is subcutaneous fat of varying thickness sitting on top of the musculature. It tends to get thicker more posteriorly.
3. The nasal tip subunit is the remaining central aspect of the nose formed by the borders of the aforementioned subunits. The nasal tip contains the lateral genu or dome of the nose formed by the lateral and medial crura of the alar cartilage.[2] The thin epidermis sits on top of thin dermis in most women, but in most men there is an abundance of sebaceous glands within a thick dermis. It is very well vascularized.
4. The soft triangle is a depression that forms at the apex of the nostril opening inferior to the alar cartilage, and

it is not supported by the alar cartilage. It has thin epidermis, thin dermis which is covered internally by thin mucosa. The vasculature is terminal and sparse, unlike the redundant and abundant vasculature of the rest of the nose.

5. The ala is formed by the lateral crus of the lower lateral cartilage and the soft tissue that extends to the nasolabial crease. It consists entirely of dense fibrous tissue with abundant sebaceous glands and has no cartilage itself.
6. The columella extends from its wide base, at the upper cutaneous lip, containing the middle and medial crura of the alar cartilages until it reaches the inferior border of the tip subunit. It also has thin epidermis and thin dermis sitting directly on the cartilaginous support of the nose.
7. The nasal sill is the soft-tissue continuation of the ala as it curves medially to join the columella, and it represents the floor of the nostril.
8. Two other important landmarks in nasal reconstruction include the alar crease, a curvilinear depression that demarcates the ala superiorly and may be more or less prominent and more or less symmetric and the upper lip triangle that defines the inferior junction of the nose with the cheek and the lip. These landmarks as well as the cosmetic subunits must be respected for reconstruction to be functionally and cosmetically appropriate.

The skin of the nose is affected by many benign and malignant processes. About 75% of nonmelanoma malignancies occur on the head and neck and, of these, ~30% occur on the nose. Tumors differ in the depth of involvement. Some subunits of the nose heal very well by granulation and re-epithelialization and some cover very well with grafts depending on the depth of the wound, while a deep wound often requires adjacent tissue rearrangement for an adequate functional and cosmetic result. It is therefore more important on the nose than on other facial sites to preserve all healthy tissue at the base of the wound in order to allow for the greatest number of repair options possible.

The primary guideline for successful nasal reconstruction is the reconstruction of the defect within the cosmetic subunit if possible. Subunit reconstruction is ideal because it ensures that the reconstructed external covering of the nose matches the color and texture of the original and remaining nasal skin. In addition, it utilizes the boundaries between the subunits to hide sutured wound edges. If a defect involves more than one cosmetic unit, it is helpful to think of each portion of the defect as a separate reconstructive issue, unifying the reconstruction only if the boundaries between subunits can be respected. For instance, if the defect encompassed part of the sidewall and extended into the ala and was fairly superficial (2 mm deep), the optimal repair may be a linear closure or Burow's advancement flap to close the defect on the sidewall and second intent or a graft for the alar crease and ala. If > 50% of a subunit is involved, excision of the entire subunit before reconstruction may be considered. This additional excision of healthy tissue may promote camouflage of the reconstruction but may also create a need for a much larger and more complex repair. The reconstructed external covering of the nose should match the color and texture of the original and remaining nasal skin. The skin over the dorsum of the nose is relatively thin and mobile as compared to the sebaceous tissue of the nasal tip and ala, which is firmly attached to the underlying framework. Therefore, the choice of tissue for reconstruction will differ based on the location of the defect.[3]

A second guideline for reconstructive procedures on the nose involves the choice of a plane for undermining to achieve the best movement of tissue possible and to allow for appropriate eversion. The ala does not move well but undermining in a mid-dermal plane will facilitate some movement. Even 1 mm of undermining in that plane helps accomplish the modest eversion required for prevention of a depressed scar. Movement of full-thickness skin from the sidewall and dorsum of the nose requires undermining in a plane deep to the muscle (Fig. 14.2). Often

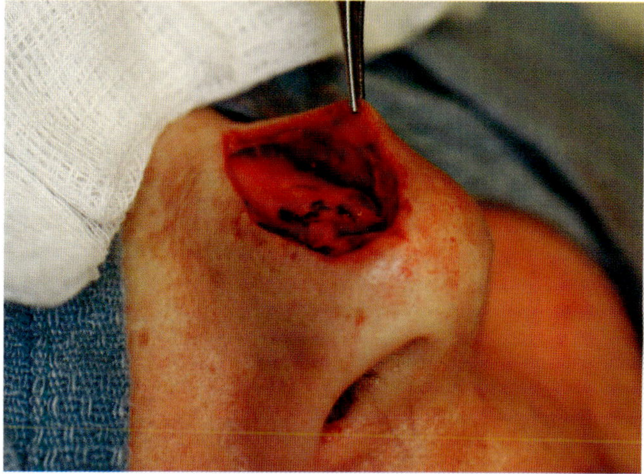

**Fig. 14.2:** Plane of undermining on the sidewall and dorsum of the nose.

called "skeletonizing," undermining in this plane not only allows ease of movement but produces a flap of full-thickness skin with excellent vascularization. In addition, this plane has fewer blood vessels and intraoperative hemostasis is easier; the surgeon mainly has to deal with perforators in the depth of the wound. The plane of undermining on the tip is more superficial than the undermining plane on the dorsum of the nose. Here the plane just superficial to the perichondrium of the two cartilage bodies works very well for tissue movement. Care must be taken to avoid undermining too deeply in between the cartilages where there is vascular support for skin as well as mucosa of the nose. The root of the nose near the glabella has thicker subcutaneous fat and numerous vessels. Undermining more superficially in a plane just under the dermis may be warranted if the resulting flap of skin is the right thickness for movement into either the primary or secondary defect.

A third guideline is to avoid placing tension on any of the free margins of the nose or adjacent structures including the nostril opening, the medial canthus, and the eyebrow to avoid deformities, but most importantly, dysfunction.

The final guideline for nasal reconstruction is to prepare the patient for possible additional procedures. Finessing the final result may require surgical revision, defatting of flaps, or surface modification with loop cautery, laser techniques or dermabrasion. In the setting of large nasal cancers with known high recurrence rates, it may be advantageous to delay repair to allow close surveillance and the early detection of recurrence. These defects may heal by second intention or be covered by a thin graft for a time before definitive reconstruction.

## INSTRUMENTATION

Fine and sharp instruments are needed to optimize excision and repair on the nose. Number 15 scalpel blades are used for full-thickness incisions. Small-toothed forceps and tissue hooks assist in grasping tissue. Scissors need to be in good condition, tightened with sharp cutting surfaces. Periosteal elevators may be useful in developing a plane between the cartilage and more superficial tissue. Hemostasis is adequately accomplished with the use of a small needle attached to an electrosurgical unit in order to cauterize the small vessels. Visualization may be assisted with use of cotton-tipped swabs rolled over the surgical site.

## NASAL REPAIR OPTIONS

### Algorithm for Nasal Reconstruction

Repair of uncomplicated surgical defects on the nose produced by the removal of benign or malignant processes is generally dictated by wound thickness and the precise site and size of the defect. An optimal surgical plan may sometimes be modified because of patient preference and acceptance of a less than optimal result or the patient's medical condition but not necessarily because of age alone. Various reconstructive options are considered in an algorithmic framework, beginning with the simplest option of second intention and progressing to more complex options for closure. This "reconstructive ladder" includes second intention healing, primary side to side closure, skin graft, local random based flap, regional flap, flaps based on a specific vascular network, and microvascular free tissue transfer. An additional consideration is whether the new cartilaginous support is required. Using the algorithm based on skin type, defect size and location assists the surgeon in determining the most appropriate repair for a given patient.[4] If the defect is superficial, away from a free margin and with intact structural support, second intention healing may give a very good result. If somewhat thicker, grafting may facilitate a better contour and prevent contraction. If the defect involves a free margin, reconstruction is often preferred to maintain both the function and the cosmetic appearance of the nose and prevent tension from distorting the nose or eyelids. Defects of the dorsum of the nose where the skin is more abundant and loose can often be closed side to side. The amount and location of donor tissue depends on the size and nasal subunit involved in the defect. Small surface defects with a well-vascularized wound bed and an intact underlying cartilaginous framework can be managed effectively with primary closure, local flaps, or skin grafts. A multi-subunit defect where the cartilaginous framework has been reconstructed will require a well-vascularized skin flap.

### Secondary Intention Healing

Small superficial defects of the nose may be allowed to heal by secondary intention with an excellent cosmetic result. The subunits of the nose that are likely to heal with cosmetically and functionally acceptable results are the tip and columella (Figs. 14.3A and B). Alar crease, dorsum, and the sidewalls of the nose may also do well. Although resulting

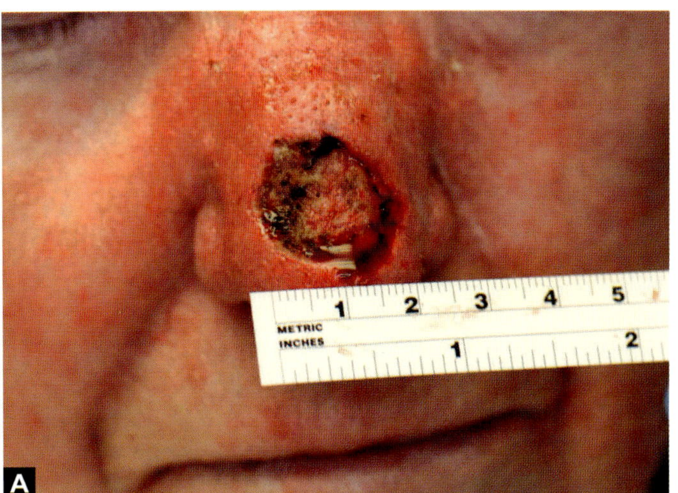


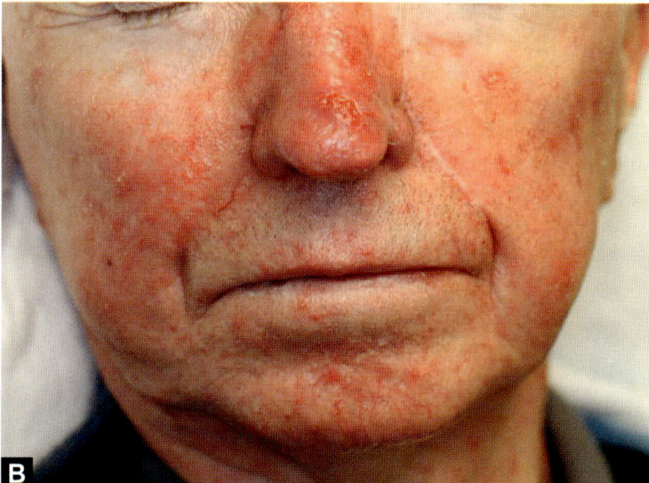


**Figs. 14.3A and B:** (A) Defect on the tip of the nose. (B) Healing by second intention with excellent results.

scars are often devoid of abundant vasculature making them somewhat whitish, the color match is often good with a gradient from the unaffected skin to the center of the scar making the scar subtle in appearance. Since the surface is smooth and whitish, it is easily coverable with light makeup for women. On the sidewall, there is often contraction yielding a somewhat linear scar suggestive of a side-to-side closure. Many patients prefer second intention healing because of their exercise or activity levels (golfing or running) and because of the ease of care.

This approach may also be considered for thicker defects in patients with thick, sebaceous skin in which other surgical alternatives would be more difficult or provide less predictable results. Augmented by use of an immediate or delayed postoperative technique in order to improve contour and reduce a sharp area of contrast between the healed wound and the unaffected skin, partial-thickness defects may heal nearly imperceptibly in this setting. Contouring techniques include dermabrasion that can be accomplished either by standard technique using a diamond fraise or simply by sanding with sterilized dry wall grid sandpaper which is rubbed over the entire subunit until fine, pinpoint bleeding is seen throughout the treatment area. Another method of modifying the wound edge involves using loop cautery. A loop can be used in cutting mode to recontour and in electrodessication mode to feather the edges. A rhinophymatous nose with a defect, even a thick defect, can be treated with the same technique as a simple rhinophyma reduction procedure, erasing the defect during the process of planning and recontouring the entire nose. For these patients, diminution of the rhinophyma can be very satisfying, and much more cosmetically and functionally appropriate than a sutured repair, which generally heals with a wide and depressed scar. Recontouring and feathering can also be done 6–12 weeks postoperatively, commonly performed with dermabrasion or laser abrasion. These techniques camouflage the surgical site, gradually blending the scar with the surrounding normal skin.

## Side-to-Side Closure

Side-to-side repair may be considered in small to medium sized defects (Figs. 14.4A to C). Midline defects found on the nasal dorsum are particularly amenable to this approach. The key issue for side-to-side closure is strict control of dog ears. A 6:1 length-to-width ratio and 15° apical angles are generally required in order to prevent the appearance of concavity or saddle nose deformity when viewed from the side. It is useful to situate the apices of closure above the area of the bony hump superiorly and below the inferior margin of the nasal tip, in the area of the infratip or columella. If the defect is slightly lateral to the midline, the inferior dog ear is displaced to midline tip in order to achieve the best contour. Small lateral sidewall defects may also be repaired in this fashion. Defects involving even a small portion of the nasal tip, ala, or free nostril margin may require dog ear displacement or more complex repairs. Defects totally within the tip, ala, or involving the free nostril margin are not generally amenable to side-to-side closure. Movement of tissue is not difficult when undermining has been accomplished widely in a

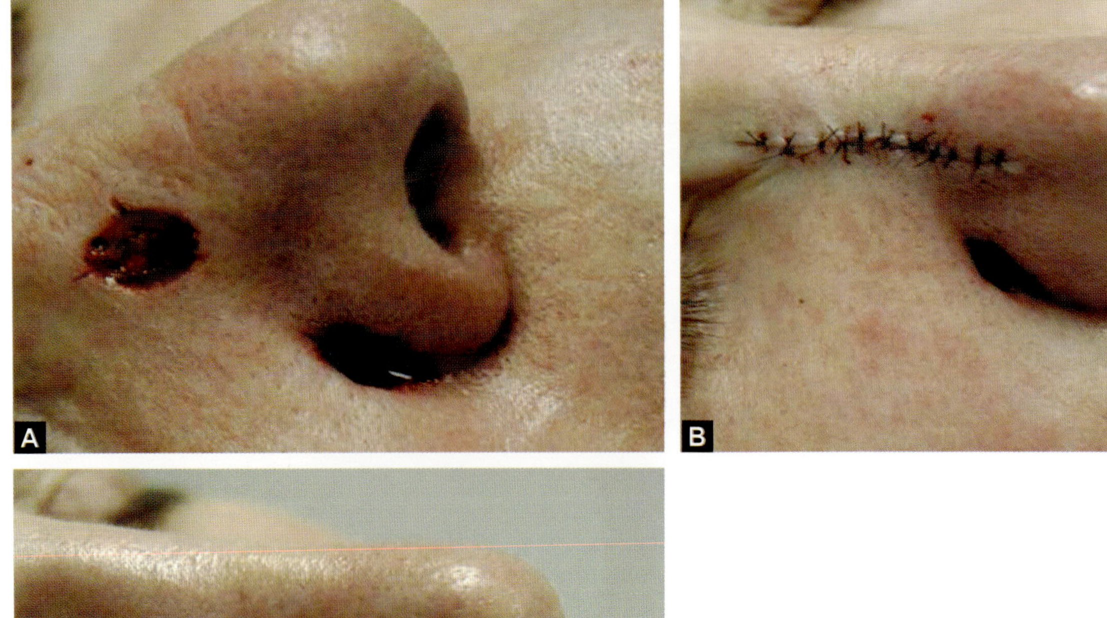


**Figs. 14.4A to C:** (A) Defect on the lateral wall of the nose. (B) Repair by primary closure. (C) Long-term follow-up with good results.

submuscular plane. Eversion of the wound edges is facilitated by wide undermining and achieved by use of buried vertical mattress sutures. A single-buried vertical mattress suture may be enough to control tension in the wound but eversion and the control of subcutaneous contraction as the wound heals require apposition of the subcutaneous tissues along the entire length of the wound.

Side-to-side closure in patients with increased nasal width is often cosmetically pleasing. A wide nose with a large defect on the mid-dorsum of the nose will be made narrower by a midline side-to-side closure, but still allow for normal respiration.

Regarding wound care, appropriate bandaging with light compression and protection of the surgical site helps to assist in preventing postoperative hemorrhage. A layered bandage of ointment such as petroleum jelly, nonstick pads, thick padding, and tape are useful to prevent stickiness of the wound to the bandage at the time of dressing change. Multiple layers are used until the site is protected and then it is secured to the cheek with tape.

## Skin Grafts

Skin grafts can be used to reconstruct small defects and, in the right setting, can provide excellent results (Figs. 14.5A to C). Skin grafting can also be an acceptable repair option for large, more complicated wounds, especially in elderly, multi-morbid patients who cannot or do not wish to undergo a more complex reconstruction. Some surgeons advocate grafting an entire subunit, even if normal skin has to be removed, in order to minimize any obvious texture and contour changes of a healed grafted site. Split-thickness skin grafts are used uncommonly because they do not prevent wound contracture which can be cosmetically and functionally disastrous for the nose. In addition, the final pigmentation of the donor skin is often unpredictable.

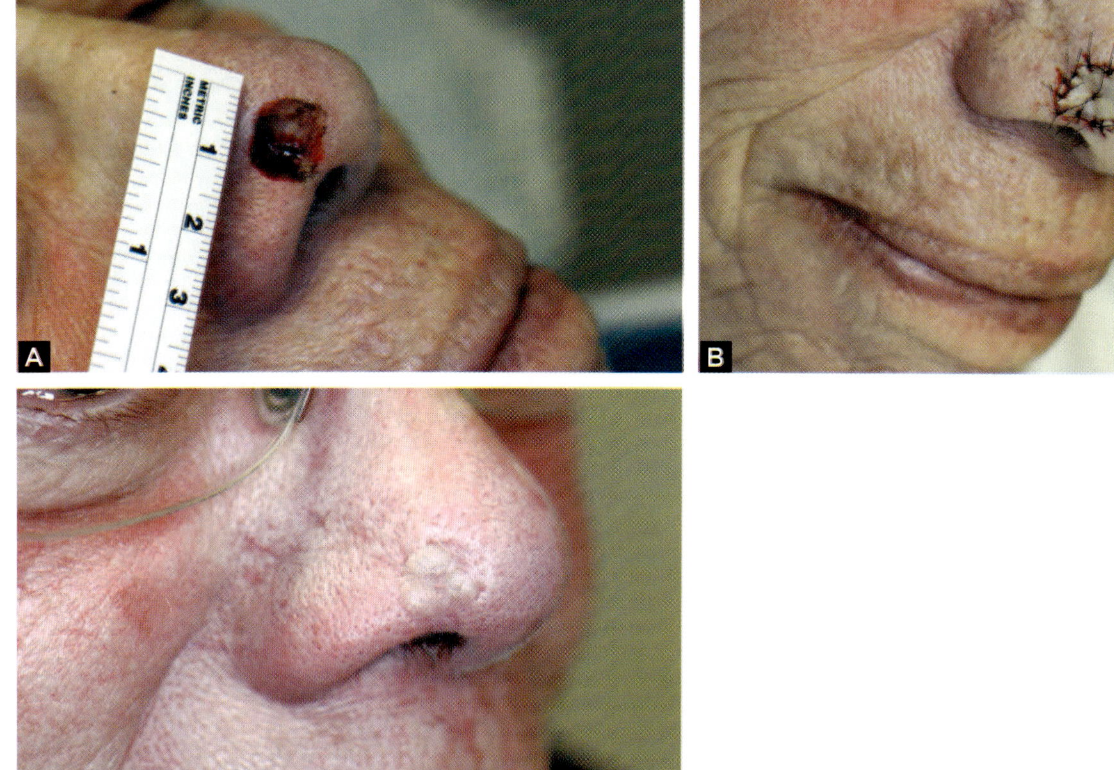

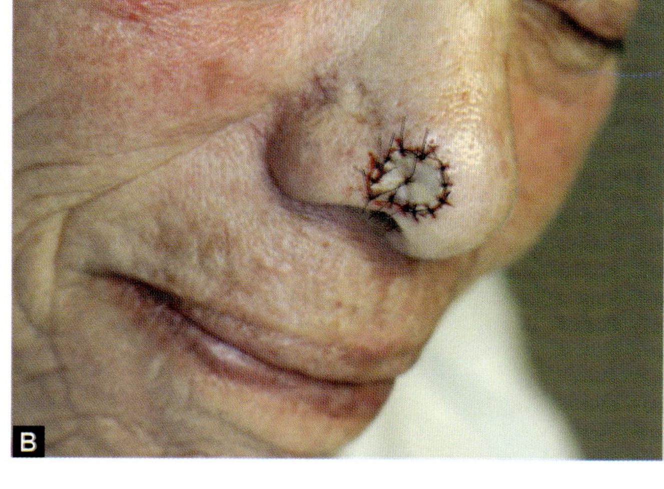

**Figs. 14.5A to C:** (A) Defect on the ala and soft triangle of the nose. (B) Repair by full thickness skin graft. (C) Long-term follow-up with good cosmetic result.

Full-thickness grafts are therefore generally preferred in nasal reconstruction. The texture and color of the skin surrounding the defect as well as the size of the graft needed and the presence or absence of hair in the proposed donor site dictates the site of skin graft harvest. Favored donor sites include the preauricular cheek, postauricular sulcus and scalp, and supraclavicular trunk and neck. In these areas, the donor site repair is cosmetically unobtrusive. Care must be taken with the preauricular site concerning transfer of sideburn hair into the defect or moving the sideburn too close to the ear with repair of the donor site. Other possible donor sites include the nasal labial fold; the donor skin is generally an excellent match but the patient's smile may suffer from some asymmetry. The skin of the conchal bowl works well for defects < 1.5 cm and the donor site heals with an unapparent scar by second intention. A supraclavicular donor site allows harvesting a larger graft, but if enough skin cannot be harvested from that site, abdominal skin, thinned aggressively, can be used. Our favorite donor skin comes from a Burow's triangle excised during partial closure of the wound; this technique allows the grafted wound to be smaller and also for the donor skin to be from adjacent nearly identical skin (Figs. 14.6A to C). This repair is particularly useful when more than one cosmetic subunit is included in the defect.[5] At times we have also used a Burow's triangle excised during repair of a second site on the face with good results, saving the patient an additional wound from repair of the donor site.

Grafting on the nose has some special considerations. Delayed grafting allowing growth of healthy granulation tissue in the wound bed increases graft survival. Even delay of as little as one day in uncomplicated wounds improves graft take. This is particularly useful when the wound bed contains exposed cartilage or bone, which may not support a skin graft. Sometimes a wound needs structure

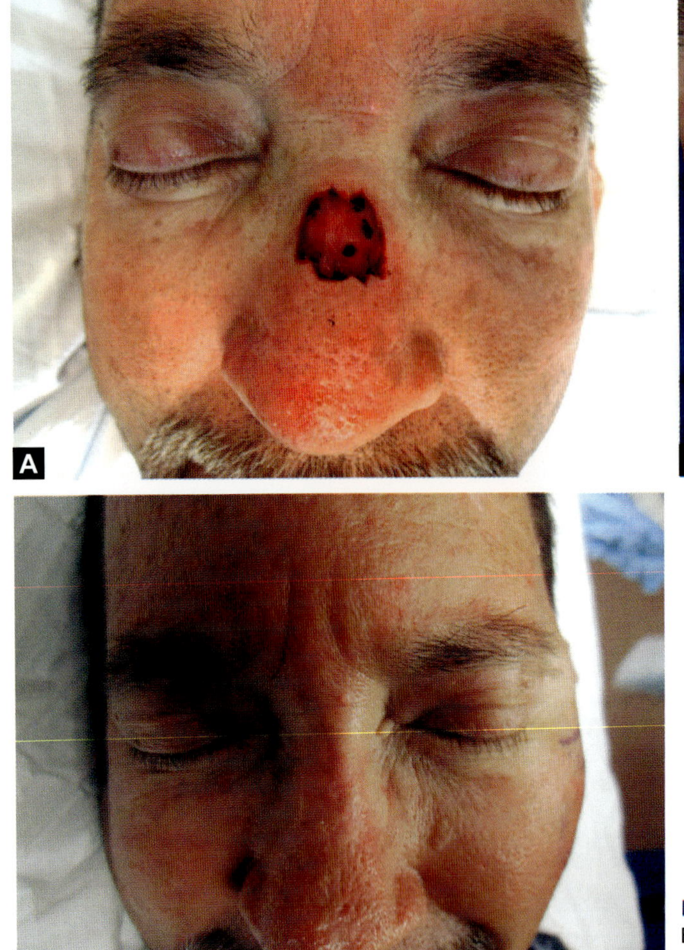

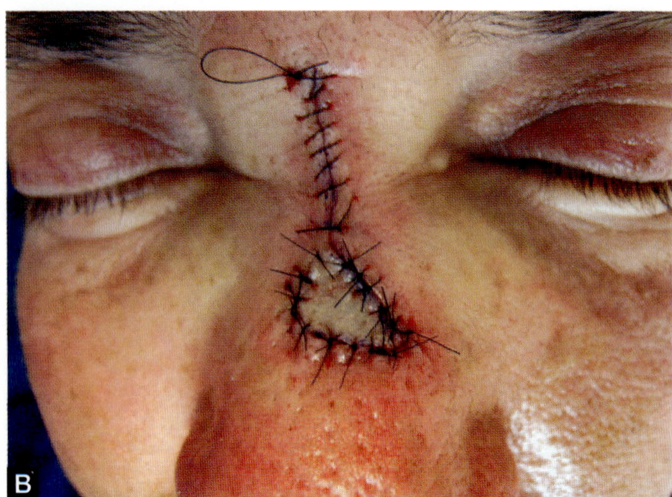

**Figs. 14.6A to C:** (A) Defect on the dorsum of the nose. (B) Repair with Burow's graft. (C) Long-term follow-up.
*Courtesy*: S Brian Jiang, MD, Sang Diego, California, USA.

that can be supplied by a cartilage graft. Cartilage can be obtained from the conchal bowl or antihelix. The antihelix offers several distinct advantages over the conchal bowl. Its flat shape and width affords the ability to cut strips of cartilage of variable size, in lengths up to 5 cm in some patients. The flat cartilage of the antihelix is also more flexible and easier to maneuver and secure into proper alignment than the curved conchal cartilage. A cartilage graft can be inserted and secured into a wound and covered on the same day with a flap or a graft.[6] Composite grafts in which skin and cartilage have been harvested together as one reconstructive unit have been used for small full-thickness defects involving the alar rim. Most often taken from the ear, composite grafts used acutely, especially in Mohs defects that have been extensively cauterized, may not revascularize adequately and may have a high failure rate.[7] An alternative procedure is to use two independent grafts of cartilage and full-thickness skin. This technique of two separate grafts is preferred over en bloc composite grafts. The higher metabolic demands of composite grafts lead to higher rates of necrosis, whereas the combination of skin and cartilage, placed as individual reconstructive components, is a more robust option.[8] However, delayed placement of a skin graft over the cartilage graft after granulating tissue has grown over the cartilage may improve survival rate for the skin graft. The editors have performed full-thickness skin grafts over cartilage grafts on the same day for nasal reconstruction with consistent results (Figs. 14.7A to D).

The main disadvantage of using a skin graft for a nasal defect is that the color and tissue texture match may not be ideal. These features can be improved with dermabrasion, laser resurfacing or even sometimes hidden with make-up. Grafts, however, often maintain contour and function very well without the morbidity of more complex reconstructive techniques.

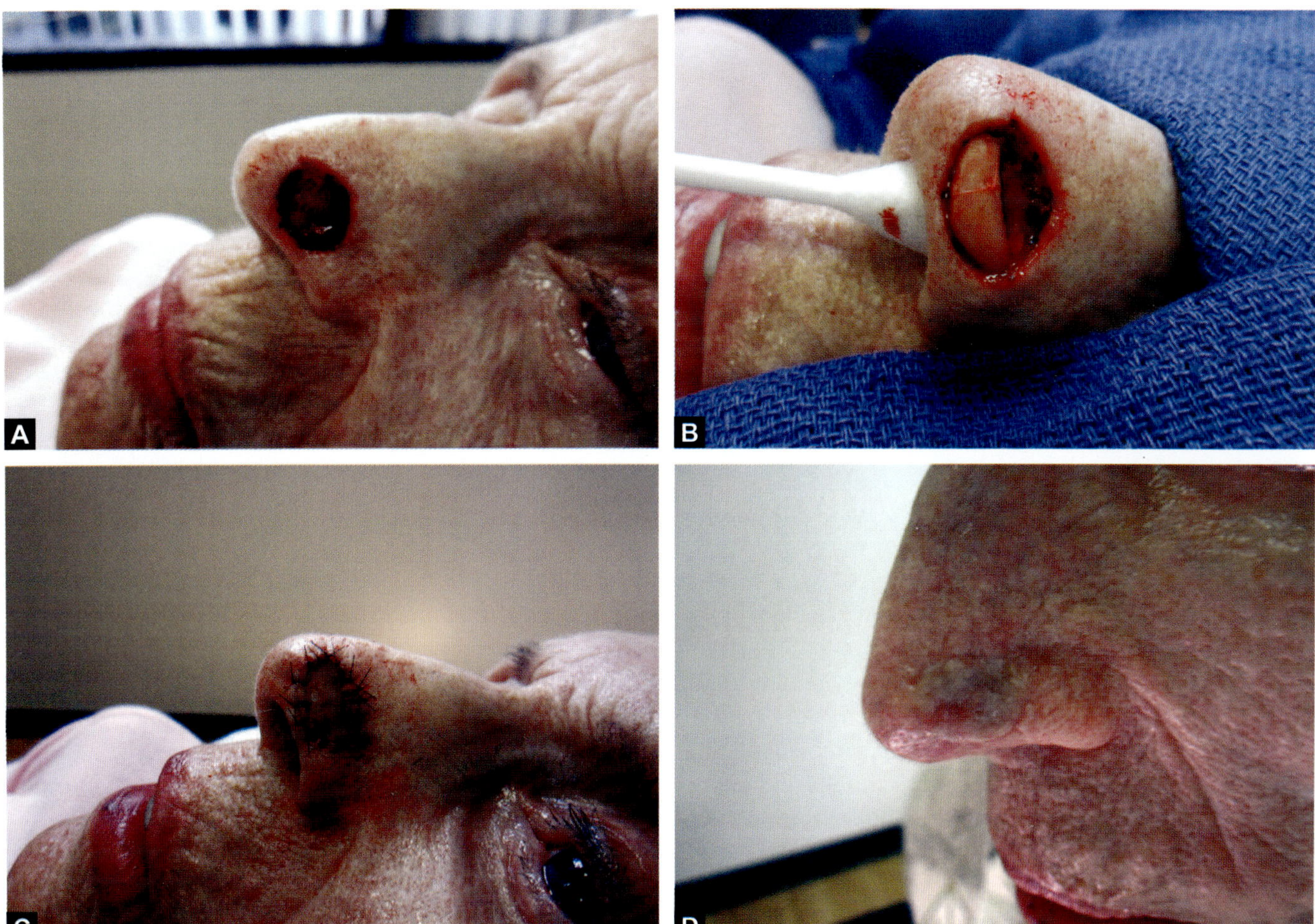


**Figs. 14.7A to D:** (A) Defect on the lateral nasal tip and ala. (B) Repair with cartilage graft. (C) Overlying full-thickness skin graft. (D) Long-term follow-up.
*Courtesy*: S Brian Jiang, MD, Sang Diego, California, USA.

## FLAP RECONSTRUCTION

Designing a flap for reconstruction of the nose follows the general principles discussed in Chapter 7. They may be categorized based on tissue movement and pedicle characteristics. More so than other larger facial sites, strict attention must be paid to the dog ears that are created in tissue movement as the nose is relatively small with small subunits. They are the least cosmetically obtrusive when their removal also abides by the principal of working within cosmetic subunits as discussed above. Dog ears must be controlled such that they do not affect the free margins. Because the nose is a full-thickness fold of skin, dog ears may not be apparent on the external surface but will still impinge on the small space in the nostril and affect breathing.

Both random-based and axial-pattern flaps are used in nasal reconstruction. Random based skin flaps are not designed around any specific vessel. They receive their blood supply from unnamed small musculocutaneous and septocutaneous vessels, running deep to the muscles or in the muscular fascia that perforate through the muscles or muscular septae to provide the blood supply for the dermal-subdermal plexus of the skin. This blood supply on the nose is redundant and feeds from both sides. The survival of these random pattern flaps is based on the perfusion pressure of the underlying vessels. Since the nose is very vascular, pedicles can be very small and tissue can be moved quite far from its original position. Care must be taken to make sure the flap is however not under any tension as that will impede perfusion of the tissues and result in necrosis.

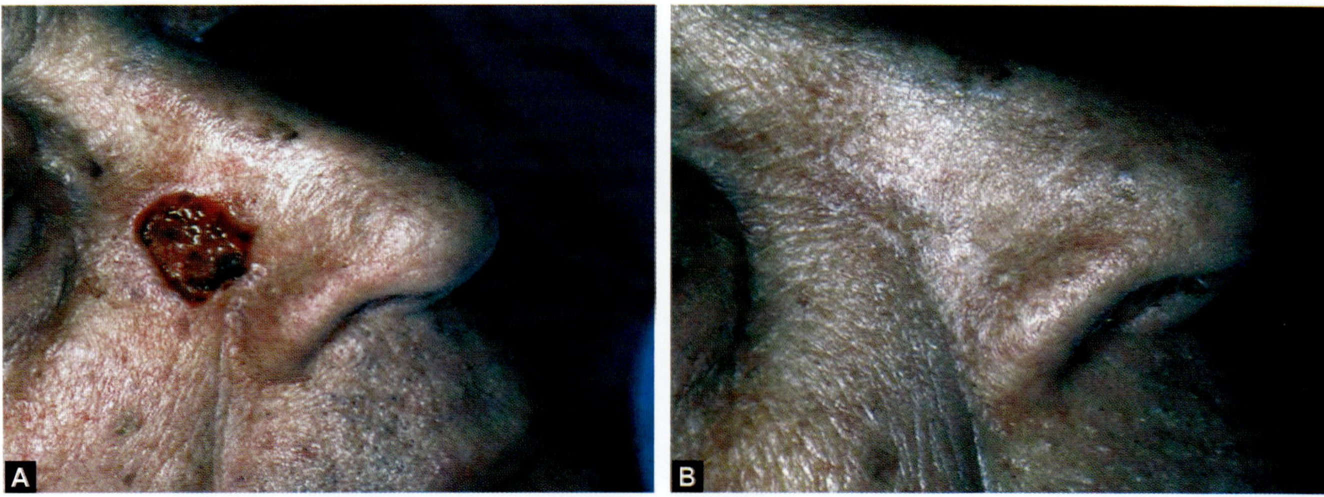


**Figs. 14. 8A and B:** (A) Defect on the sidewall of the nose. (B) Repair by cheek advancement flap.

Axial pattern flaps, on the other hand, have a blood supply that comes from large named arteries in the subcutaneous tissue. The flap is designed along the directional axis of the vessel in order to maintain the integrity of the blood supply in that basin. The flap can be large and can be taken from a site distant from the defect as long as the vascular bed is intact. The rich and reliable vascular supply provided by this axial blood supply makes these flaps more amenable to primary thinning and contouring. Primary defatting of the flap is another principle that improves results and decreases the number of operative stages. By removing deep subcutaneous fat while preserving the subdermal plexus, there is low incidence of flap necrosis that may require revision.

Flaps can be categorized based on tissue movement into the following types: advancement, rotation, transposition, and pedicle/interpolation flaps.

## Advancement Flaps

### *Cheek Advancement Flap*

Defects of the lateral nasal sidewall can be effectively covered using a cheek advancement flap from the adjacent cheek skin (Figs. 14.8A and B). A large volume of tissue can be moved from the reservoir in the medial cheek after undermining widely adjacent to the sidewall defect and a smaller amount of tissue from the nasal side of the defect. Dog ear removal can be performed with incisions along the nasolabial fold, hiding the scar in an already concave boundary between the cosmetic units. The flap must be large and loose to drape into the defect or there can be bridging and loss of the lateral nasal sulcus. Some surgeons will use a deep subcutaneous anchoring stitch to prevent bridging if the flap is too tight to drape well.

This flap can also be used in conjunction with other repairs for a single defect that includes more than one cosmetic unit. We commonly use the dog ear as a Burow's graft to fill residual defect after optimal movement of the flap. The design of these flaps provides excellent scar placement along the nasolabial crease and junction of the dorsum and nasal sidewall.

### *V-Y Flap*

Defects involving the ala, sidewall, and/or dorsum may be closed by a single V-Y advancement flap (Figs. 14.9A to C). The superiorly based island pedicle flap is an excellent option for repair of small but deep alar defects. Asgari and Odland[9] described a laterally based nasalis myocutaneous island pedicle flap to repair small and deep defects of the nasal ala. This important advancement allowed the island pedicle flap to be completely freed from its base below and receive its vascular supply from the lateral nasalis muscles. Therefore, the flap could swing on its muscular slings. A superiorly designed island pedicle flap with a laterally based nasalis muscle sling offers a one-stage reconstruction with an excellent cosmetic outcome for wounds on the nasal ala. It easily addresses the need to fill the depth of the wound. Potential complications seen with this flap include pincushioning and compromise of the nasal valve. In 2008, Zeikus and co-workers reported the dog ear island pedicle flap, which is a combination flap consisting of

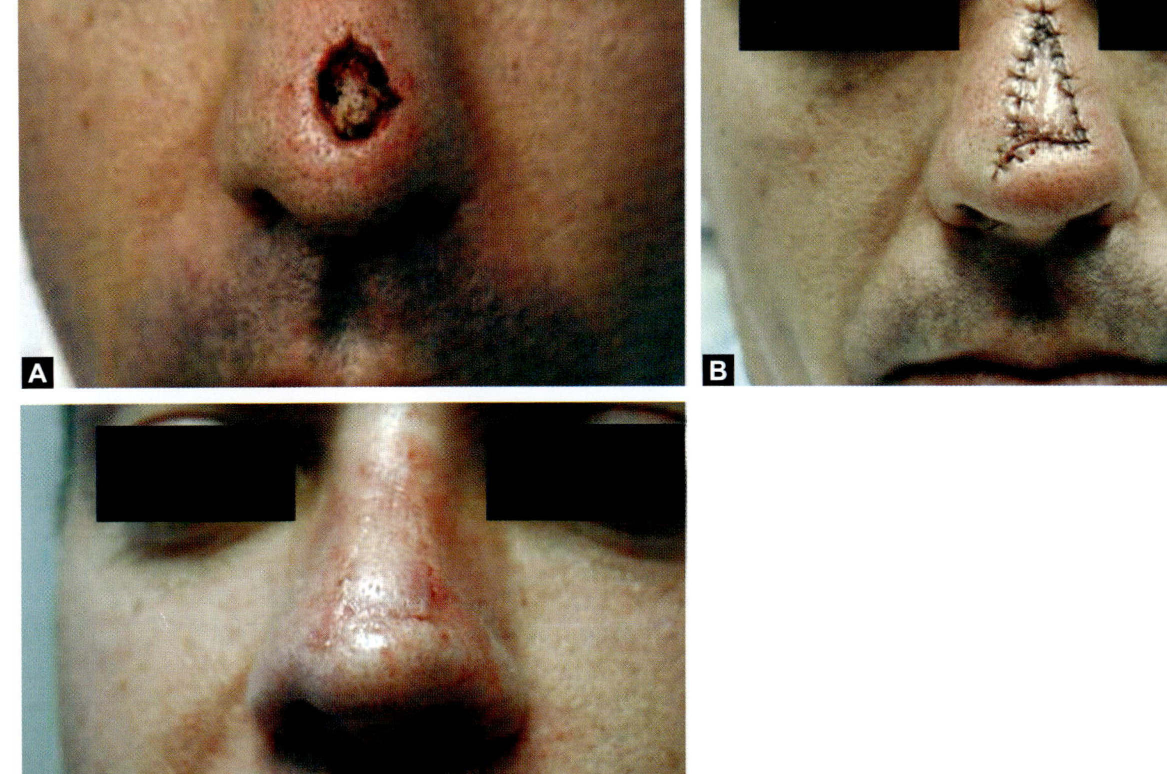

**Figs. 14.9A to C:** (A) Defect on the dorsum of the nose. (B) Repair by island pedicle (V-Y advancement) flap. (C) Long-term follow-up.

a cheek advancement flap and a rotated dog ear island pedicle flap.[10] This full-thickness pedicle flap extending down to perichondrium advances adequate tissue into place. The color and texture match of the skin is nearly perfect, because it comes from skin immediately adjacent to the wound. This repair is also relatively simple to perform and offers the patient a one-stage procedure.

## Rotation Flaps

### *Dorsal Nasal Flap*

The dorsal nasal flap, originally described by Rieger, can alternatively manage tip and dorsal defects from 1 to 2 cm (Figs. 14.10A to C). This flap has the advantage of a single large sweeping movement, large pedicle, and excellent drape over the dorsum and supratip sidewall of the nose with the ability to hide most of the lines of closure in the sulcus or other cosmetic boundaries. Care must be taken to avoid elevation of the nose or an increase in the nasolabial angle, generally managed by assuring that all tension is in a completely horizontal direction, depending on the laxity of the cheek skin to lessen tightness. Although the flap can be used for defects that are close to the alar rim and those that extend over the domes, other options may preserve the normal contour more easily. For smaller defects on the nasal dorsum or sidewall, a conventional rotation flap on the dorsal or lateral nose is also frequently performed with excellent results (Figs. 14.11A and B).

### *Spiral Flap*

The spiral flap is best used for nasal alar reconstruction (Figs. 14.12A to C). It has the advantage of being a one-stage flap. It is indicated for small to medium-sized defects of the nasal ala and alar groove. Spiral flap produces topographic restoration with low risk of aesthetic or functional complication.[11]

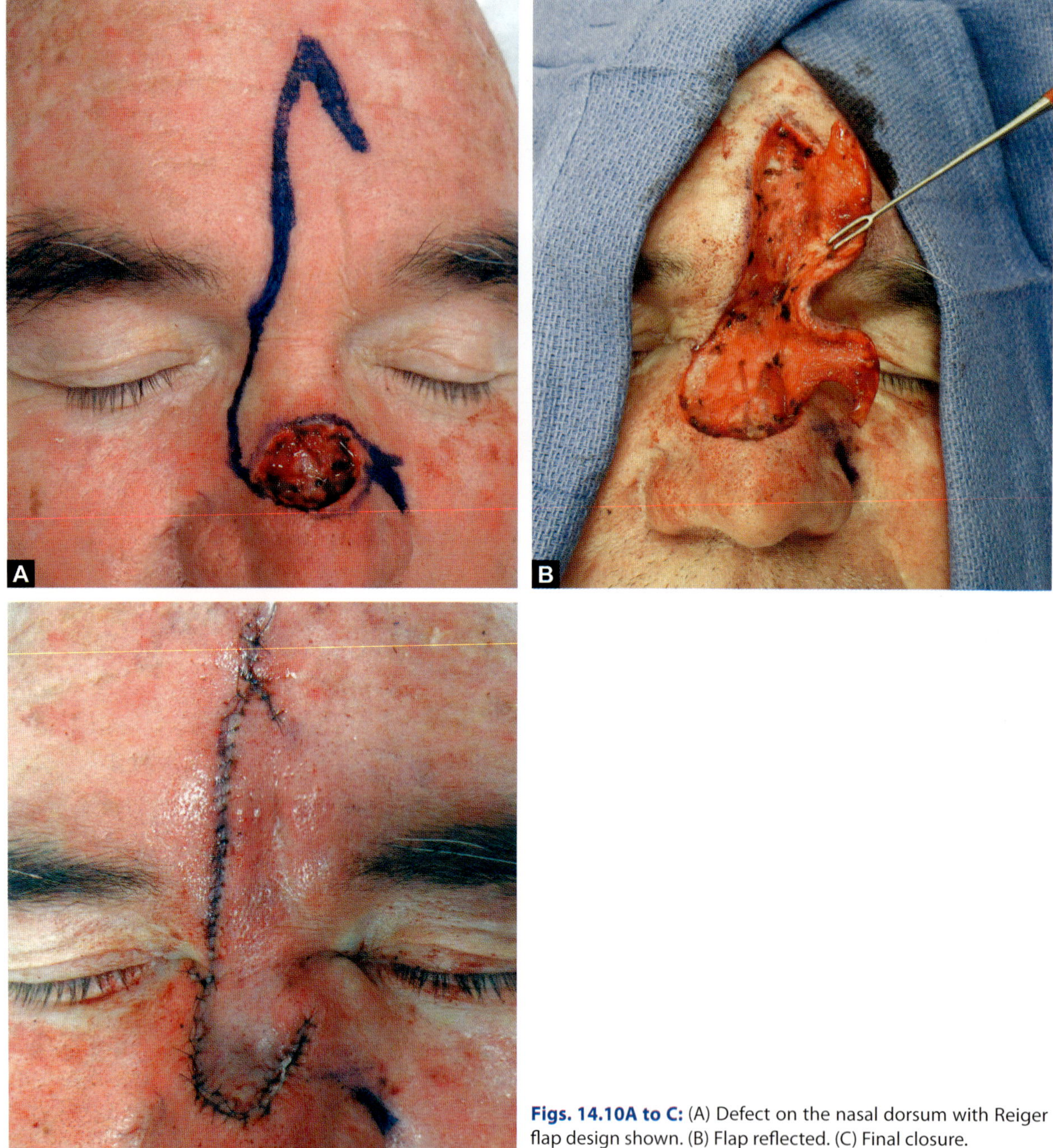

**Figs. 14.10A to C:** (A) Defect on the nasal dorsum with Reiger flap design shown. (B) Flap reflected. (C) Final closure.
*Courtesy*: S Brian Jiang, MD, Sang Diego, California, USA.

## Transposition Flaps

### *Banner Flap*

The banner flap can manage small defects of the dorsum and tip (Fig. 14.13). This flap is useful only in defects up to 1.2 cm. Beyond this size, the local nasal distortion is too great to justify use of this flap. The benefit of this flap is that it can be designed to orient the scar with the transverse wrinkle lines of the nose.

### *Bilobed Flap*

The bilobed flap is often used to reconstruct small defects of the lower two-thirds of the nose (Figs. 14.14A to C).

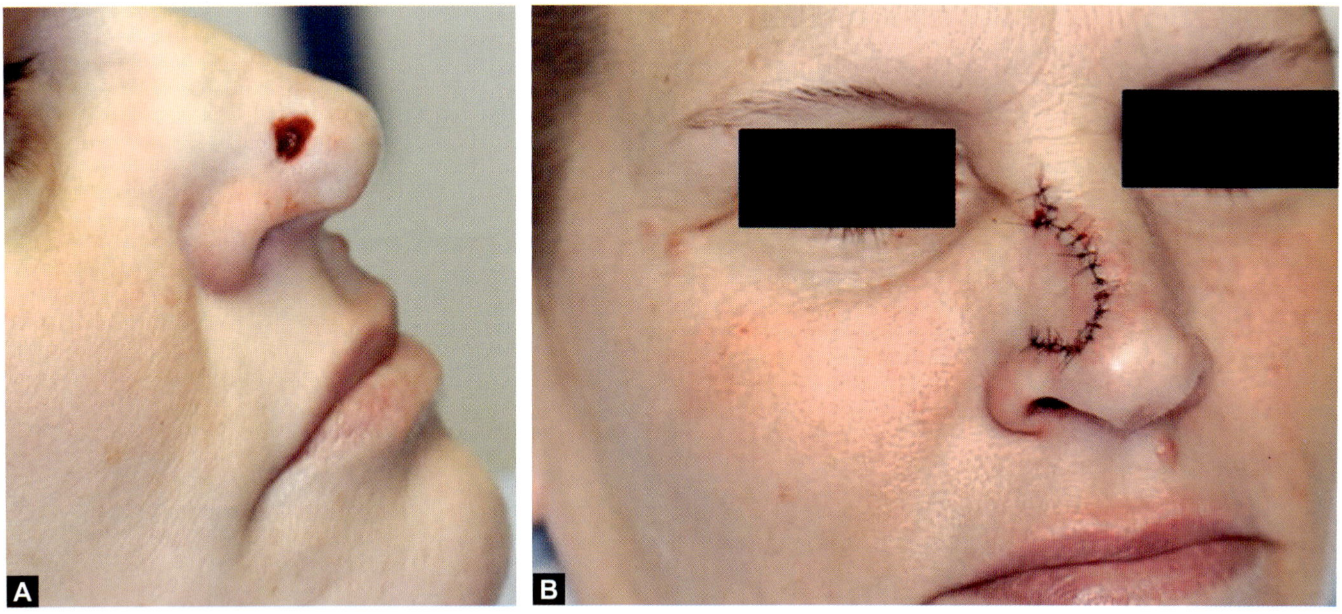

**Figs. 14.11A and B:** (A) Defect on the right tip of the nose. (B) Repaired by rotation flap.

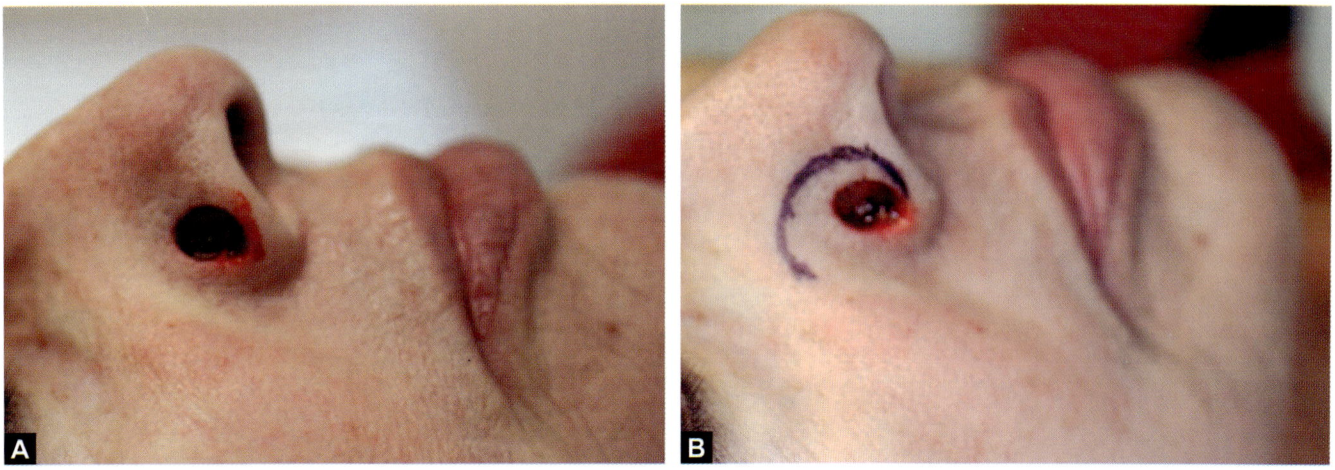

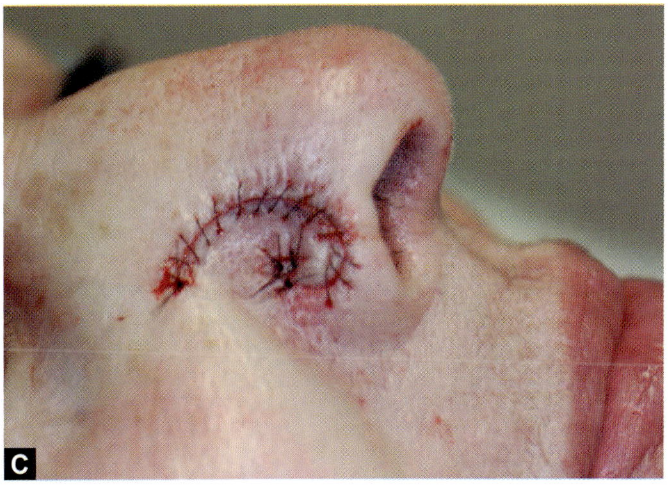

**Figs. 14.12A to C:** (A) Defect on the ala of the nose. (B) Spiral flap design shown. (C) Final closure of spiral flap.

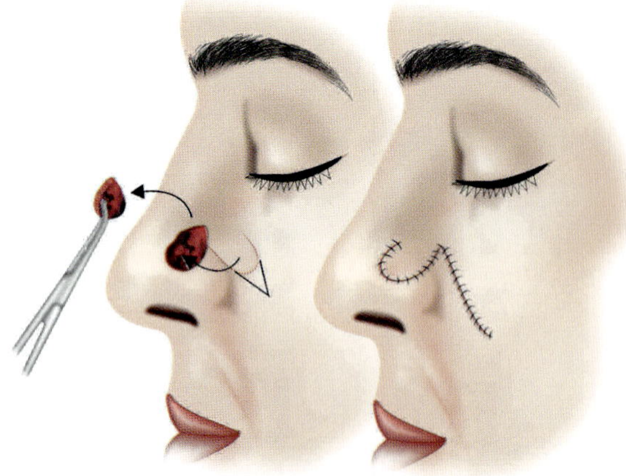

**Fig. 14.13:** Design of a banner flap on the nose.

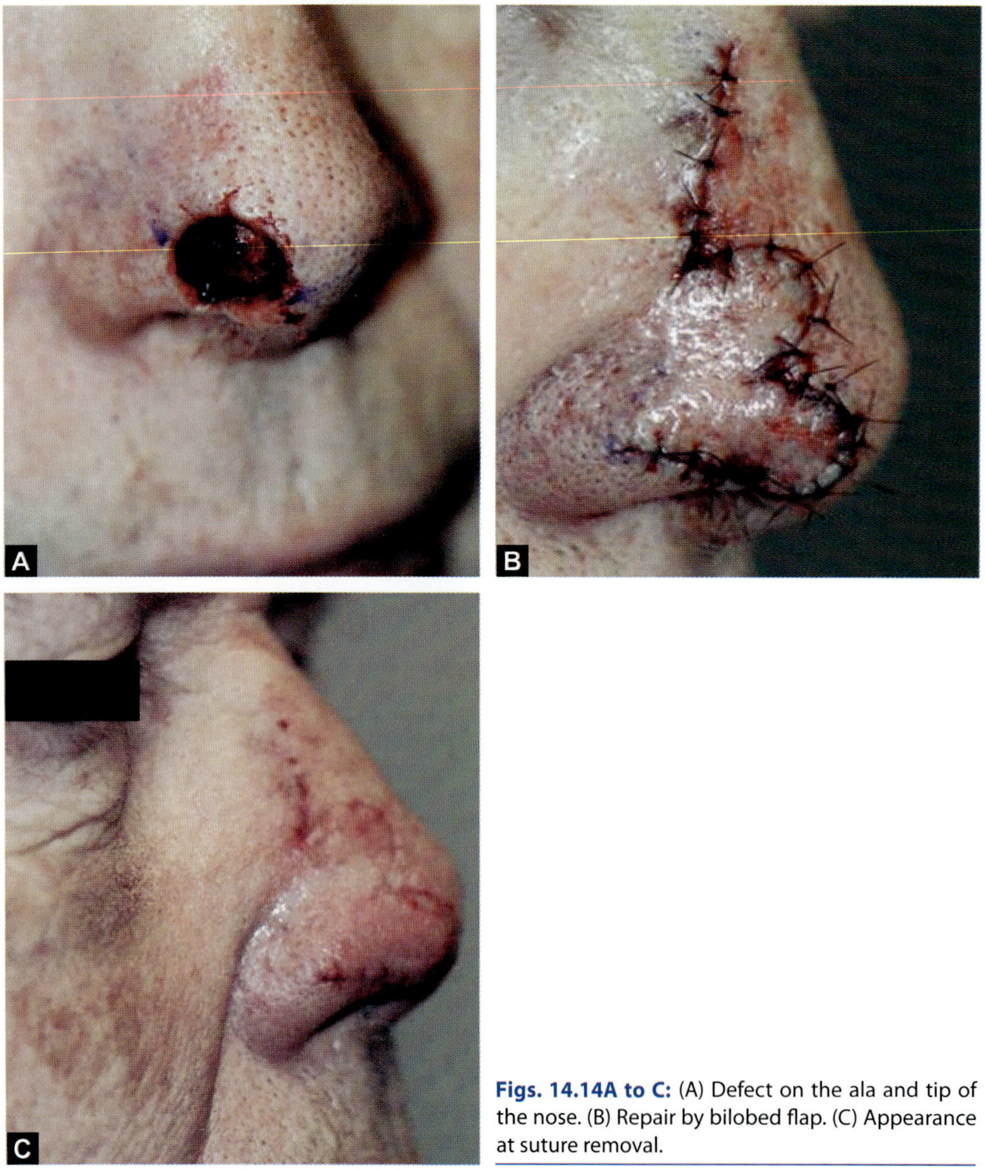

**Figs. 14.14A to C:** (A) Defect on the ala and tip of the nose. (B) Repair by bilobed flap. (C) Appearance at suture removal.

The design consists of two lobes of tissue; the first lobe rotates to fill the defect while the second flap rotates to fill the donor site of the first lobe. The defect left by the second lobe is closed primarily. The flap must be carefully designed. Design of the bilobe begins with drawing two arcs; one being equal to two times the radius of the defect with the arc passing through the center point of the defect site. The bilobe is drawn with the first lobe equal to the same width of the defect, while the second lobe is drawn in a cone shape with the height twice the length of the first lobe. The axis of the defect and the two lobes of the flap are 45° apart. The bilobe flap is transposed into the defect site.[12] Tip and dorsum defects from 1 to 2 cm maximum may be addressed with the bilobed flap. At times a third lobe is needed to fill the second lobe without contour distortion and tension. This is an especially useful repair for a large medium thickness defect in the ala where the boundary between the defect and the first lobe is the alar crease. When the first lobe is moved into the second lobe, the alar crease is recreated. This flap is very versatile. However, it is still subject to similar local nasal contour distortion especially if it is not sized appropriately. The size and angle of movement of the second lobe is also important as a dog ear impinging on the nostril can result if it is too small or too tight and the patient will experience difficulty breathing.

## Pedicle/Interpolation Flaps

### *Melolabial Flap*

The redundant skin of the cheek, adjacent to the nasolabial crease, should be considered in the reconstruction of partial or complete alar defects (Figs. 14.15A to D). Designed either as a random flap or on the perforators from the angular and facial arteries, this rotational flap can be designed to match the color, texture, and contour of the ala. Importantly, the donor defect on the cheek can be closed primarily, leaving an inconspicuous scar along the nasolabial crease. Three weeks later, the pedicle is divided, and the flap is thinned according to the contour of the ala. A revision may be considered at a later time if necessary.

### *Paramedian Forehead Flap*

The paramedian forehead flap is an axial flap based on the supratrochlear artery. Sidewall defects at or larger than 2 cm are usually managed with the paramedian forehead flap. It can provide an excellent functional and aesthetic outcome in the reconstruction of large nasal defects particularly involving the nasal tip and/or alae. The forehead donor site can be closed primarily in small defects; however, if left to heal by secondary intention the donor site heals within 6 weeks and often leaves an imperceptible scar that can be well concealed. This flap can be defatted and thinned and contoured to preserve the nose–cheek junction. Each stage takes place at ~3-week intervals to allow neovascularization, which ensures flap viability. It may take several revision surgeries to obtain a symmetrical and aesthetically pleasing result; however, the outcome can be outstanding.[13]

The columella is a difficult area to reconstruct. Thankfully, it is rarely involved in skin cancer extirpation. Options for repair include unilateral or paired nasolabial flaps. When a columellar defect is paired with a larger tip defect, a paramedian forehead flap can be used to resurface the tip and columella together.[14]

Smokers are a special consideration. They are usually healthy enough to tolerate multi-stage reconstruction; however, because of compromised skin vascularity, adjustments must be made for these patients to avoid flap complications. Smokers who require paramedian forehead flaps may benefit from a delay in the procedure before flap transfer, also, to double the time between flap transfer and division and inset.

## Restoring Nasal Lining

A common cause for aesthetic failure in nasal reconstruction is disregard for lining. The nasal vestibule is lined by a strip of thin skin (stratified squamous keratinized epithelium). This epithelium loses its keratinizing nature and transitions into the nasal mucosa (pseudostratified columnar ciliated epithelium) as it moves further into the nose. This epithelium, called the respiratory epithelium, lines the sinonasal cavity with the exception of the area covered by the olfactory epithelium. The nasal mucosa has a rich vascular supply, which makes it an attractive option for either second intention healing or flaps in reconstructing the inner lining of full-thickness nasal defects. In full-thickness defects, all components of the nose need to be reconstructed, including the nasal lining. There are two important considerations when selecting the appropriate lining. It must be well vascularized, to nourish cartilage and bony grafts, and it must be thin enough to avoid airway obstruction. Improper tissue selection in lining reconstruction can lead to poor results from either collapse of framework secondary to poor perfusion or as a result

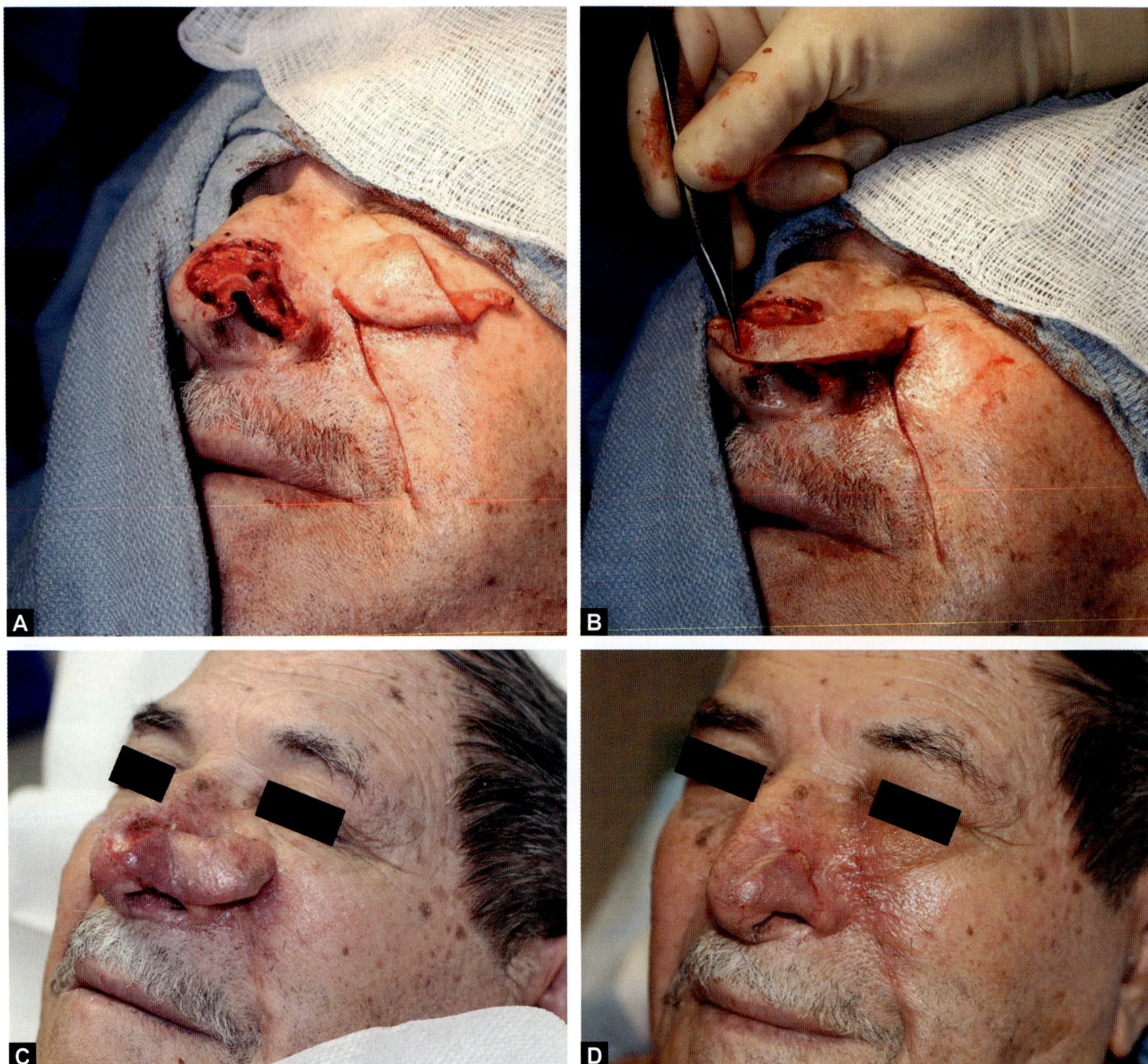

**Figs. 14.15A to D:** (A) Defect on the tip and ala of the nose. (B) Melolabial interpolation flap put in place. (C) Three weeks after placement the pedicle is divided and thinned. (D) Final appearance.

of obstruction of the nostril from thick intranasal flaps. Meticulous attention to lining deficits is essential to a stable, aesthetic result in nasal reconstruction. For small vestibule lining defects, and in cases where there is insufficient local mucosa full-thickness skin grafts, turn-in flaps from skin adjacent to the defect are adequate. However, blood supply to these small, random flaps is sometimes an issue.[2]

## COMPLICATIONS

A consequence of the rich vascular supply of the nose, perioperative bleeding is the most common complication (please see Chapter 24 for details about complications). Bleeding can generally be controlled by appropriate attention to hemostasis during the procedure. This is important because blood collecting under a graft or flap will cause necrosis of the overlying skin. If intraoperative bleeding is problematic, the defect can be allowed to heal by second intention and definitive reconstruction performed at a later date. Appropriate bandaging with light compression and protection of the surgical site can assist in preventing postoperative hemorrhage. A layered bandage of ointment, nonstick pads, thick padding, and tape can be useful. Multiple layers are used until the site is protected and then it is secured to the cheek with tape.

Infection may occur following surgery on the nose but is very rare.[15] Pain and tenderness developing 7–10 days postoperatively are reliable signs of early infection. While the usual skin bacteria such as *Staphylococcus aureus* and *Streptococci* are most common, *Pseudomonas* infections may occur in both normal and diabetic patients.[16] A particularly effective preventative measure is to ask the patient to perform daily wound care by washing the wound first with mild soap and water, then white vinegar diluted in half with tap water. After cleansing, the wound should be covered with ointment and dressed. If signs of infection develop, a culture should be taken prior to instituting antibiotic therapy so that if there is no response to treatment, the sensitivities are available to change the antibiotic as needed.

Graft and flap reconstruction may be complicated by necrosis. Graft necrosis may be related to a poor wound bed, compromised by bleeding or excessive cautery. The graft itself must be defatted and thinned because if it is too thick, it cannot be adequately nourished in the early stages of attachment. Some grafts will have full-thickness necrosis, but epidermal necrosis alone is also common. As long as the dermal component of the graft survives, reepithelialization will occur with excellent cosmetic outcome if the wound is kept clean, moist, and protected.

Flaps may have partial necrosis, particularly in areas of tension. Flaps should always be designed large enough and be elevated and undermined such that they can be draped into the primary defect, not pulled and tugged, with no tension on the sutured edges. While the rich nasal vasculature allows the surgeon to design flaps with small pedicles, tension on the pedicle will also compromise distal perfusion. The soft triangle is an area that is poorly vascularized normally and is particularly prone to necrosis with any kind of repair. Necrosis of the soft triangle gives rise to a notch in the normal contour of the rim of the nostril. An obvious notch is difficult to repair but may be amenable to full-thickness z-plasty.[17]

Reconstruction of the distal sidewall, alar crease, and superior ala of the nose may give rise to a functional malformation in which there is poor air movement on inspiration. The complaint of patients is that they cannot breathe through that side of their nose. On physical examination, there is a fullness to the inside lateral and superior aspect of the distal nostril accentuated during inspiration. Sometimes there is visible collapse of the ala during inspiration. Although this is described in the literature as nasal valve dysfunction, there is no anatomic valve identifiable in the normal state. Most commonly, this complication is related to undersizing of the repair such that there is redundant tissue folded underneath the flap or graft creating a narrowed or weak passageway. Attention to creating a flap that drapes across the defect will prevent most complications. However, at times, a structural support such as the alar batten graft or cartilage graft may be helpful. Placing a buttressing suspension suture across alar defects to maintain alar patency and contour has also been described.[18]

Because smokers have compromised vascular supplies, they are at significantly increased risk for flap and donor-site complications. Therefore, we advocate more conservative defatting and accept more operative stages in nasal reconstructions performed on smokers.[19]

## CONCLUSION

Closure of surgical defects on the nose is challenging. The full range of repair options should be considered in every case. The goal should be the reestablishment of a normal nasal contour; scarring will occur as part of the reconstruction but is much more tolerable than contour abnormalities of the nose. Creativity is warranted for nose reconstruction, rewarding both the patient and the surgeon with excellent cosmetic and functional results.

## REFERENCES

1. Bloom JD, Antunes MB, Becker DG. Anatomy, physiology, and general concepts in nasal reconstruction. Facial Plast Surg Clin North Am. 2011;19:1-11.
2. Michelotti B, Mackay D. Nasal reconstruction. Clin Anat. 2012;25:86-98.
3. O'Quinn B Jr, Thomas JR, Patton TJ. Classification of nasal defects: a practical guide for reconstruction. Otolaryngol Head Neck Surg. 1986;95:5-9.
4. Parrett BM, Pribaz JJ. An algorithm for treatment of nasal defects. Clin Plast Surg. 2009;36:407-20.

5. Weathers WM, Bhadkamkar M, Wolfswinkel EM, et al. Full-thickness skin grafting in nasal reconstruction. Semin Plast Surg. 2013;27:90-5.
6. Zopf DA, Iams W, Kim JC, et al. Full-thickness skin graft overlying a separately harvested auricular cartilage graft for nasal alar reconstruction. JAMA Facial Plast Surg. 2013; 15:131-4.
7. Zilinsky I, Farber N, Haik J, et al. Nasal ala reconstruction with a crus helix composite graft: a stepladder approach. J Drugs Dermatol. 2012;11:376-81.
8. Olazagasti J, Kleinerman R, Eisen DB. Composite full-thickness skin and fat graft for nasal reconstruction. Dermatol Surg. 2014;40:337-40.
9. Asgari M, Odland P. Nasalis island pedicle flap in nasal ala reconstruction. Dermatol Surg. 2005;31:448-52.
10. Zeikus P, MacCormack M, Olbricht S. Dog ear island pedicle flap for repair of alar and nasal wall defects. Dermatol Surg. 2008;34:1697-700.
11. Mahlberg MJ, Leach BC, Cook J. The spiral flap for nasal alar reconstruction: our experience with 63 patients. Dermatol Surg. 2012;38:373-80.
12. Zitelli JA. Design aspect of the bilobed flap. Arch Facial Plast Surg. 2008;10:186.
13. Correa BJ, Weathers WM, Wolfswinkel EM, et al. The forehead flap: the gold standard of nasal soft tissue reconstruction. Semin Plast Surg. 2013;27:96-103.
14. Faris C, Vuyk HD. Reconstruction of nasal tip and columella. Facial Plast Surg Clin North Am. 2011;19:25-62.
15. Lutz ME, Otley CC. Rhinophyma and coexisting occult skin cancers. Dermatol Surg. 2001;27:201-2.
16. Alam M, Ibrahim O, Nodzenski M, et al. Adverse events associated with mohs micrographic surgery: multicenter prospective cohort study of 20,821 cases at 23 centers. JAMA Dermatol. 2013;149:1378-85.
17. Sand M, Sand D, Brors D, et al. Cutaneous lesions of the external ear. Head Face Med. 2008;4:2.
18. Thornton JF, Griffin JR, Constantine FC. Nasal reconstruction: an overview and nuances. Semin Plast Surg. 2008;22: 257-68.
19. Wang JH, Finn D, Cummins DL. Suspension suture technique to prevent nasal valve collapse after Mohs micrographic surgery. Dermatol Surg. 2014;40:345-7.

# CHAPTER 15

# Eyelid and Periorbital Reconstruction

*Ian A Maher, Joseph Kallini, Jeremy S Bordeaux*

## INTRODUCTION

The eyelids and periorbital area play an important role in the function and aesthetic perception of the face.[1] The eyelids function to protect the orbit and produce the tear film to hydrate the globe.[2,3] Disruption of eyelid function can cause keratitis and even blindness.[4] Furthermore, the eyes and eyelid are some of the most important facial structures in terms of visual recognition of the face. Studies show that the eyes are the most "looked at" part of the face.[5] Thus, reconstruction of the eyelids and periorbital area is of utmost functional and aesthetic importance. Much like the lower nose, the eyelid is a multilaminar structure serving as lining, structural support, and cutaneous coverage. Prior to undertaking any periorbital reconstruction, the impact of the eyelid defect on the above three parameters must be carefully analyzed.

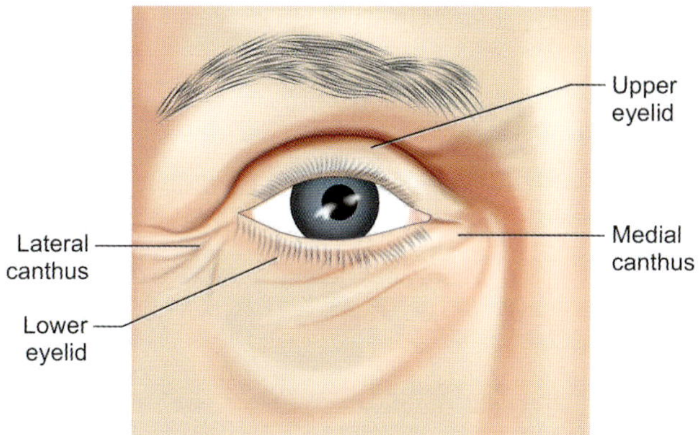


**Fig. 15.1:** An illustration depicting the cosmetic subunits of the eyelid.

## ANATOMY

### Surface Anatomy

The eyelid cosmetic unit is one of the most important on the face.[6] The lid unit is bounded by the eyebrow superiorly, the orbital rim laterally, the nasal bone medially, and the lower lid fold inferiorly. The cosmetic subunits of the eyelids are outlined in Figure 15.1.

### Structural Support of the Lids

The complex anatomy of the eyelid is inextricably linked to its aesthetic appearance. The eyelids are suspended by the medial and lateral canthal tendons, which are the condensation of the orbicularis oculi muscle.[2,3] The canthal tendons originate on the tarsal plates of the upper and lower lid. The tarsal plates are cartilaginous structures that provide structural integrity to the lid margins and house the Meibomian glands of the lids. The tarsal plate of the lower lid is ~5 mm in vertical height, whereas the tarsal plate of the upper lid is 1 cm in height. The lateral canthal tendon bifurcates as it travels laterally. The superficial limb merges with the temporalis fascia, while the deep limb inserts on Whitnall's tubercle on the inner surface of the lateral orbital rim.[7] The medial canthal tendon also bifurcates as it travels medially and inserts on the surface of the nasal bone. Importantly, the lacrimal collection system can be found between the superficial and deep limbs of the medial canthal tendon. The structural support system of the lids is shown in Figure 15.2.

### Muscular Anatomy, Innervation, and Lamellar Structure

The eyelid is divided into its anterior and posterior lamina.[1] The anterior lamina is composed of delicate, thin lid skin, and the orbicularis oculi muscle. The orbicularis oculi is innervated by the facial nerve and functions to close the

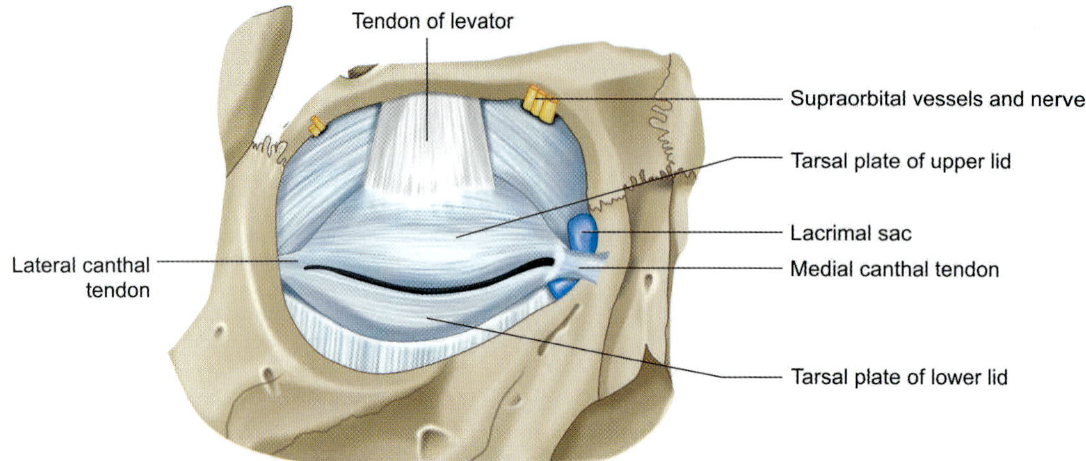


**Fig. 15.2:** An illustration depicting the structural support system of the eyelids.

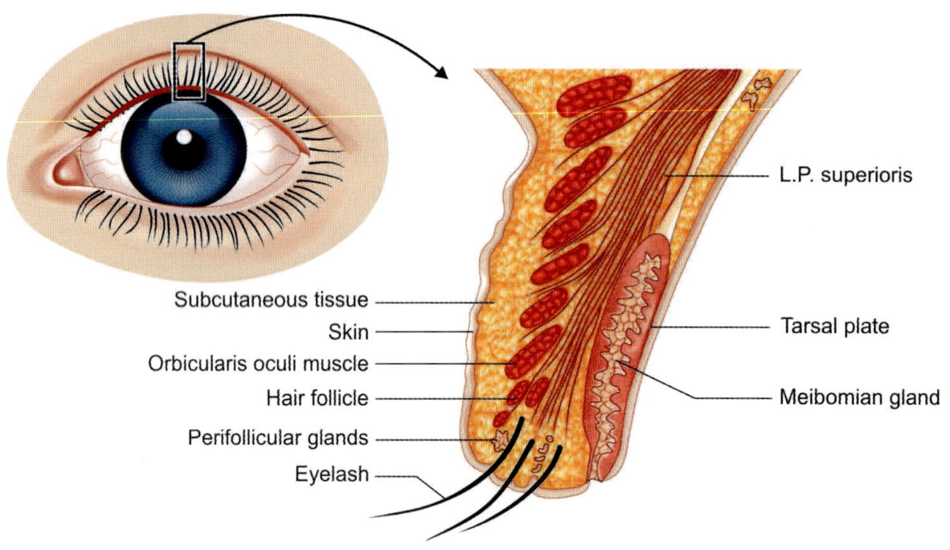


**Fig. 15.3:** An illustration depicting the cross-sectional anatomy of the upper and lower eyelids.

eye. The anterior lamina is separated from the posterior lamina by the orbital septum. Near the lid margins, the posterior lamina is composed of the tarsal plates, which are covered posteriorly by mucosa. Moving away from the lid margins, the eyelid fat pads can be found deep to the orbital septum, with the lid retractors and lid mucosa still deeper. The upper eyelid is elevated by the levator palpebrae superioris, innervated by cranial nerve III, with a minor contribution from the sympathetically innervated Mueller's muscle. The lid elevators insert on the superior surface of the tarsal plate of the upper lid. The cross-sectional anatomy of the lids can be seen in Figure 15.3.

## Vascular Supply

The eyelids have a rich and highly anastomosing vascular supply derived from the internal carotid circulation.[8] The medial and lateral palpebral arteries derive from the ophthalmic artery and give rise to a series of vascular arcades that provide blood supply to the lids. The marginal arcade runs along the tarsus near the lid margin just deep to the orbicularis. The peripheral arcades run along the edge of the tarsal plate distant to the lid margin. These arcades anastomose with one another freely. In addition, the palpebral arcade of the upper lid anastomoses with

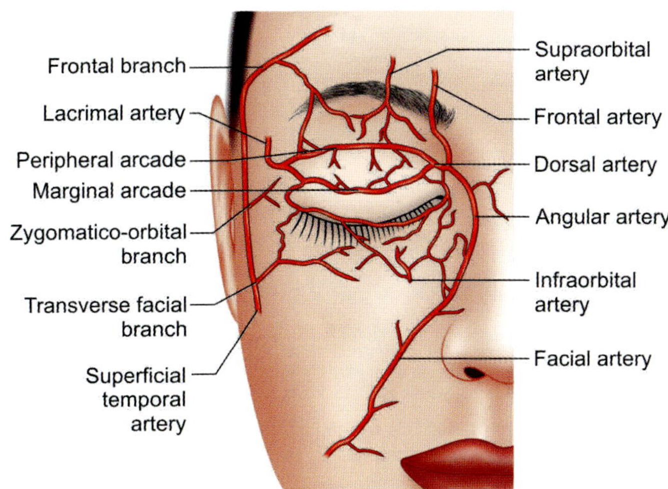


**Fig. 15.4:** An illustration depicting the arterial blood supply of the eyelids.

branches of the supraorbital artery, while the palpebral arcade of the lower lid anastomoses with the external carotid circulation via branches of the angular and infraorbital arteries. A schematic of the lid vasculature can be seen in Figure 15.4.

## ASSESSMENT OF THE WOUND

As mentioned above, the eyelid is a bilaminar structure with its own structural support system. Like the distal nose, the eyelid is composed of an interior lining, structural support system, and cutaneous covering. If disrupted, all three of these layers must be reconstructed in order to reestablish the functional and aesthetic integrity of the lid. In addition, the inherent properties of the eyelid should be examined both before surgery and prior to reconstruction. One should be particularly careful at noticing preoperative presence of ectropion, lid laxity, and/or upper lid ptosis. In patients with presurgical lid laxity, a concomitant tightening procedure may be considered.[9]

## RECONSTRUCTION OF ANTERIOR LAMELLAR DEFECTS

Partial-thickness defects of the lid are those that involve only skin and orbicularis oculi. These defects are generally less challenging to reconstruct and are amenable to a wider range of reconstructive possibilities than defects that involve the structural components, or full thickness of the lid. It is imperative that tension on the lid margin be avoided to prevent ectropion. Likewise, all undermining should be performed anterior to the orbital septum. The lower lid, upper lid, and medial canthus will be discussed as separate subunits, due to their distinct properties, tissue reservoirs, and reconstructive needs.

### Lower Lid Anterior Lamellar Defects

There are a broad range of options for the closure of lower lid anterior lamellar defects due to the nearby tissue reservoirs of the cheek and temple. The choice of reconstructive technique is determined by the size of the defect, mobility of the surrounding tissue, and the availability of nearby tissue reservoirs. Granulation of anterior lamellar defects is rarely possible as scar contracture can cause lid ectropion.

#### *Primary Closure*

Primary closure is a technically simple, reliable, and commonly used tool in cases when the defect is distant from the lid margin.[10] Depending on the amount of tissue laxity wounds of $\leq$ 2 cm can generally be closed primarily. In order to allow for primary closure without wedge resection of the eyelid, there must be sufficient space between the superior margin of the wound and the lash margin to allow for excision of a standing cutaneous deformity (SCD). The extreme pliability of lower lid skin allows for the successful execution of elliptical closures with angles much more obtuse than the typical 30° (Figs. 15.5A to C).

It is imperative that all tension vectors be kept parallel to the lid margin. To facilitate this, primary closures are best designed on the lower lid as a "lazy-S." The superior limb should be verticalized so the line of closure is perpendicular to the direction of the lid margin. The lengthening vector from closure of the ellipse provides support to the lid margin helping to minimize the risk of ectropion. The inferior SCD can then be designed to conform to the relaxed skin tension lines (RSTL) of the cheek to aid in scar camouflage. The wound should be undermined in the supraorbicularis plane. All tension bearing sutures should be oriented parallel to the lid margin.

#### *Full-Thickness Skin Grafts*

Full-thickness skin grafts (FTSG) are a reasonable closure option for the repair of anterior lamellar lower lid defects. Lid skin is the thinnest on the body.[4] As such, the ideal donor site in order to obtain skin of similar quality is eyelid skin.[11]

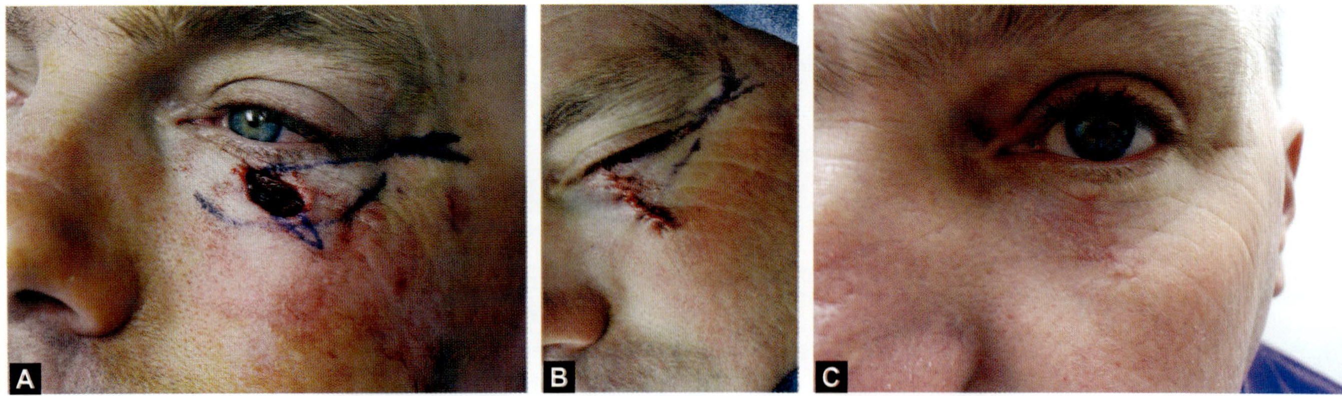

**Figs. 15.5A to C:** (A) A middle-aged Caucasian man is shown after an excision of a lesion on the left lower eyelid. (B) The defect on the left lower eyelid of this man was repaired via elliptical primary closure, with an obtusely-angled cone removal. (C) Eight weeks following primary closure of the lower eyelid defect.

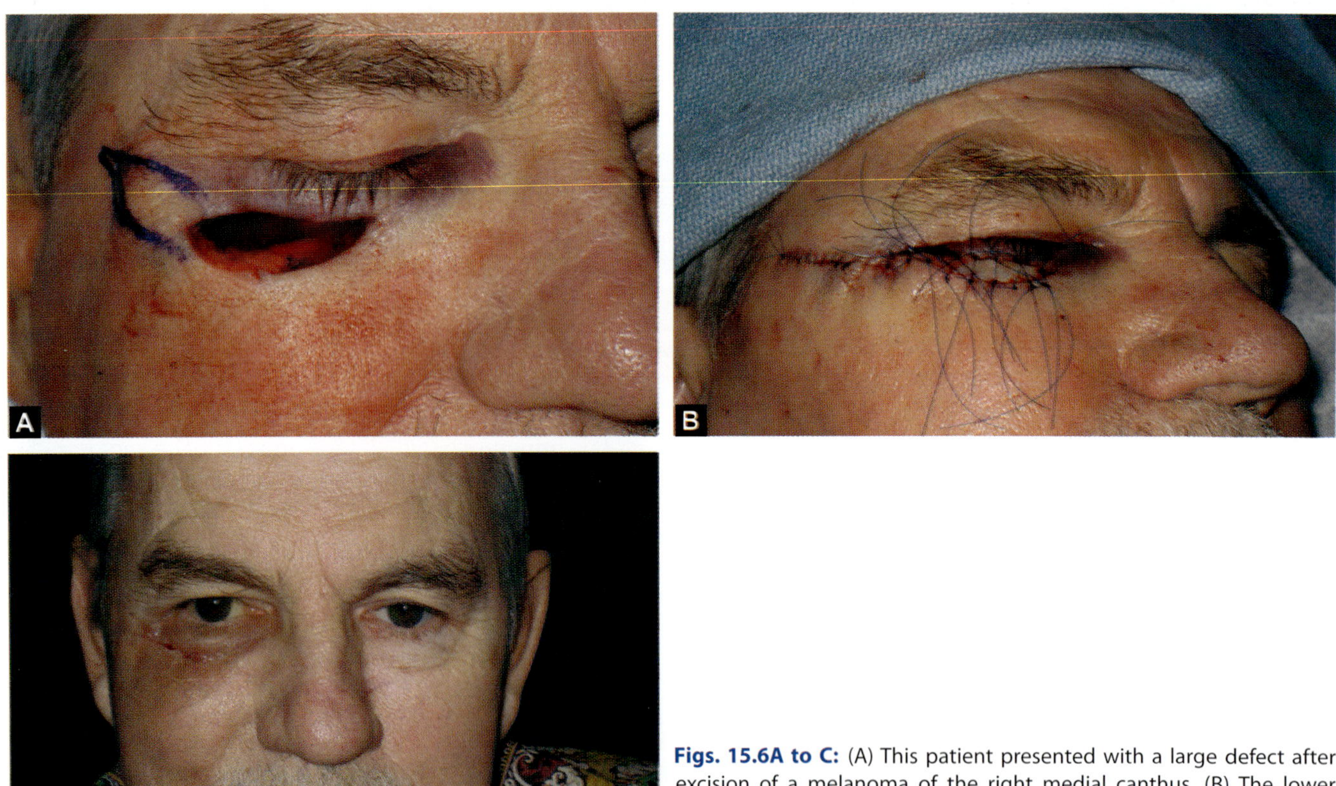

**Figs. 15.6A to C:** (A) This patient presented with a large defect after excision of a melanoma of the right medial canthus. (B) The lower eyelid was reconstructed with a free tarsoconjunctival graft from the contralateral upper lid (as well as a Mustardé flap). (C) Aesthetic result at 8-week follow-up.

In patients with substantial upper lid laxity, a skin-only blepharoplasty can provide sufficient tissue to resurface many anterior lamellar defects (Figs. 15.6A to C).[12] Thicker-skinned areas such as preauricular or supraclavicular skin may be used. However, our experience suggests that grafts from thicker-skinned areas have a greater tendency to contract and lead to a greater risk of ectropion.

When designing an FTSG for placement on the lower lid, the graft should be oversized by ~10% to allow ample tissue to prevent downward traction on the lid margin.

A Frost suture may be used to provide upward support for the lower lid during the early healing process.[13] There is wide variability in the execution of the Frost suture, but all modifications involve passing of a suture through the tarsal plate of the lower lid. Upward tension is applied to the suture to lift the lower lid and the suture is affixed to the forehead.[14] The Frost suture is placed prior to FTSG placement and the graft should be designed to fit the expanded wound produced by the Frost suture.

## Rotation Flaps

Rotation flaps are a standby for the repair of lower lid defects.[15-17] They recruit laxity from the cheek or temple to resurface eyelid defects. They may be based on an inferolateral, or less commonly, a superolateral pedicle. The incision lines of rotation flaps on the cheek and eyelid tend to conform well with the natural lines of the face, lending to good aesthetic results.

Inferolaterally-based rotation flaps for defects of the anterior lamella beneath the lash margin should be designed with the following parameters in mind. The flap incision should be made laterally from the superolateral edge of the primary defect. If the superior edge of the primary defect is beneath the lash margin, additional normal tissue can be excised to allow for camouflage of the flap incision in the subciliary line—although this step is not strictly necessary. The flap incision should proceed laterally until it reaches the vertical line extending through the lateral canthus at which time it should extend superolaterally above the level of the intercanthal line.[18] The flap incision can be continued out to the hairline and down the preauricular sulcus as necessary to achieve the amount of flap movement required to close the primary defect. Extending the flap beyond the lateral canthus and above the intercanthal line prevents formation of a secondary defect in the infraorbital area with flap movement, and consequently minimizing the risk of ectropion.

The flap is undermined in the suprafascial plane on the eyelid and subcutaneous plane on the cheek and temple. While the authors have had very few cases of flap necrosis with subcutaneous undermining, some studies have shown lower rates of distal flap necrosis with sub-superficial muscular aponeurotic system (SMAS) undermining.[17] It is important to note that even with sub-SMAS undermining of the area, overlying the temple and parotid should always be undermined in the subcutaneous plane to avoid injury to the facial nerve. The SCD is excised in the RSTL of the cheek as the flap is rotated medially (Figs. 15.7A to D).

As the flap is rotated medially, a secondary defect forms in the temple region. The flap can then be tacked upward to the temporal fascia to close the secondary defect and support the flap. Periosteal tacking sutures can be placed from the dermal undersurface of the flap to the periosteum of the orbital rim to further support the flap against contraction and its resulting ectropion.

For lower lid wounds near the medial canthus, the flap incision can be made down the nasofacial sulcus, continuing into the melolabial fold to create a superolaterally-based rotation flap. This flap is most useful for wounds that are relatively wide—thus making tissue movement from lateral to medial difficult—but with a limited vertical height (Figs. 15.8A to C). This approach is reliant upon the use of tacking sutures placed from the flap to the nasal sidewall and orbital rim to prevent downward traction on the lid margin. The SCD is excised in the lid crease. It is best to be conservative and excise a smaller standing cone in this setting. This closure option does have the advantage of placing all scar lines in cosmetic unit junction lines.

## V–Y Advancement Flap

V–Y flaps, also known as island pedicle flaps, are random pattern flaps based on a deep subcutaneous pedicle. The lengthening effect of V–Y closures can be applied to the repair of lower eyelid defects to help prevent postoperative ectropion.[19] In fact, V–Y closures have been found to be equivalent to Mustardé style rotation flaps in the prevention of ectropion.[20] These flaps are an excellent solution for broad wounds of limited vertical height. Compared to cheek rotation flaps they have a relatively modest undermined area. However, the disadvantage of the V–Y is that its incision lines do not conform to the RSTL and cosmetic unit lines of the face in the same way as a rotation flap. Thus, the surgeon is reliant upon fastidious suturing technique to deliver the desired result.

The V–Y flap should be designed as a long, tapering triangle. As much as possible, the lateral flap incision should conform to the RSTL of the cheek (Figs. 15.9A to C). Once the flap is designed it is incised to the level of deep fat or fascia. The leading edge and tail of the flap almost always need to be undermined to allow flap movement—thus the importance of making the flap long and tapered so that a robust central pedicle is maintained. The skin surrounding the flap and primary defect is then undermined in the subcutaneous plane to allow further flap movement and minimize postoperative pincushion deformity.

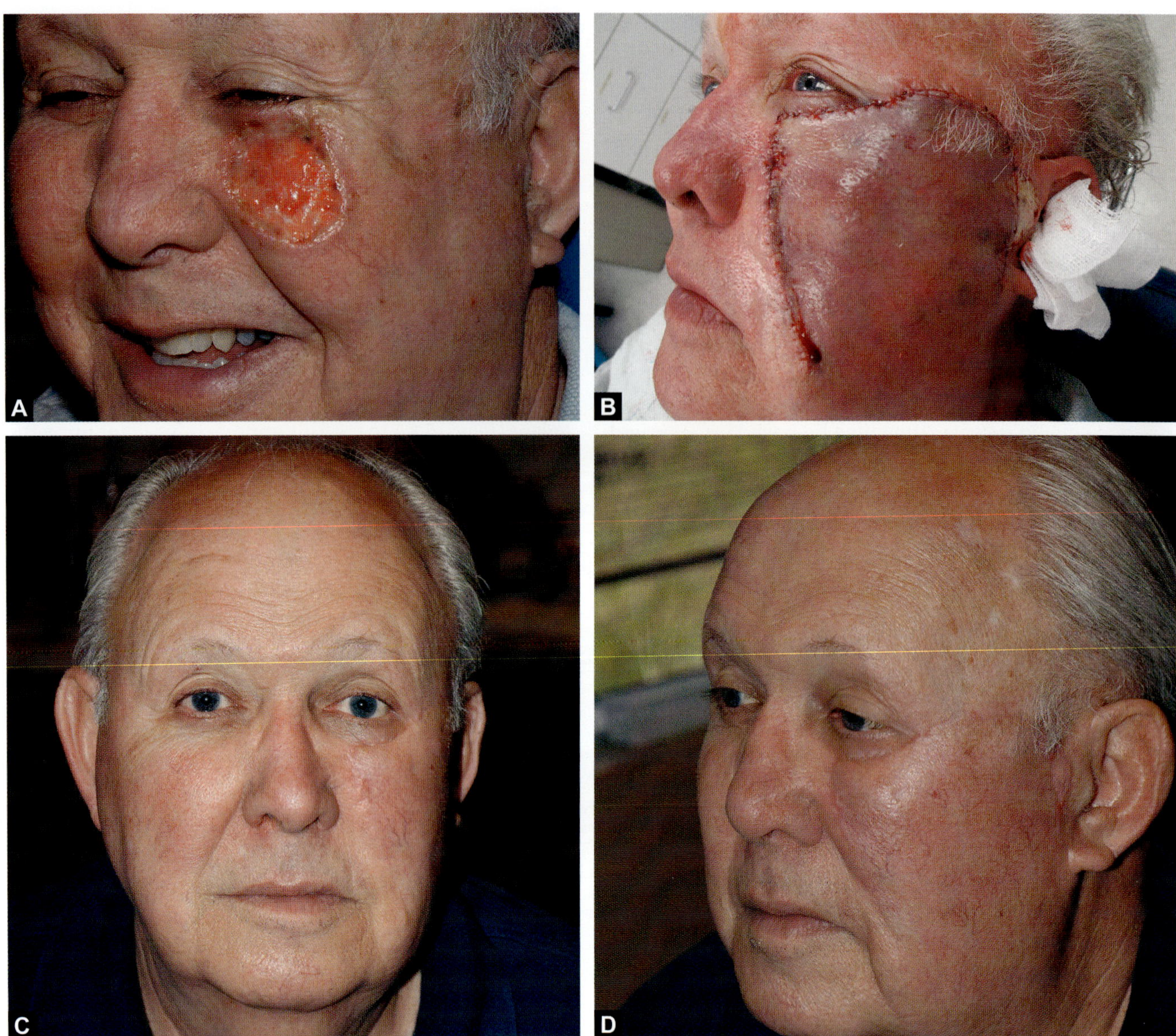

**Figs. 15.7A to D:** (A) A 4 × 3.5 cm defect of the cheek and lower eyelid following staged excision of a melanoma-in-situ. (B) The defect was repaired with a cheek rotation flap. A small burrow's graft was used to repair the secondary defect in the preauricular area. (C) A frontal view of the well-healed flap at 8 weeks. (D) A side view at 8 weeks.

If resistance is felt when advancing the flap into the primary defect, it can be helpful to "strum" the edges of the flap with the tips of a scissors to feel the origin of the restraint. Further undermining can be performed in the needed areas until sufficient movement is achieved.

When performing a V-Y closure on the lower lid, downward traction on the lid margin is avoided in one or more of the following three ways; placement of periosteal tacking sutures to pull the flap upward into the primary defect, placement of all tension bearing sutures from the sides of the flap to the medial and lateral edges of the primary defect, and finally aggressive closure of the donor site to force the flap upward into the primary defect (Figs. 15.10A to C). With these steps taken the leading edge of the flap should meet the superior edge of the primary defect obviating the need for any downward tension vector on the lid margin.

## Transposition Flaps

Transposition flaps are frequently used tools for defects of the anterior lamella of the lower lid.[21-23] Transposition

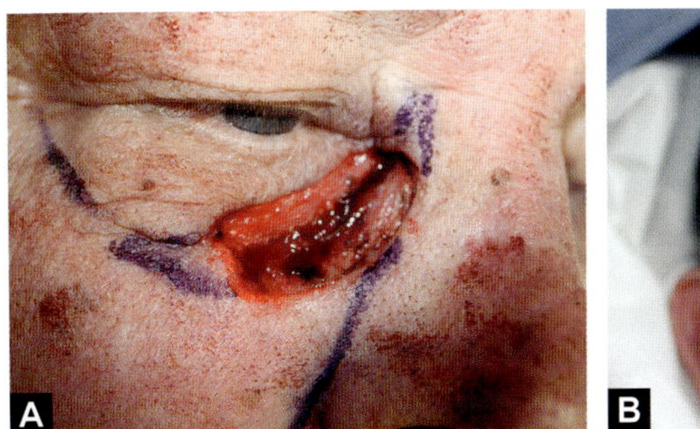

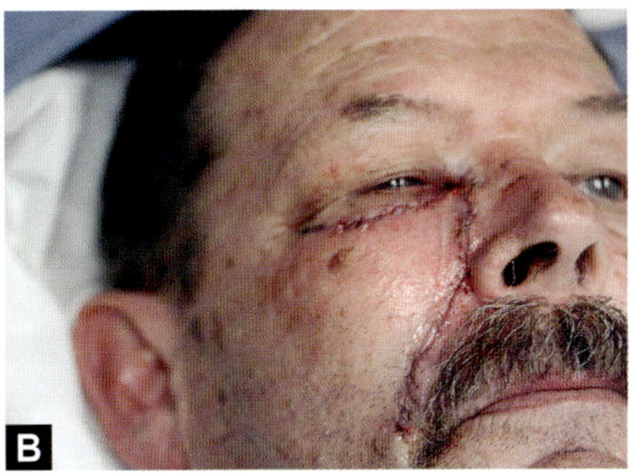

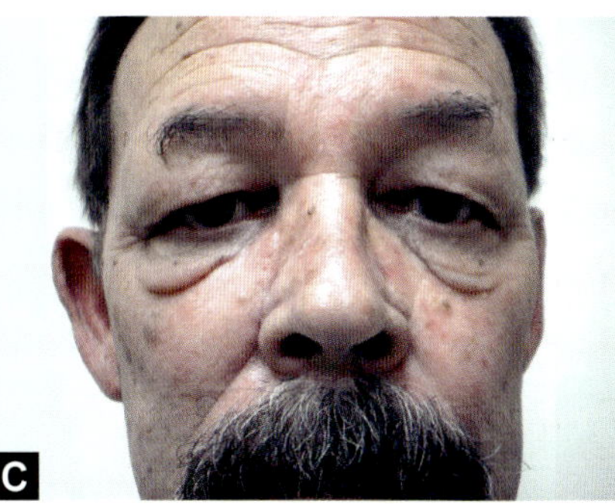


**Figs. 15.8A to C:** (A) A patient with a relatively wide defect on the right inferior eyelid near the medial canthus. A inferiolaterally-based rotation flap was designed. (B) The inferiolaterally-based rotation flap sewn in place. (C) Aesthetic result at 8-week follow-up.

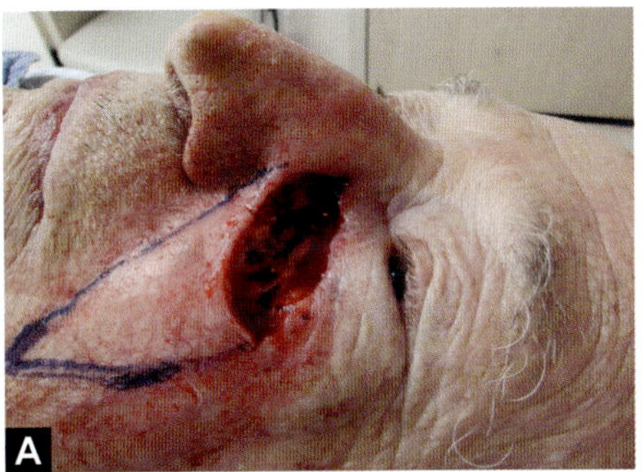

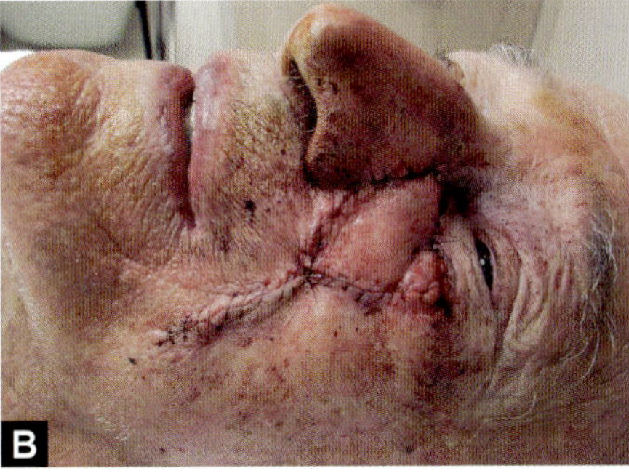

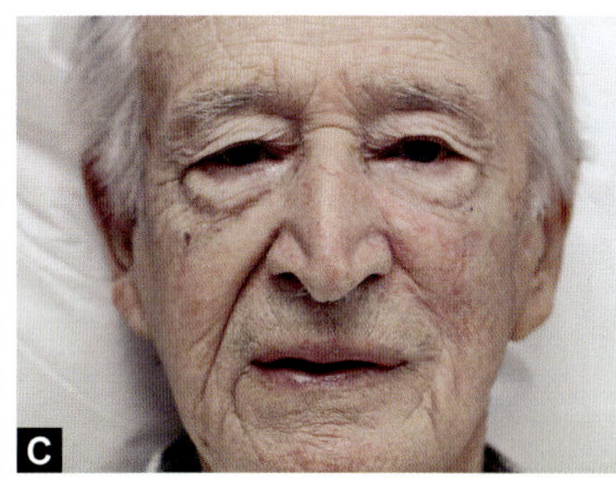


**Figs. 15.9A to C:** (A) A V–Y flap was designed for this elderly man with a relatively large wound beneath the left eye. (B) Immediate post-V–Y reconstruction. (C) Aesthetic result at 6-month follow-up.

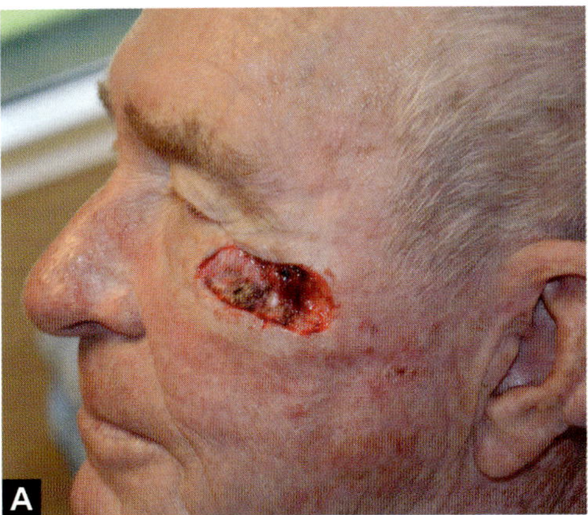

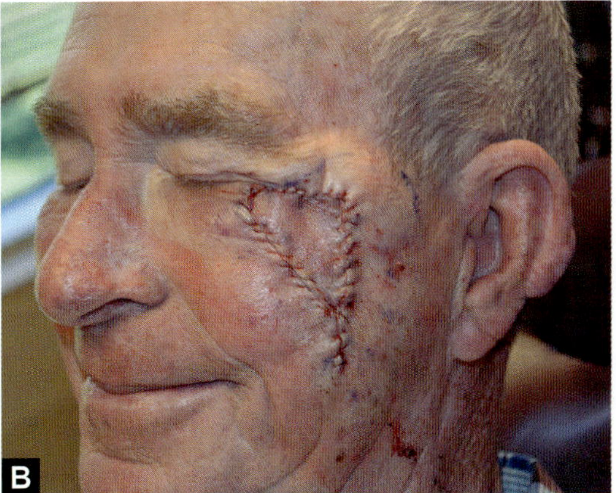

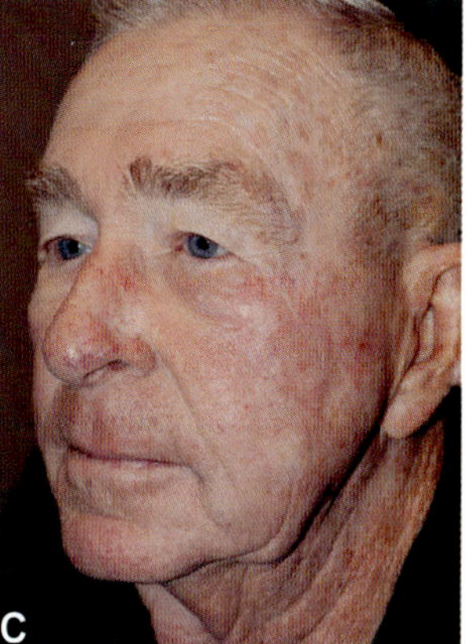


**Figs. 15.10A to C:** (A) A defect on the left malar region after excision. (B) After V–Y flap construction, the patient demonstrates no downward tension on the left lid margin. (C) Aesthetic result at 8-week postoperative photograph.

flaps, whether single lobed rhombic modifications or bilobed flaps, have the advantage of causing Z-plasty-like lengthening to support the lower lid.[24]

Medially based Dufourmental style rhombic flaps are a reasonable option for small-medium defects of the lower lid. By using a medially based flap the secondary defect is placed in the RSTL of the cheek, easing closure of the tension bearing defect, and contributing to better scar camouflage (Figs. 15.11A to C). Care should be taken to make sure that the flap is designed at least as wide as the primary defect is tall to prevent downward pull on the lid margin once the flap is sutured in place.

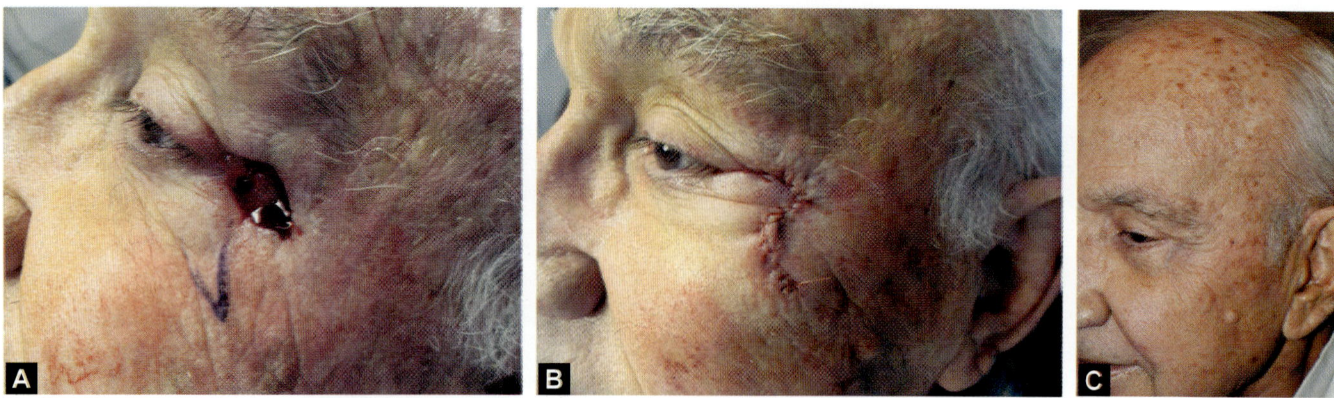


**Figs. 15.11A to C:** (A) A defect near the left lateral canthus to be closed with a medially based rhombic flap. (B) Rhombic flap sutured into place. (C) Aesthetic result at 8-week follow-up.

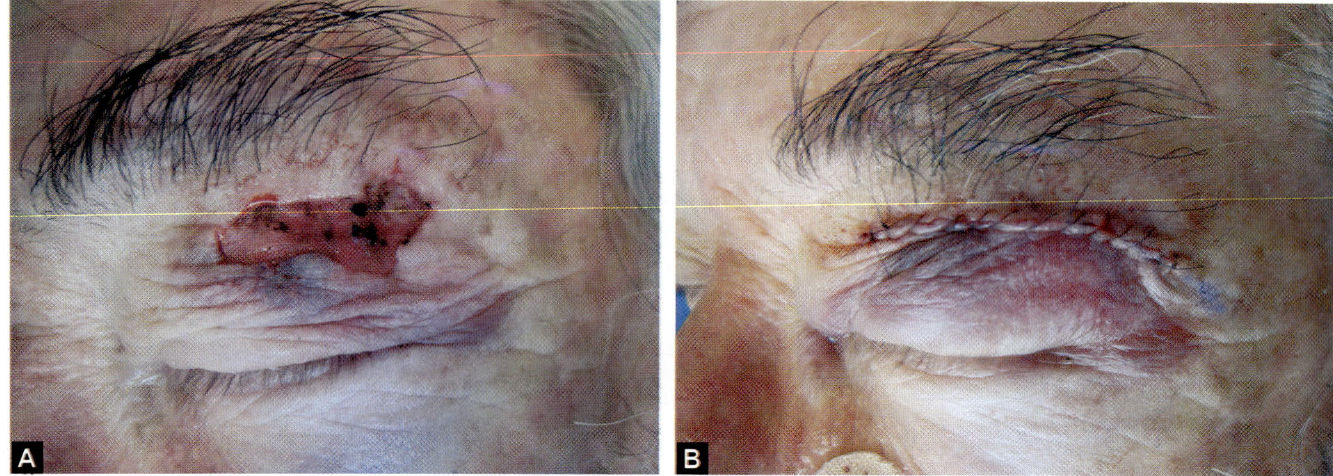


**Figs. 15.12A and B:** (A) Defect on the upper lid to be closed primarily. (B) Immediate postoperative result.
*Courtesy*: S Brian Jiang, MD, Sang Diego, California, USA.

Bilobed flaps have also been reported for closure of a number of anterior lamellar lower lid defects. The design aspects of these flaps vary from report to report.[22,23] However, the principles of careful design to minimize secondary movement of the lid are unchanged from the single lobed transposition flaps.

## Upper Lid Anterior Lamellar Defects

Unlike the lower lid, the upper eyelid is isolated from nearby tissue reservoirs by the presence of the brow.[3] Moreover, the forehead and glabella skin are not as good of a texture match for the eyelid area compared to the cheek. These two factors combined restrict the repair options for upper lid defects. Fortunately, skin cancers of the upper lid are much rarer than lower lid cancers.[25]

### *Primary Closure*

In patients with redundant upper eyelid skin and small primary defects, a blepharoplasty type primary closure may be possible (Figs. 15.12A and B). The patient should be asked to open and close their eye with the wound pulled shut to insure that full eyelid closure is still possible with wound approximation. For patients with less redundant skin, or small, narrow defects, a vertical primary closure can be performed. This option is restricted due to the lack of space in the upper lid subunit.

### *Full-Thickness Skin Grafts*

Full-thickness skin grafts are an excellent option for the closure of upper lid defects.[4,25] The favored donor site is

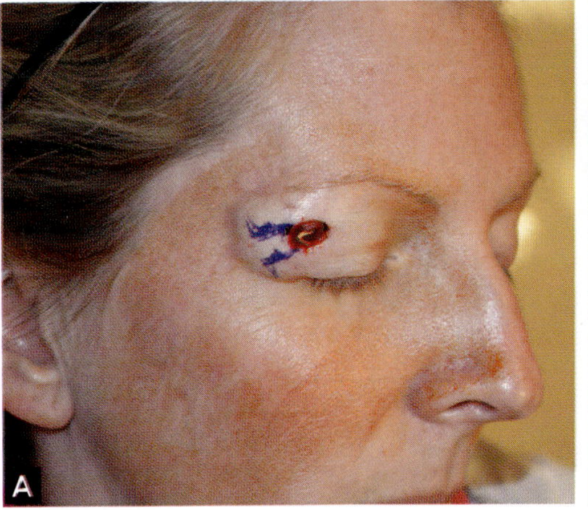

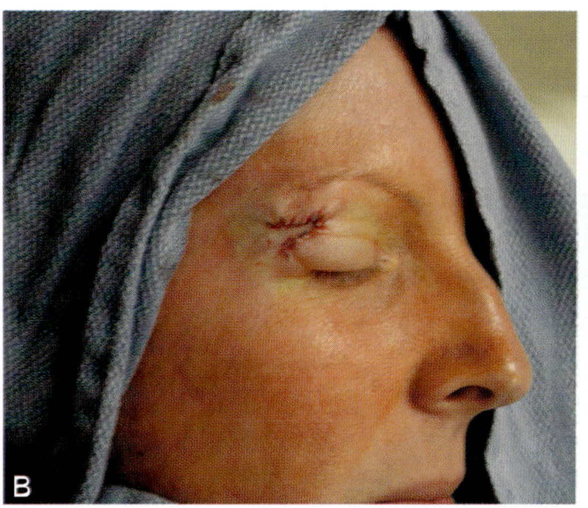

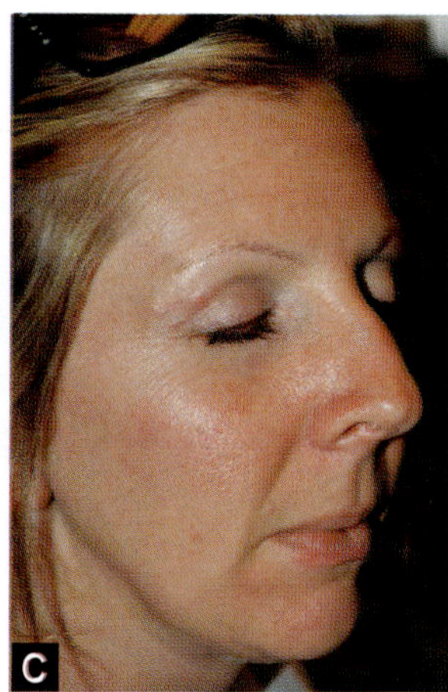


**Figs. 15.13A to C:** (A) The O–U double tangent advancement flap was chosen to repair the defect of the right upper eyelid of this young Caucasian woman. The O–U flap recruits laxity from the lateral upper lid and temple. (B) After the completion of the O–U advancement flap. (C) Aesthetic result at 8-week follow-up.

the contralateral upper eyelid.[1] As with FTSG for the lower lid, if the contralateral upper lid does not provide a sufficient reservoir, other donor sites must be considered. The thinnest possible skin should be selected to maximize texture match and minimize the risk of graft contraction.

### Advancement Flaps

Advancement flaps are useful tools for reconstruction of upper lid defects. These horizontally moving flaps allow importation of tissue via the only points of access into this restricted anatomic space. O-U flaps, double tangent advancement flaps, are a viable option for upper lids. They allow recruitment of laxity from the temple laterally (Figs. 15.13A to C), and to a lesser extent the glabella medially. V-Y closures based on the underlying orbicularis muscle can also be performed. If oriented horizontally, they should be designed with a slow taper and a very acute apical angle to minimize upward pull on the lid margin with secondary defect closure.

### Transposition Flaps

The use of transposition flaps on the upper lid is fairly limited by the brow superiorly and the lid margin inferiorly. For small defects, rhombic flaps may be designed to recruit superior lid skin. As with any other lid closure, all tension vectors should be kept parallel to the lid margin. Larger defects may be repaired with inferiorly based, Banner type transposition flaps. Flaps from the glabella and temple allow closure of lid defects without distortion of either the lid margin or brow (Figs. 15.14A to C). However, in many patients, these donor sites will provide suboptimal tissue match for native eyelid skin.

## Medial Canthal Wounds Not Involving the Full Thickness of the Lid

The medial canthal subunit is an aesthetically important concave area at the junction of the superolateral nasal sidewall and the medial lid margins. Wounds in this area often require more tissue than is immediately apparent to recreate the natural contour of the area. Patients should be asked to raise their eyebrows to reveal the full size of the wound. Restoration of sufficient tissue to fill the expanded wound apparent on eyebrow elevation is of the utmost importance to avoid formation of a medial canthal web. If insufficient length is supplied and scar contracture occurs, the skin takes the “short cut” across the top of the concave region producing a web.

The wound should be subdivided into the portions above and below the intercanthal line. In order to obtain optimal cosmesis, the portions of the wound above and below the intercanthal line often must be repaired separately (Figs. 15.15A and B). Additionally, in order to fully resurface the full length of the canthal concavity, “lengthening closures” such as transposition flaps, and V-Y flaps are favored.[26,27]

### Granulation

Concave areas are normally amenable to granulation.[28,29] However, in large medial canthal wounds, webbing will

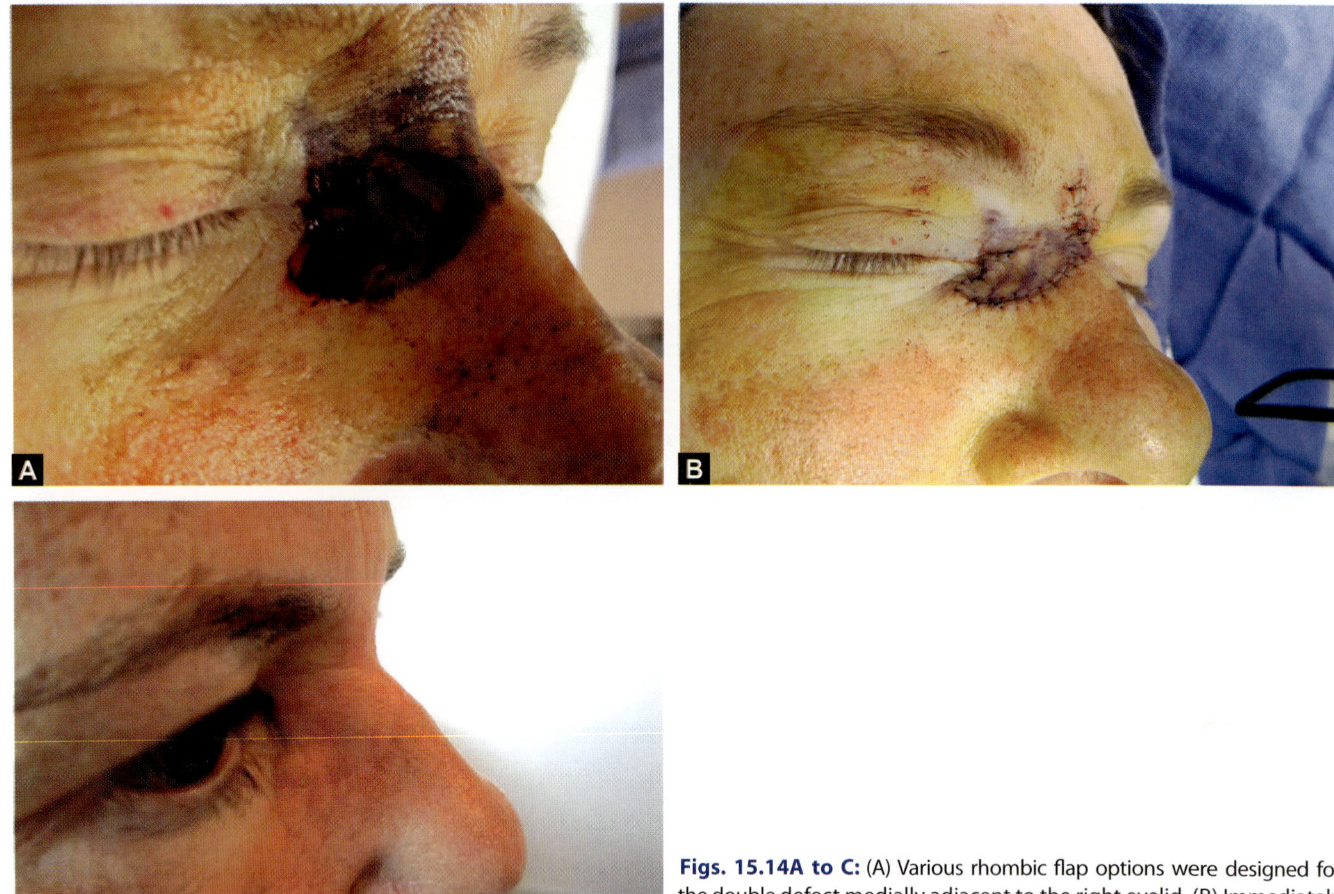

**Figs. 15.14A to C:** (A) Various rhombic flap options were designed for the double defect medially adjacent to the right eyelid. (B) Immediately postrepair. (C) Aesthetic result at 4-month follow-up.
*Courtesy*: S Brian Jiang, MD, Sang Diego, California, USA.

**Figs. 15.15A and B:** (A) A large defect in the areas both above and below the intercanthal line. These portions were to be closed separately. (B) Immediate postrepair result.

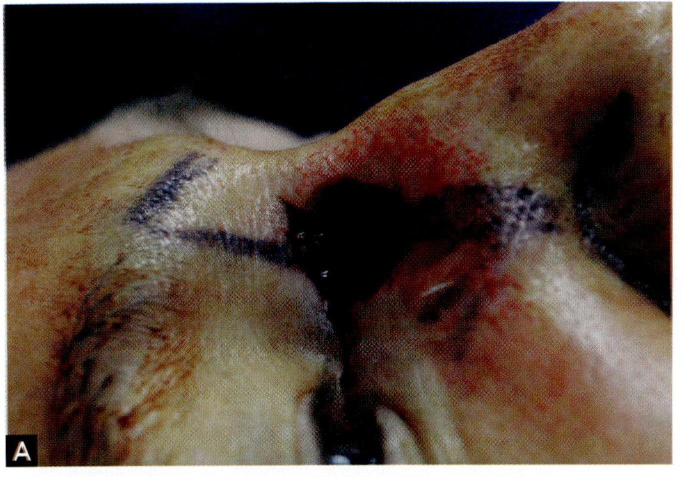
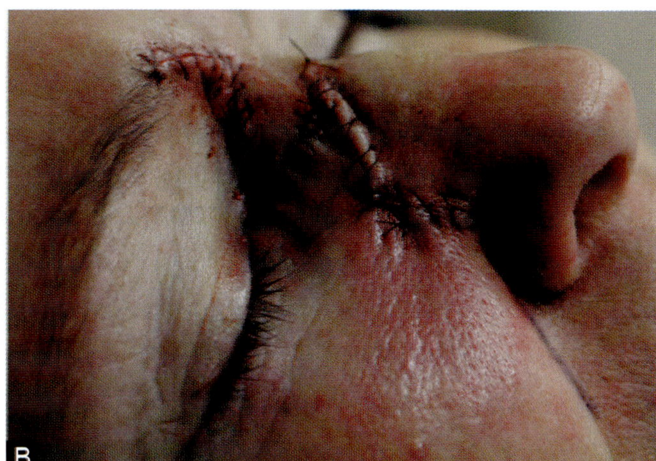
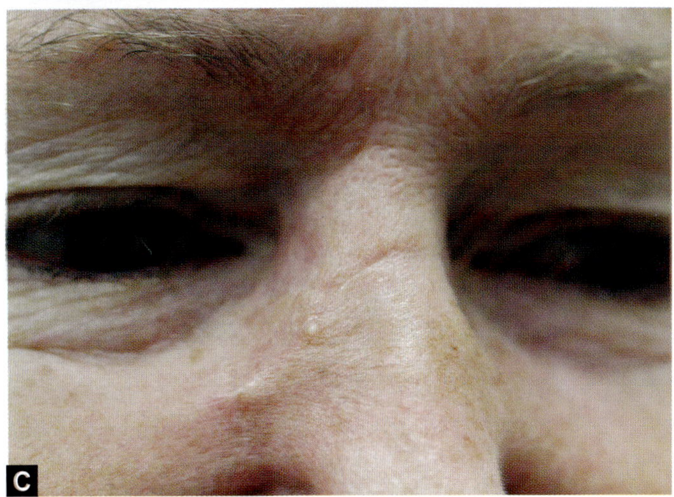

**Figs. 15.16A to C:** (A) This patient's defect on the right nasal bridge encompasses the intercanthal line. A paired rhombic flap was designed for repair. (B) Immediately following repair. (C) Aesthetic result at 8-week follow-up.

occur with granulation. Wounds most amenable to granulation are those that are evenly divided by the intercanthal line—to avoid asymmetrical pull on the lids—and ≤ 1 cm in diameter.

## Full-Thickness Skin Grafts

Full-thickness skin grafts are an excellent option for medial canthal repair in the presence of a well-vascularized wound bed.

## Transposition Flaps

Rhombic type transposition flaps are a reliable option for medial canthal repair. The Z-plasty-like lengthening effect of the transposition flap helps protect against contraction mediated canthal webbing.[24] Additionally, vertical orientation of the donor site (or sites) prevents pulling of the lid off the globe.

For defects above the intercanthal line, the senior author often designs a laterally based flap without removing the SCD. The residual tissue from the SCD can then be draped into the concavity.

Large transposition flaps can often lend a bulky appearance to the medial canthus, especially if the primary defect straddles the intercanthal line. In these cases, paired rhombic flaps can be used to resurface the defect (Figs. 15.16A to C).

## V–Y Advancement Flaps

Similar to transposition flaps, V–Y advancement flaps provide a lengthening effect that is desirable in the medial canthal region.[27,30] Design and undermining techniques are similar to that used in other locations. As with transposition flaps, it is best to subdivide the wound at the intercanthal line and repair the superior and inferior portions

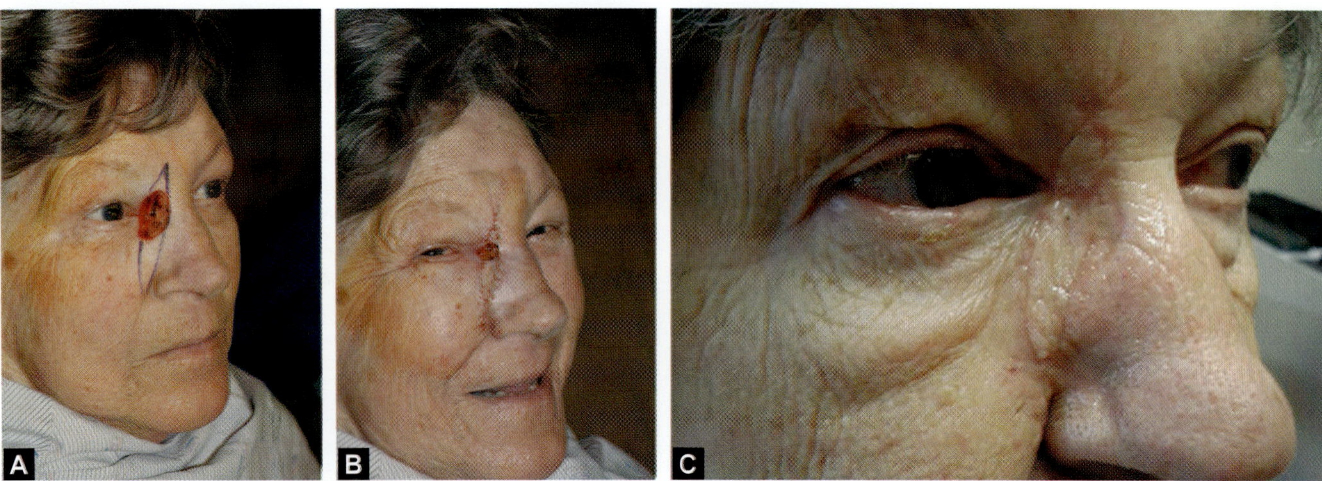


**Figs. 15.17A to C:** (A) A combination of paired V–Y advancement flaps and granulation were used to close this tall medial canthal defect. (B) The flaps were advanced to create a small defect centered on the intercanthal line. (C) Granulation of the defect centered on the intercanthal line allowed for reformation of the canthal concavity as can be seen in this 8-week follow-up photograph.

separately to avoid a bulky appearance at the medial canthus (Figs. 15.17A to C).

## RECONSTRUCTION OF FULL-THICKNESS EYELID DEFECTS

Full-thickness defects of the eyelid can be intimidating, but most can be safely repaired under local anesthesia as long as several important principles are abided by:

- The eyelid is a bilaminar structure.[2-4] In order to execute a successful repair, tissue deficits from each lamina must be fully addressed.
- The eyelid has its own structural support system that must be repaired if it has been compromised during tumor excision. The contiguity of the tarsal plate must be re-established and the tarsal plate should be anchored to the medial and lateral canthal tendons (or to the insertion of these tendons if the tendons are obliterated).
- The eyelids, especially the upper lid, are dynamic structures. For large upper lid defects, the repair should be anchored to the lid elevators to allow for opening of the eye.
- Tension on the free lid margin must be avoided to prevent ectropion.
- The lacrimal drainage system is formed by the lacrimal punctate on the medial lids, which drain into the lacrimal collecting system just deep to the anterior crus of the medial canthal tendon. Wounds extending through the medial canthal tendon can destroy the lacrimal collecting system and lead to epiphora if not repaired. However up to 40% of patients have some degree of asymptomatic lacrimal obstruction,[31] and patients can have epiphora with a patent lacrimal system,[32] so the likelihood of postoperative epiphora can be difficult to predict.

Full-thickness lid defects are most often divided based on their size in proportion to the total width of the lid. The size cut-offs given below are approximate. Patients with less lid laxity, or who have undergone previous eyelid tightening surgery, will often be less amenable to more simple closure options. Conversely, patients with abundant eyelid laxity and wounds less than a third of the lid may be amenable to direct closure.

### Full-Thickness Wounds Involving <25% of the Lid

Most wounds encompassing <25% of the lid margin are amenable to closure with a pentagonal wedge closure. This is a simple and reliable closure method that provides excellent cosmetic results with minimal morbidity. First, two pairs of forceps should be used to ensure that the wound can be pulled together without undue tension, pressure on the orbit, or "bow-stringing of the reapproximated eyelid beneath the globe. The pentagonal wedge should be designed such that it widens slightly as it moves away from the lid margin before converging to a single point (Figs. 15.18A to C). By making the nonmarginal portion of

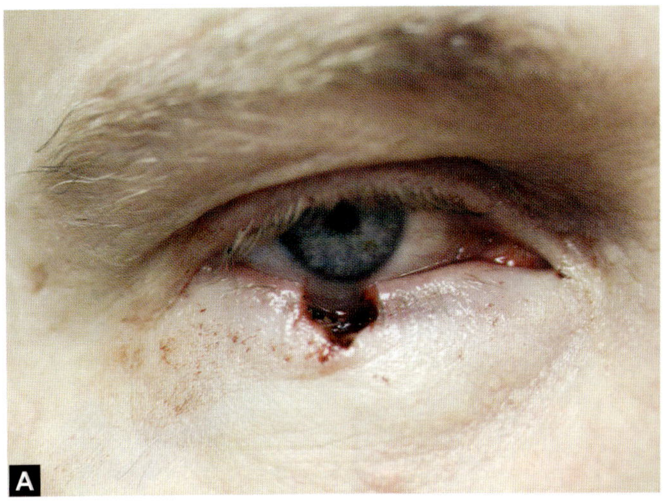


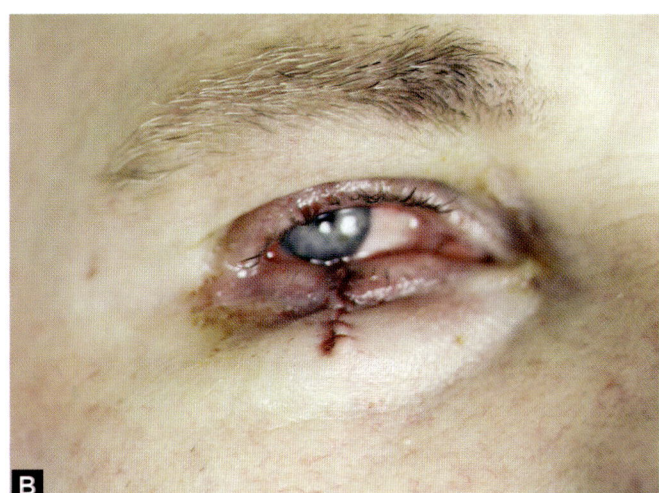


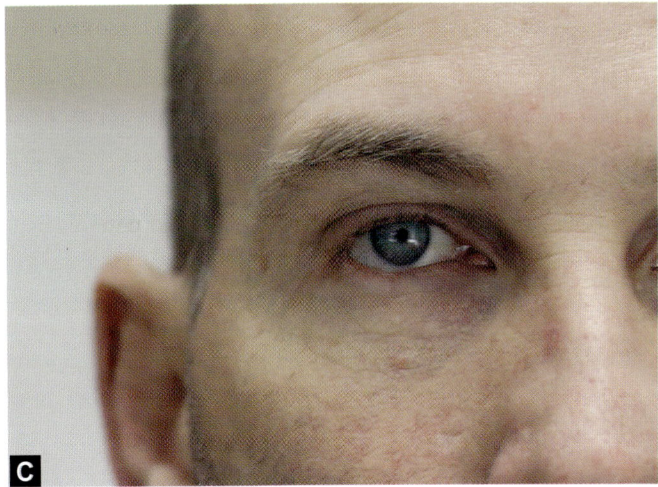


**Figs. 15.18A to C:** (A) A pentagonal wedge prior to wound closure. (B) The pentagonal wedge immediately after closure. (C) Aesthetic result at 8-week follow-up.

the wound slightly wider, an upward pushing vector is applied to the lid margin with wound closure.

Generally, reapproximation of these wounds can be assured with a single key suture. A single diagonal tarsal suture is placed[33] to reapproximate the tarsal plate and lid margin. This suture technique has greatly simplified marginal closures obviating the need for the technically difficult top sutures on the lid margin that are a frequent cause of discomfort for patients. Depending on the size of the wound, one or two buried sutures may be placed to reapproximate the orbicularis. Epidermal sutures can then be placed from the lash margin to the end of the cutaneous closure. No top sutures are placed on the lid margin, and no sutures are placed on the mucosal surface.

For small defects involving the lateral margin of the lid, the lateral tarsal plate should be sutured to the lateral canthal tendon remnant or the periosteum of Whitnall's tubercle if there is no remaining lateral canthal tendon (Figs. 15.19A to C). Small thickness defects of the medial lid that involve the lacrimal punctum may be evaluated for canalicular reconstruction. This will be discussed in slightly more detail below.

In some cases, a relatively modest full-thickness portion of the defect will be accompanied by a larger anterior lamellar portion. In these cases, the full-thickness defect can be repaired by a pentagonal wedge, and the residual anterior lamellar defect repaired as discussed earlier in the chapter (Figs. 15.20A to C). Full-thickness defects involving the lacrimal puncta should be considered for stenting and canalicular repair.

## Full-Thickness Defects Involving 25–50% of the Lid Margin

The addition of lateral canthotomy and cantholysis allows closure of most eyelid defects of this size.[1,4,12,25] To perform

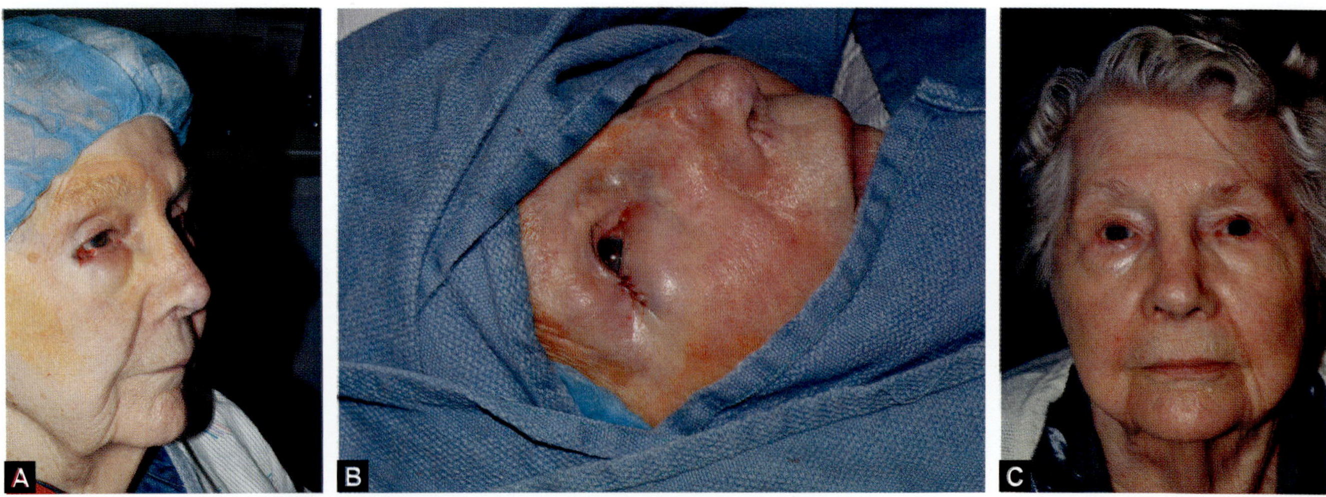


**Figs. 15.19A to C:** (A) Right lateral lid margin defect prior to wedge closure. (B) Immediately following primary closure. (C) Aesthetic result at 8-week follow-up.

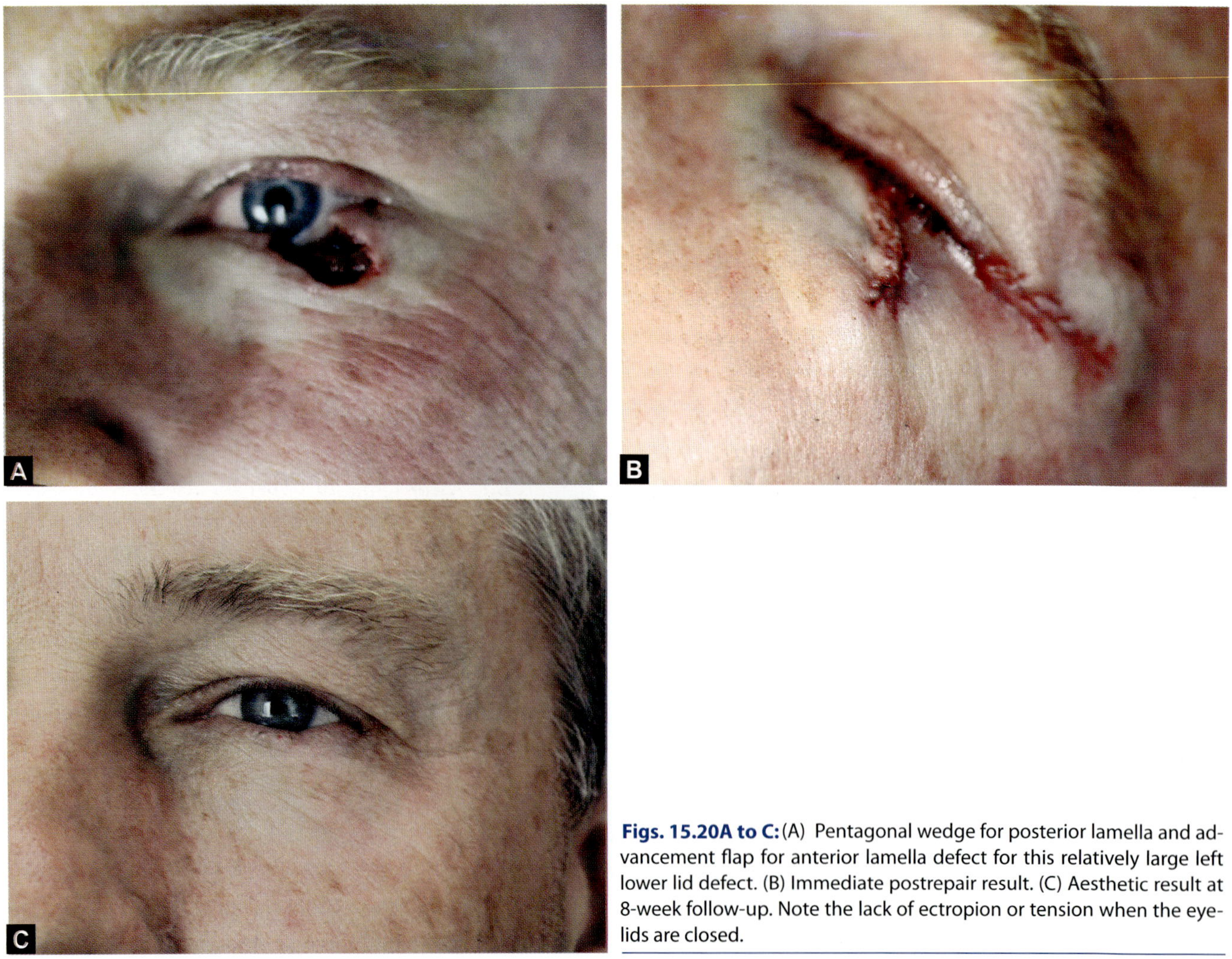

**Figs. 15.20A to C:** (A) Pentagonal wedge for posterior lamella and advancement flap for anterior lamella defect for this relatively large left lower lid defect. (B) Immediate postrepair result. (C) Aesthetic result at 8-week follow-up. Note the lack of ectropion or tension when the eyelids are closed.

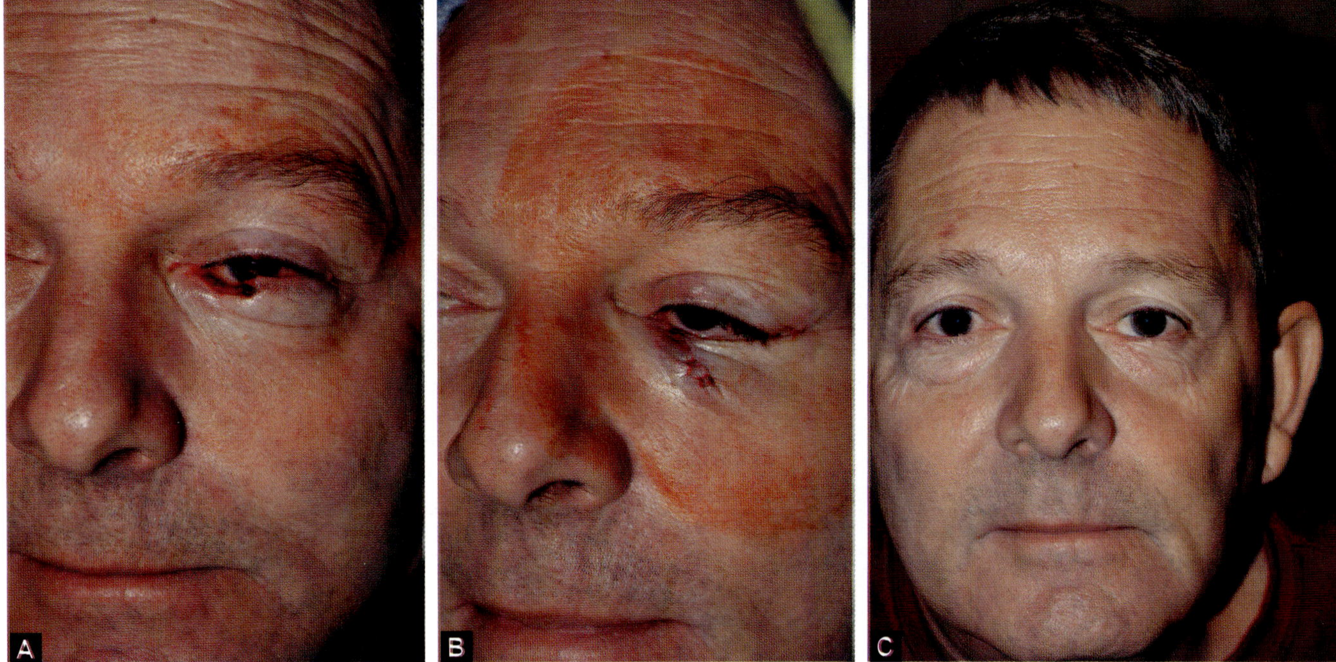

**Figs. 15.21A to C:** (A) Full-thickness defect involving >25% of the left lower lid margin. (B) Immediately following lateral canthotomy and cantholysis. (C) Aesthetic result at 8-week follow-up.

the canthotomy, a pair of scissors is inserted into the lateral canthus and an incision is made through the lateral canthus oriented slightly toward the lid opposite the defect (e.g. for an upper lid defect, the canthotomy should be oriented a few degrees superior of horizontal). Scissors tips can be used to strum the lateral canthus to palpate the canthal tendon. The scissors should then be oriented toward the lid that contains the defect and the canthal tendon snipped until sufficient movement is achieved. The tarsus is then reapproximated in the same manner as a pentagonal wedge closure (Figs. 15.21A to C). The skin of the canthotomy incision can then be reapproximated. If the lateral canthus appears ptotic, it can be resuspended to the temporal periosteum using deep sutures.

The Tenzel semicircular flap is an adjunct to direct closure with lateral cantholysis.[15] The flap is designed as a U-shape rotation flap emerging from the lateral canthus that classically is restricted within the orbital rim.

## Defects of > 50% of the Lid

Defects encompassing >50% of the full thickness of the eyelid margin often require more tissue than can be replaced by local tissue rearrangement alone. As these procedures are not commonly performed by dermatologic surgeons, they will only be discussed briefly. They are often repaired by one of two approaches:

- Staged lid sharing procedure:
  - *Hughes flap for lower lid defects*: A tarsoconjunctival flap from the upper lid is used to replace the posterior lamella of the lid.[34] The larger tarsal plate of the upper eyelid allows for harvesting of a tarsal flap while not compromising the structural integrity of the donor lid. The anterior lamella is resurfaced either with a cheek rotation flap or an FTSG.
  - *Cutler-Beard flap for upper lid defects*: A full-thickness rectangular skin muscle flap harvested from the lower lid inferior to the tarsal plate. This flap is sewn to the residual tarsus and lid elevators of the upper lid. A cartilage graft is placed at takedown to replace the missing upper lid tarsus.
- *Combination of tarsoconjunctival graft and myocutaneous flap*: A tarsoconjunctival graft can be harvested from the ipsilateral upper lid for lower lid defects or contralateral upper lid for upper lid defects. The tarsoconjunctival graft is affixed to the remaining tarsus or canthal tendon system. An inferiorly based myocutaneous advancement (cheek lift) flap or a cheek rotation flap can be used to resurface the anterior lamella and provide vascular support to the tarsoconjuntival graft.

## CONCLUSION

The eyelids are one of the most functionally and aesthetically important areas of the face. Careful analysis of the defect prior to reconstruction should be performed to assess the need for conjunctival lining, structural support, and cutaneous covering. Any proposed reconstructive plan should address any needs necessary. With careful planning and execution, eyelid reconstruction can consistently yield rewarding results for both the patient and surgeon.

## REFERENCES


1. Alghoul M, Pacella SJ, McClellan WT, et al. Eyelid reconstruction. Plast Reconstr Surg. 2013;132(2):288e-302e.
2. Kakizaki H, Malhotra R, Madge SN, et al. Lower eyelid anatomy: an update. Ann Plast Surg. 2009;63(3):344-51.
3. Kakizaki H, Malhotra R, Selva D. Upper eyelid anatomy: an update. Ann Plast Surg. 2009;63(3):336-43.
4. Stein JD, Antonyshyn OM. Aesthetic eyelid reconstruction. Clin Plast Surg. 2009;36(3):379-97.
5. Ishii L, Carey J, Byrne P, et al. Measuring attentional bias to peripheral facial deformities. Laryngoscope. 2009;119(3):459-65.
6. Gonzalez-Ulloa M, Castillo A, Stevens E, et al. Preliminary study of the total restoration of the facial skin. Plast Reconstr Surg (1946). 1954;13(3):151-61.
7. Knize DM. The superficial lateral canthal tendon: anatomic study and clinical application to lateral canthopexy. Plast Reconstr Surg. 2002;109(3):1149-57; discussion 58-63.
8. Erdogmus S, Govsa F. The arterial anatomy of the eyelid: importance for reconstructive and aesthetic surgery. J Plast Reconstr Aesthet Surg. 2007;60(3):241-5.
9. Georgescu D, Anderson RL, McCann JD. Lateral canthal resuspension sine canthotomy. Ophthal Plast Reconstr Surg. 2011;27(5):371-5.
10. Ibrahim AM, Rabie AN, Borud L, et al. Common patterns of reconstruction for Mohs defects in the head and neck. J Craniofac Surg. 2014;25(1):87-92.
11. Tuncali D, Ates L, Aslan G. Upper eyelid full-thickness skin graft in facial reconstruction. Dermatol Surg. 2005;31(1):65-70.
12. Kakizaki H, Madge SN, Mannor G, et al. Oculoplastic surgery for lower eyelid reconstruction after periocular cutaneous carcinoma. Int Ophthalmol Clin. 2009;49(4):143-55.
13. Sharabi SE, Hatef DA, Hollier LH Jr, et al. Opening eyes to the Frost suture. J Oral Maxillofac Surg. 2010;68(6):1430-1.
14. Desciak EB, Eliezri YD. Surgical pearl: temporary suspension suture (Frost suture) to help prevent ectropion after infraorbital reconstruction. J Am Acad Dermatol. 2003;49(6):1107-8.
15. Tenzel RR, Stewart WB. Eyelid reconstruction by the semicircle flap technique. Ophthalmology. 1978;85(11):1164-9.
16. Kroll SS, Reece GP, Robb G, et al. Deep-plane cervicofacial rotation-advancement flap for reconstruction of large cheek defects. Plast Reconstr Surg. 1994;94(1):88-93.
17. Jacono AA, Rousso JJ, Lavin TJ. Comparing rates of distal edge necrosis in deep-plane vs subcutaneous cervicofacial rotation-advancement flaps for facial cutaneous Mohs defects. JAMA Facial Plast Surg. 2014;16(1):31-5.
18. Chong KK, Goldberg RA. Lateral canthal surgery. Facial Plast Surg. 2010;26(3):193-200.
19. van Niekerk WJ, Taggart I. The size of the Y: the multiple Y-V plasty revisited. Burns. 2008;34(2):257-61.
20. Sugg KB, Cederna PS, Brown DL. The V-Y advancement flap is equivalent to the Mustarde flap for ectropion prevention in the reconstruction of moderate-size lid-cheek junction defects. Plast Reconstr Surg. 2013;131(1):28e-36e.
21. Nelson AA, Cohen JL. Modified Tripier flap for lateral eyelid reconstructions. J Drugs Dermatol. 2011;10(2):199-201.
22. Cohen AJ. Lateral bilobed flap for anterior lamellar eyelid reconstruction. Ophthal Plast Reconstr Surg. 2010;26(2):77-9.
23. Perry JD, Taban M. Superiorly based bilobed flap for inferior medial canthal and nasojugal fold defect reconstruction. Ophthal Plast Reconstr Surg. 2009;25(4):276-9.
24. Kirkland EB, Zitelli JA. The bilobed flap versus the AIRNS flap for repair of distal nose defects. J Am Acad Dermatol. 2013;68(4):684-5.
25. O'Donnell BA, Mannor GE. Oculoplastic surgery for upper eyelid reconstruction after cutaneous carcinoma. Int Ophthalmol Clin. 2009;49(4):157-72.
26. Ng SG, Inkster CF, Leatherbarrow B. The rhomboid flap in medial canthal reconstruction. Br J Ophthalmol. 2001;85(5):556-9.
27. Skaria AM. Island pedicle flaps for medial canthus repair. Br J Dermatol. 2012;166(6):1270-4.
28. Zitelli JA. Secondary intention healing: an alternative to surgical repair. Clin Dermatol. 1984;2(3):92-106.
29. Zitelli JA. Wound healing by secondary intention. A cosmetic appraisal. J Am Acad Dermatol. 1983;9(3):407-15.
30. Lee BJ, Elner SG, Douglas RS, et al. Island pedicle and horizontal advancement cheek flaps for medial canthal reconstruction. Ophthal Plast Reconstr Surg. 2011;27(5):376-9.
31. Cervelli V, Gravante G, Colicchia GM, et al. Asymptomatic lacrimal flow abnormalities in patients with septal deviations and turbinate hypertrophy. Aesthet Plast Surg. 2008;32(1):72-6.
32. Guzek JP, Ching AS, Hoang TA, et al. Clinical and radiologic lacrimal testing in patients with epiphora. Ophthalmology. 1997;104(11):1875-81.
33. Willey A, Caesar RH. Diagonal tarsal suture technique sine marginal sutures for closure of full-thickness eyelid defects. Ophthal Plast Reconstr Surg. 2013;29(2):137-8.
34. Ooms LS, Beets MR, Grosfeld EC, et al. Reconstruction of the lower eyelid using Hughes' tarsoconjunctival flap: follow up of 28 cases. J Plast Reconstr Aesthet Surg. 2014;67(7):e177-9.

CHAPTER

16

# Reconstruction of the Lip/Perioral

G Richard Nichols, T Minsue Chen, J Ramsey Mellette

## INTRODUCTION

### Anatomy and Function

The lips and perioral region occupy the lower third of the face. This region is one of the major focal points of the face and reconstruction demands attention to aesthetic detail. Basic functions include portal to the digestive tract, speech, and emotion.

The midline upper lip contains the philtrum and cupid's bow. The nasolabial (melolabial) fold is the lateral boundary between the cheek and perioral cosmetic units. The vermillion border is the junction between the skin and vermillion of the lip (dry mucosa). The white roll of the upper lip is just superior to the vermillion border. Much of the perioral skin up to the vermillion border is hair bearing. The vermillion or red lip can contain sebaceous glands without hair follicles. The red hue of the vermillion lip is due to the lack of keratinization and vascular plexus below.

**Table 16.1:** Perioral musculature.

| *Function* | *Muscles* |
|---|---|
| Labial elevators | Zygomaticus major<br>Zygomaticus minor<br>Levator labii superioris<br>Levator labii superioris alaeque nasi<br>Levator anguli oris<br>Risorius |
| Labial depressors | Depressor labii inferioris<br>Depressor anguli oris<br>Mentalis |
| Force cheek against teeth and food into the oral cavity | Buccinator |

The orbicularis oris muscle comprises the bulk of the lip. It is arranged as a sphincter around the mouth and works together with adjacent facial musculature to elevate, depress, and provide lateral movement of the lips and perioral region (Table 16.1). The region is supplied by the superior and inferior labial arteries, which are branches of the facial artery (Fig. 16.1). The infraorbital and mental branches of the trigeminal (V) cranial nerve provide sensation. Buccal and marginal mandibular branches of the facial (VII) cranial nerve supply sensation and motor function, respectively. Lymphatic drainage is generally inferior toward the submental and submandibular nodal areas.[1-4]

### Aging and Anatomic Variation

Aging and normal anatomic variations include nasolabial fold deepening and lengthening, philtrum and cupid's

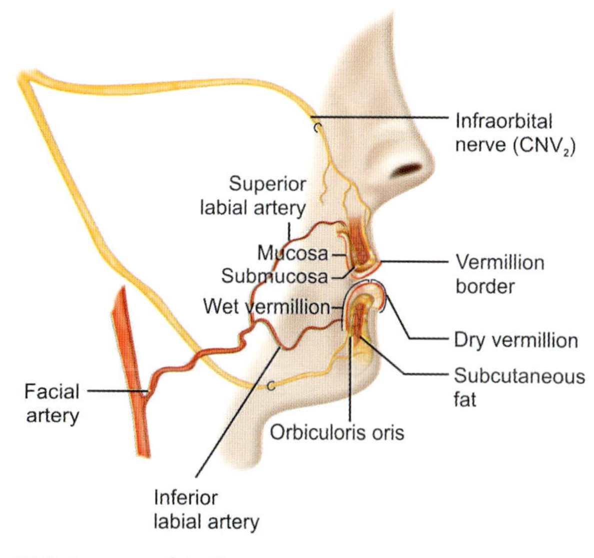


**Fig. 16.1:** Anatomy of the lip.

bow flattening, downward drooping of the lateral commissures, vermillion lip volume loss, prominence of perioral rhytides, facial hair predisposition, as well as dental issues that impact the cutaneous lip and perioral function and aesthetic. In younger individuals, the vermillion lip is the most protuberant, giving the appearance of a fuller, youthful lip. As people age, the nonglabrous portion of the upper lip becomes more prominent leading to the appearance of a thinner vermillion lip.[2,5]

## RECONSTRUCTION PLANNING

### Defect Etiology and Loss of Function

Cutaneous defects of the lips and perioral region occur with numerous conditions and traumatic events including birth defects (cleft lip), birthmarks (hemangiomas), trauma (dog and human bites), and excision of cutaneous neoplasms (skin cancer).[6-9] These defects as well as inadequate reconstruction result in abnormal facial form and asymmetry. Resultant abnormalities include drawing unwanted attention, microstomia, lip biting, eclabium, lip notch or depression, oral incompetence (drooling), speech difficulties (faulty articulation), and cryptic emotions (inability to smile or frown).[2]

### Reconstructive Principles

Careful reconstructive planning and meticulous technique are required for optimal outcomes. Basic reconstructive principles are similar to other cosmetic regions. The clinician should tailor care to each patient and strive for an aesthetic that approaches the original appearance of the patient. When applicable, enlarge the defect to replace the entire cosmetic subunit for more optimal scar camouflage. Recruit reservoirs of lax skin from the adjacent nasolabial fold, cheek, neck, and oral mucosa. When possible, plan for incisions to be located in normal anatomic boundaries and relaxed skin tension lines. An exception is a horizontal incision from the commissure toward the cheek to access the regional laxity of the medial cheek. This allows for adequate flap movement and decreased wound tension. Consider marking the vermillion border preoperatively with suture, surgical marker or a shallow skin nick to facilitate alignment during reconstruction. Consider aligning the wet lip border for full-thickness reconstructions prior to vermillion border alignment as vermillion lip step-off and "fat-lip" deformities can occur. Z-plasty variations may be used to align the vermillion border after aligning the wet lip border.[5] Excise and undermine widely with caution. For instance, as patients age, the labial arteries can become tortuous and more superficially located, especially in the setting of a thin and atrophic mouth. Risk of paralytic nerve damage is rare as nerves are located deep under the muscles. Consider nerve blocks to minimize facial form distortion that might result with excessive local anesthesia infiltration. Ensure visualization and access with a well-trained assistant, hemostasis, and clamps.

### Repair Options

Surgical defects of the lip and perioral region provide opportunities to utilize a multitude of reconstructive options.[10] Granulation is an appropriate option for small defects that have minimal contour irregularity (superficial shave biopsy), as well as lesions of the vermillion lip. Granulation and skin substitutes can be considered for larger wounds of the lip and perioral region, although healing is prolonged and can lead to unpredictable scarring and postoperative bleeding.[11,12] Abundant laxity and wide undermining will often indicate that a linear closure is the best option, especially with defects involving up to one-third of the lip. Defects involving more than one-third of the lip often require tissue rearrangement for optimal cosmesis and function. Advancement flaps, island (V-to-Y) advancement flaps, rotation flaps, and primary linear closures are the workhorses to repair wounds located in this cosmetic unit. Although rarely used due to potential color and texture discrepancies, full-thickness skin grafts are an option for concave areas of the lip and perioral region (philtrum, apical triangle of the upper cutaneous lip). Large, complex wounds could require multispecialty care, such as consultation with a reconstructive, microvascular surgeon and/or orodental/maxillofacial expert.

### Technique Pearls

The lip is an area of constant movement with eating, drinking, talking, and facial expressions. The constant movement can lead to scar spread and scar depression.[13] Meticulous dermal and wound edge approximation and superficial vertical mattress sutures maximize wound edge eversion on the lip and often prevent depressed scar formation.[14]

### Aftercare

Postoperative care instructions should include eating soft, bland, and nonchewy foods. Minimize talking, consider a liquid diet, and advance as tolerated. Although bathing the wound in saliva is acceptable, it is important to continue an oral hygiene regimen. Rinse the oral cavity four times per day with salt water (one half teaspoon salt in warm water) or dilute hydrogen peroxide (dilute hydrogen peroxide half-strength with water). Alcohol-based oral rinses often cause pain until the wound is sutured closed or healed. Brush the teeth when tolerated. Avoid dentures if denture insertion and removal might cause wound separation. Moisturize with petrolatum, lip balms, mineral oil, or glycerin. Dressing size is dependent on size and location. Warn patients of expected postoperative swelling, bruising, and bleeding. The first week is usually the worst and will continue to improve over the next several months.[13]

## Complications, Revision, and Camouflage

If a wound dehisces, consider conservative management. Notching or depression can be revised once healed, if necessary. Lip contractures alter the vermillion border and require revision such as a Z-plasty tissue rearrangement. Men can consider additional scar camouflage with facial hair growth. Women can consider low shine (matte) lip makeup.

# LOCATION

## Upper Cutaneous and Vermillion Lip

### *Linear Closure*

Large (Figs. 16.2A to C), medium (Figs. 16.3A to C), and small-sized (Figs. 16.4A to C) medial defects of the upper cutaneous lip and vermillion lip can be closed primarily. Scar orientation follows vertical rhytides of the upper cutaneous lip. Extension through the vermillion allows for excision of a portion of orbicularis oris muscle to prevent a bulldozing effect and depression of the upper vermillion lip. This depression of the lip is most apparent when smiling.

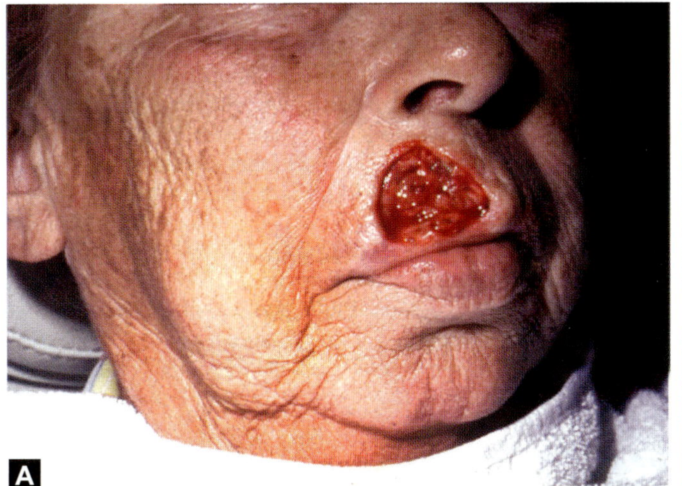

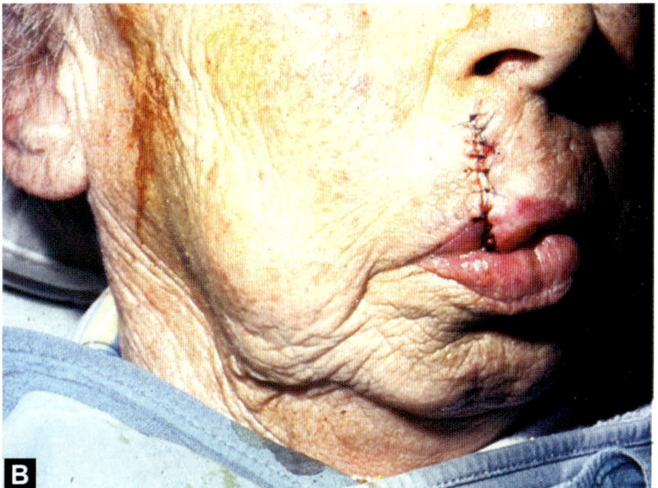

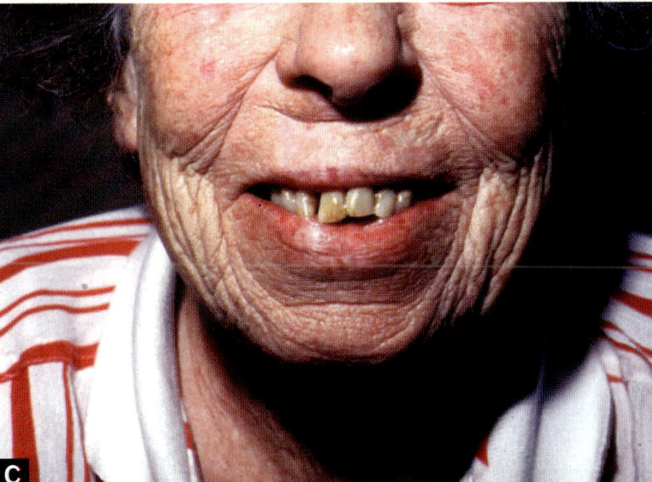

**Figs. 16.2A to C:** (A) Large off-midline defect involving the philtral border, philtral column, and lateral upper cutaneous lip. (B) Repaired with a linear closure with extension through the vermillion border and excision of a portion of orbicularis oris muscle to prevent downward displacement of the lip. (C) Note alignment of the wet lip border and vermillion border.

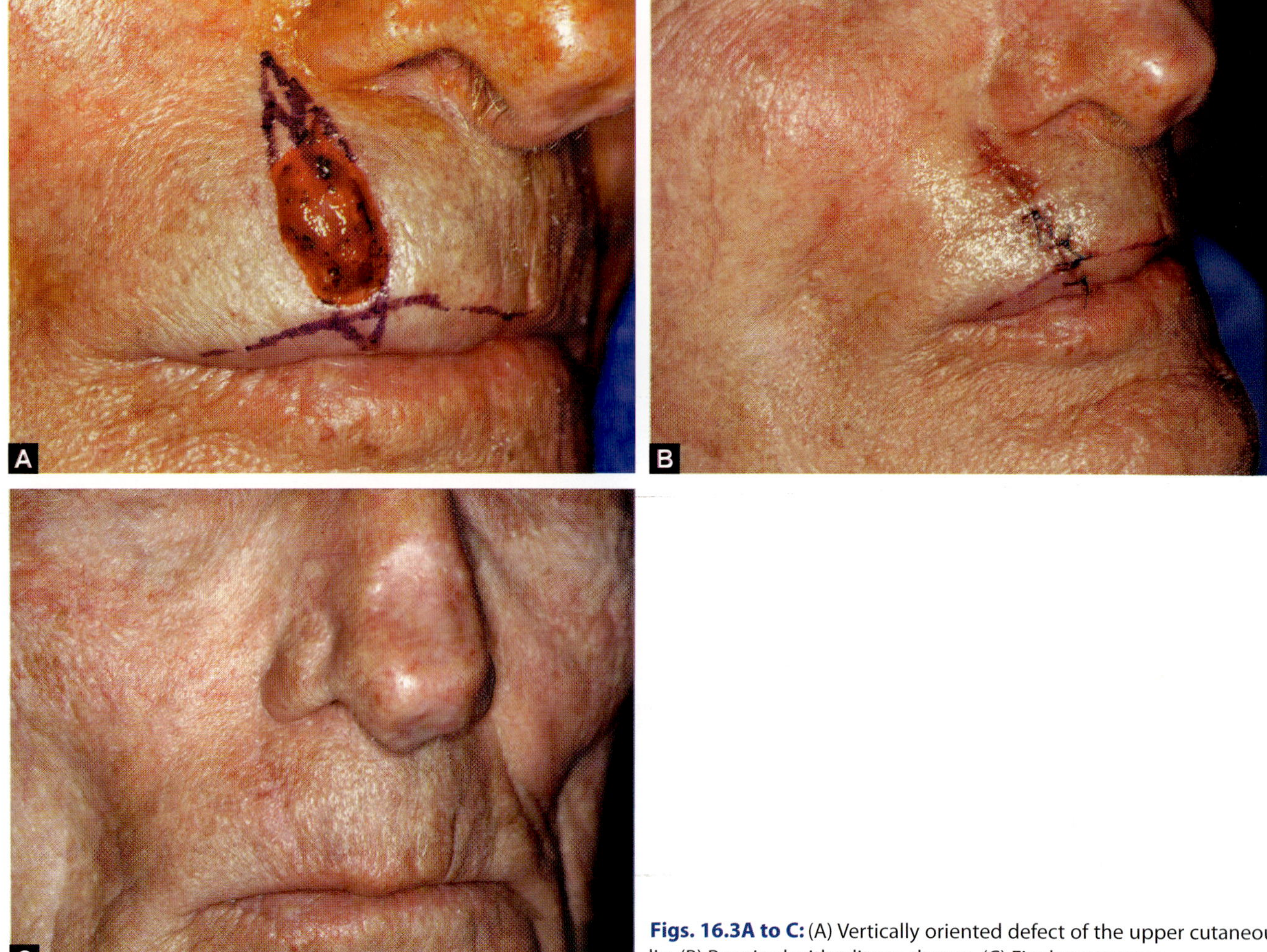


**Figs. 16.3A to C:** (A) Vertically oriented defect of the upper cutaneous lip. (B) Repaired with a linear closure. (C) Final appearance.

**Figs. 16.4A and B**

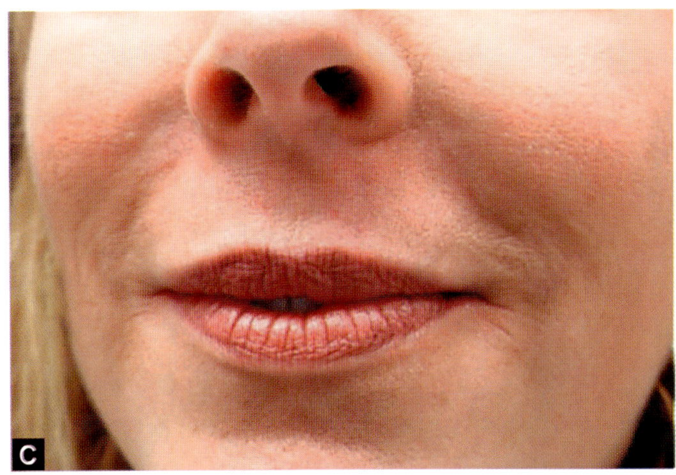


**Figs. 16.4A to C:** (A) Small off-midline defect of the upper cutaneous lip. (B) Repaired with a linear closure. (C) Final appearance.

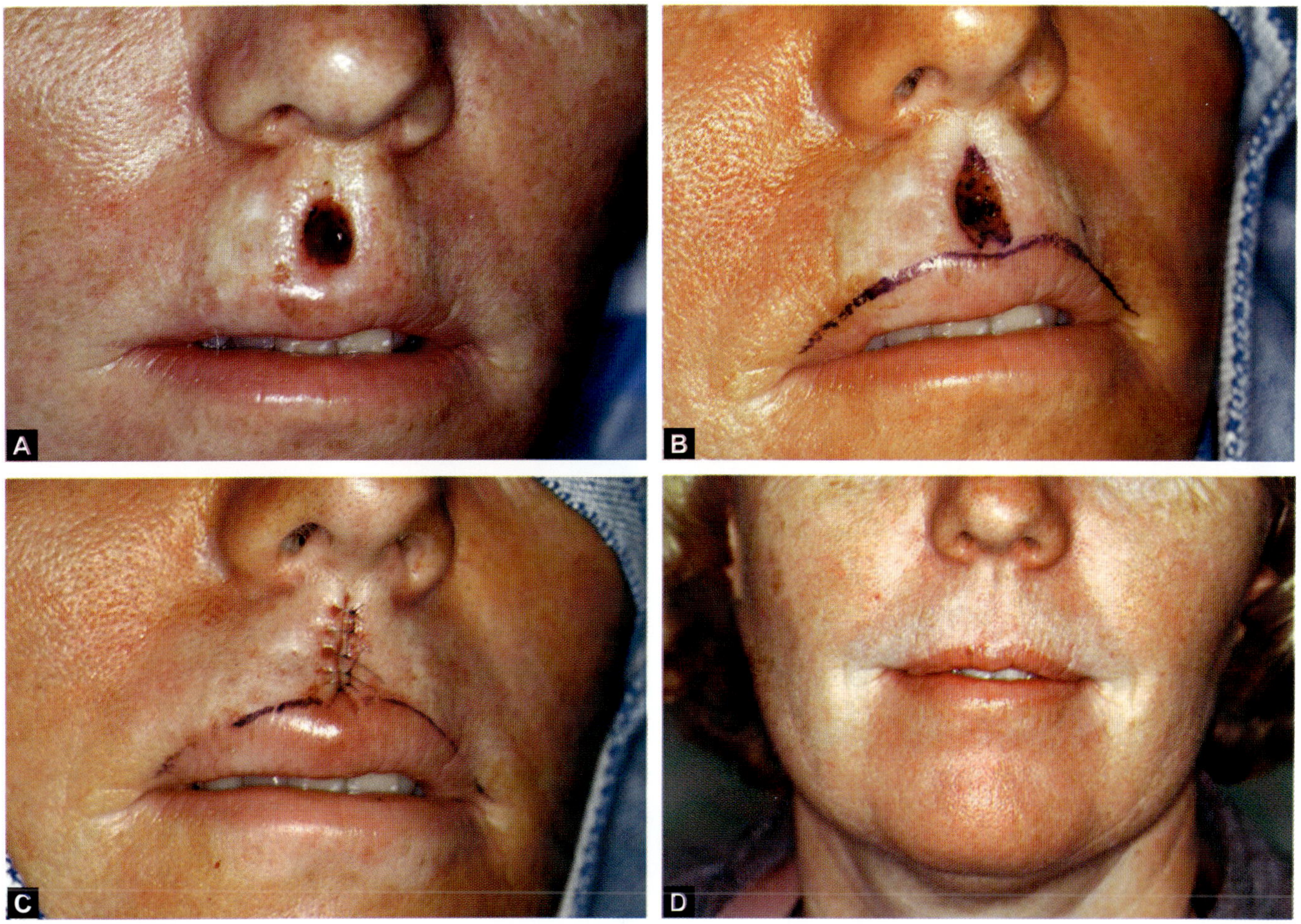

**Figs. 16.5A to D:** (A) Small midline defect involving the philtral column. (B and C) Repaired with a linear closure with M-plasty to shorten wound closure length. (D) Final appearance.

Though the bulldozing effect will diminish with time, the depression of the lip often does not fully resolve.[13,15] A linear closure with M-plasty can be used to shorten the length of a wound closure (Figs. 16.5A to D).

## Cupid's Bow Repair (Gull-Wing Flap, Seagull Flap)

Defects of the cupid's bow of the upper cutaneous lip and vermillion lip can be repaired with the cupid's bow repair, also reported as a gull-wing flap or seagull flap (Figs. 16.6A to D).[16] This reconstruction preserves the natural shape and contour of the cupid's bow cosmetic subunit by recreating the shape of the cupid's bow on the inferior border of the philtrum of the upper cutaneous lip and advancing the vermillion lip superiorly. The cupid's bow repair relies on mucosal advancement with excision of lateral standing tissue cones of the vermillion and upper cutaneous lip. This repair works well with defects of smaller vertical height. Defects of greater vertical height will require additional lateral excision and increased vertical mucosal advancement of the upper vermillion lip. This creates a larger, more prominent upper vermillion lip (Figs. 16.7A to D). This repair also works well with defects of the upper cutaneous and vermillion lip immediately lateral to the cupid's bow (Figs. 16.8 and 16.9).[16]

## Island (V-to-Y) Advancement Flap

Defects of relatively increased vertical height can also be reconstructed with the addition of an island (V-to-Y) advancement flap to a traditional cupid's bow repair (Figs. 16.10A to F). For medial lip defects, the island (V-to-Y) advancement flap design can extend up to the columella of the nose to provide optimal inferior tissue advancement and prevent excessive vertical advancement of the vermillion lip. The island (V-to-Y) advancement flap is

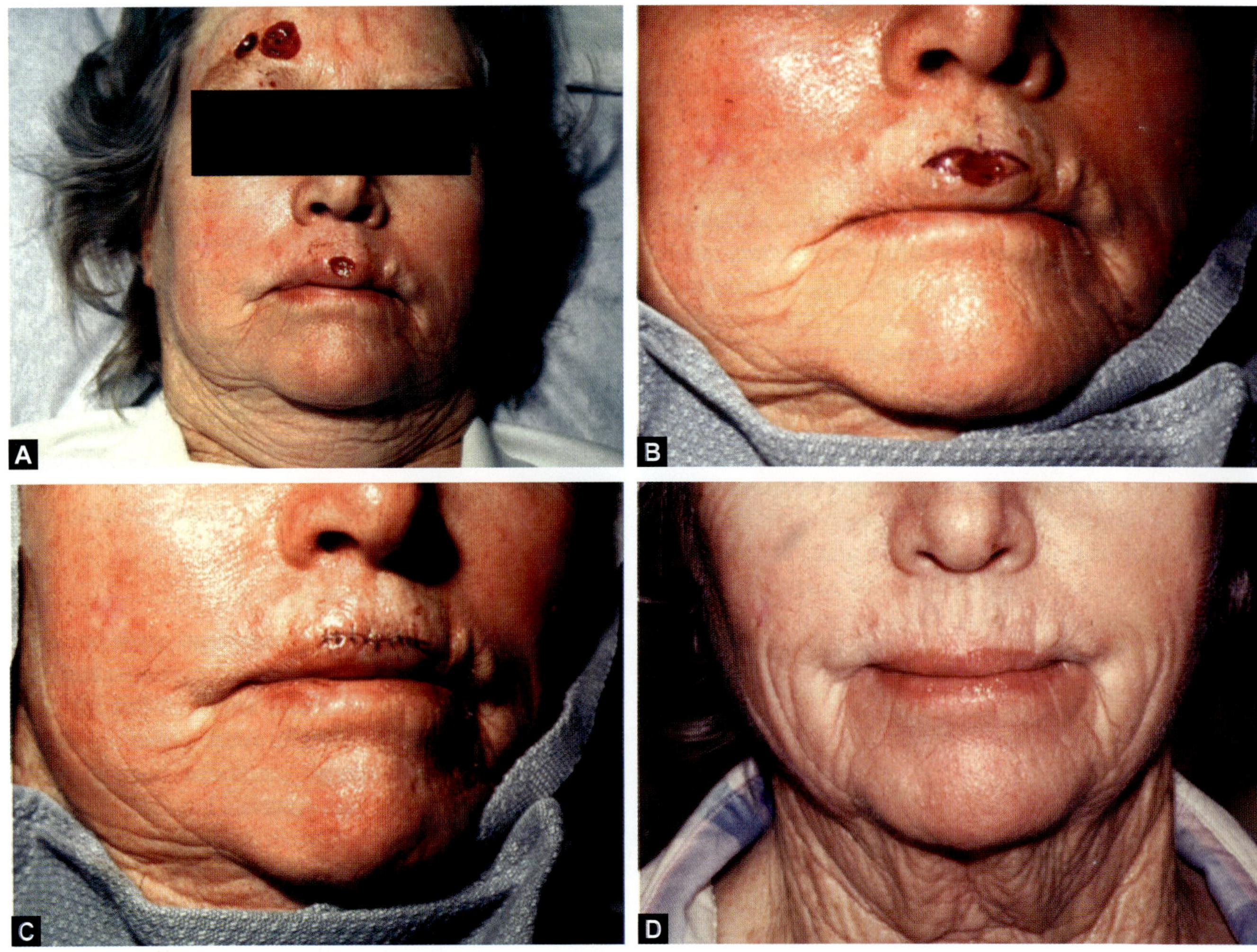

**Figs. 16.6A to D:** (A) Small midline defect spanning the cutaneous and vermillion lip. (B and C) Repaired with a cupid's bow repair (gull-wing repair, seagull flap). (D) Final appearance.

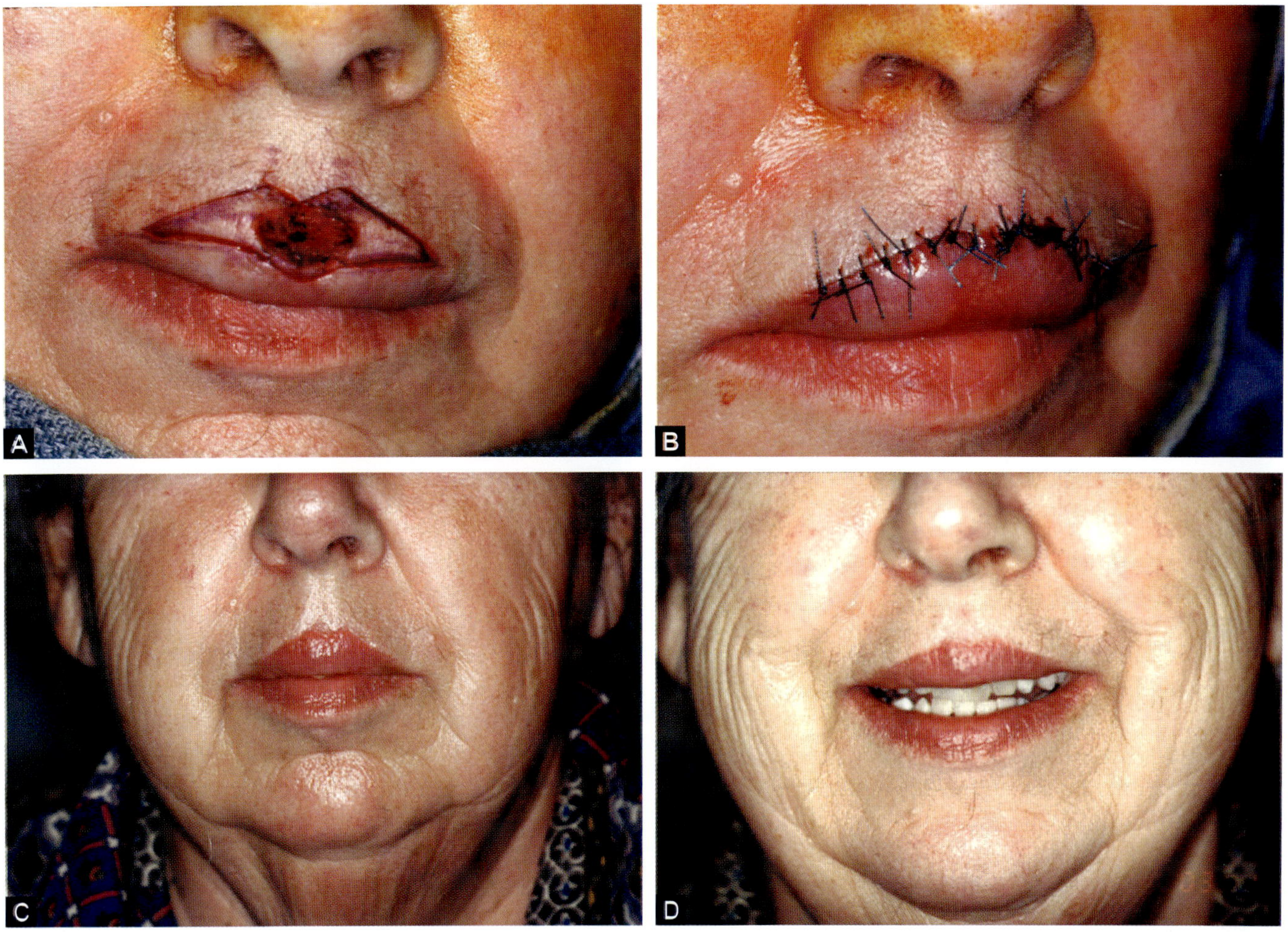

**Figs. 16.7A to D:** (A) Midline philtral defect isolated to the cutaneous upper lip. (B) Repaired with a cupid's bow repair (gull-wing repair, seagull flap). (C and D) The mucosa is advanced superiorly in this reconstruction; note downward movement of the vermillion border in long-term follow-up.

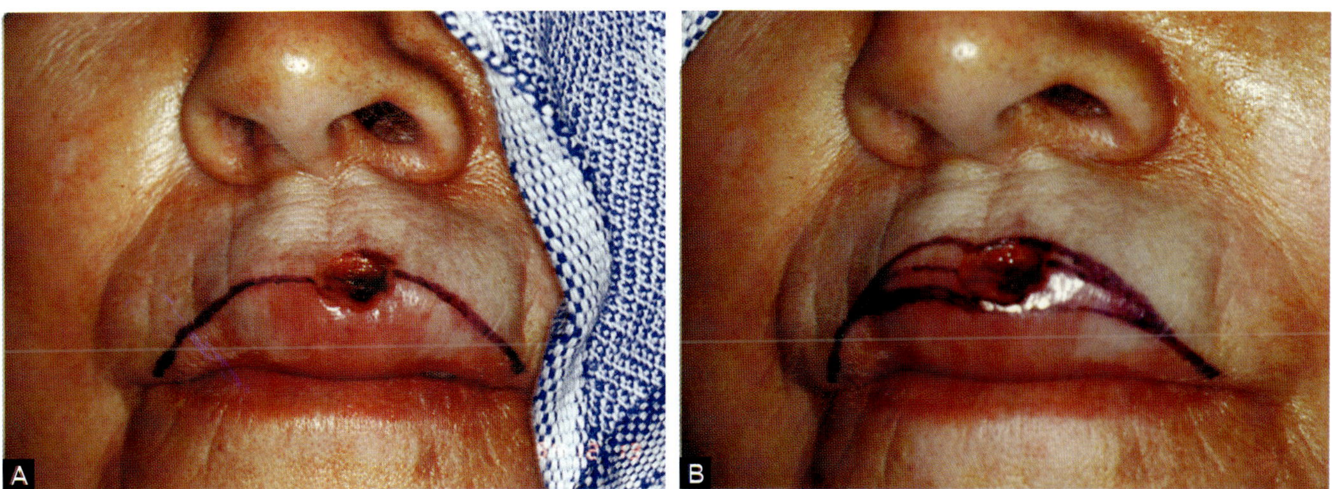


**Figs. 16.8A and B**

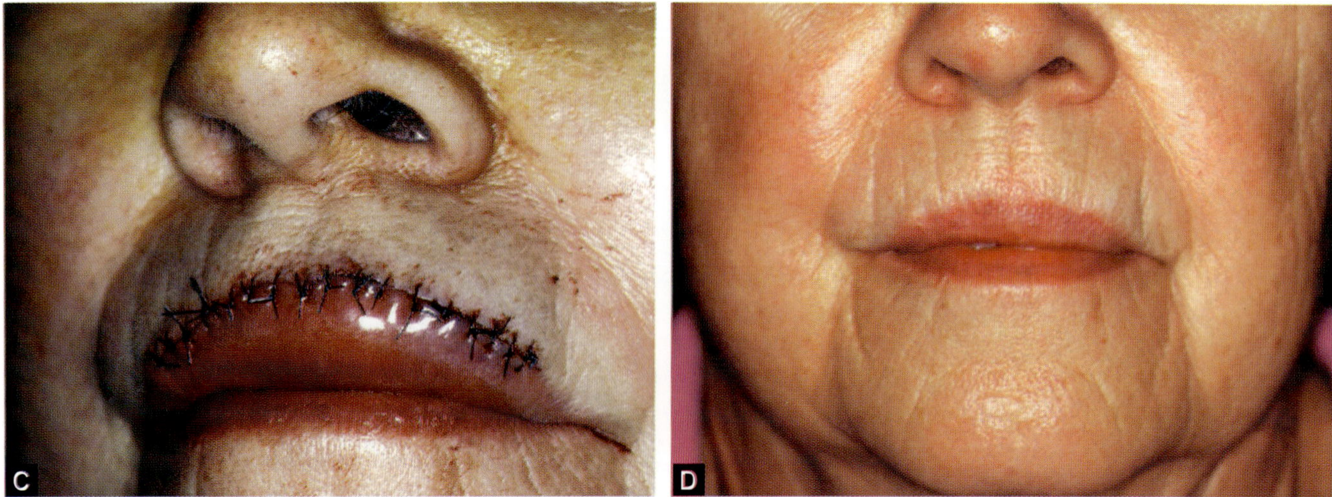


**Figs. 16.8A to D:** (A) Small off-midline defect spanning the cutaneous and vermillion lip. (B and C) Repaired with a cupid's bow repair (gull-wing repair, seagull flap). (D) Final appearance.

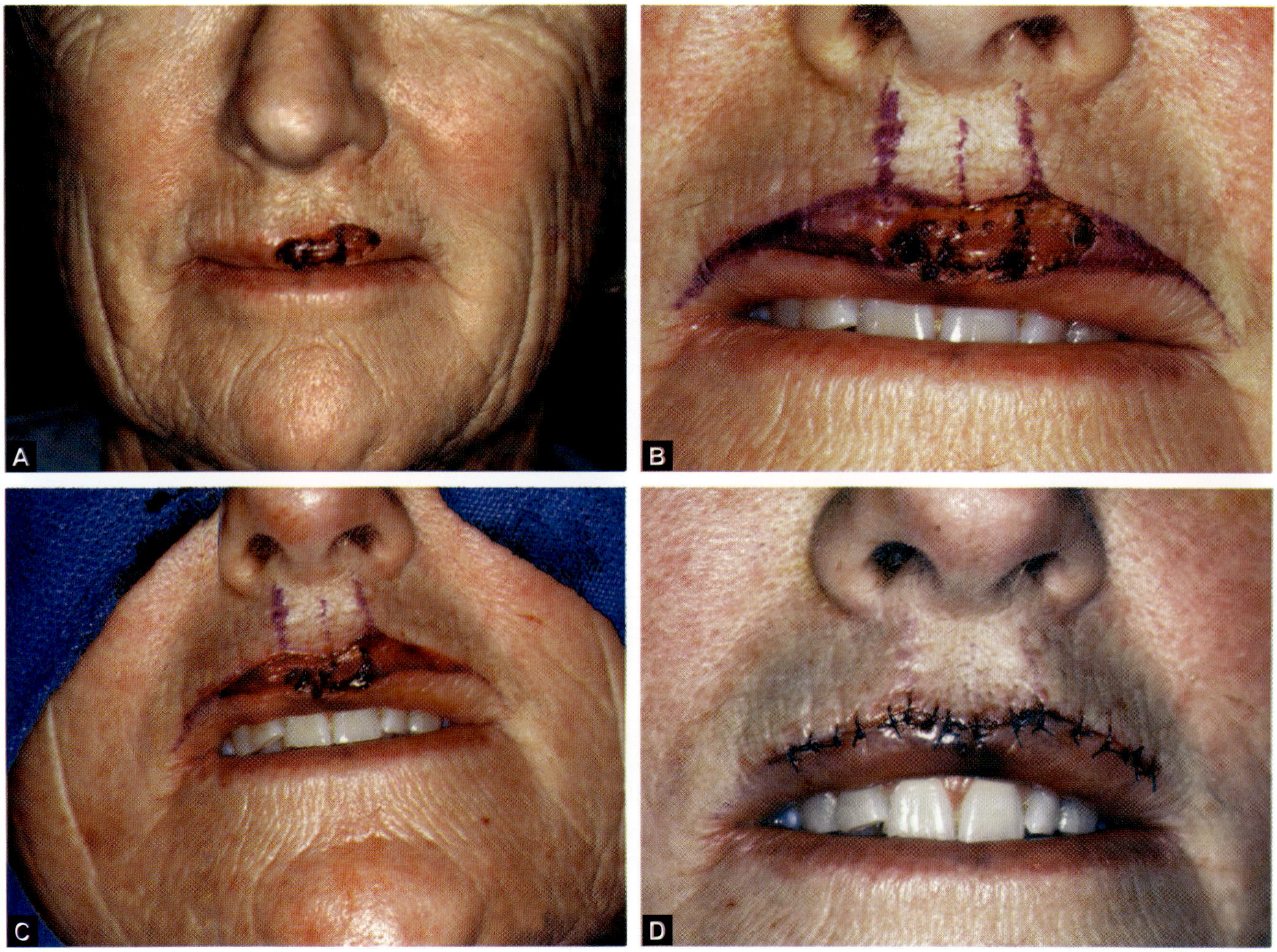

**Figs. 16.9A to D**

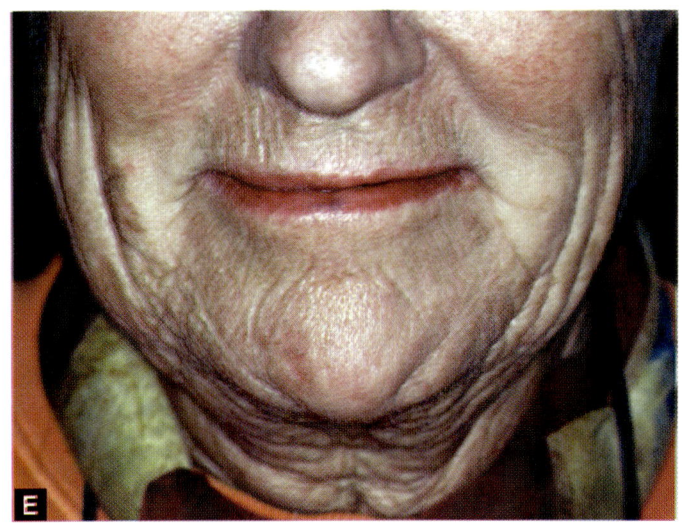


**Figs. 16.9A to E:** (A) Horizontally oriented off-midline defect spanning the cutaneous and vermillion lip. (B to D) Repaired with a cupid's bow repair (gull-wing repair, seagull flap). (E) Final appearance.

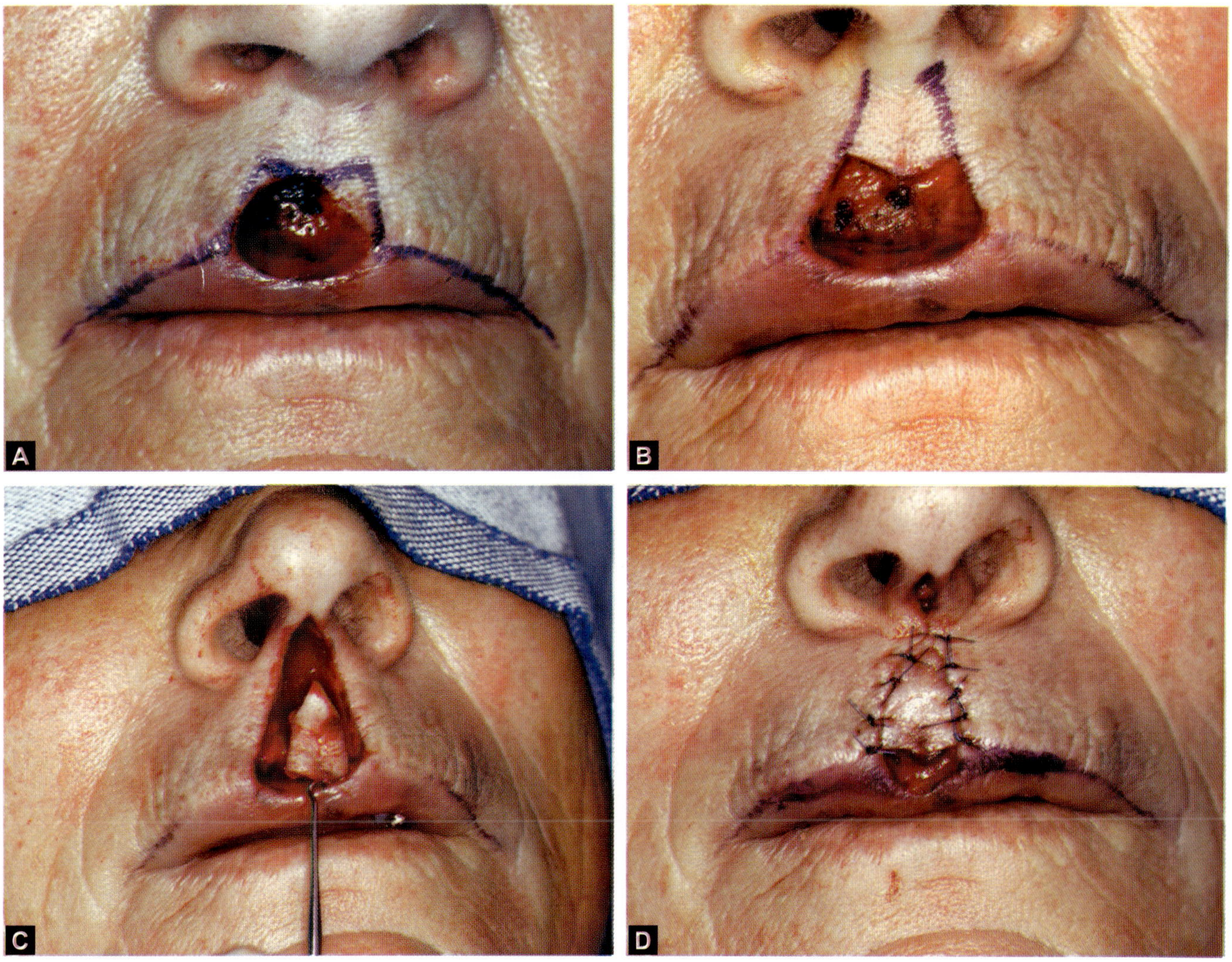

**Figs. 16.10A to D**

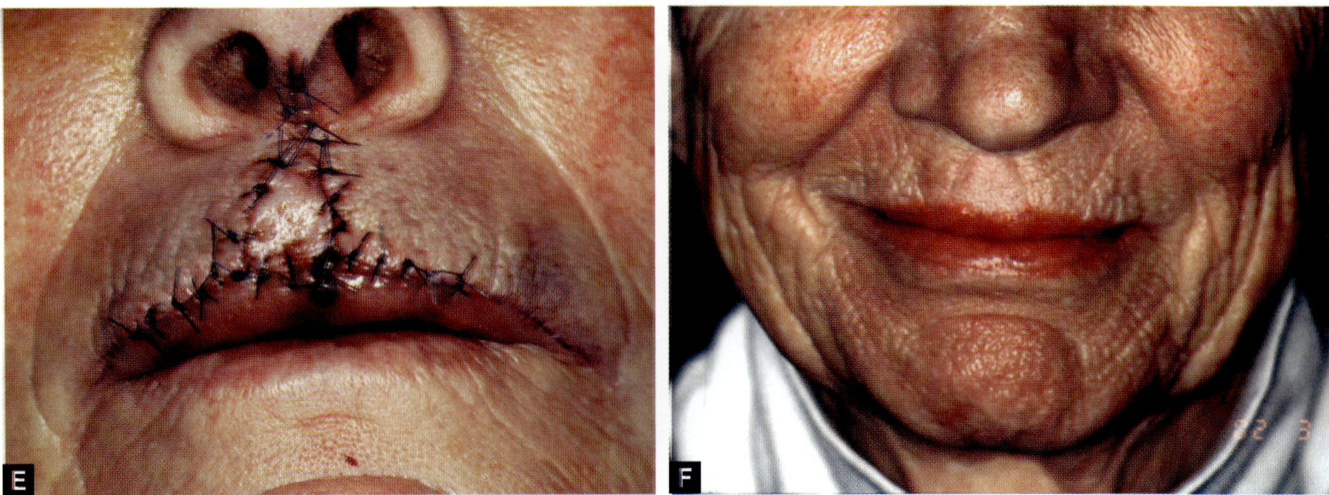

**Figs. 16.10A to F:** (A) Tear-drop shaped, midline defect spanning the cutaneous and vermillion lip. (B) Defect was enlarged to approximate the borders of the cosmetic subunit and (C) repaired with an island (V-to-Y) advancement flap maintaining the cupid's bow. (D) The island (V-to-Y) advancement flap is advanced to the vermillion border (E) and the remaining vermillion defect is repaired with a mucosal advancement flap. (F) Final appearance.

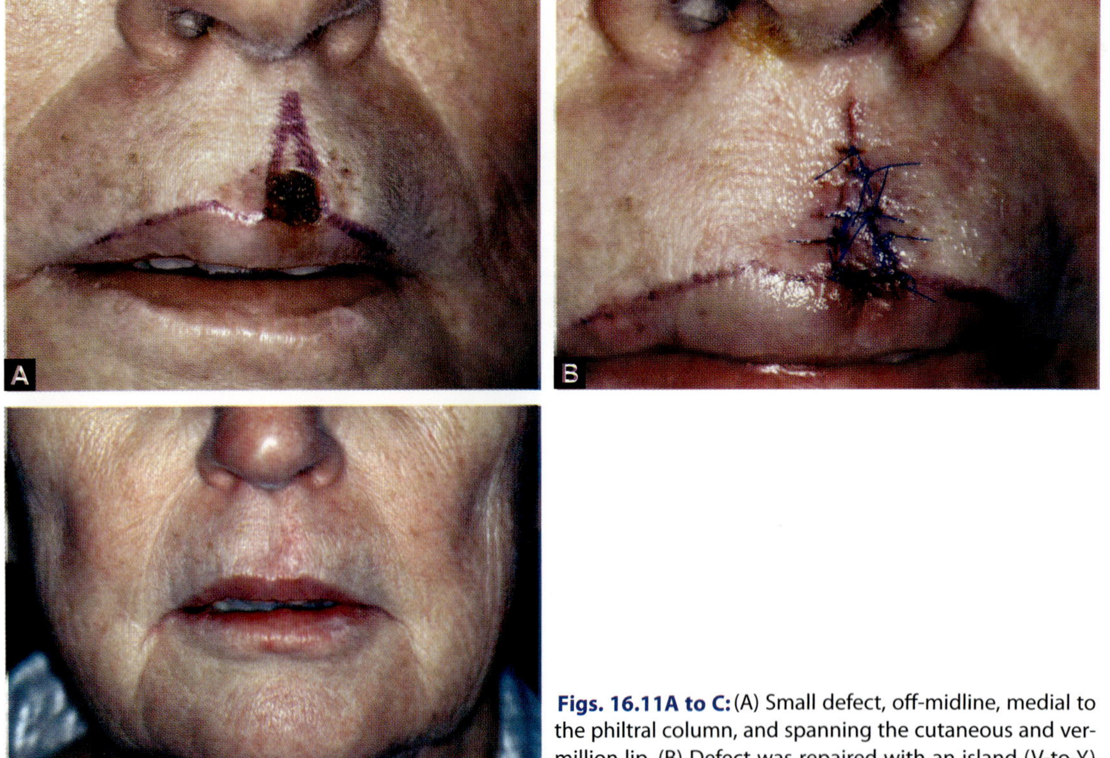

**Figs. 16.11A to C:** (A) Small defect, off-midline, medial to the philtral column, and spanning the cutaneous and vermillion lip. (B) Defect was repaired with an island (V-to-Y) advancement flap. (C) Final appearance.

also useful for defects that are adjacent to but do not involve the cupid's bow (Figs. 16.11A to C). Horizontally oriented defects can be repaired with a laterally based island (V-to-Y) advancement flap (Figs. 16.12A to E). Defects adjacent to the nasolabial fold can be repaired with the island (V-to-Y) advancement flap. This repair yields excellent scar camouflage when the incision can be concealed within the nasolabial fold[13] (Figs. 16.13A to D).

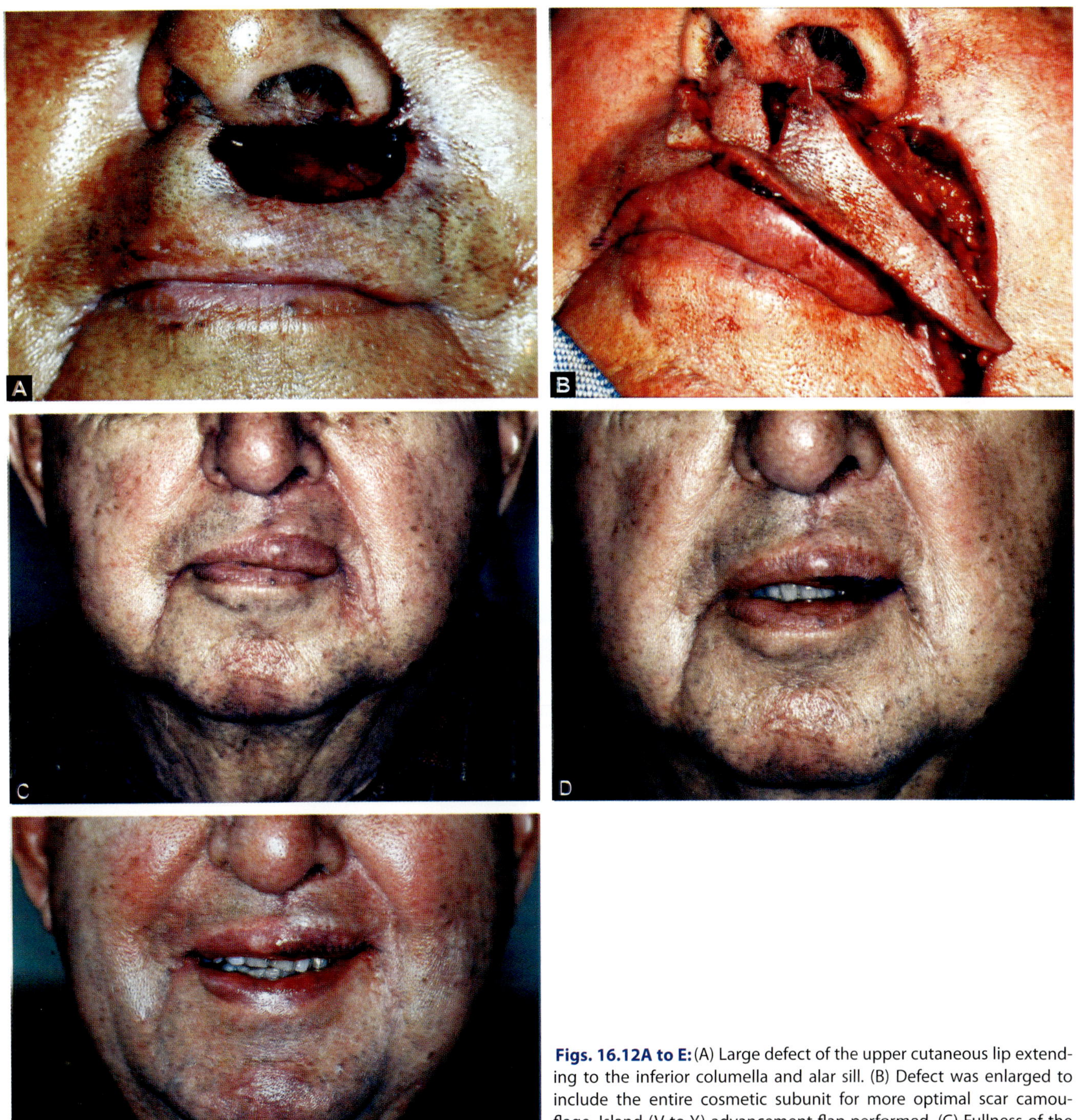

**Figs. 16.12A to E:** (A) Large defect of the upper cutaneous lip extending to the inferior columella and alar sill. (B) Defect was enlarged to include the entire cosmetic subunit for more optimal scar camouflage. Island (V-to-Y) advancement flap performed. (C) Fullness of the upper vermillion lip presented in the postoperative period (D and E) and this was revised with a linear excision of the redundant upper vermillion lip.

## *Advancement Flap Variations*

Adjacent tissue laxity can be recruited with various tissue rearrangement designs. Wide undermining is necessary to ensure adequate flap movement. Flap designs include A-to-T flap design and incisions along the vermillion border (Figs. 16.14A to F), L-shaped unilateral flap design

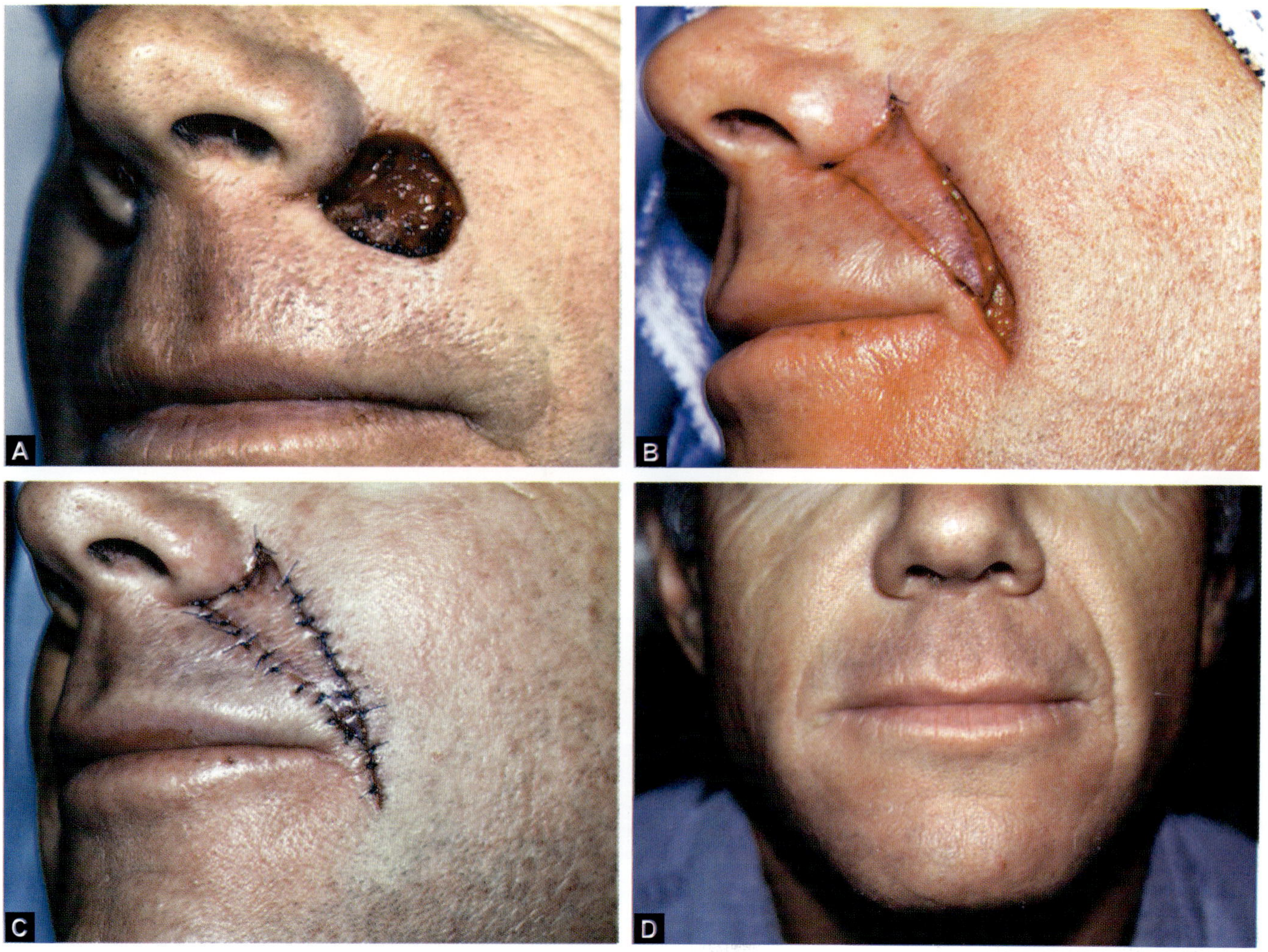

**Figs. 16.13A to D:** (A) Upper cutaneous lip defect involving the apical triangle of the upper cutaneous lip and medial cheek. (B and C) Repaired with an island (V-to-Y) advancement flap. (D) Note this reconstructive option produces a horizontal suture line on the upper cutaneous lip.

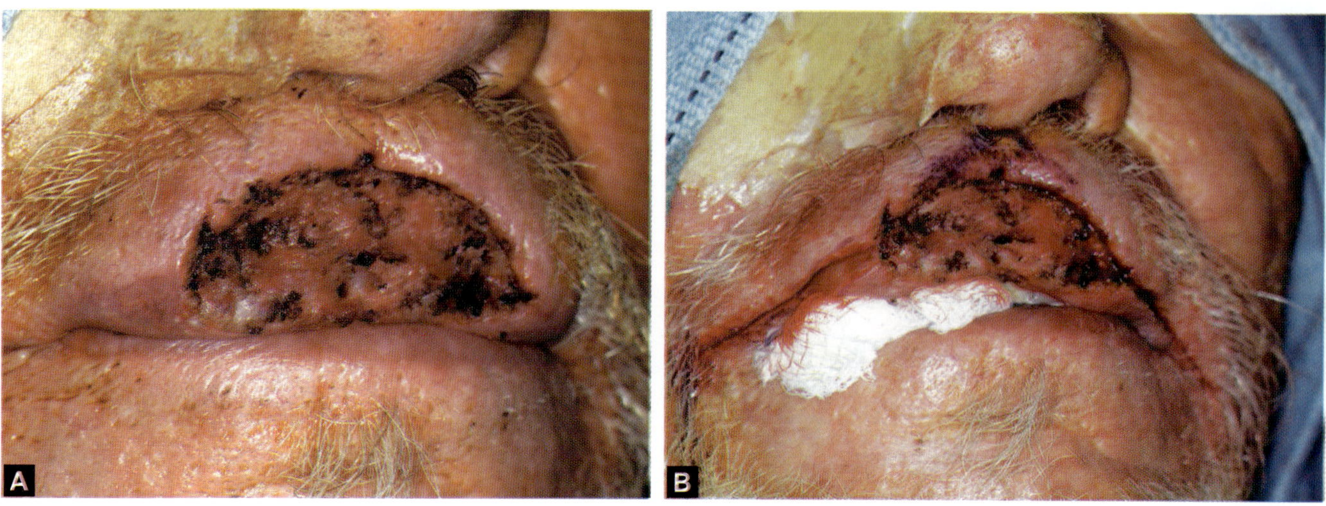

**Figs. 16.14A and B**

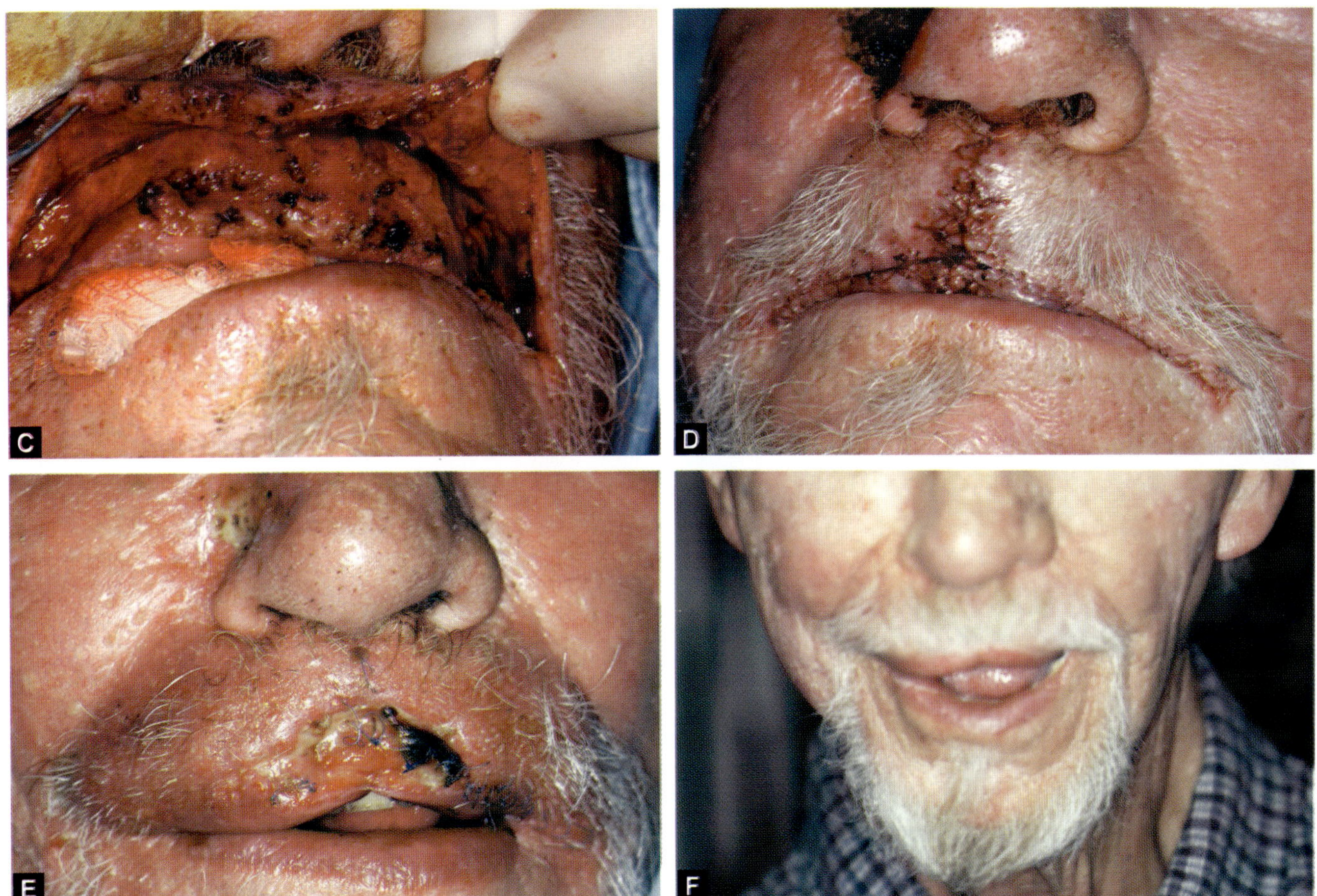


**Figs. 16.14A to F:** (A) Large, superficial, horizontally oriented defect spanning the upper cutaneous and vermillion lip. (B to E) Repaired with an A to T advancement flap. Wide and extensive undermining used to maximize tissue mobilization. (F) Final appearance.

(Figs. 16.15 to 16.17), L-shaped unilateral flap design extending to involve the oral commissure (Figs. 16.18 and 16.19), U-shaped unilateral flap design (Figs. 16.20A to F), and a perialar crescentic advancement flap design (Figs. 16.21 to 16.28].

*Editor's note:* These advancement flap variations efficiently recruit adjacent cheek tissue to repair the wound, but they will sometimes have limitations such as blunting of the melolabial folds or misplacement of the isthmus of the upper cutaneous lip. Depending on technical preferences of the surgeon, island (V-to-Y) advancement flaps may sometimes be preferred over unilateral or perialar crescentic flaps in order to prevent distortion of the melolabial fold or the isthmus of the upper cutaneous lip.

## Rotation Flap

If the wound can be triangulated, a rotation flap can be designed to repair the wound (Figs. 16.29 and 16.30).

## Banner Transposition Flap

Transposition flaps from the adjacent cheek predictably pincushion (Figs. 16.31 and 16.32). This might be useful in an area where convexity is desired. If not, thinning of the mature flap is often required to improve contour.

## Interpolation Flap

Complex and large wounds often necessitate a staged reconstructive approach. Options include an adjacent melolabial interpolation flap (Figs. 16.33A to H).

## Graft

Combined defects of the upper cutaneous lip and vermillion lip can be reconstructed with a full-thickness skin graft (Figs. 16.34A to D). Color and texture discrepancies are potential long-term cosmetic issues. The clavicular

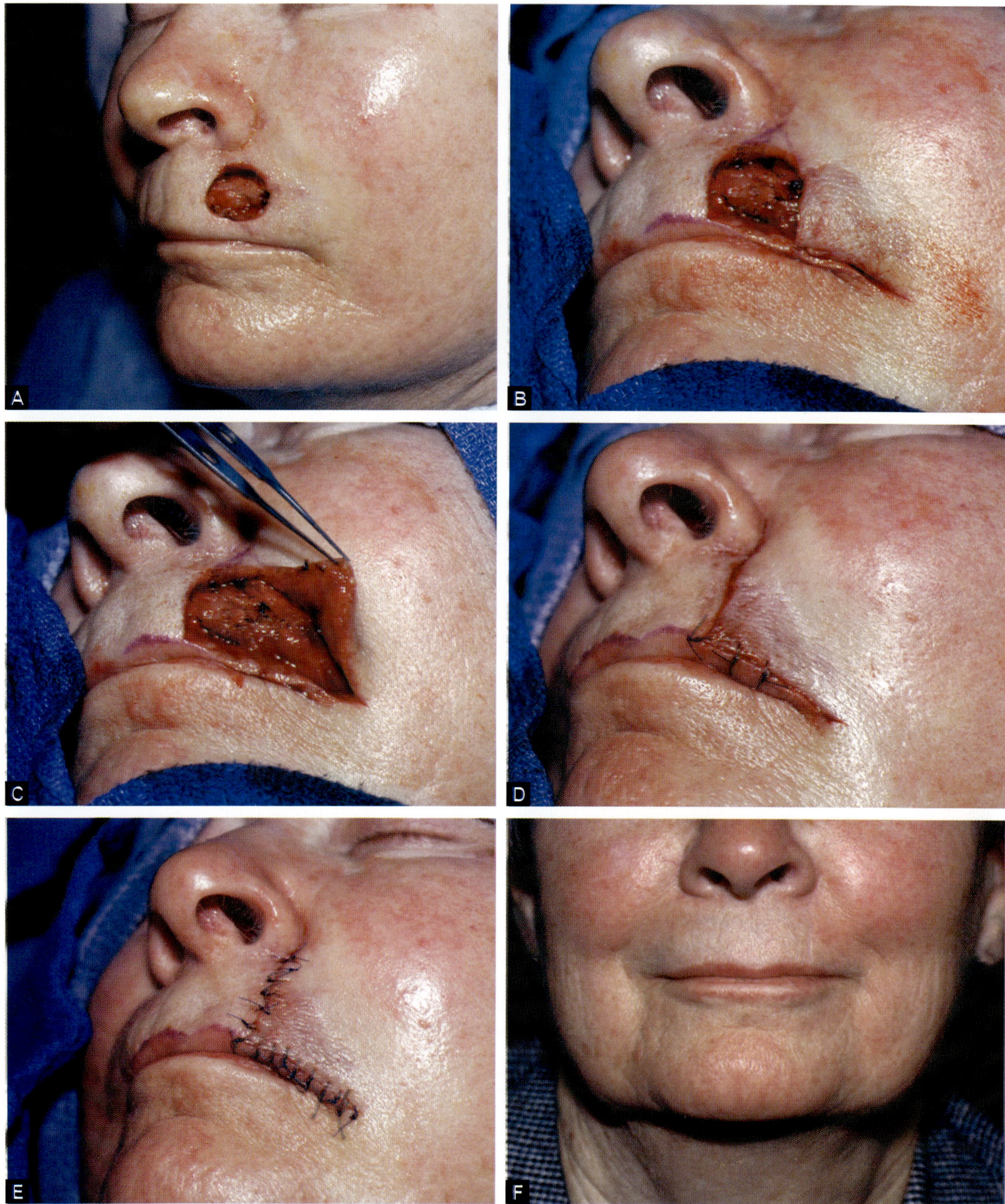


**Figs. 16.15A to F:** (A) Defect of the lateral upper cutaneous lip. (B to D) Repaired with a unilateral advancement flap after the defect was enlarged to the vermillion border. The flap is extended inferolateral to the oral commissure to utilize the laxity of the cheek. (F) Final appearance.

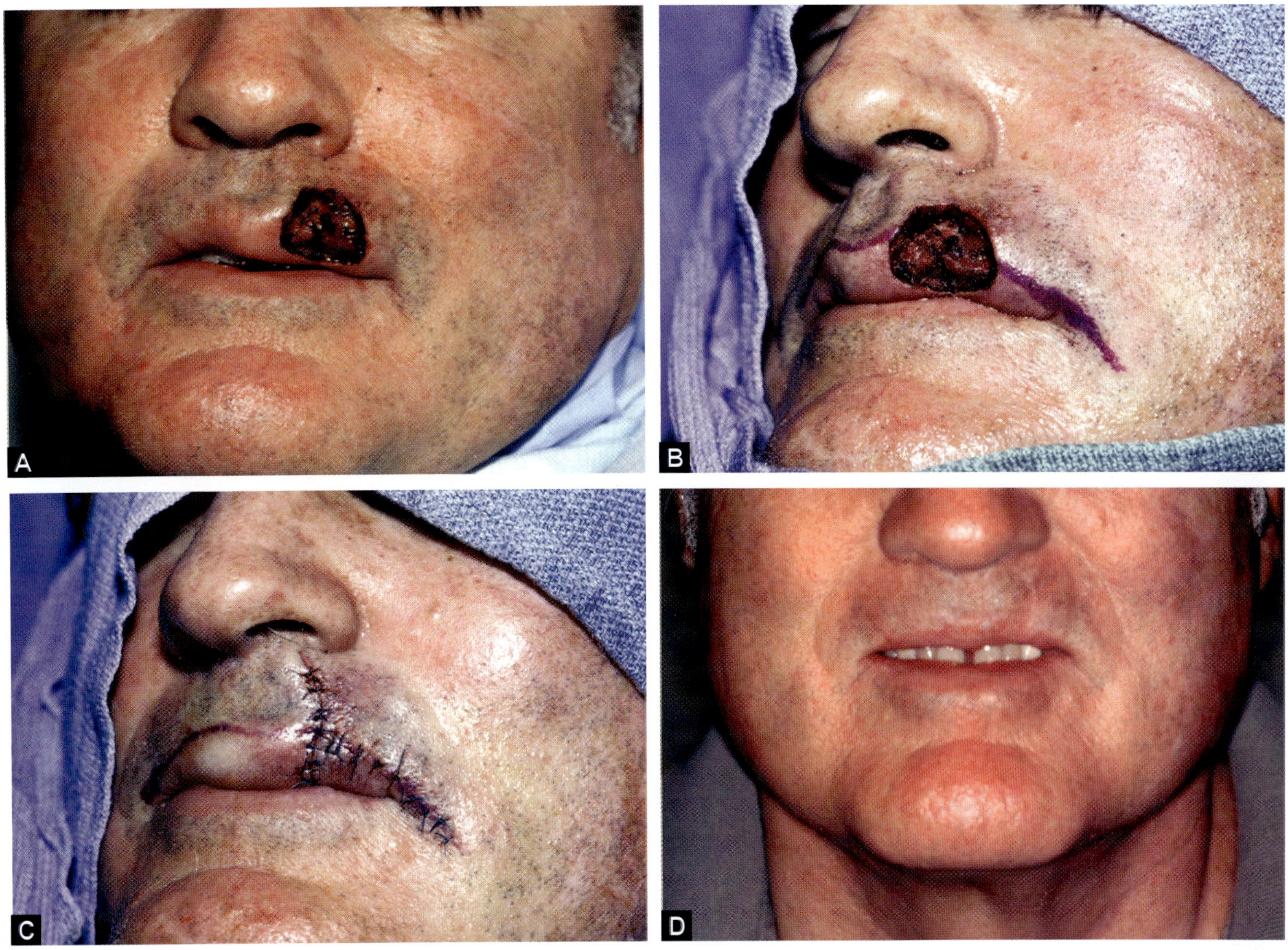

**Figs. 16.16A to D:** (A) Defect involving the upper cutaneous lip and vermillion lip. (B and C) Repaired with a unilateral advancement flap and partial mucosal advancement flap. The unilateral advancement flap extended beyond the oral commissure to utilize the lax tissue of the cheek. (D) Final appearance.

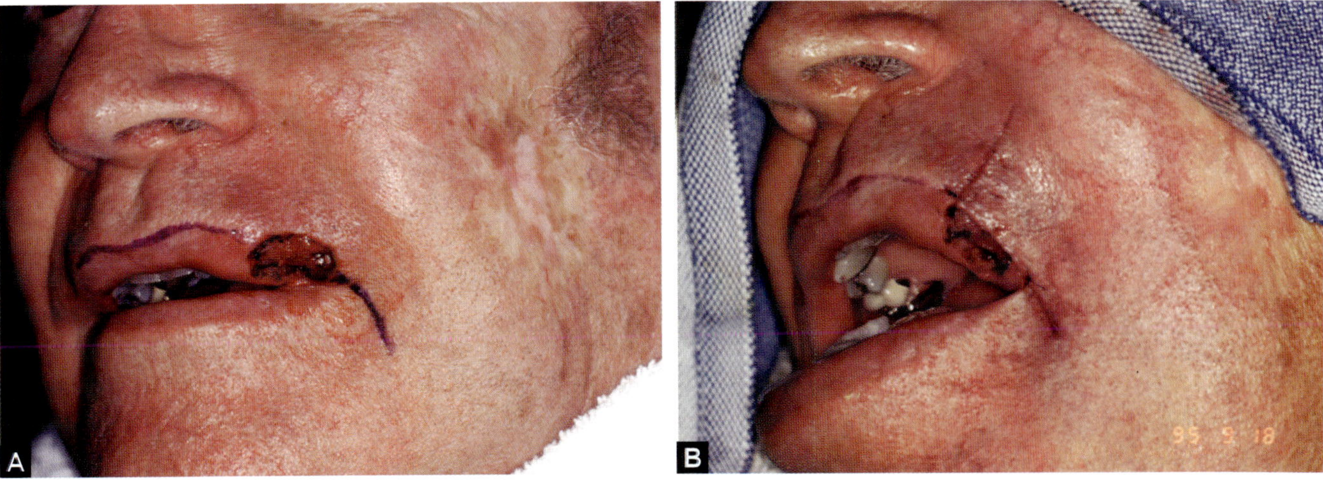

**Figs. 16.17A and B**

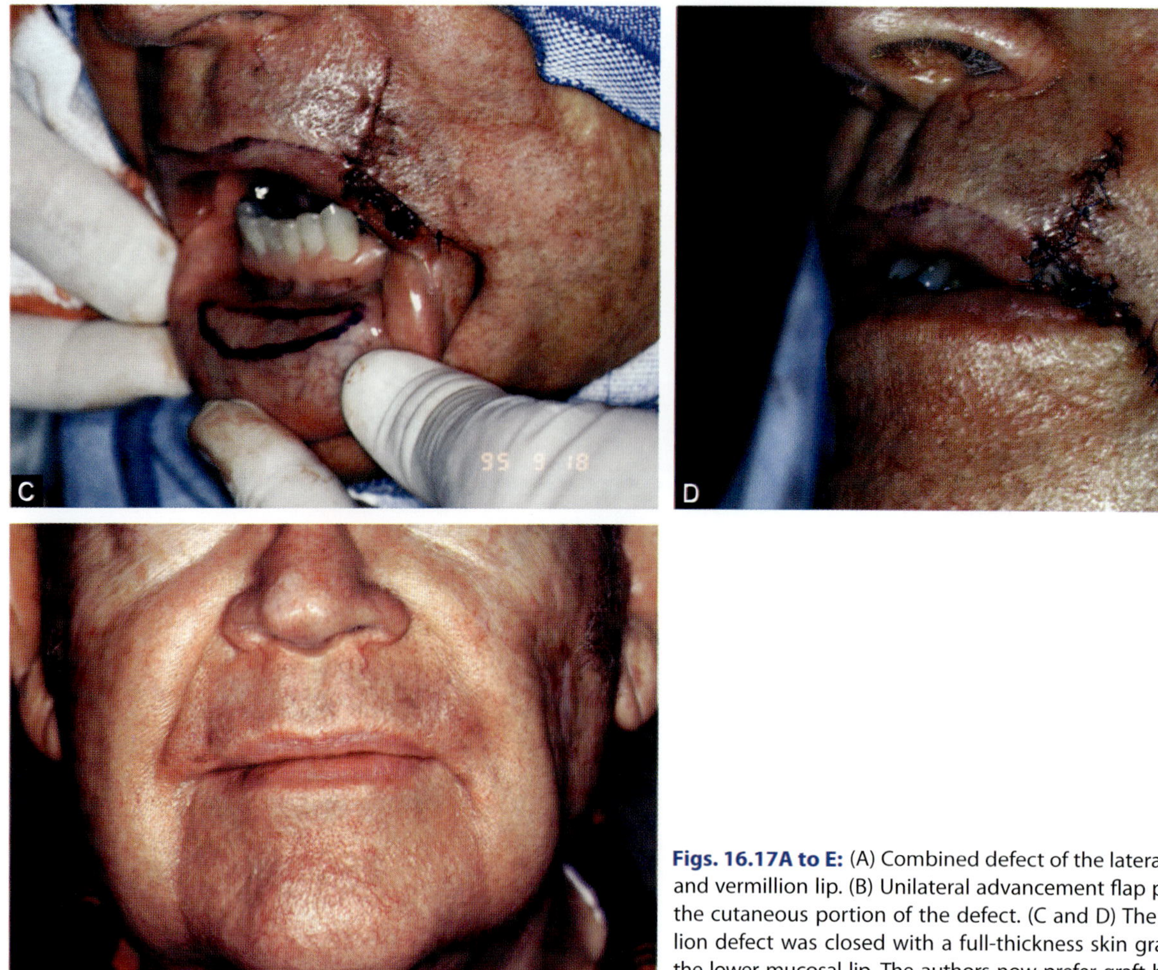

**Figs. 16.17A to E:** (A) Combined defect of the lateral upper cutaneous and vermillion lip. (B) Unilateral advancement flap performed to close the cutaneous portion of the defect. (C and D) The remaining vermillion defect was closed with a full-thickness skin graft harvested from the lower mucosal lip. The authors now prefer graft harvest in a vertical orientation as it facilitates donor site wound closure. (E) Final appearance.

**Figs. 16.18A and B**

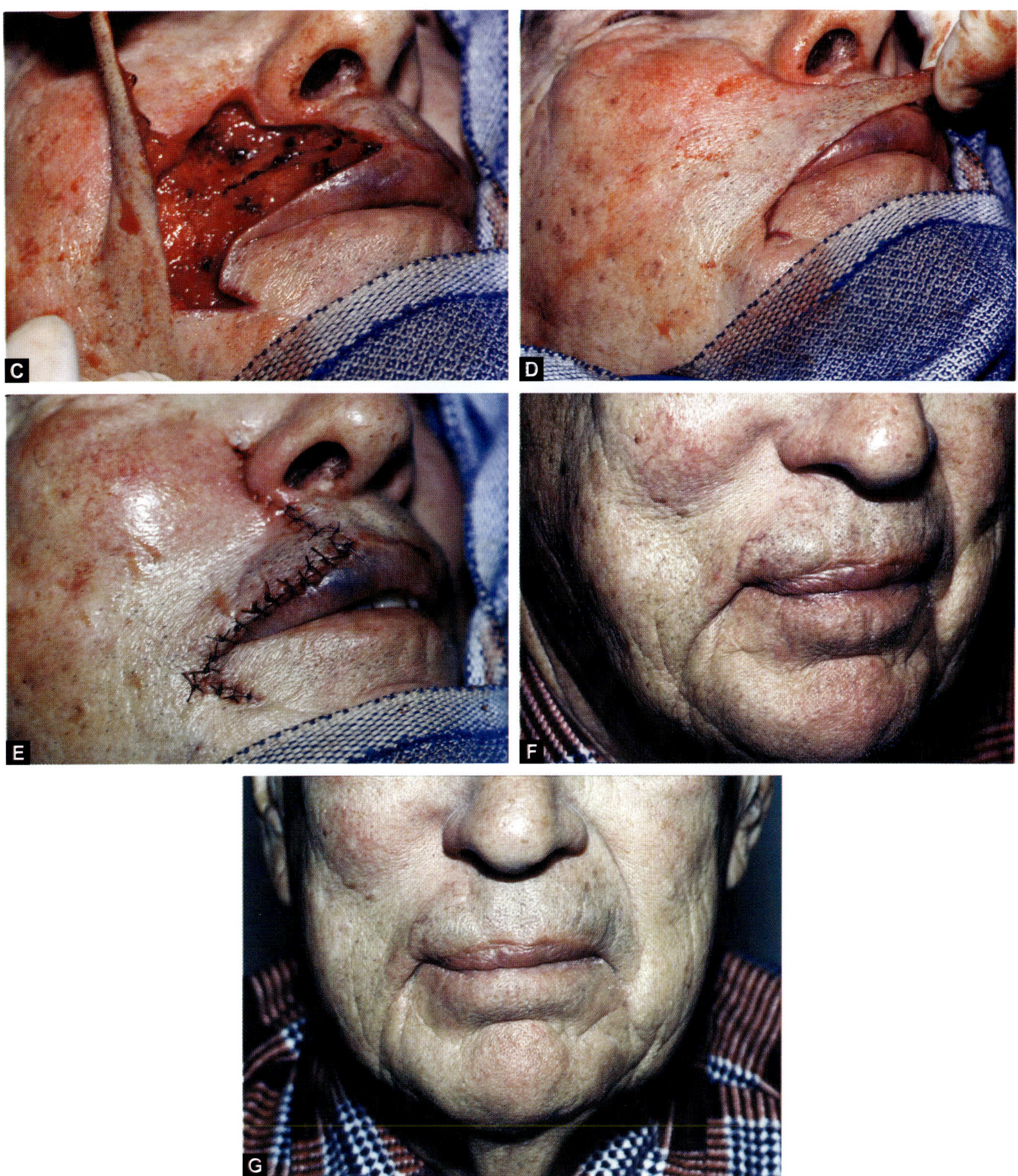


**Figs. 16.18A to G:** (A) Large deep defect of the upper cutaneous lip with a small area of full-thickness loss. (B) Upper vermillion marked and defect enlarged to the vermillion and philtral borders. (C to E) Unilateral advancement flap developed extending inferior and lateral to the oral commissure to utilize the lax skin of the cheek. (F) Mild postoperative pincushioning is often responsive to intralesional steroid injection. (G) Tumor extirpation compromised a branch of the buccal nerve resulting in partial paralysis.

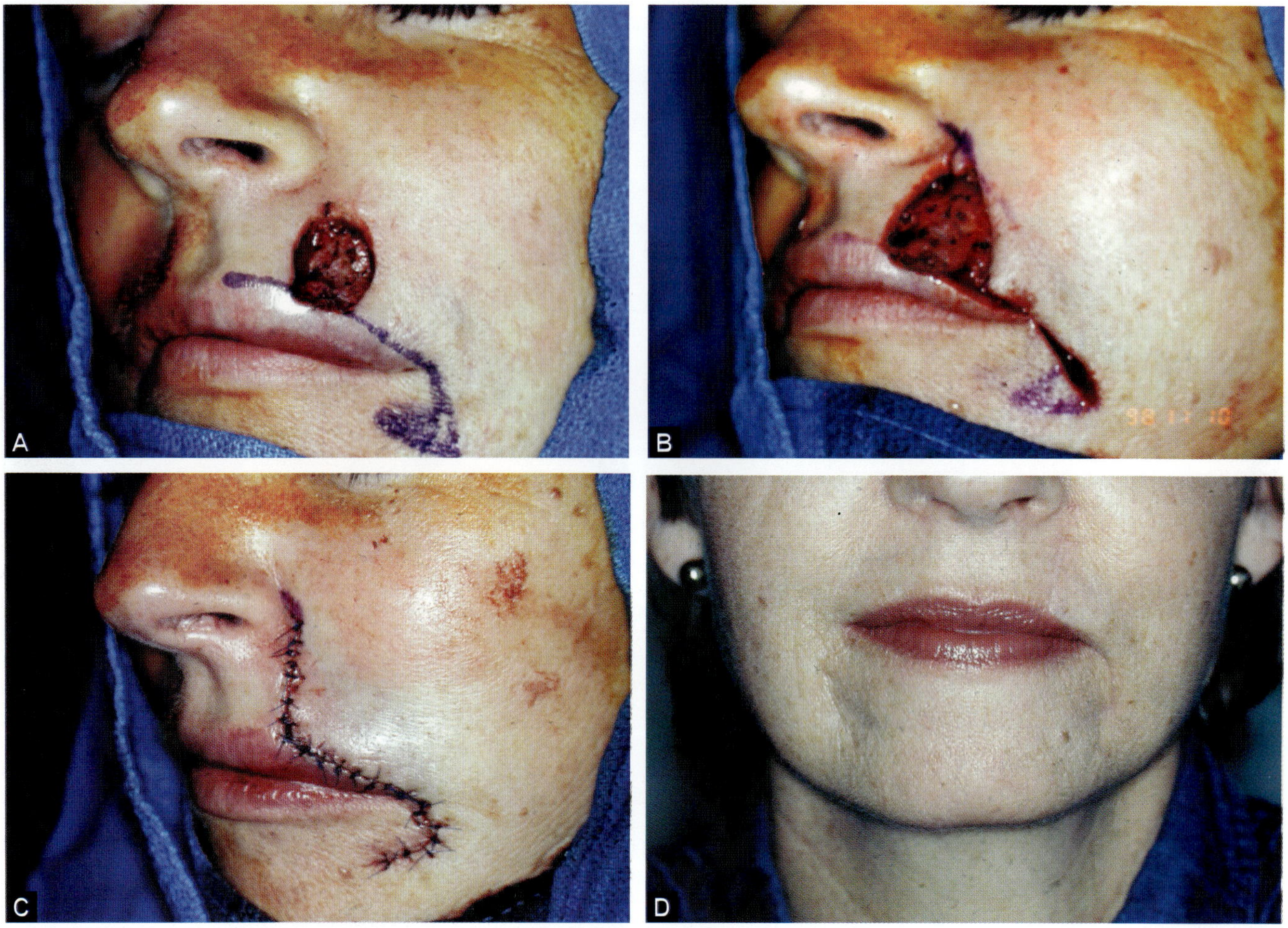

**Figs. 16.19A to D:** (A) Upper cutaneous lip defect involving the vermillion border. Advancement flap planned with incision extending lateral to the oral commissure. (B and C) Advancement flap developed with the incision made along the vermillion border with preservation of the white roll of the upper cutaneous lip. (D) Slight hooding of lateral upper lip could have been prevented with a larger Burow's triangle or revised with additional excision of redundant tissue.

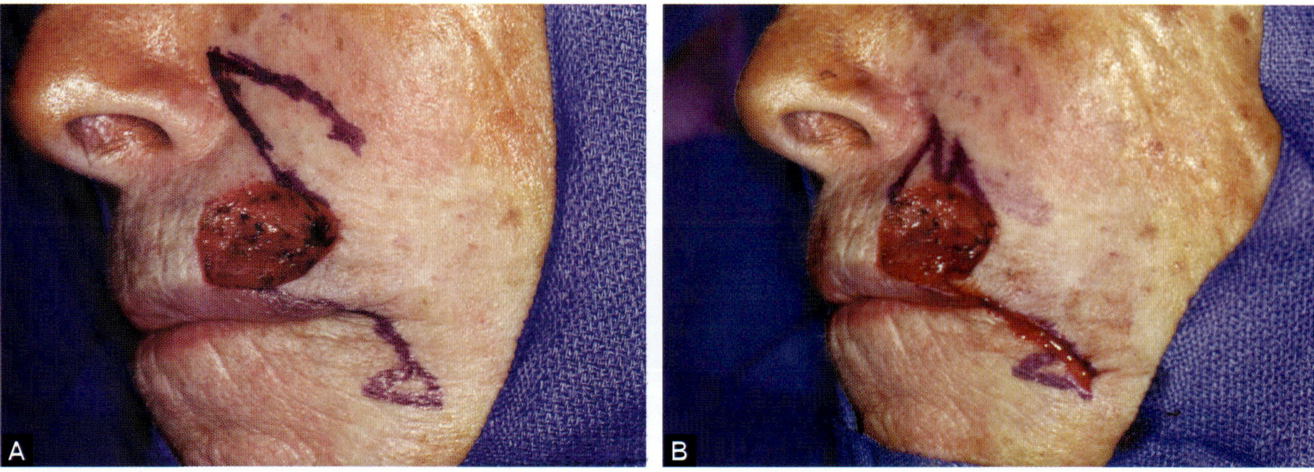

**Figs. 16.20A and B**

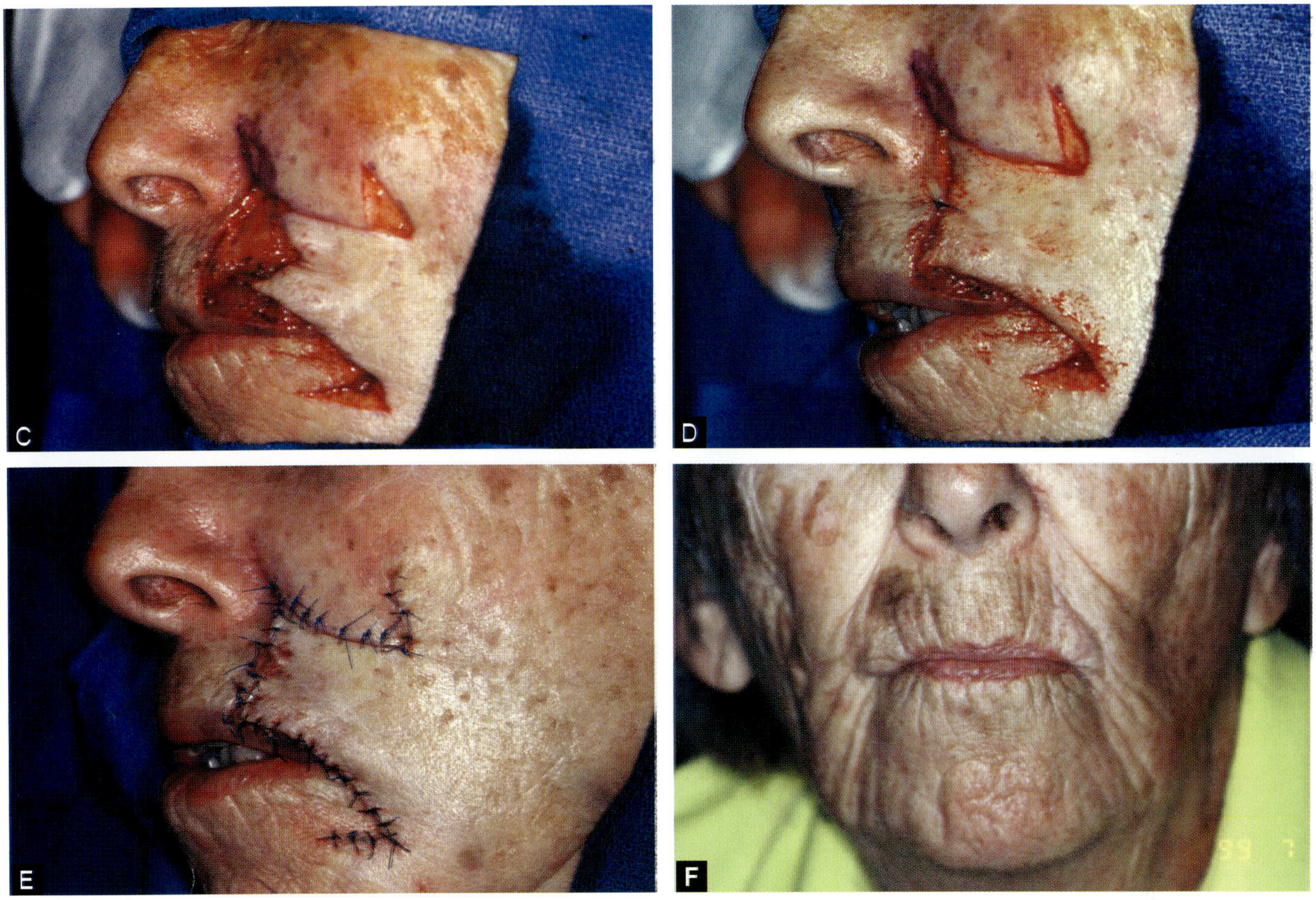

**Figs. 16.20A to F:** (A) Larger upper cutaneous lip defect. Repair options include a transposition flap and advancement flap. (B) Mobility was limited with an M-plasty and Burow's triangle design. (C) Therefore, a unilateral advancement flap was performed with the superior incision extending across the melolabial fold onto the cheek. Generally, it is unwise to extend an excision across cosmetic subunits. In this severely elastotic skin, placing Burow's triangles in natural dynamic rhytides allows for acceptable scar camouflage. (D) A polypropylene guiding suture was utilized at the leading edge to ensure proper placement of the flap. (E) The guiding suture is repositioned as necessary during incremental closure. (F) Final appearance.

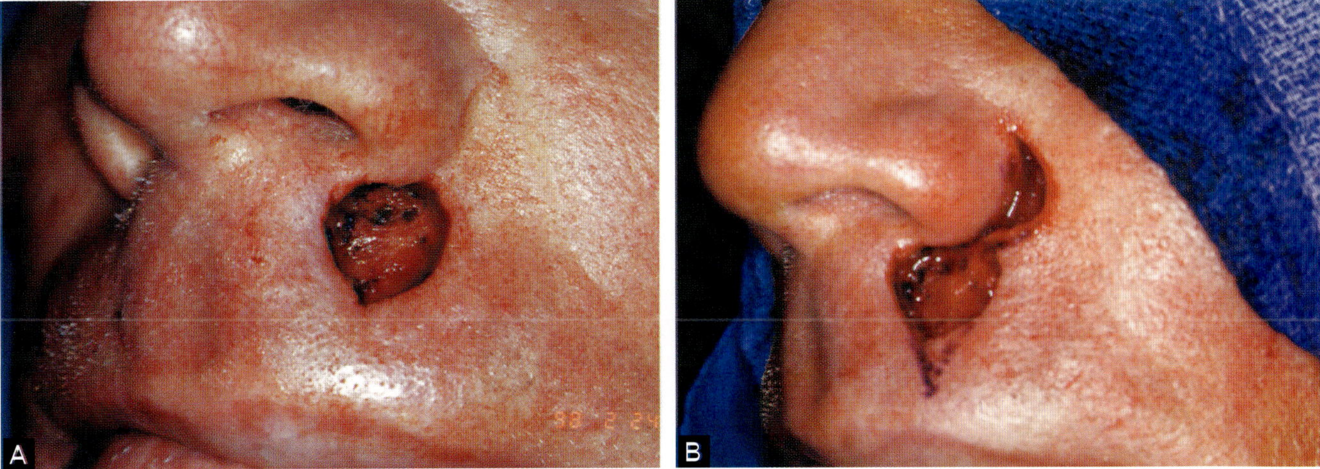


**Figs. 16.21A and B**

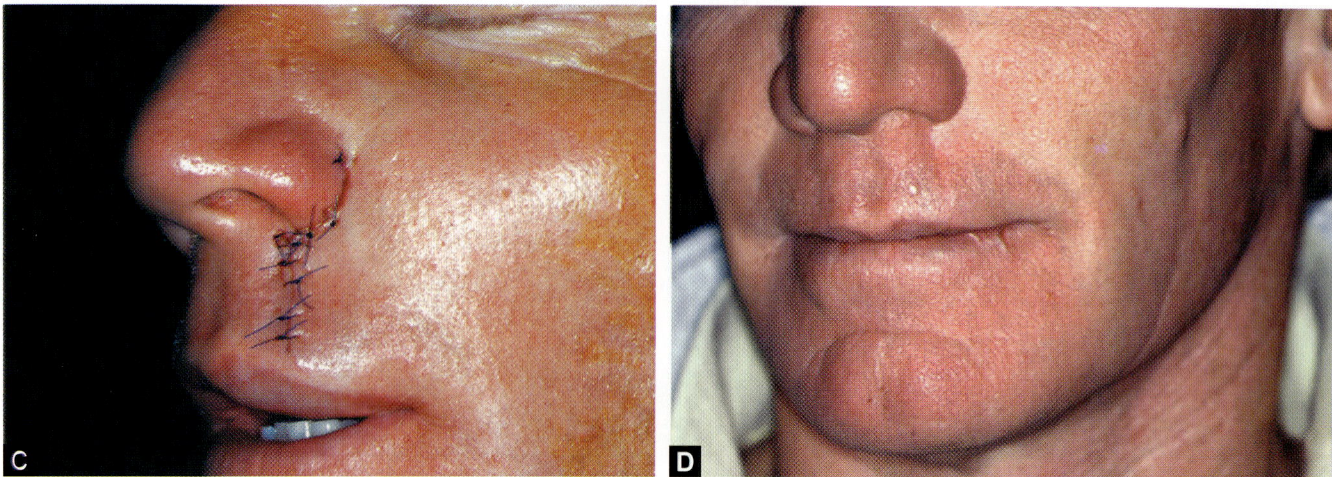

**Figs. 16.21A to D:** (A) Upper cutaneous lip defect abutting alar sill and the apical triangle of the upper cutaneous lip. (B and C) Curvilinear closure planned around the alar crease. Removal of a small crescentic tissue cone preserves the concave surface of the apical triangle of the upper cutaneous lip. (D) Final appearance.

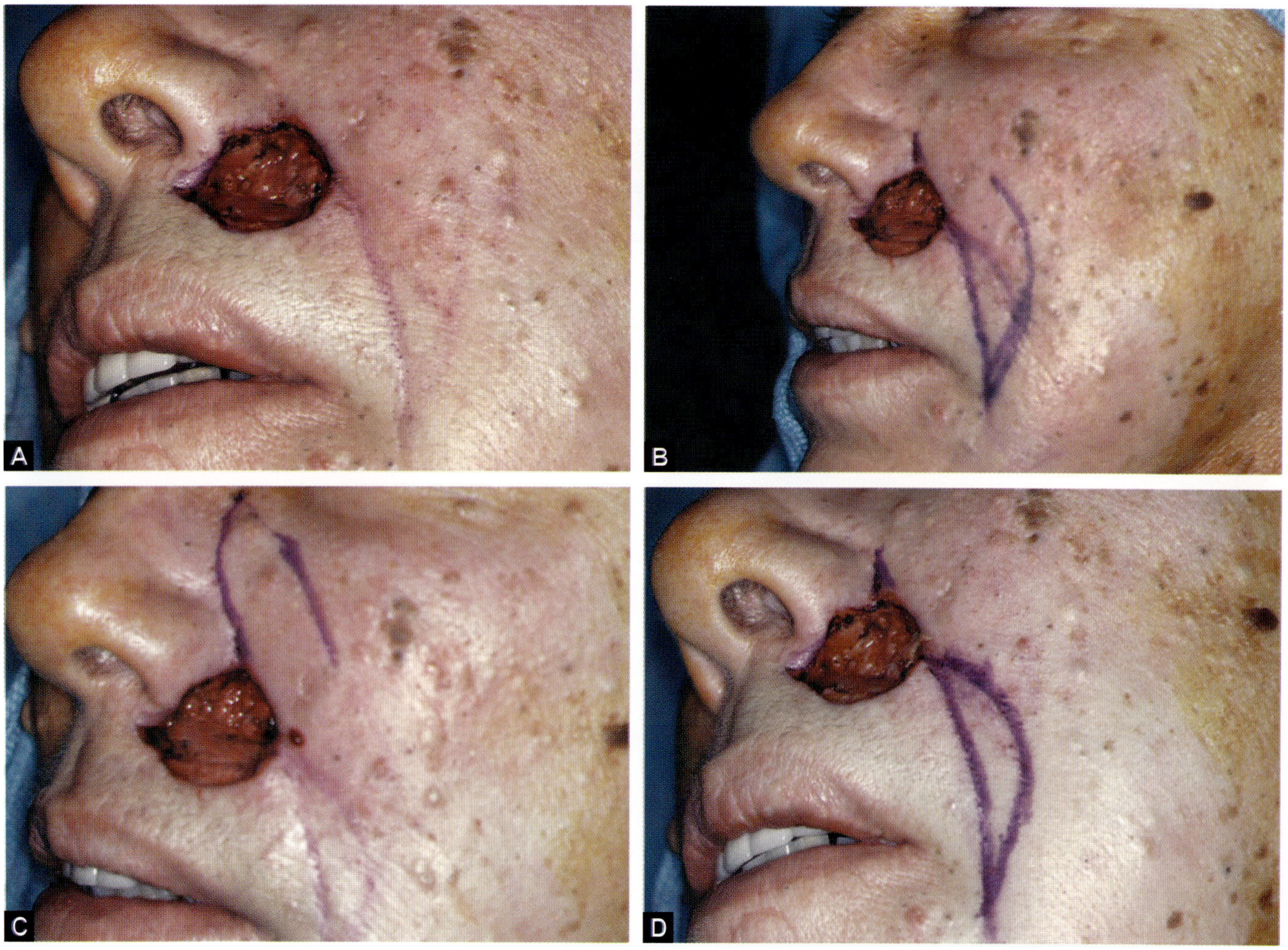

**Figs. 16.22A to D**

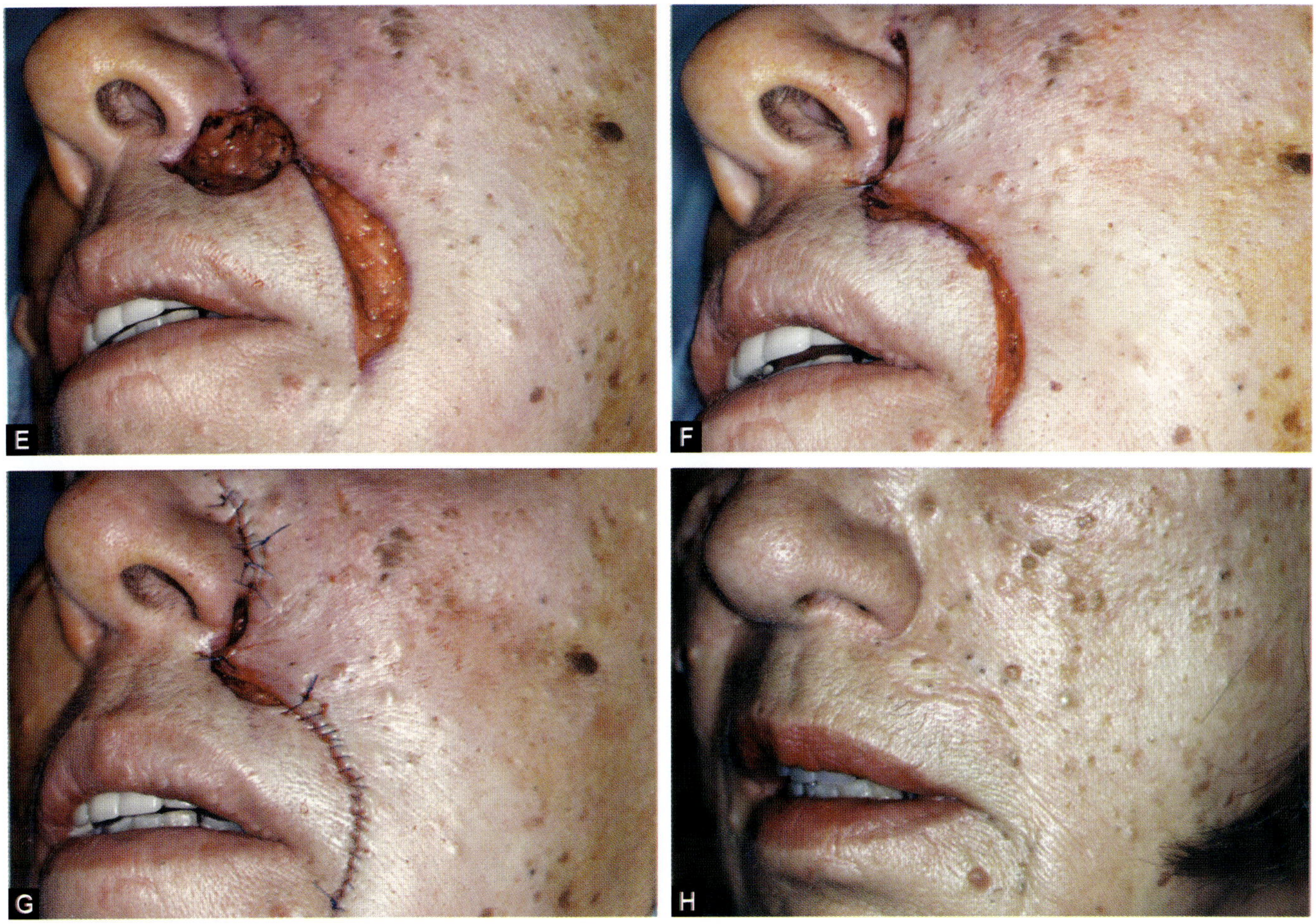

**Figs. 16.22A to H:** (A) Combined alar and apical lip defect. Multiple reconstructive options were considered: (B) inferior banner transposition flap and (C) superior banner transposition flap. (D) Repaired with a perialar crescentic advancement flap. (E and F) Removal of the crescent of tissue facilitates symmetrical repair of the defect and alleviates limb length discrepancy of the advancement flap. This minimizes long-term fullness and tissue redundancy of the cheek. (G and H) Partial second intention wound healing to maintain the alar crease and on the upper cutaneous lip to prevent partial eclabium.

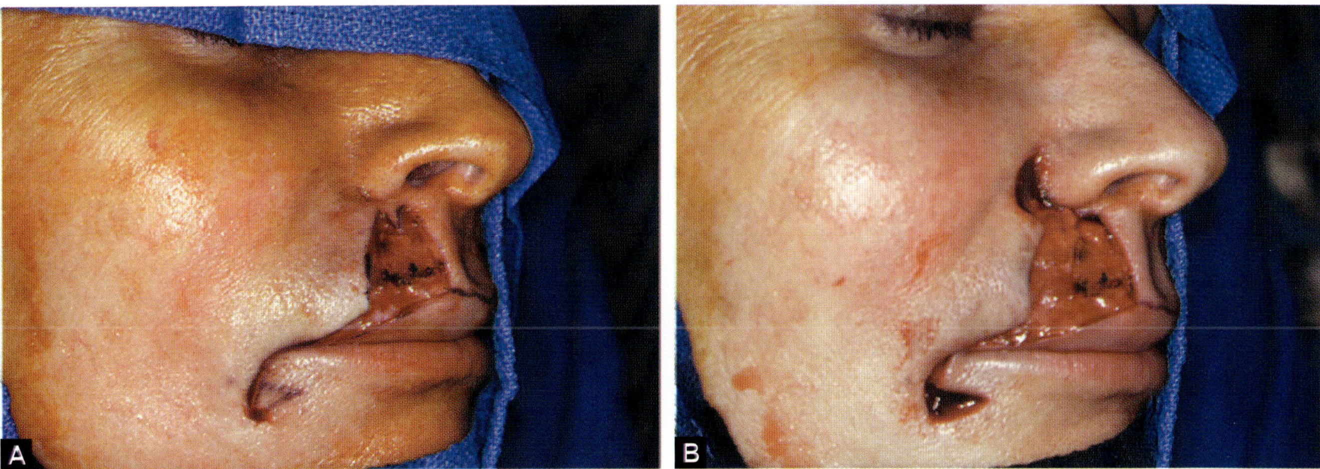


**Figs. 16.23A and B**

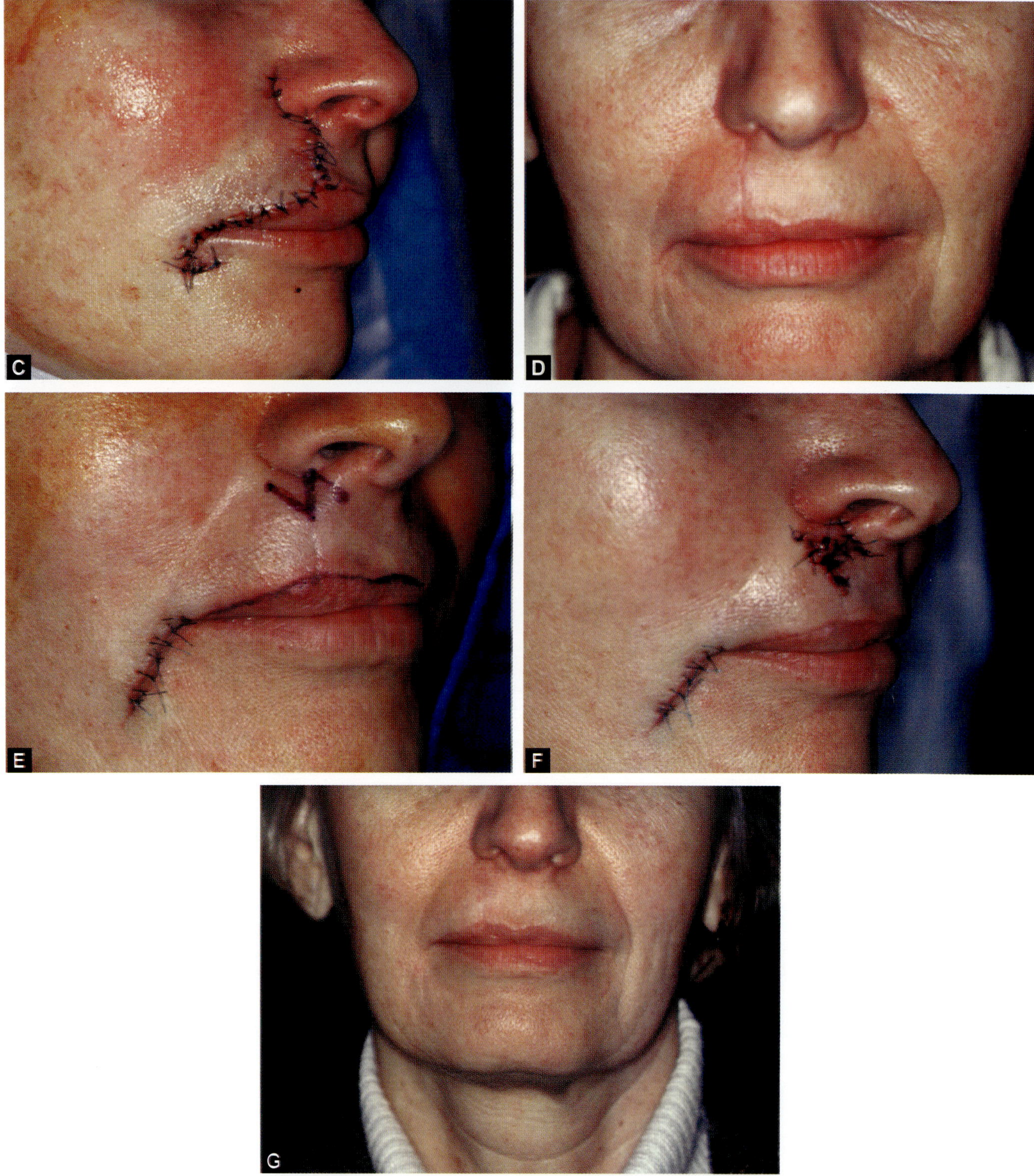


**Figs. 16.23A to G:** (A) Defect of the upper cutaneous lip just lateral to the philtrum. An advancement flap was planned along the vermillion border with a superior M-plasty. (B) The superior portion of the reconstruction was converted to excision of a perialar crescent to facilitate additional tissue movement. (C) Mild postoperative eclabium improved with Z-plasty performed on the upper cutaneous lip inferior to the alar sill. (D) Tissue redundancy lateral to the oral commissure resulted in trough formation and the appearance of a slight frown. (E to G) This was revised with simple excision of redundant tissue.

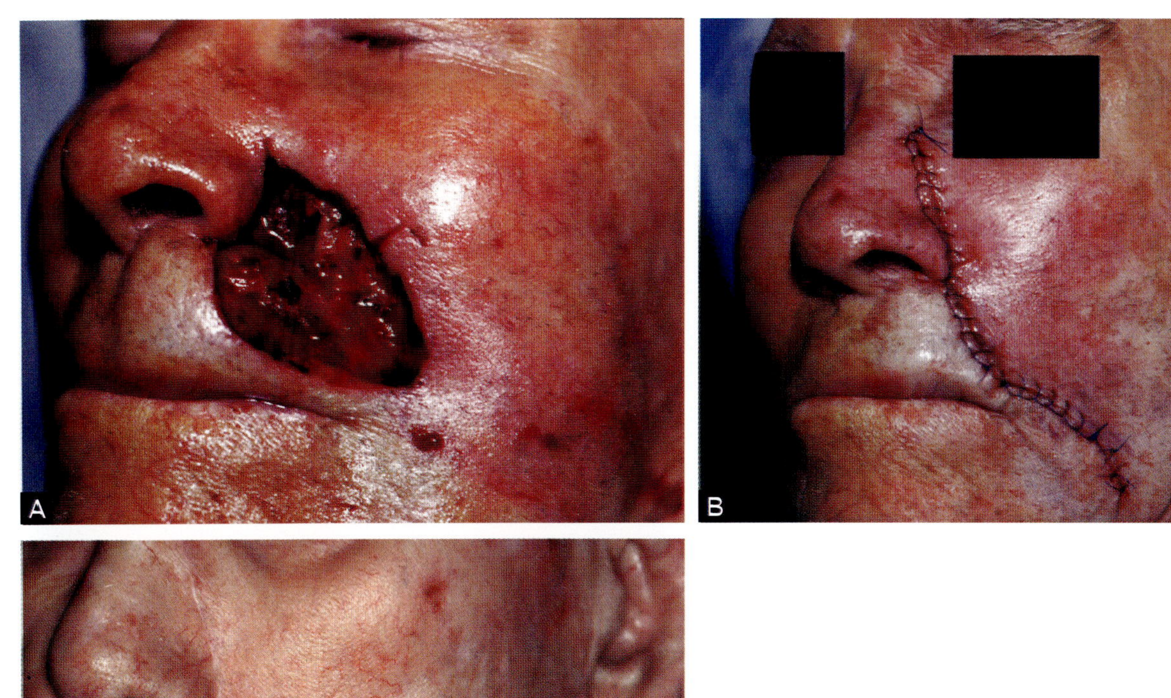


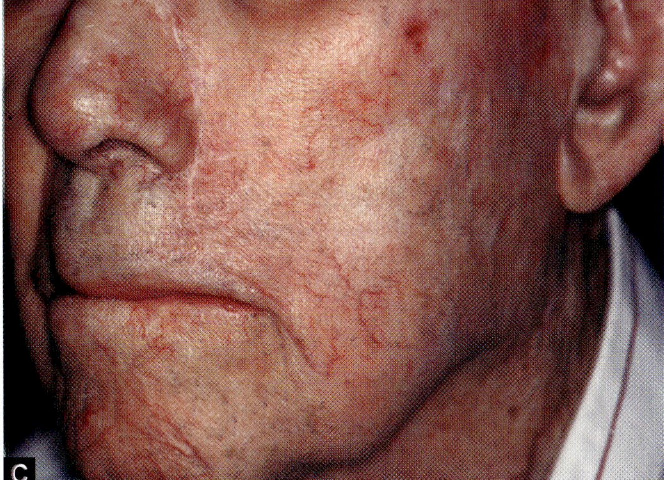


**Figs. 16.24A to C:** (A) Large complex defect that involved multiple cosmetic units: lip, cheek, and ala. (B) Repaired with a perialar crescentic advancement flap. Wide undermining mobilizes tissue from the cheek and jowls. Note the incision extends superiorly to medial canthus and inferiorly to the ramus of the mandible. (C) Final appearance.

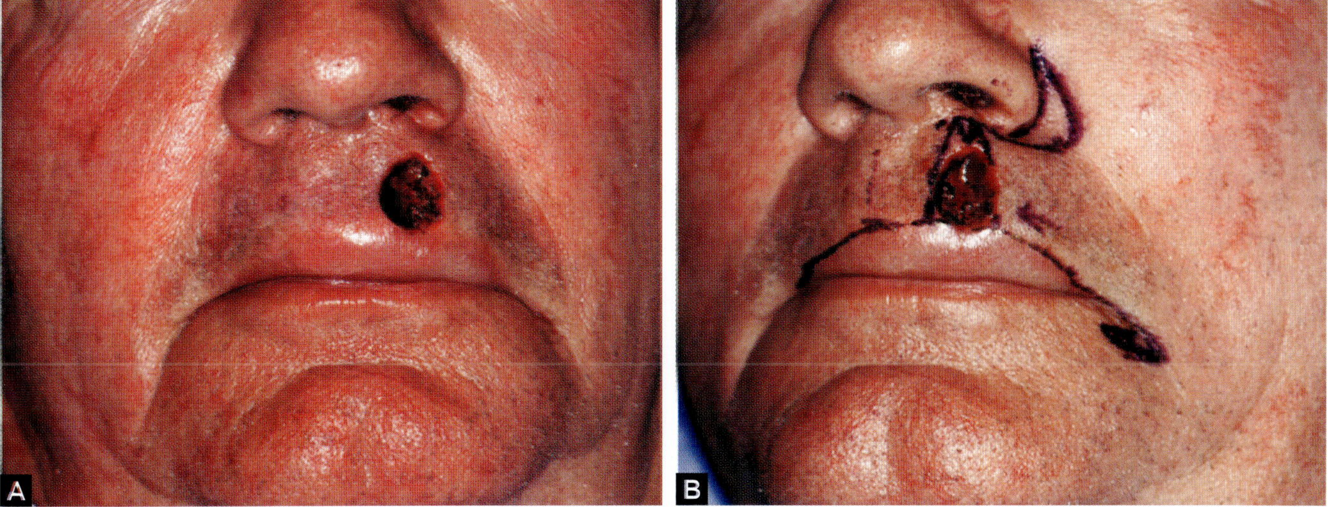


**Figs. 16.25A and B**

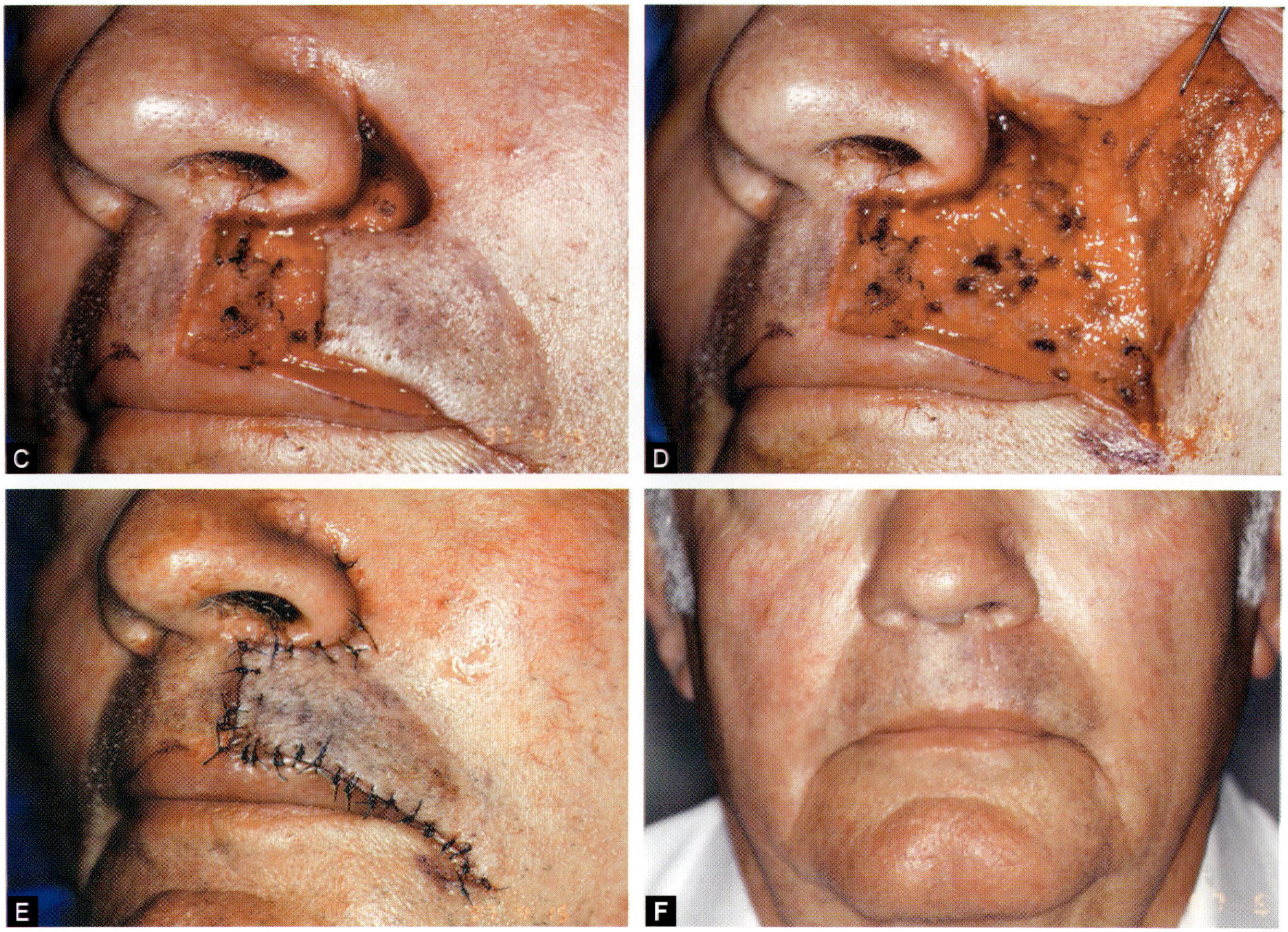

**Figs. 16.25A to F:** (A) Defect involving the philtral columns. (B and C) Repaired with a unilateral advancement flap after the defect was enlarged to the entire cosmetic subunit. (D and E) Wide undermining performed to minimize wound tension. Excision of a perialar crescent performed at the superior border of the flap. Note extension inferolateral to the oral commissure to utilize the laxity of the cheek. (F) Final appearance.

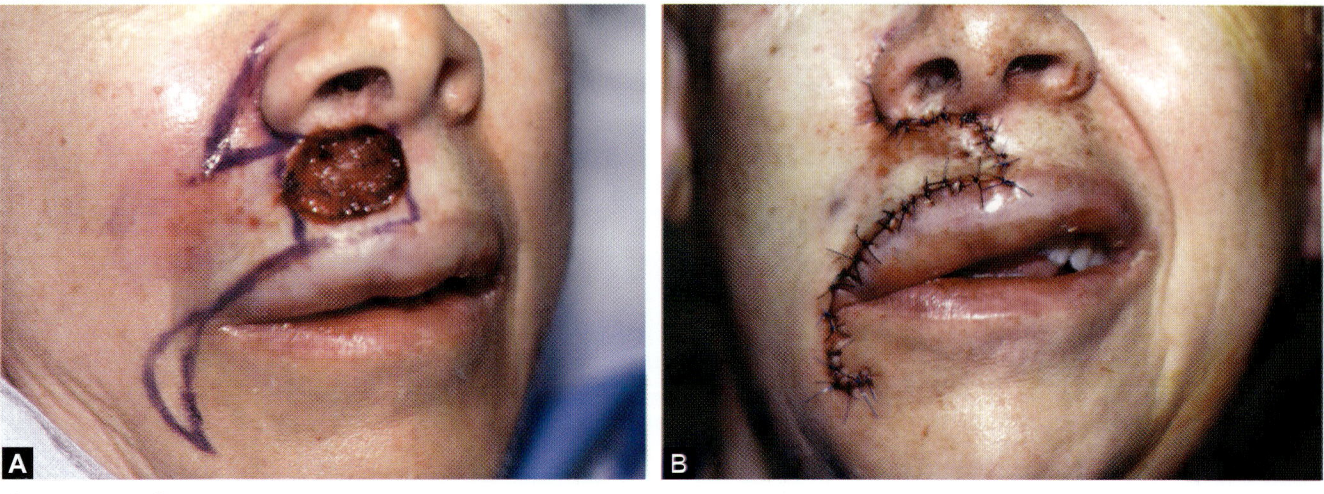


**Figs. 16.26A and B**

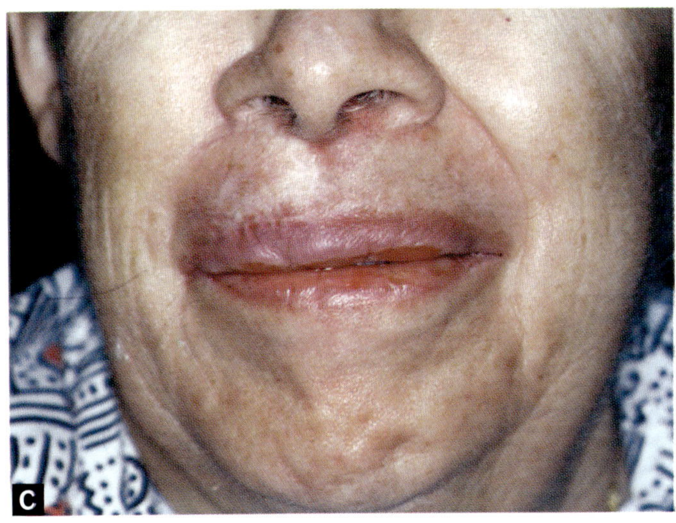

**Figs. 16.26A to C:** (A and B) Upper cutaneous lip defect with advancement flap planned. Patient's upper lip fullness and thick sebaceous skin predicts a challenging repair with poor tissue mobilization. Large perialar crescent excised. (C) Final appearance.

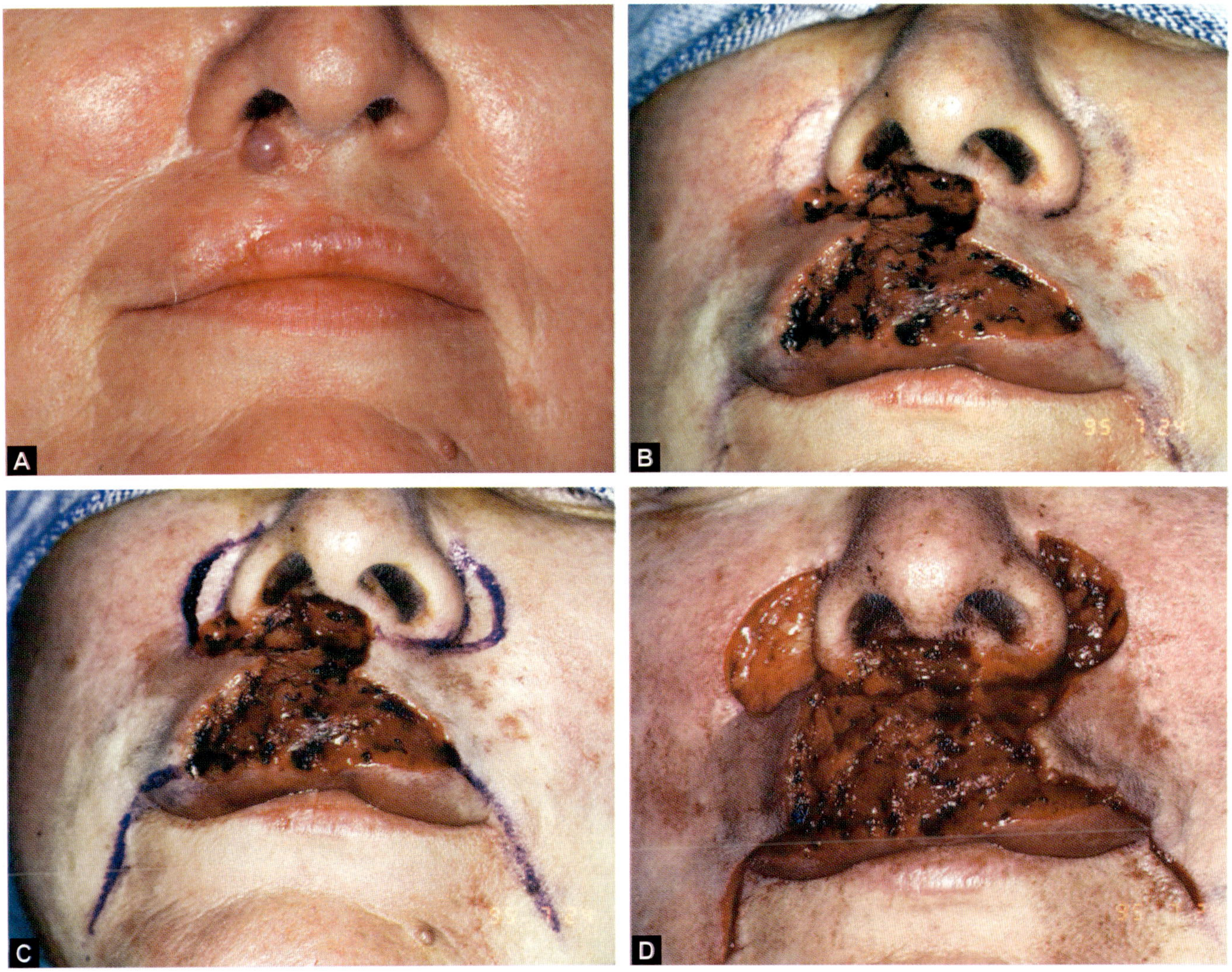

**Figs. 16.27A to D**

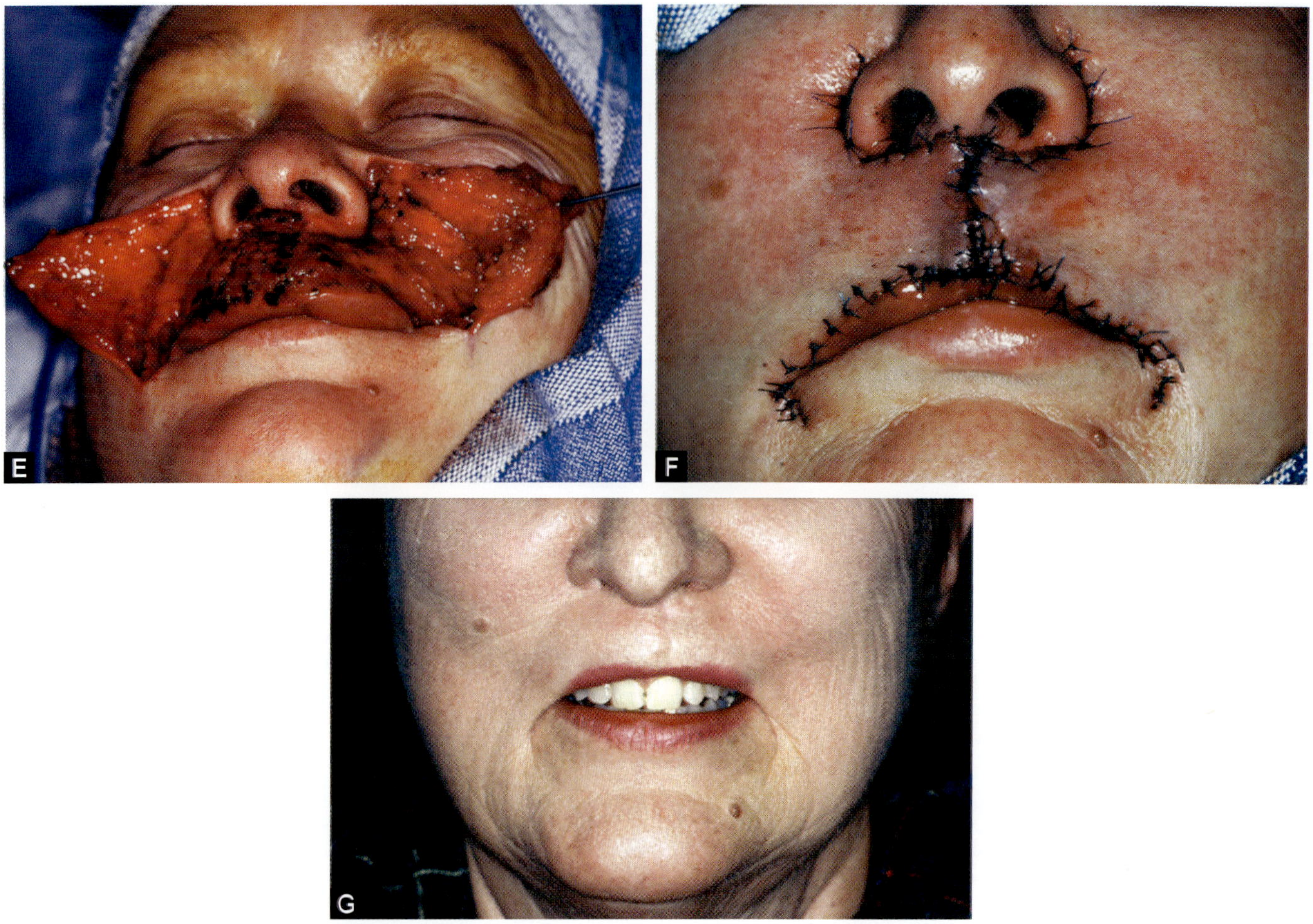

**Figs. 16.27A to G:** (A) Multiply recurrent basal cell carcinoma and (B) post-Mohs surgery defect involving multiple cosmetic subunits of the upper cutaneous lip, columella, alar sill, and apical triangle of the upper cutaneous lip. (C and D) Bilateral advancement flap with excision of perialar crescents. The inferior flap incisions are made along the vermillion border and extend inferolateral to the oral commissures to utilize the laxity of the cheek. (E) Wide and extensive undermining performed to facilitate movement and reduce flap tension. (F) Central suture line placed to approximate the philtrum. (G) Final appearance.

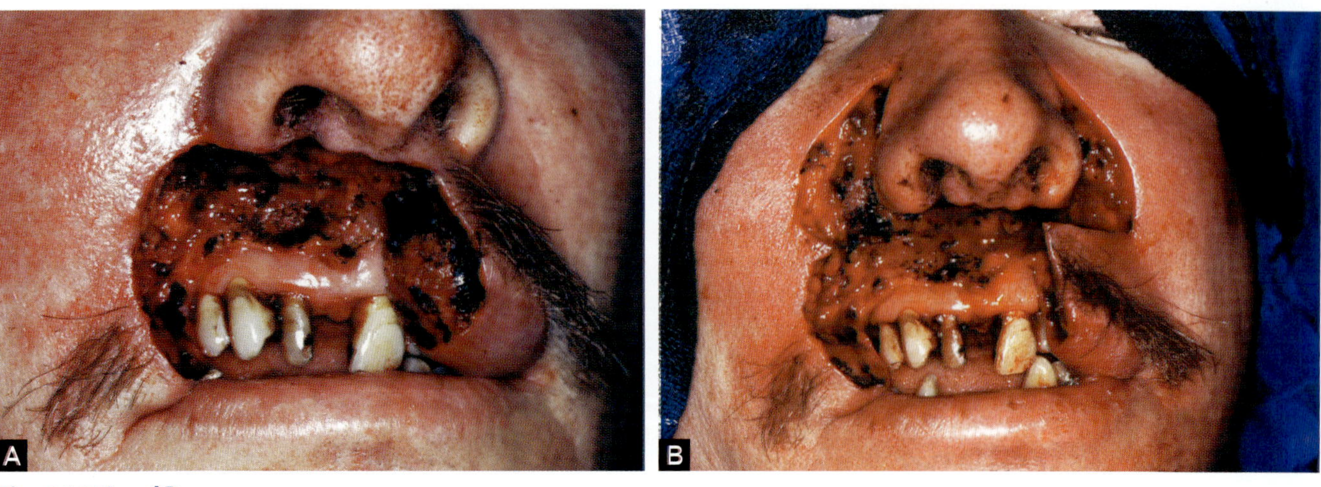

**Figs. 16.28A and B**

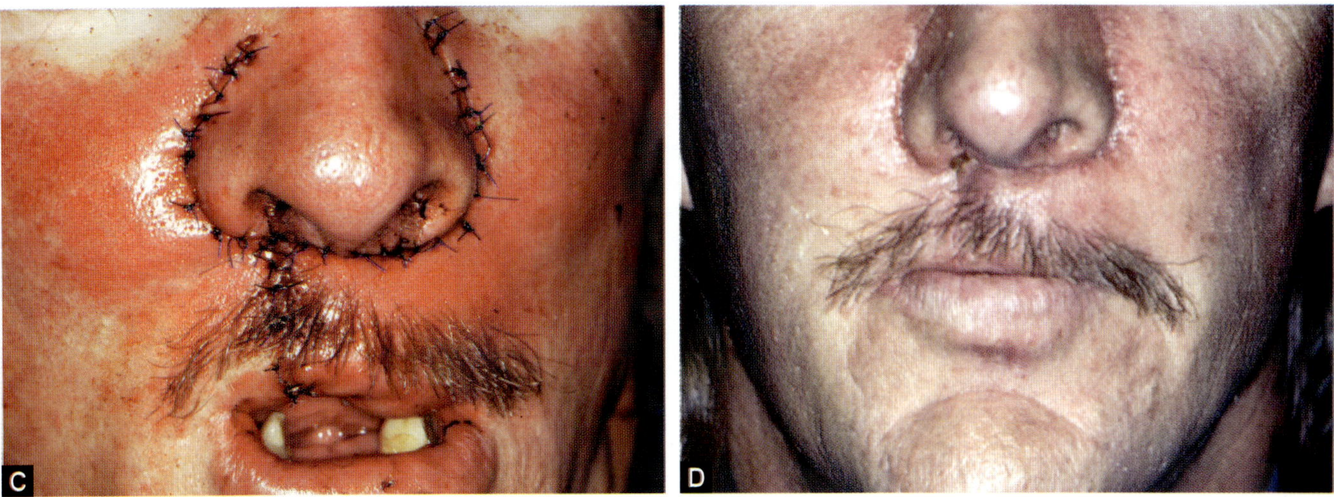

**Figs. 16.28A to D:** (A) Full-thickness defect after aggressive squamous cell carcinoma resection. (B and C) Repair with a single-stage bilateral crescentic advancement flap to preserve facial hair. An Abbe lip-switch staged repair could be considered as an alternate repair option. Excision of large perialar crescents allowed for adequate medial movement of the bilateral advancement flap and reapproximation of mustache. (D) Final appearance.

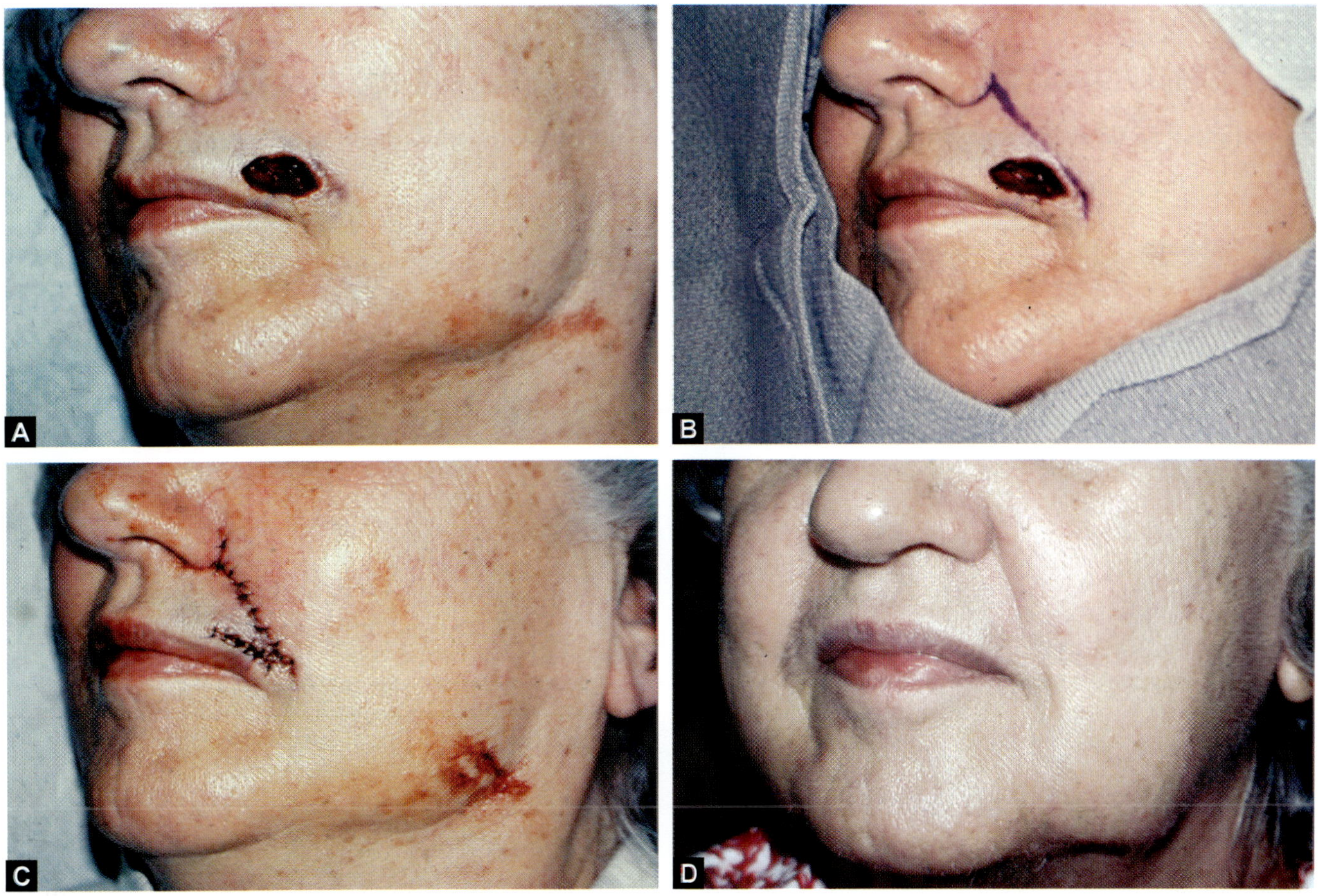

**Figs. 16.29A to D:** (A) Lateral upper cutaneous lip defect, longer in horizontal dimension. (B) Melolabial fold marked as landmark. (C) Rotation flap with incision following the melolabial fold and Burow's triangle concealed within the alar crease. (D) Note slight postoperative eclabium of the lateral lip. Minimal eclabium resolves with time.

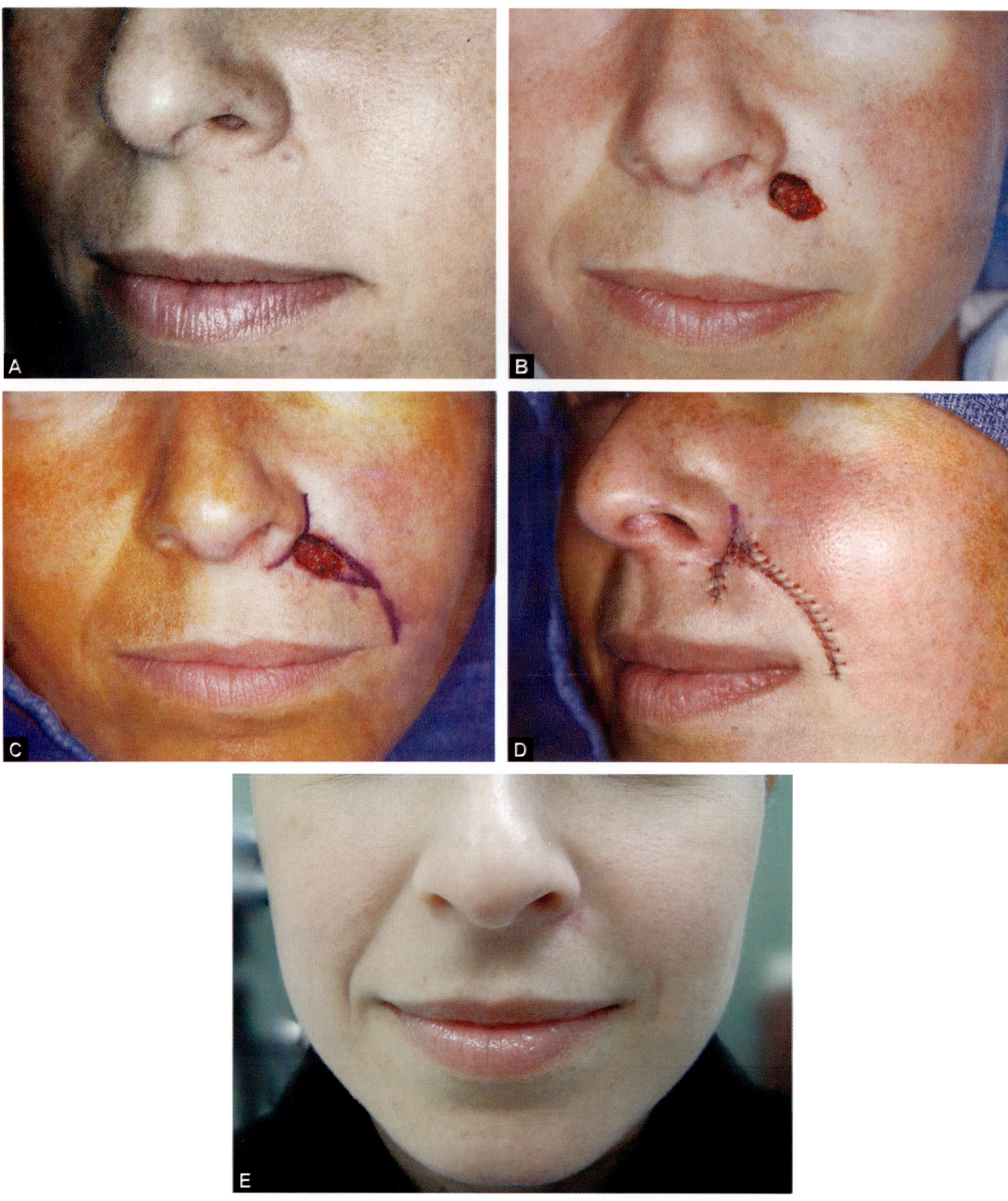


**Figs. 16.30A to E:** (A and B) Upper cutaneous lip defect. (C) Numerous reconstructive options considered. Linear reconstruction deemed to promote excessive vermillion lip elevation. (D) Rotation flap performed in the melolabial crease. (E) Long-term follow-up with subtle blunting of left melolabial crease.

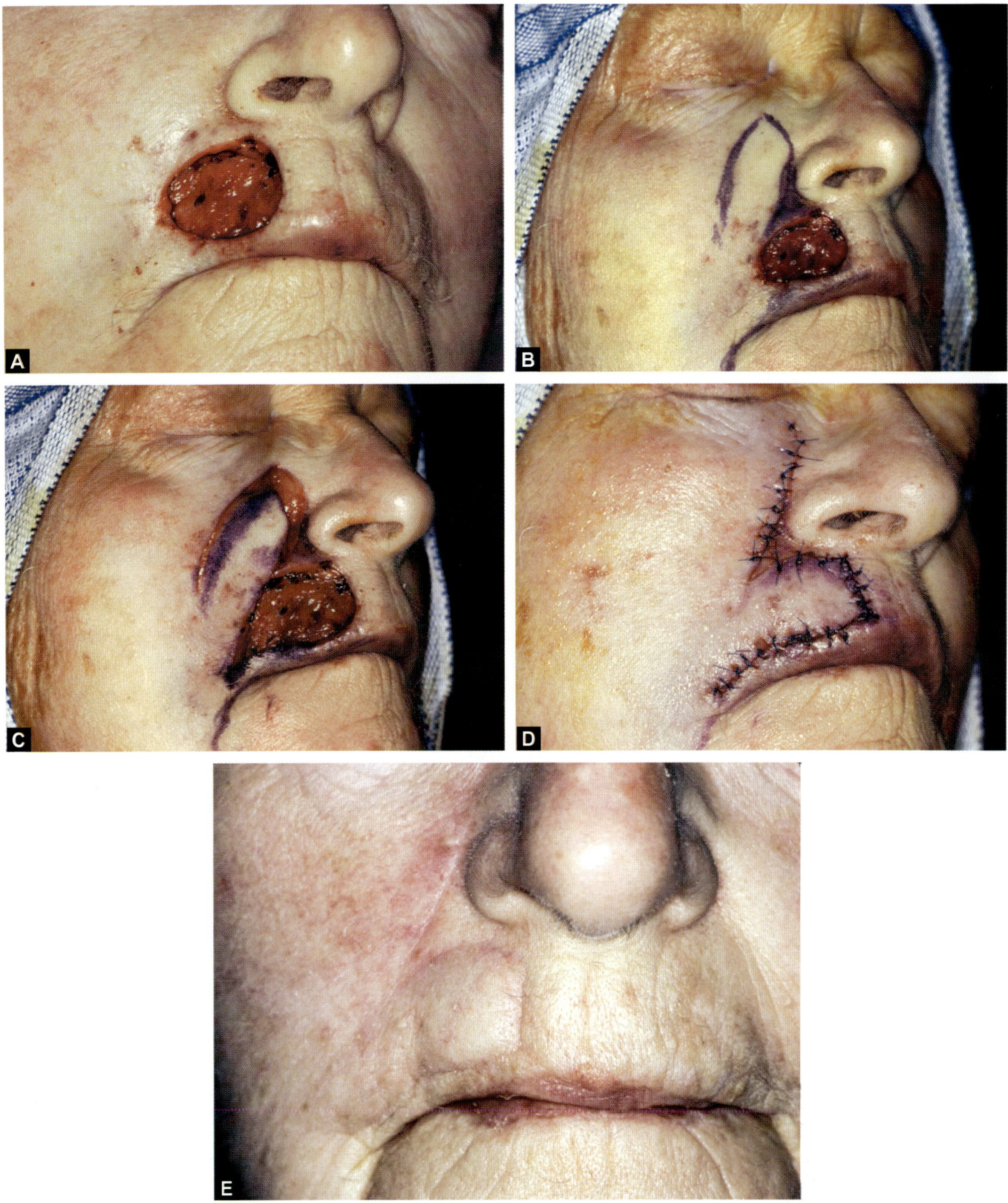


**Figs. 16.31A to E:** (A to D) Large upper cutaneous lip defect repaired with a banner transposition flap. (E) Note pincushioning of the flap as the convexity of the cheek is transposed to the upper cutaneous lip.

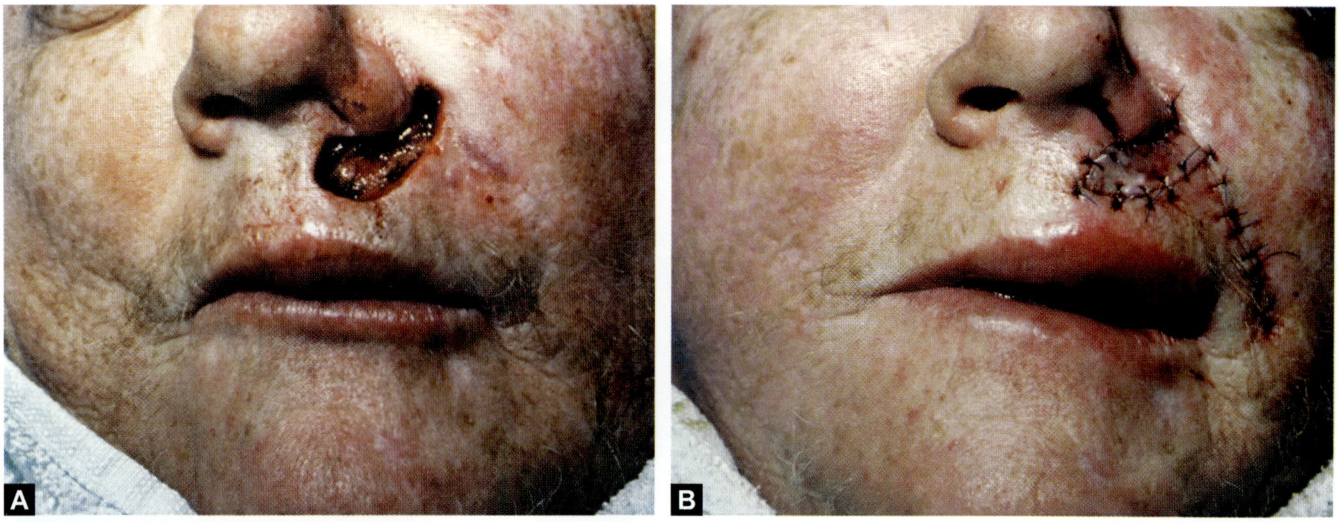

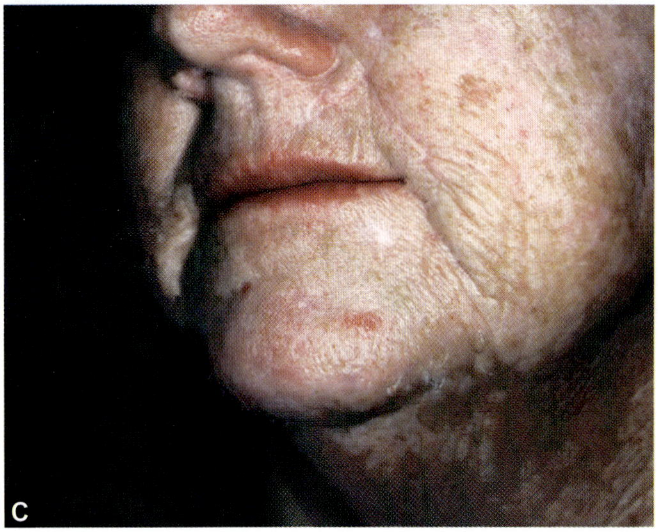

**Figs. 16.32A to C:** (A) Irregularly shaped upper cutaneous lip and cheek defect (B and C) repaired with a banner transposition flap.

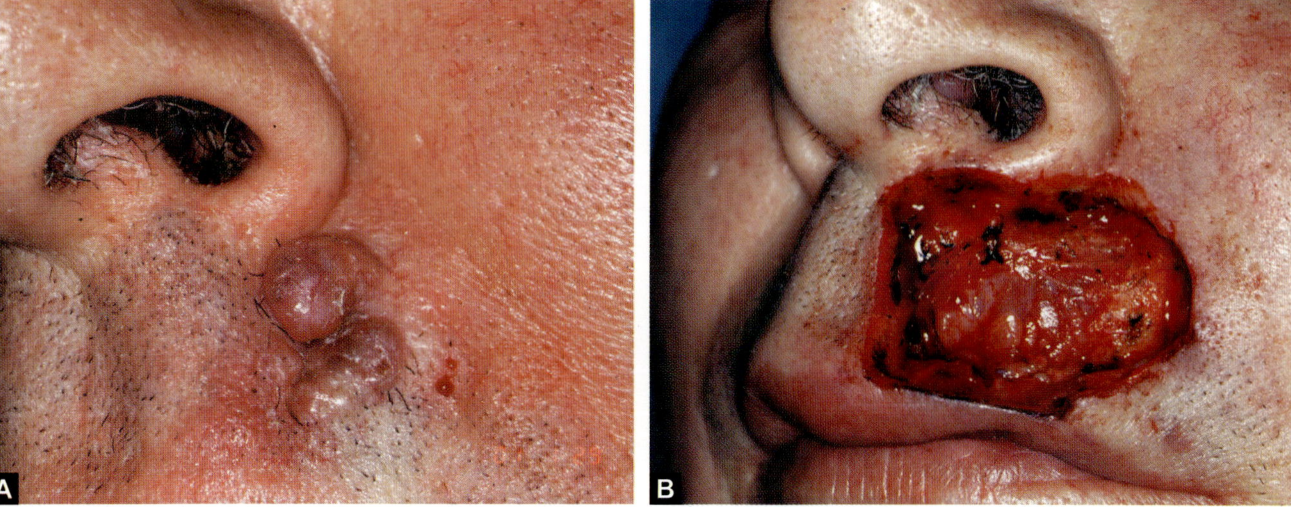

**Figs. 16.33A and B**

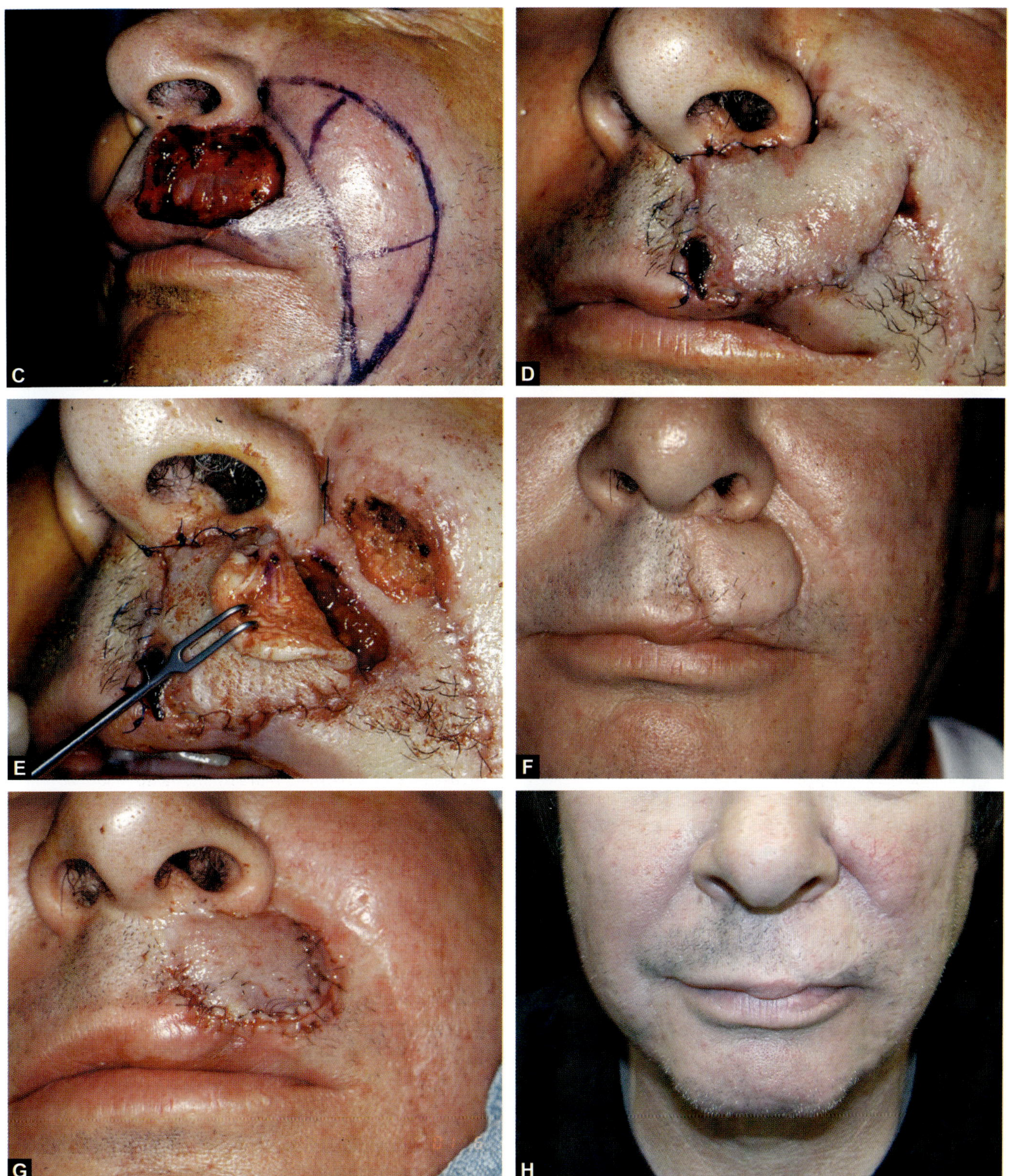


**Figs. 16.33A to H:** (A and B) Large neglected basal cell carcinoma results in an extensive upper cutaneous lip and vermillion lip defect after tumor removal. (C to E) Repaired with a melolabial interpolation flap. (F and G) Pincushioning necessitated flap thinning. (H) Note loss of upper cutaneous lip facial hair.

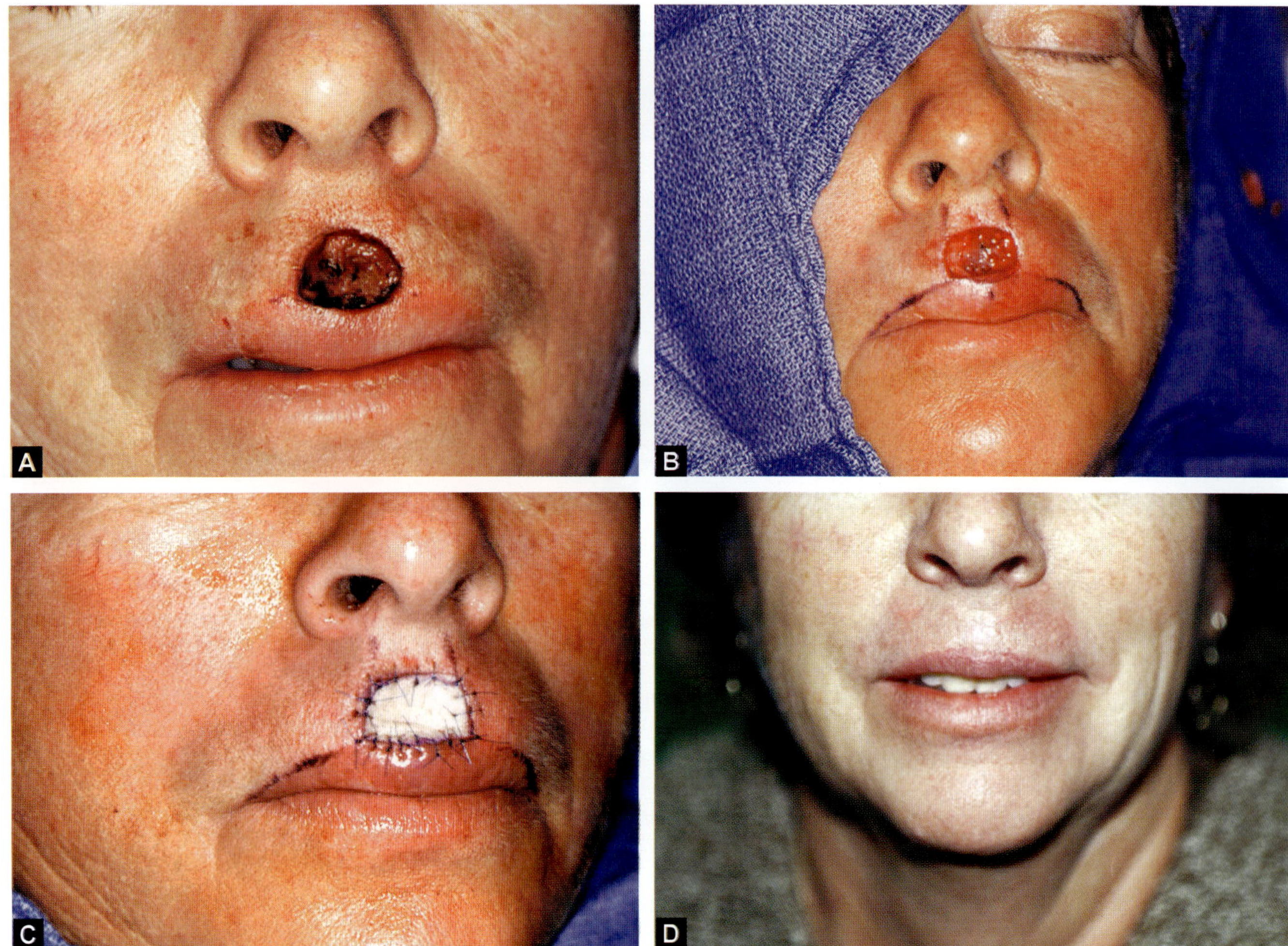

**Figs. 16.34A to D:** (A) Midline defect abutting but not involving the vermillion lip. (B) Defect enlarged to the philtral ridges and (C) repaired with a full-thickness skin graft. (D) Final appearance.

donor site offers abundant tissue for larger defects[17] (Figs. 16.35A to E).

## Lower Vermillion and Cutaneous Lip

### *Second Intention*

Second intention wound healing is often an option on the vermillion lip and can yield acceptable cosmetic results[11,12] (Figs. 16.36A to C).

### *Mucosal Advancement*

Mucosal advancement flap can resurface the entire lower vermillion (dry mucosa) (Figs. 16.37 and 16.38). Extending the incision across the oral commissure and onto the upper vermillion lip minimizes contracture and microstomia. Undermining is performed in a plane between the minor salivary glands and the posterior border of the orbicularis oris muscle.[18] Undermining can be performed to the gingiva-labial sulcus to allow for adequate advancement of the mucosa. Precisely approximate the vermillion to the cutaneous lip. Wound edges of a full-thickness defect with irregular contour can be sharply freshened into a smooth line approximating a new vermillion border (Figs. 16.39A to E).

### *Linear Repair*

Lower lip defects involving one-third of the lip can be repaired with a linear closure design.[19] Defects larger than one-third of the lip may be reconstructed with a wedge excision repair with appropriate patient selection. Clinically significant microstomia is a consideration with wedge

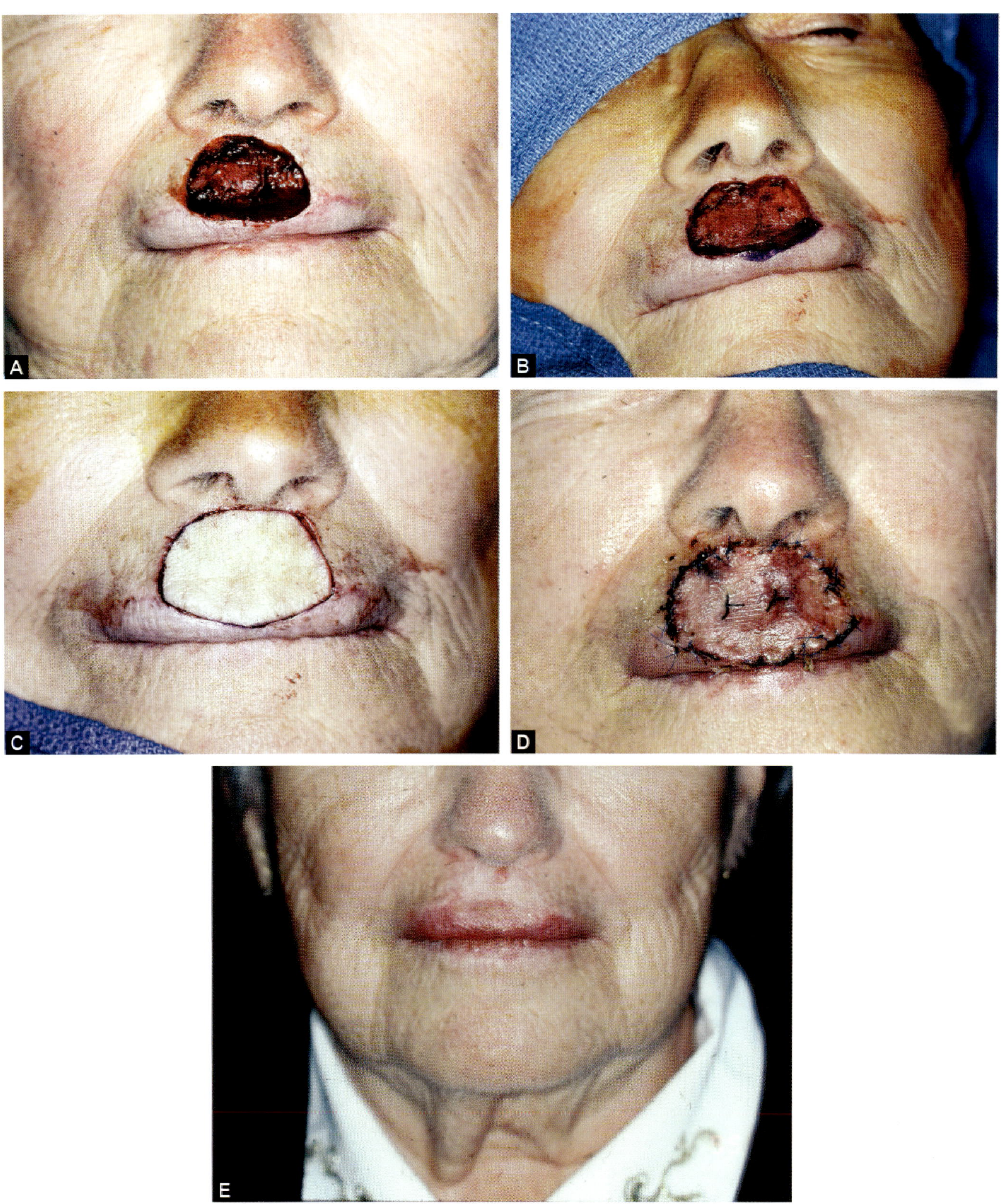


**Figs. 16.35A to E:** (A) Large defect involving the upper cutaneous, vermillion, and philtrum. (B) The defect was enlarged for more effective scar camouflage. (C and D) Repaired with a full-thickness skin graft, clavicular donor site. (E) Note hypopigmentation.

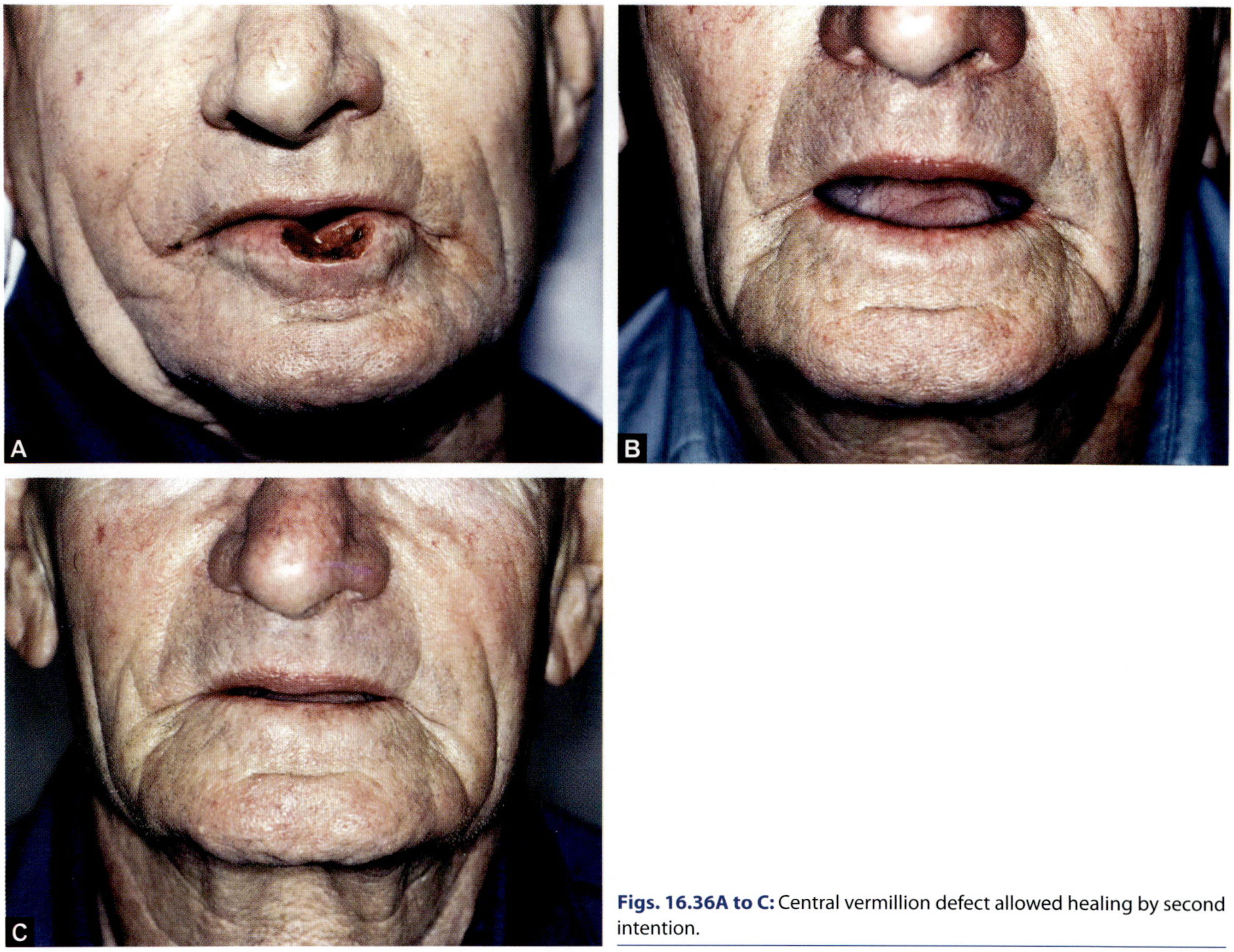

**Figs. 16.36A to C:** Central vermillion defect allowed healing by second intention.

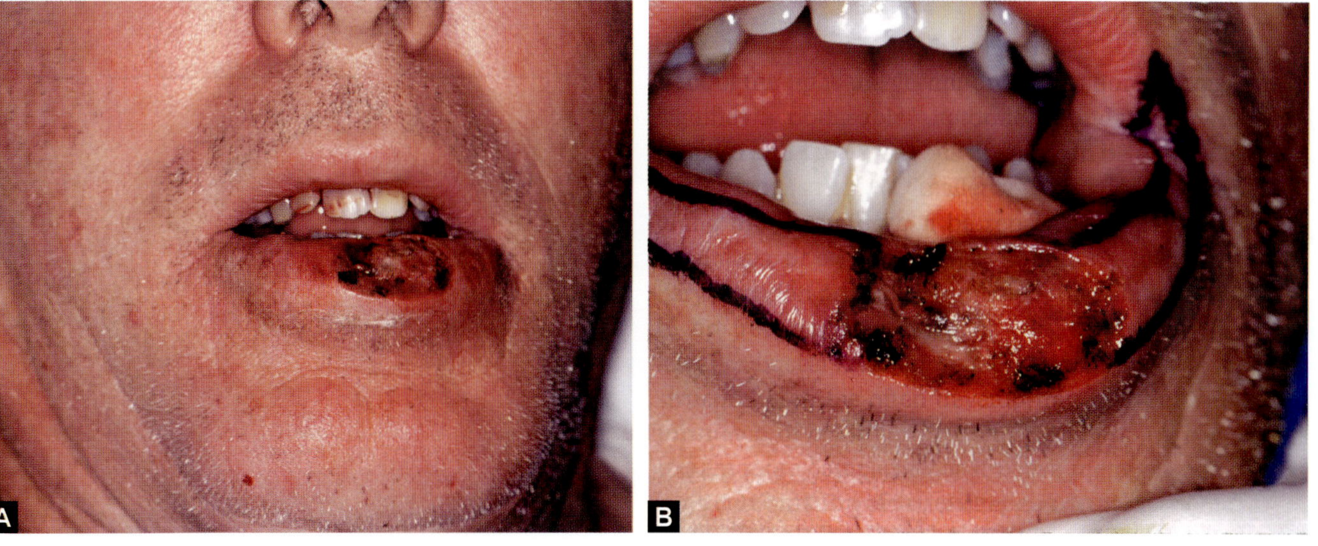


**Figs. 16.37A and B**

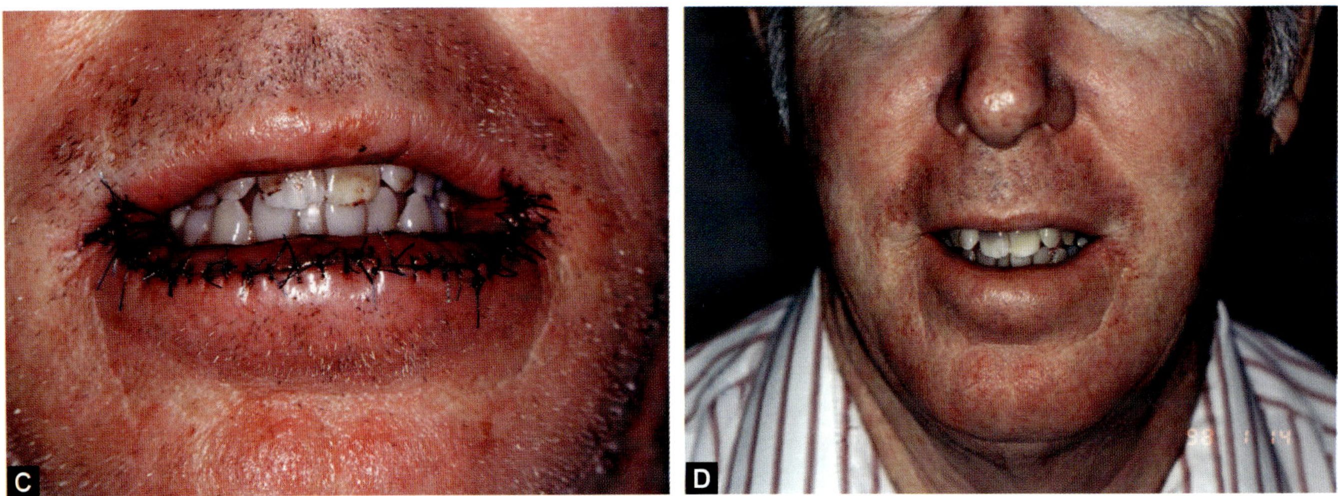


**Figs. 16.37A to D:** Central vermillion defect with surrounding actinic cheilitis repaired with mucosal advancement flap.

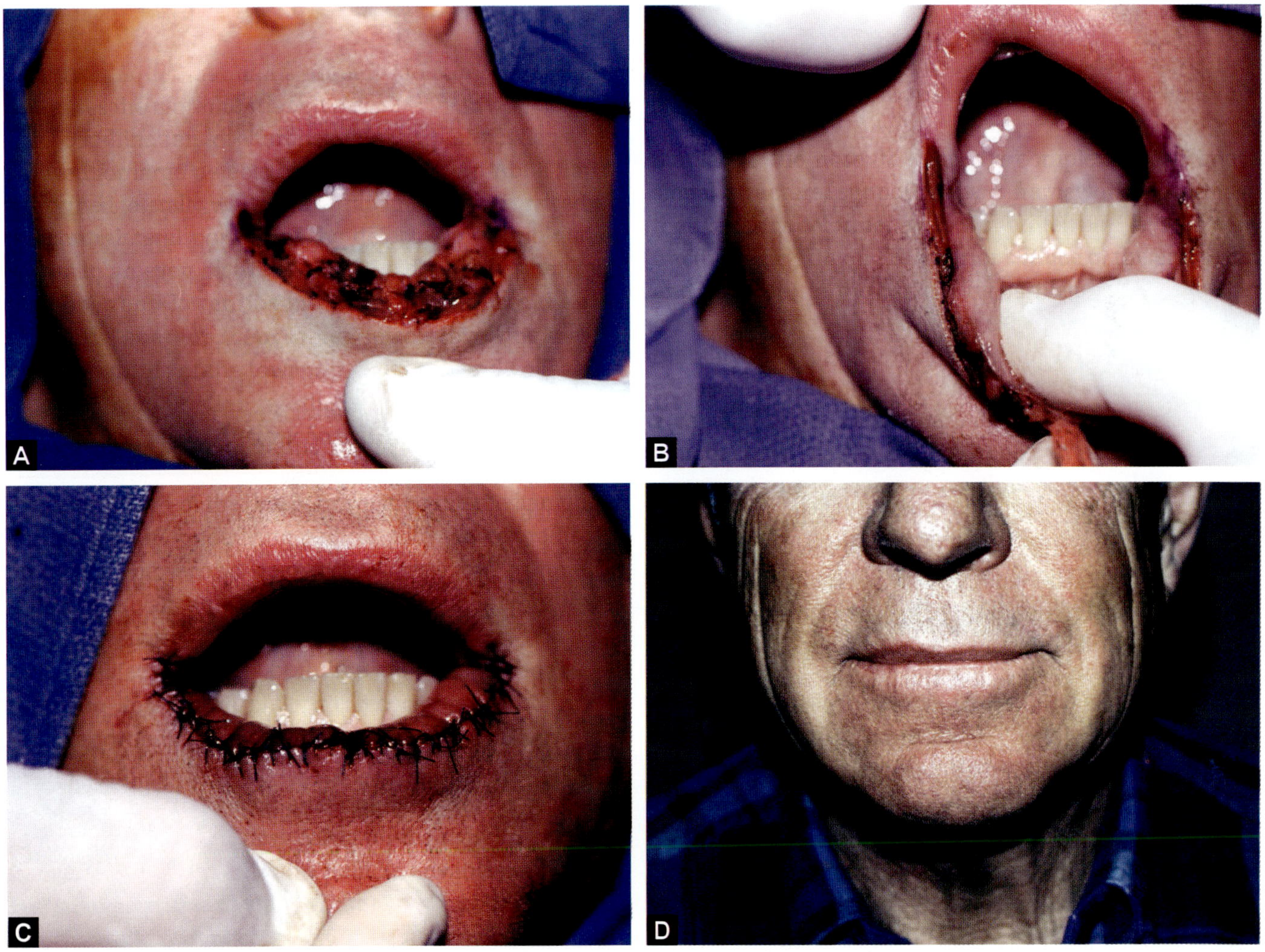

**Figs. 16.38A to D:** (A) Extensive defect of the lower vermillion lip. (B and C) Repaired with mucosal advancement flap. Note extension beyond the commissures to the upper lateral vermillion lip. (D) Final appearance.

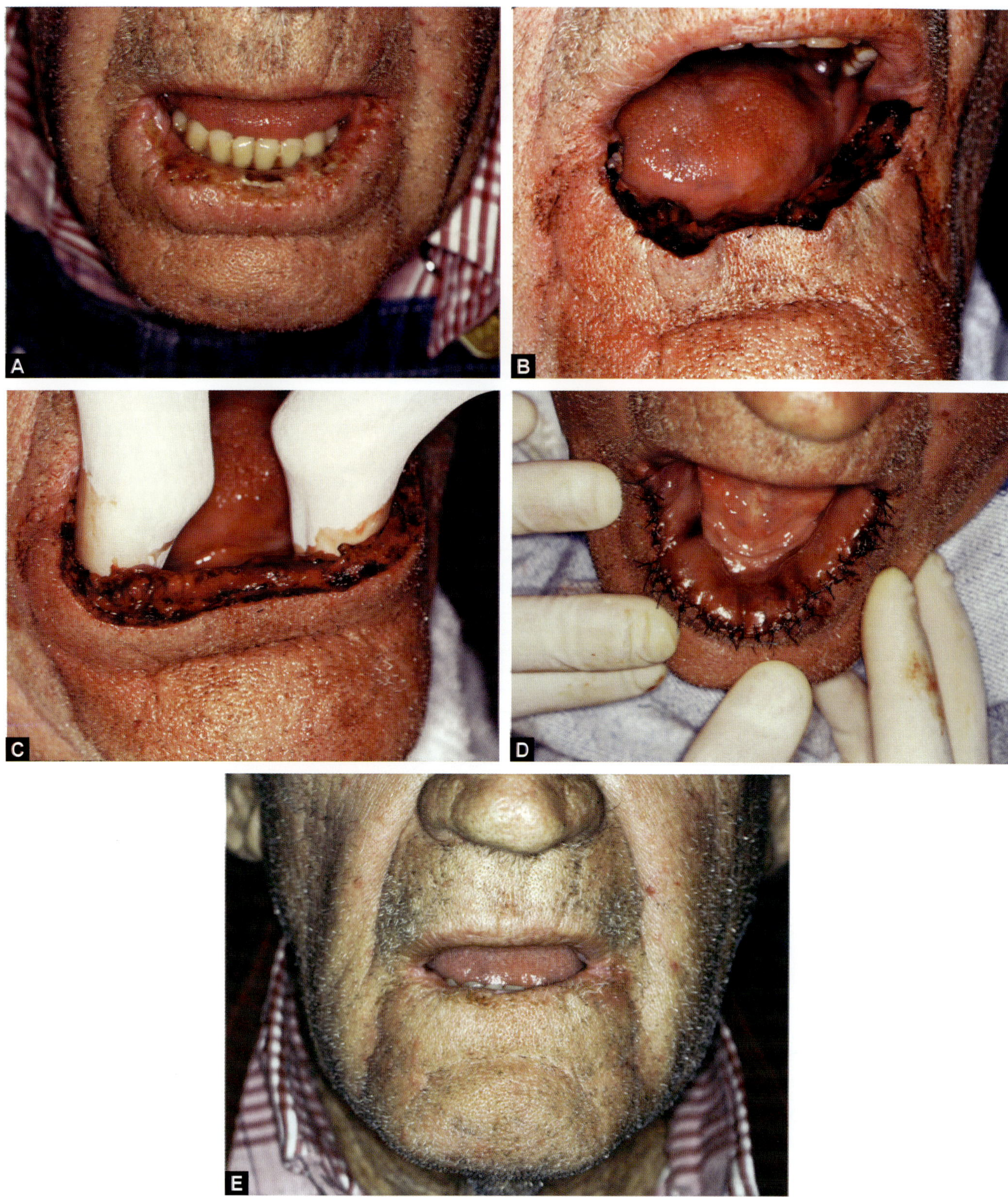


**Figs. 16.39A to E:** (A) Squamous cell carcinoma with extensive in situ component extending from the vermillion to the cutaneous lip. (B to D) Full-thickness defect with irregular contour is repaired with a mucosal advancement after the wound edges are sharply freshened to form a new smooth vermillion border. (E) Final appearance.

excision repairs, especially in patients who wear dentures.[20] If a wound defect is full-thickness, the internal portion of the wedge excision of mucosa can be shorter in vertical height than the external cutaneous portion of the wedge thus preserving additional muscle, submucosa, and mucosa.[15] The wound is closed in multiple layers beginning with buried vertical mattress sutures to close the mucosa. Orbicularis oris muscle is reapproximated with buried sutures. Dermal buried vertical mattress sutures are placed to maximize wound edge eversion. The vermillion border and wet lip mucosal internal borders are meticulously reapproximated with superficial guiding sutures followed by superficial sutures to provide additional eversion (Figs. 16.40A to L). If necessary, vertical mattress sutures can be placed to maximize wound edge eversion. M-plasty can be added to a linear closure if the incision length needs to be shortened (Figs. 16.41A to D).

## Advancement Flap Variations

Tissue laxity from the lateral lower cutaneous lip can be recruited with an A-to-T flap (Figs. 16.42 and 16.43), unilateral advancement flap (Figs. 16.44A to C), a unilateral advancement flap displaced to the melolabial fold utilizing the laxity of the cheek beyond the oral commissure (Figs. 16.45A to C), or an island (V-to-Y) advancement flap (Figs. 16.46A to C). Note that wide undermining is necessary to ensure adequate flap movement. Camouflage is enhanced with the incision placed along the vermillion border.

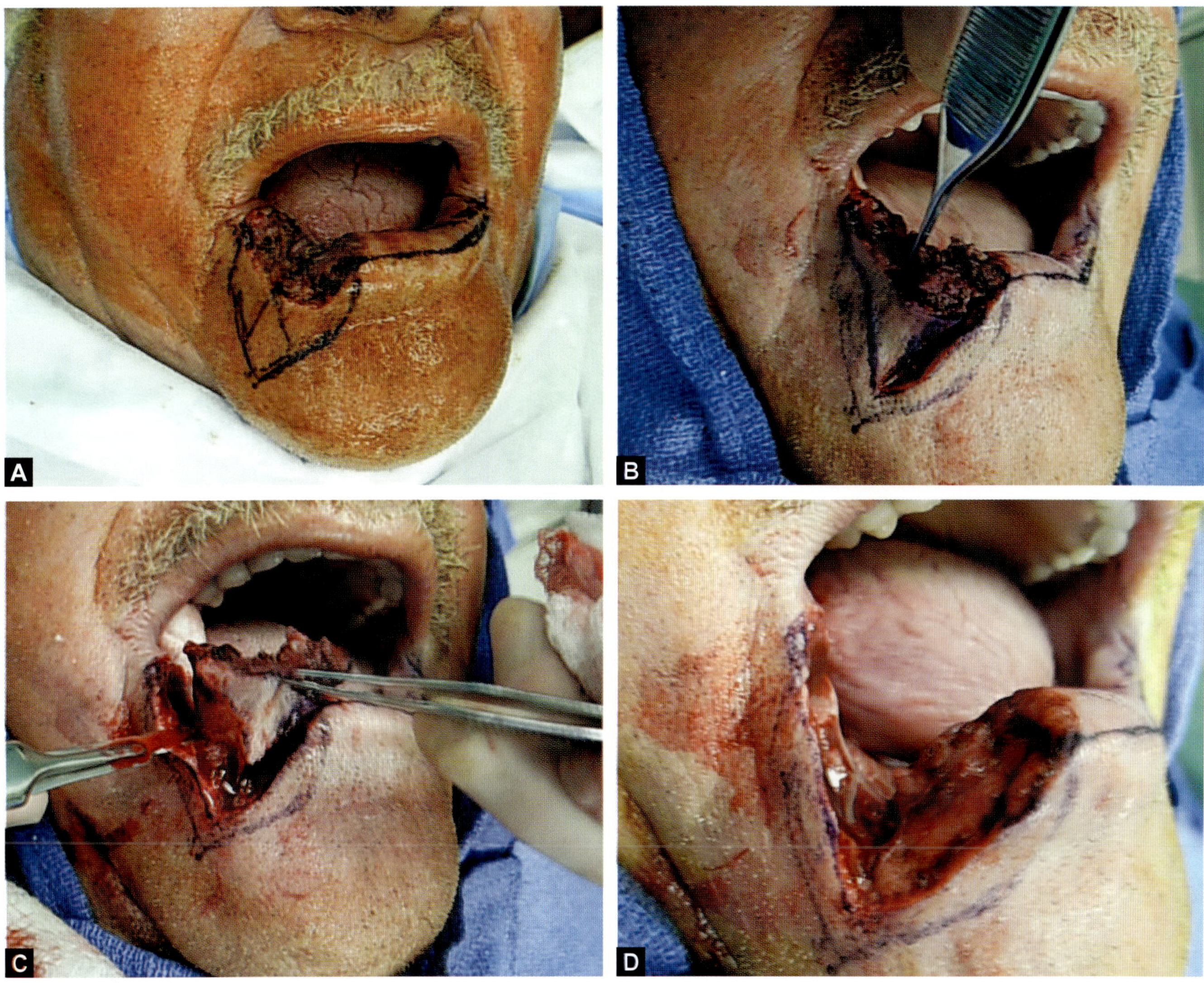


**Figs. 16.40A to D**

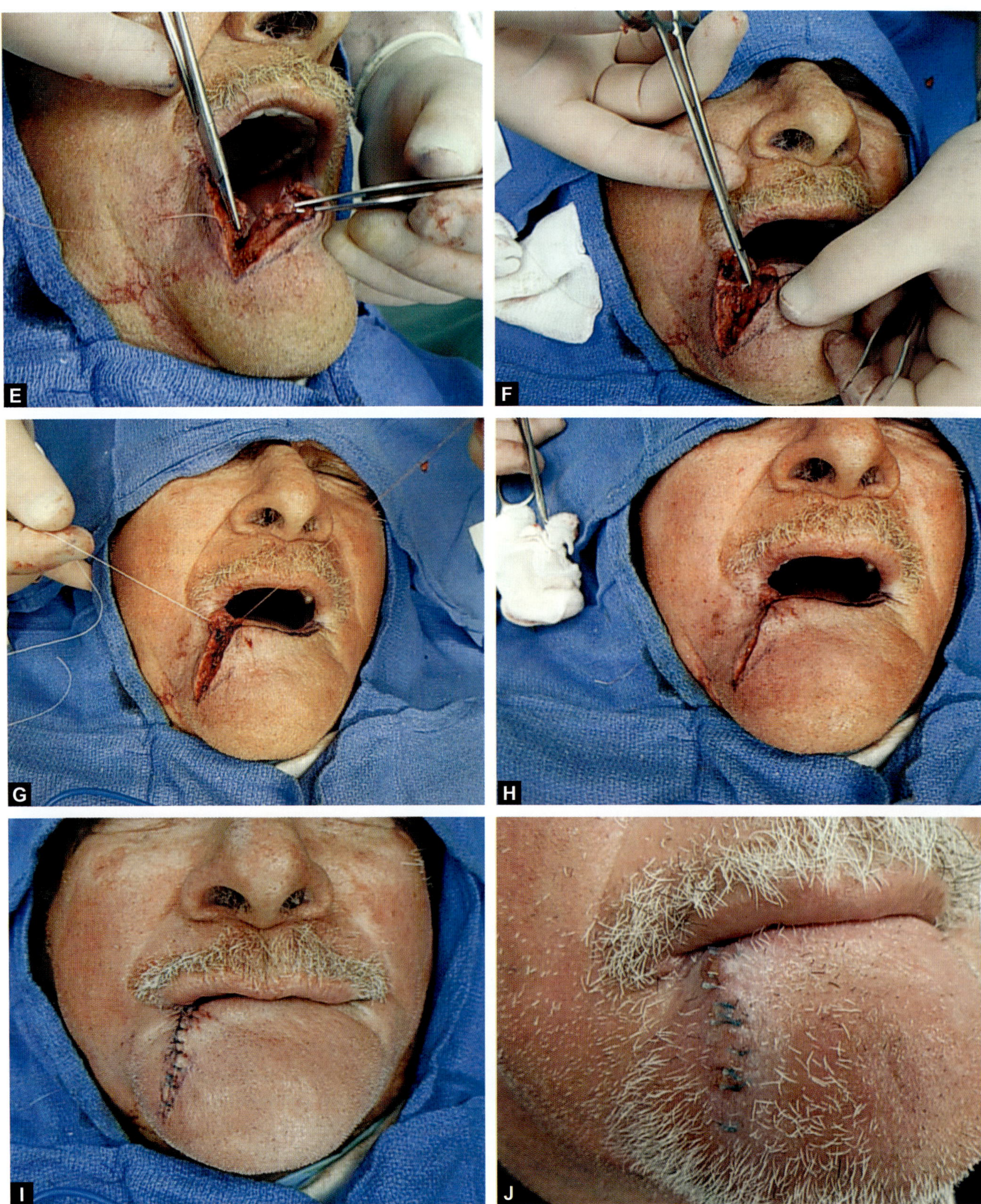


**Figs. 16.40E to J**

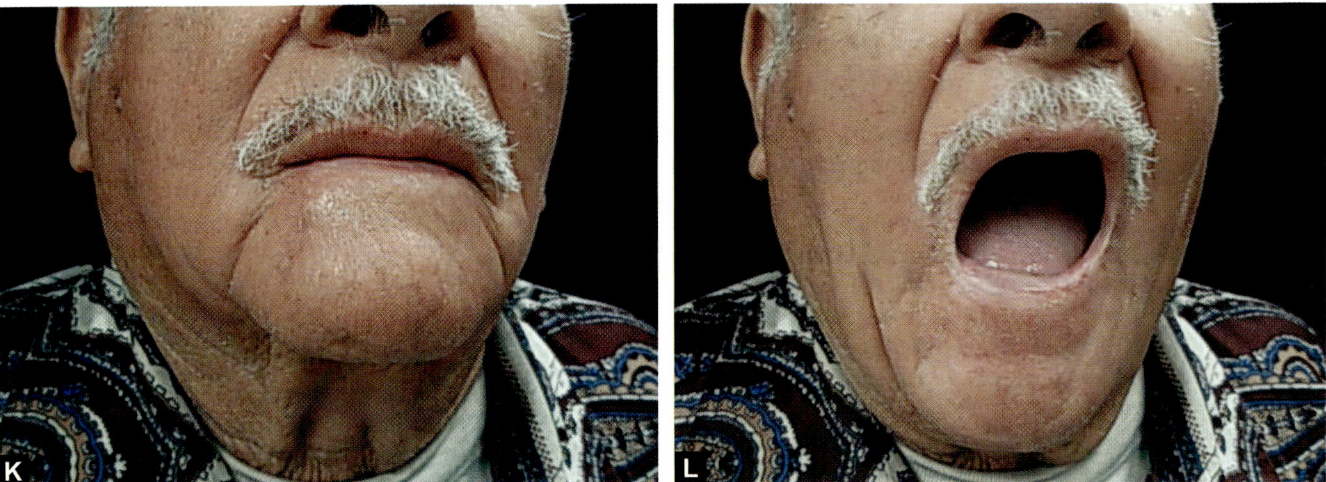


**Figs. 16.40A to L:** (A) Lower vermillion and cutaneous lip defect of approximately one-third the lower lip. (B to J) A full-thickness wedge of skin, subcutaneous fat, orbicularis oris muscle, submucosa, and mucosa was excised and repaired with a multilayered linear wound closure design. (K and L) Long-term follow-up with adequate opening of the oral aperture.

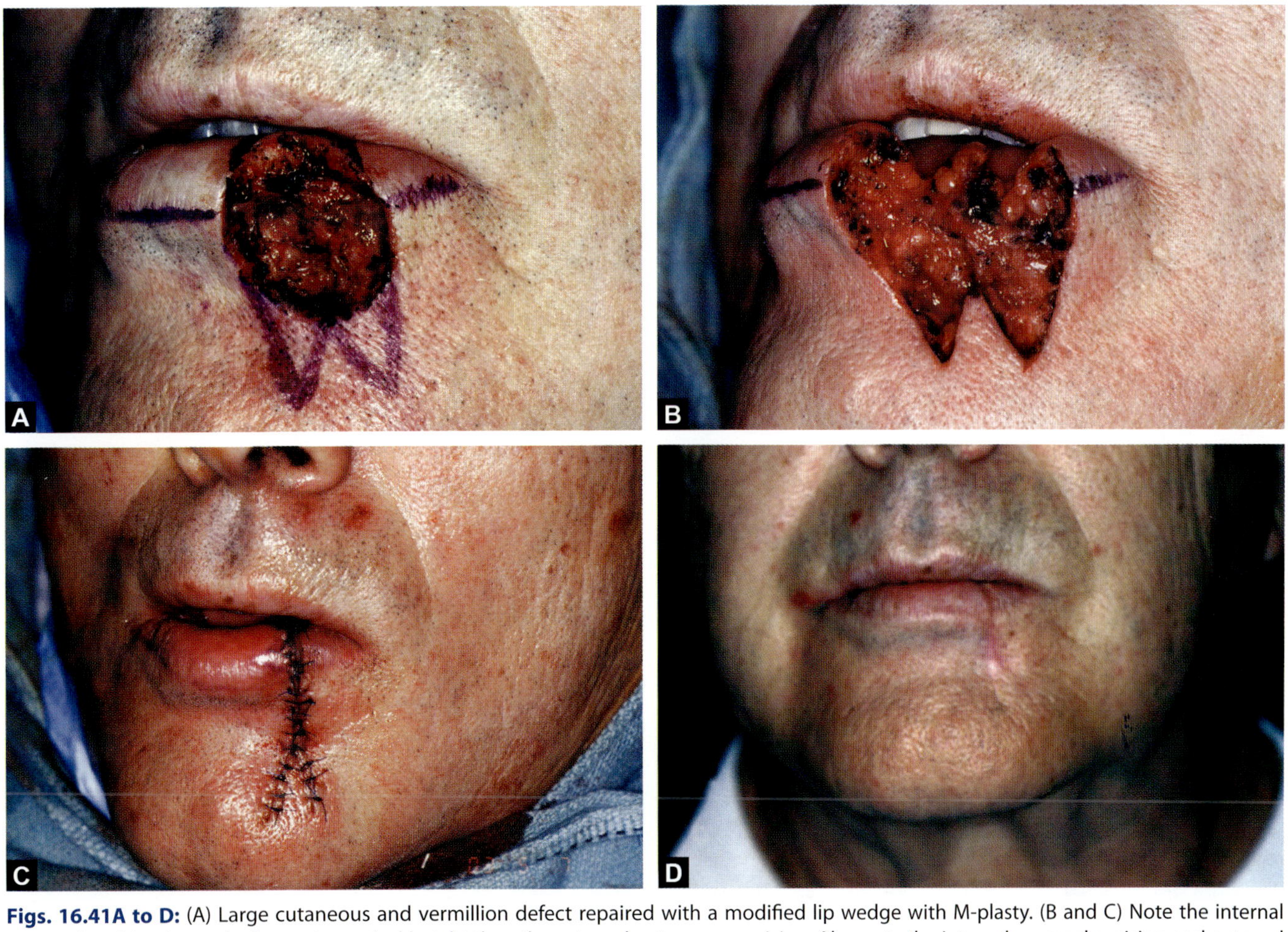

**Figs. 16.41A to D:** (A) Large cutaneous and vermillion defect repaired with a modified lip wedge with M-plasty. (B and C) Note the internal mucosal excision is much shorter in vertical height than the external cutaneous excision. Also note the internal mucosal excision and external cutaneous excision were both performed as M-plasties. (D) Final appearance.

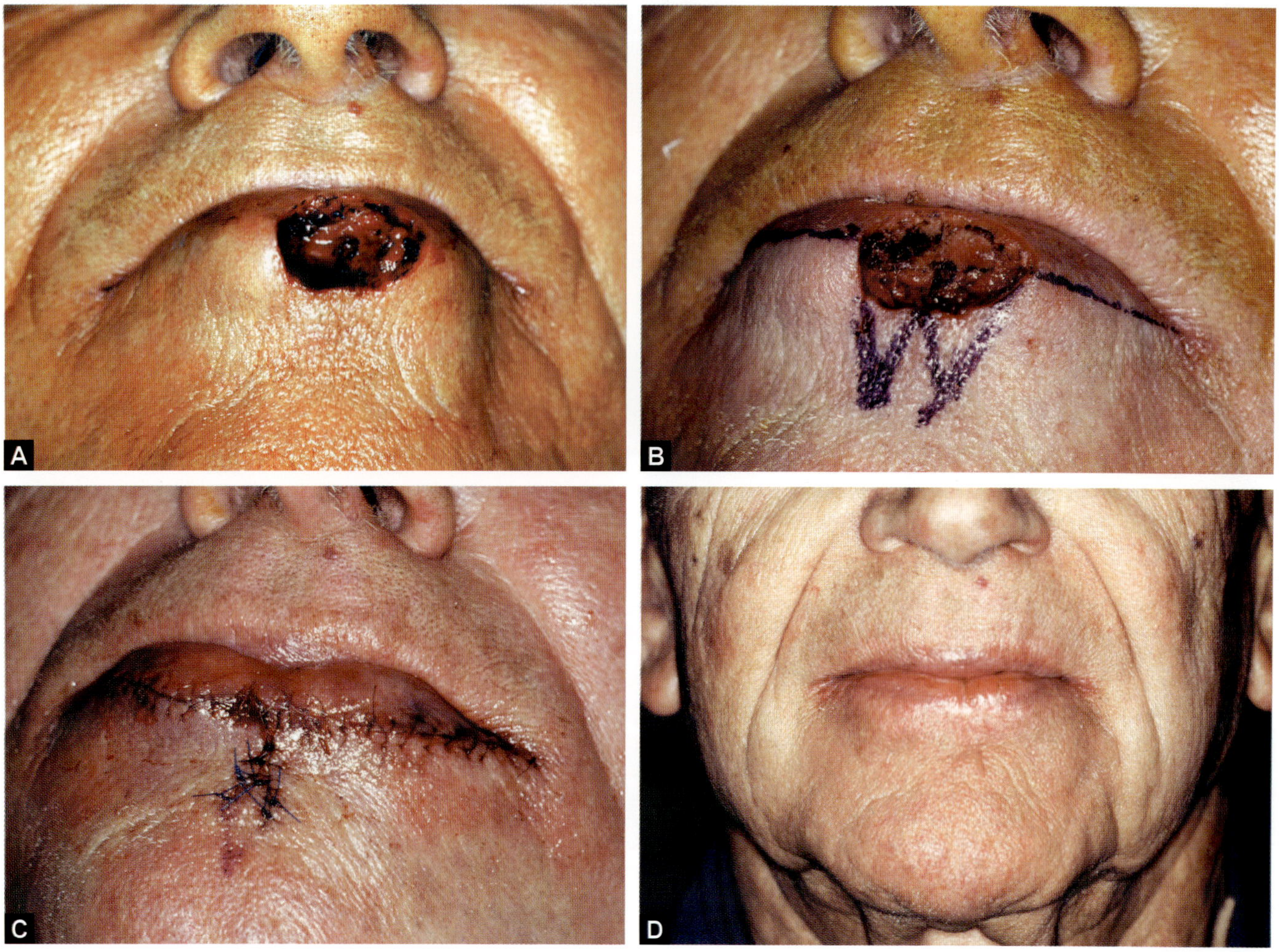

**Figs. 16.42A to D:** (A) Left of midline defect involving cutaneous and vermillion lip. The defect is superficial and does not involve underlying musculature. (B and C) Repaired with an A to T advancement flap with mucosal advancement. M-plasty used for inferior standing tissue cone to decrease suture length. (D) Final appearance.

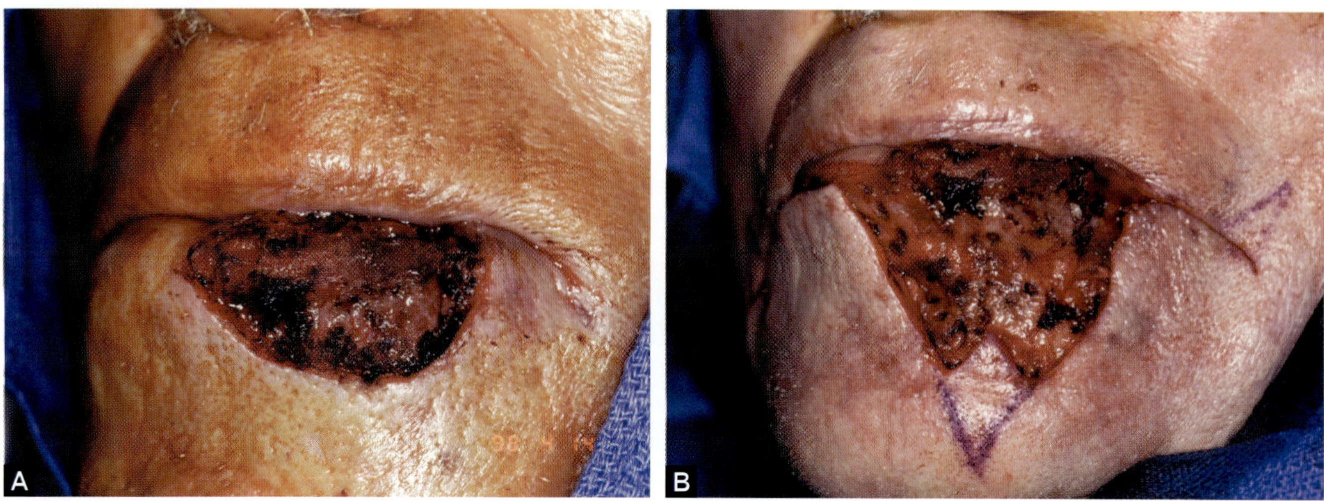


**Figs. 16.43A and B**

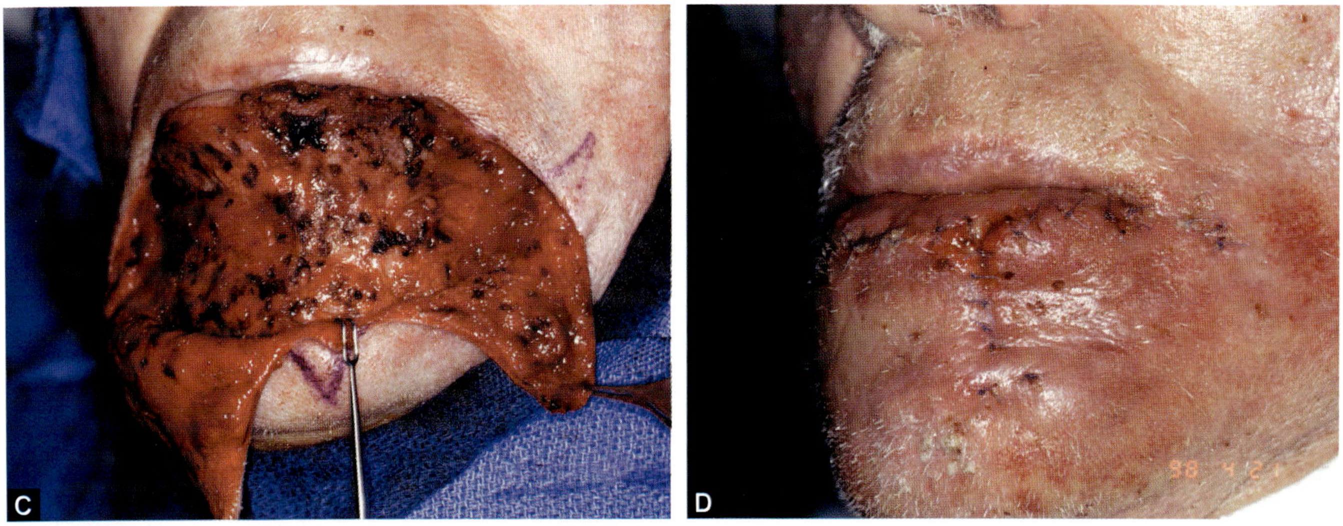

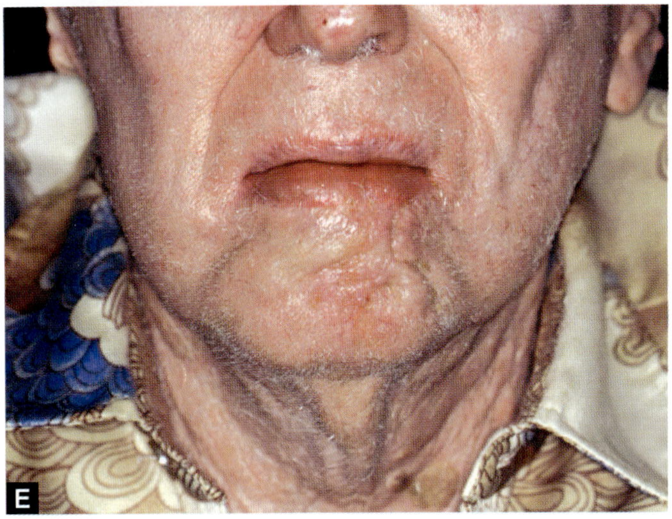

**Figs. 16.43A to E:** (A) Large cutaneous and vermillion defect with relative preservation of orbicularis oris muscle. (B to D) Repaired with an A to T advancement flap with M-plasty. (E) Final appearance.

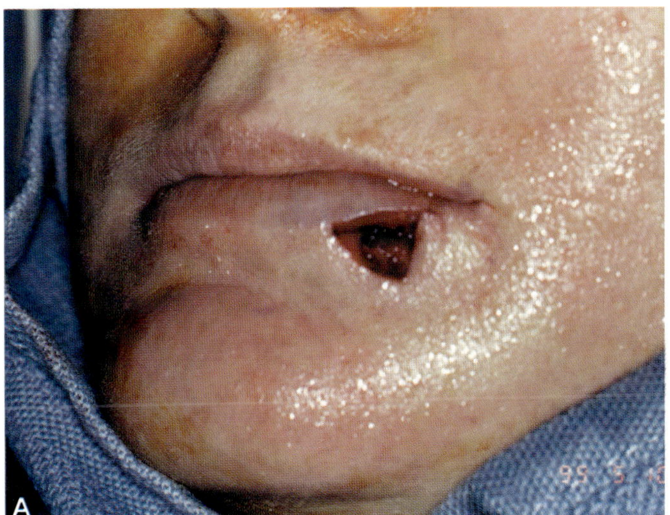

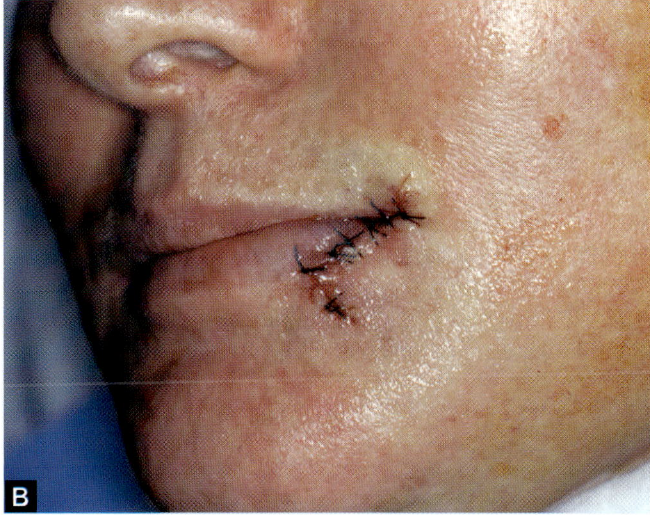

**Figs. 16.44A and B**

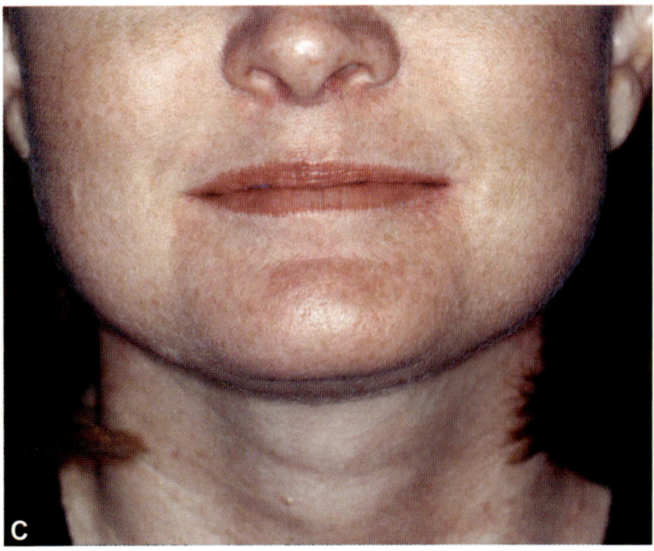

**Figs. 16.44A to C:** Lateral lower cutaneous lip defect repaired with a unilateral advancement flap with incision placed along vermillion border.

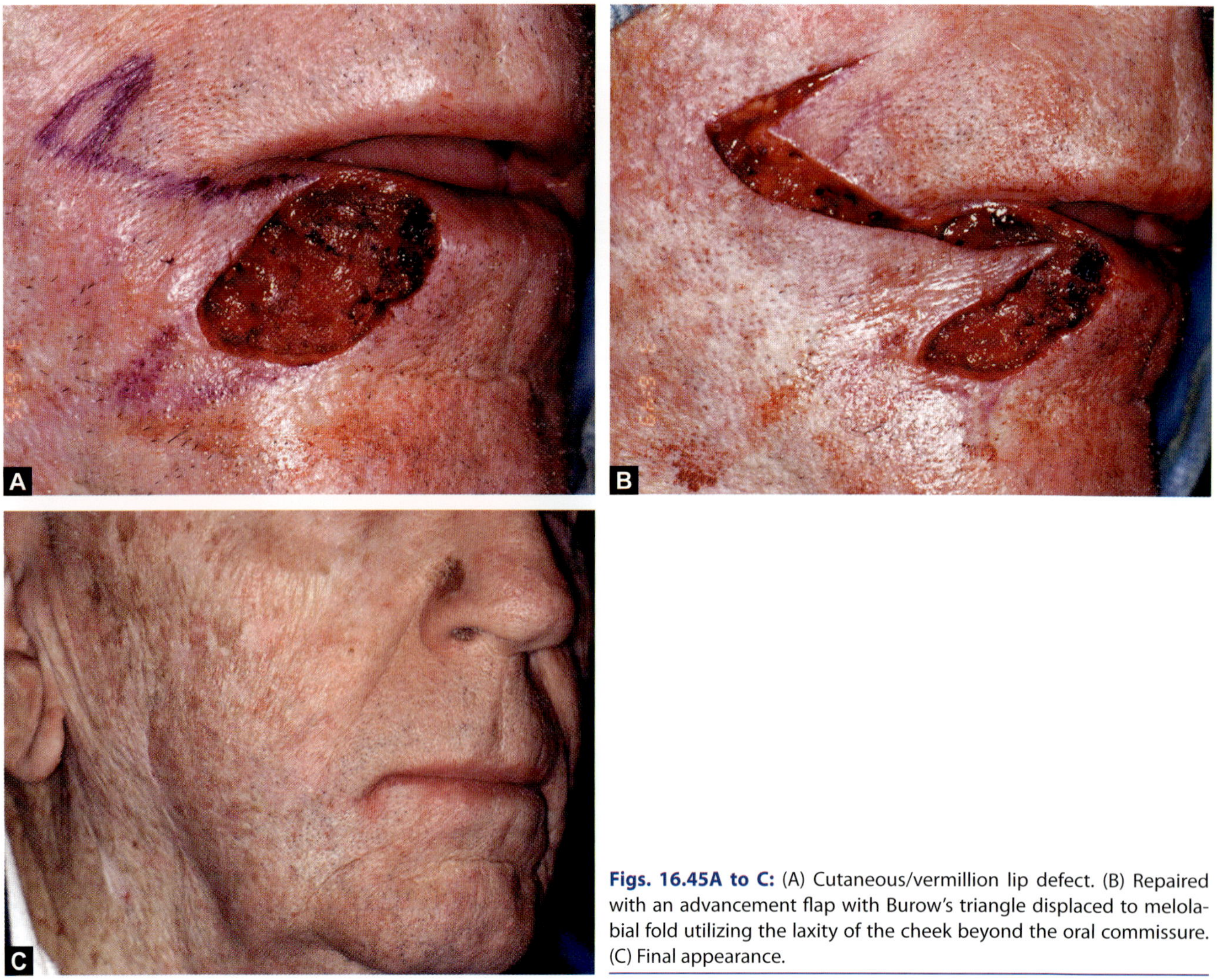

**Figs. 16.45A to C:** (A) Cutaneous/vermillion lip defect. (B) Repaired with an advancement flap with Burow's triangle displaced to melolabial fold utilizing the laxity of the cheek beyond the oral commissure. (C) Final appearance.

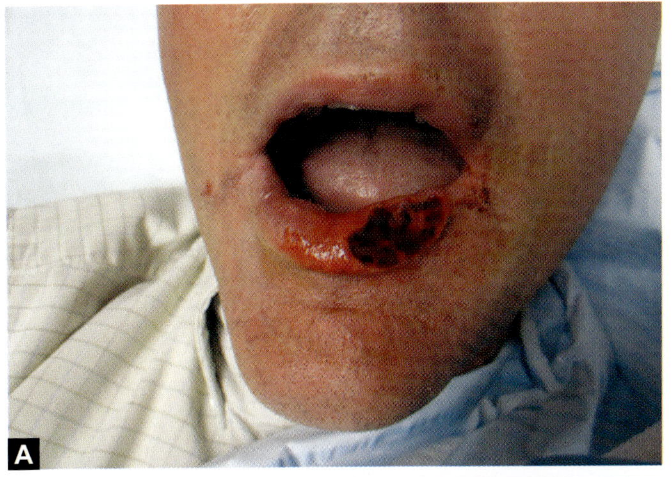
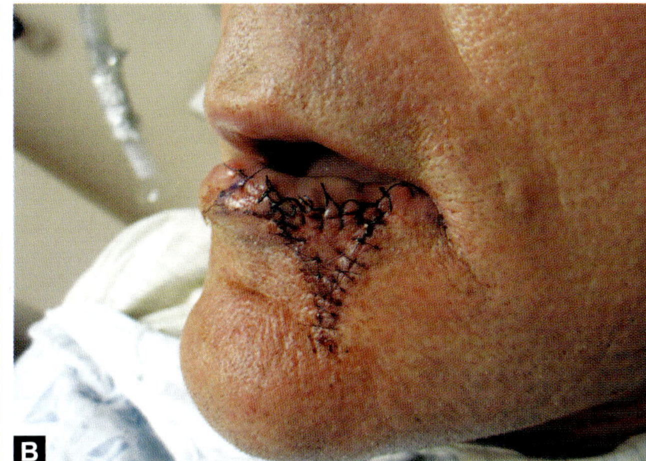
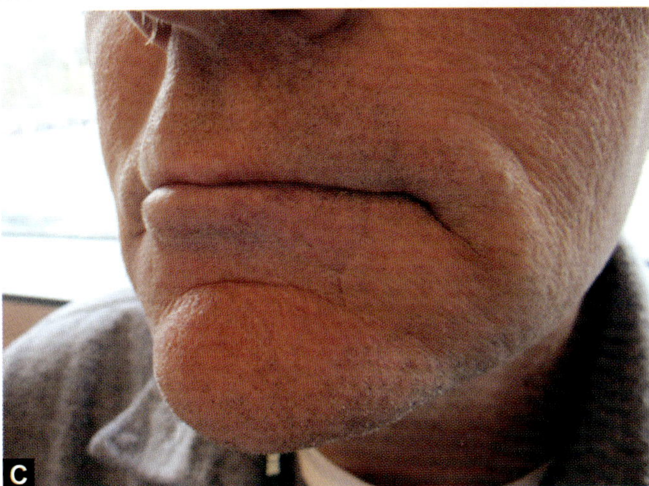

**Figs. 16.46A to C:** (A) Large defect involving the lower vermillion and cutaneous lip. (B) Repaired with combined Island (V-to-Y) advancement flap and mucosal advancement flap. (C) Final appearance.
*Courtesy*: S Brian Jiang, MD, Sang Diego, California, USA.

## SUMMARY

The lip and perioral cosmetic region is a vital component of the central face. Aesthetic and functional reconstruction of this region is challenging yet rewarding. Failure to restore function, cosmesis, symmetry, and shape can be distressing to the patient. Understanding the anatomy, reconstructive principles, and postoperative care is vital for optimal outcomes.

## REFERENCES

1. Baker S, Swanson N. Local Flaps in Facial Reconstruction. St Louis, MO: Mosby; 1995.
2. Epstein E, Epstein EJ. Skin Surgery. Springfield, IL: Charles C Thomas Pub Ltd; 1982.
3. Jackson I. Local Flaps in Head and Neck Reconstruction. St Louis, MO: Quality Medical Publishing Inc; 2002.
4. Nabili V, Knott PD. Advanced lip reconstruction: functional and aesthetic considerations. Facial Plast Surg. 2008;24: 92-104.
5. Wentzell JM, Lund JJ. Z-plasty innovations in vertical lip reconstructions. Dermatol Surg. 2011;37:1646-62.
6. Daraei P, Calligas JP, Katz E, et al. Reconstruction of upper lip avulsion after dog bite: case report and review of literature. Am J Otolaryngol. 2014;35:219-25.
7. Harris L, Higgins K, Enepekides D. Local flap reconstruction of acquired lip defects. Curr Opin Otolaryngol Head Neck Surg. 2012;20:254-61.
8. Liliav B, Zaluzec R, Hassid VJ, et al. Lip replantation: a viable option for lower lip reconstruction after human bites, a literature review and proposed management algorithm. J Plast Reconstr Aesthet Surg. 2012;65:e197-9.
9. O TM, Scheuermann-Poley C, Tan M, et al. Distribution, clinical characteristics, and surgical treatment of lip infantile hemangiomas. JAMA Facial Plast Surg. 2013; 15:292-304.
10. Mellette JR Jr, Chapman JT. Practical perioral closures. Semin Cutan Med Surg. 2003;22:255-62.
11. Gloster HM Jr. The use of second-intention healing for partial-thickness Mohs defects involving the vermilion and/or mucosal surfaces of the lip. J Am Acad Dermatol. 2002;47: 893-7.

12. Leonard AL, Hanke CW. Second intention healing for intermediate and large postsurgical defects of the lip. J Am Acad Dermatol. 2007;57:832-5.
13. Zitelli JA, Brodland DG. A regional approach to reconstruction of the upper lip. J Dermatol Surg Oncol. 1991;17:143-8.
14. Roenigk R, Roenigk H. Dermatologic Surgery Principles and Practice. New York, NY: Marcel Dekker Inc; 1988.
15. Goldman G, Dzubow L, Yelverton C. Facial Flap Surgery. New York, NY: McGraw-Hill; 2013.
16. Paniker PU, Mellette JR. A simple technique for repair of Cupid's bow. Dermatol Surg. 2003;29:636-40.
17. Matheson BK, Mellette JR Jr. Surgical pearl: clavicular grafts are "superior" to supraclavicular grafts. J Am Acad Dermatol. 1997;37:991-3.
18. Cook JL. Reconstruction of the lower lip. Dermatol Surg. 2001;27:775-8.
19. Wheeland RG. Reconstruction of the lower lip and chin using local and random-pattern flaps. J Dermatol Surg Oncol. 1991;17:605-15.
20. O'Quinn RP, Stasko T. Repair of the lower lip after Mohs micrographic surgery. Dermatol Surg. 2001;27:845-7.

# CHAPTER 17

# Reconstruction of the Cheek

*Daniel Y Sugai, Daihung V Do*

## INTRODUCTION

The cheek is the largest cosmetic subunit of the face, and occupies most of the middle third of the face. The cheek provides a large surface area susceptible to developing defects from trauma, burns, or neoplasm. As the largest cosmetic subunit of the face, proper reconstruction of the cheek is crucial for optimal cosmesis. Repair of the cheek should involve preserving symmetry, skin color, and skin texture. In addition, maintaining anatomical function is paramount given that the cheek aids in multiple functions such as speech and bolus formation. In planning for repair of the cheek, multiple factors should be considered including location, size and depth of the defect, patient age, subcutaneous fat distribution, and tissue quality and laxity.

## ANATOMY OF THE CHEEK

The cheek is a multilayered structure composed of superficial to deep layers: epidermis, dermis, subcutaneous tissue, and the superficial musculoaponeurotic system (SMAS). The underlying deep structures of the cheek include the branches of the facial nerve, the parotid gland, the buccal fat pad, and the mandible. The SMAS is confluent with the galea layer on the scalp, with the temporoparietal fascia in the temporal region, and continues as the superficial cervical fascia in the neck. In general, motor nerves are found deep to the SMAS and sensory branches are located superficial to it.

Anatomically, the cheek is defined superiorly by the infraorbital rim and zygomatic arch, laterally by the preauricular crease, inferiorly by the mandible, and medially by the nasofacial junction, nasolabial folds, and labiomandibular crease[1,2] (Fig. 17.1).

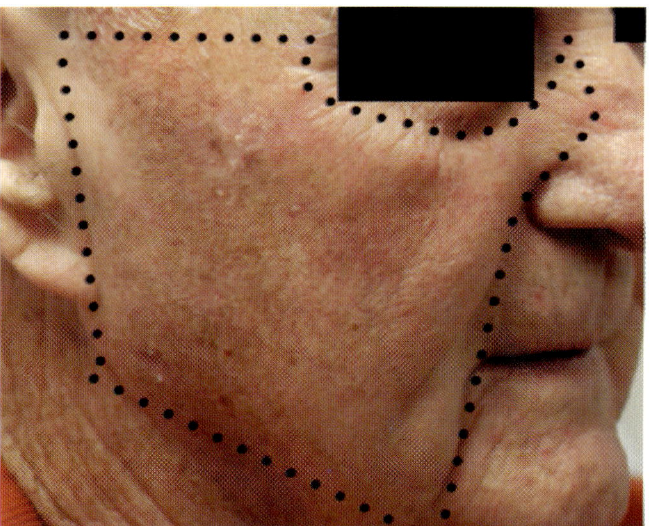

**Fig. 17.1:** Borders of the cheek. The cheek is bordered by (1) the infraorbital rim and zygomatic arch superiorly, (2) the preauricular crease laterally, (3) the mandible inferiorly, and (4) the nasofacial junction, nasolabial folds, and labiomandibular crease medially.

### Sensory Innervation

Sensory innervation is provided by the maxillary and mandibular divisions of the trigeminal nerve, which run above the SMAS. Medial and zygomatic cheek sensory innervation is provided by the maxillary division via the infraorbital, zygomaticofacial, and zygomaticotemporal branches. The lateral and buccal subunits are supplied by the mandibular division through the buccal and auriculotemporal branches, and the mental nerve innervates the inferomedial cheek.[2]

### Motor Innervation

Superficial facial muscles are innervated by the facial nerve and its branches. The facial nerve exits the stylomastoid

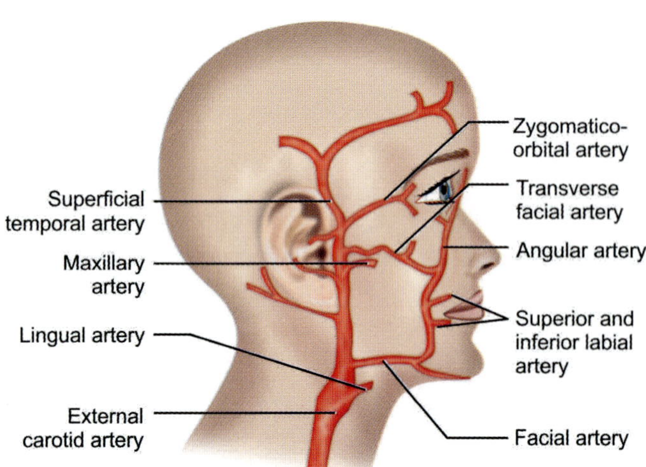


**Fig. 17.2:** Arterial vasculature of the cheek. The arterial supply of the cheek is provided by branches of the external carotid artery, including the superficial temporal artery which gives rise to the transverse facial artery that terminates into the angular artery.

foramen, and branches within the parotid gland. It is protected by the superficial lobe of the parotid gland. At the anterior border of the parotid gland, the facial nerve becomes superficial and is at risk of injury when raising local flaps in this region.[3] The facial nerve branches traverse deep to the SMAS before reaching the facial muscles. The marginal mandibular branch of the facial nerve is vulnerable over the lateral mandible; transection of this branch can lead to permanent weakness of the corner of the mouth.[4,5] The masseter and temporalis muscles are innervated by the trigeminal nerve.

## Vascular Supply

The arterial supply of the cheek (Fig. 17.2) is provided by branches of the external carotid artery, including the transverse facial artery, which arises from the superficial temporal artery and terminates into the angular artery. There is a small contribution from the infraorbital artery, which is a continuation of the maxillary artery, and supplies the mid cheek with anastomotic connections with the facial artery. The superficial temporal artery typically enters the parotidomasseteric fascia ~1 cm anterior and 1.75 cm superior to the external auditory canal, and breaks off into parietal and frontal branches.[6] The transverse facial artery branches off from the superficial temporal artery deep to the parotid gland and runs along the superficial surface of the masseteric fascia.[6] In the lateral face, septocutaneous perforators from the transverse facial artery connect to a dense subdermal plexus.[7] The random vasculature of the subdermal plexus feeds most local cheek reconstruction flaps.[8] In general, the venous drainage primarily runs with the arterial vasculature.

## Reconstruction Planning

The first consideration when approaching a cheek defect is the overall surgical context and whether resurfacing or reconstruction is more clinically appropriate. For tumors in which there is a high risk of recurrence, simply resurfacing the defect via second intention healing or a skin graft may be preferred to facilitate monitoring for recurrence. Timing of flap surgery is also important in overall success of reconstruction. Delayed complex flap reconstruction is warranted when adequacy of histological margins needs to be confirmed, especially for melanocytic tumors or tumors with aggressive features (perineural spread, microsatellitosis).[3] If there is a low likelihood that the tumor will recur, as for most nonmelanoma skin cancer following Mohs surgery, then reconstruction with the most aesthetically pleasing outcome while maximally preserving function is desired.

The second consideration is the depth and size of the defect. Deeper defects and defects which are large in size are more likely to pose functional problems. There is an increased risk for facial nerve involvement. In addition, the surgeon must consider the need for soft tissue bulk or intraoral lining. In through-and-through defects, most lining defects can be closed primarily or with small local flaps but sometimes a second regional or a microvascular free flap is required. Composite defects are addressed differently (i.e. scapular/parascapular free flap) as these defects extend beyond soft tissues and involve bone.[9] Multidisciplinary consultation with ear, nose and throat (ENT) or plastic surgery should be considered for extensive defects to ensure the best possible outcome for the patient.

Patient factors may influence the choice of repair. Some patients (particularly the elderly) may value a shorter operative time and care less about the cosmetic outcome. For these patients, second intention healing or more straightforward repair options should be selected. In patients who smoke, the risk of graft and flap failure should be considered.[10] Smoking cessation or reduction should be encouraged. For patients on anticoagulant therapy or who have intrinsic bleeding disorders, the risk of postoperative hemorrhage or hematoma formation should be considered. Minimizing undermining to what is necessary and placing postoperative drains may mitigate this risk. Patients with a prior history of radiation treatment in the operative area have impaired healing and have increased skin fibrosis depending on the radiation dose received, the number of fractions, and the length of time that has passed since the radiation treatment occurred.[11,12] Unless skin flaps originate from nonirradiated areas, flaps tend to fare poorly due to increased skin fibrosis resulting in little to no secondary flap movement, decreased flap mobility, and impaired vascularity of irradiated skin. Split-thickness skin grafts and second intention healing are preferred for defects on previously irradiated skin. Similarly, these types of repairs are preferred for patients with other fibrotic skin disorders such as scleroderma and chronic graft-versus-host disease.

Finally, the location and shape of the defect should be considered when designing an operative plan. It is often helpful to consider the reconstructive ladder. When possible, primary closure is preferred for its simplicity, quick healing time, and lower health care cost. If primary closure will result in tissue distortion or functional impairment, second intention healing should be considered, particularly in areas that tend to heal well with such an approach. In cases where a defect cannot be closed primarily or by second intention, closure alternatives include local flaps, free flaps, or skin grafts.

The design, position, and orientation of the flap are dictated by many factors including defect location, size, shape, and depth; regional skin laxity; and presence of nearby free margins.

## Second Intention

Second intention healing is the simplest form of reconstruction and involves three processes: wound contraction, re-epithelialization, and scar formation.[13] It is appropriate for small (< 1 cm), superficial defects on concave surfaces such as the preauricular sulcus. Facial regions with concave contours (nose, ears, temple) allow high rates of mechanical contraction leading to favorable results with just local wound care.[14] Defects in these areas heal with excellent cosmetic outcomes, especially if they are < 2 cm in size.[13,15] Because the cheek is predominantly a convex surface, there will be less contraction of the wound. The wound surface area that is not covered by contraction will fill in with scar tissue, and thus lead to surface and color irregularities as well as contour irregularities, which can be accentuated by the overall convex shape of the cheek.[1] Moreover, incision lines over convex surfaces typically become tethered and depressed. Thus, second intention healing is usually not employed for large cheek defects, especially in the preauricular region as scar contraction could put tension on the free margins of the ear.[16] Situations in which second intention healing would be considered include defects < 1 cm and defects close to the canthi. Primary closure adjacent to the canthi runs the risk of deforming the contour of the eye and causing ectropion.[9]

Healing by second intention can be considered in buccal mucosal defects < 2 cm. If the buccal mucosal defect is > 2 cm, scar contracture from secondary healing can yield significant trismus and visible external dimpling.[9]

## Primary Intention

Primary closure should be considered for small to medium cheek defects, especially in elderly patients who have excess skin laxity (Figs. 17.3A to C). In elderly patients, defects up to 4 cm in width can be closed primarily after wide undermining, especially in the buccal subunit.[17] This approach is also favorable in patients with pronounced rhytides. Scars should be hidden in rhytides, relaxed skin tension lines, or natural creases and folds. In the zygomatic subunit, primary closure with an ellipse within crow's feet rhytides is desired[2] (Figs. 17.4A to C).

The infraorbital rim, nasolabial fold, preauricular crease, and inferior mandibular margins are useful anatomic structures in camouflaging scar lines. Extension of the ellipse into the lateral canthus can be avoided with an M-plasty, and thus prevent distortion of the lower lid or canthus.[2] Small defects (< 1 cm) in the lateral subunit are often amenable to primary closure with a vertically oriented scar in the preauricular crease.[2] Defects > 30% of the cheek unit are not suitable for primary closure and usually require transposition or rotation of residual cheek and neck skin.[18]

## Local, Regional, Distant/Free Flaps

Local cheek flaps involve tissue adjacent to the primary defect being used for advancement, transposition, and rotation. Local flaps are best used for small to medium sized cheek defects, which are not amenable to primary closure. Because local flaps are in close proximity to the defect, they excel at providing matches in skin color, texture, and thickness through the principle of "replacing like with like."[17] The choice of flap is often determined by

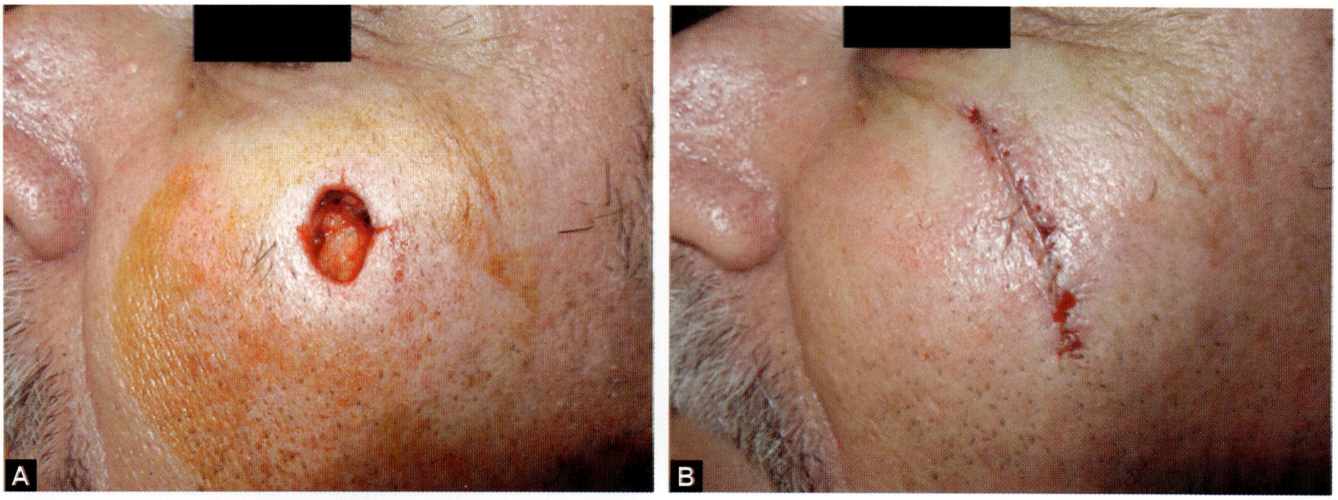

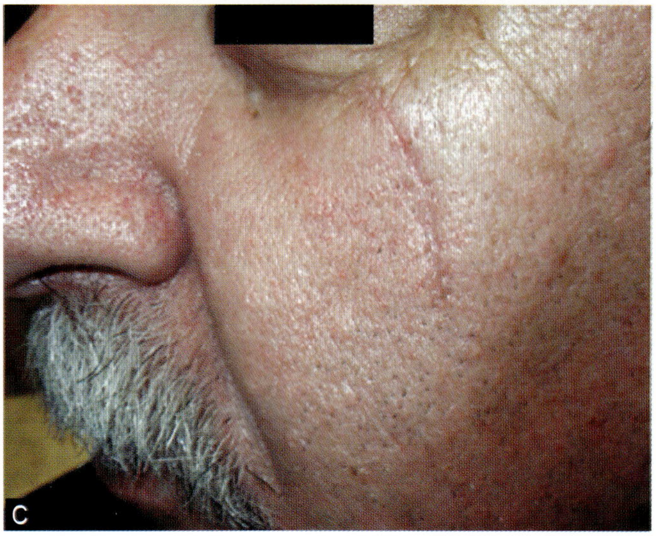

**Figs. 17.3A to C:** Primary closure should be oriented within pre-existing folds or rhytides. (A) Mohs defect of the left zygomatic cheek. (B) Primary closure. (C) Repair at 3 weeks.

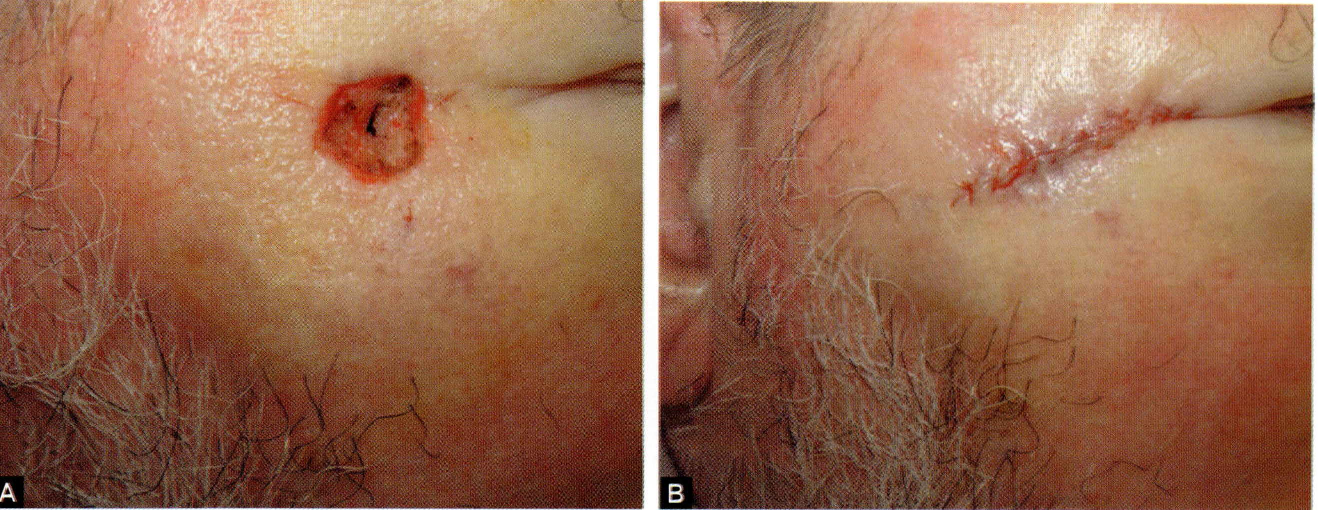


**Figs. 17.4A and B**

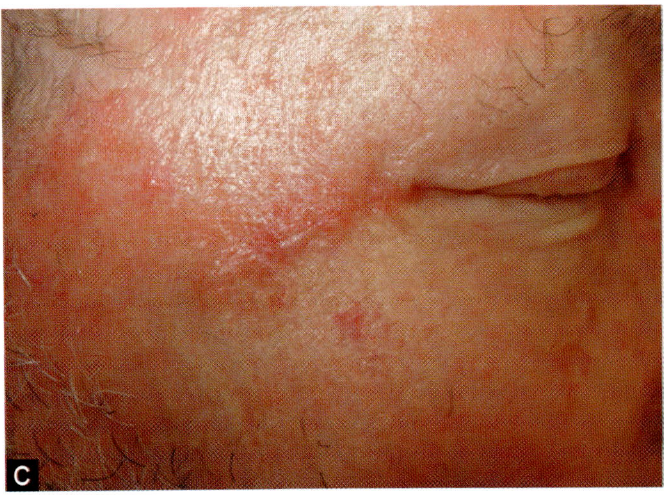

**Figs. 17.4A to C:** Primary closure utilized near the eye without distortion of the lateral canthus. (A) Mohs defect of the upper right zygomatic cheek adjacent to the lateral canthus. (B) Primary closure. (C) Repair at 3 weeks.

the defect location: lateral, medial, zygomatic, and buccal subunits.

Often, there is a choice in terms of the location from which tissue is recruited. Designing flaps properly to recruit skin with the best match for color and texture will optimize cosmesis. Common sites from adjacent units in relation to the cheek include the neck, submental area, or chest. Flaps taken from these locations can be anterior- or posterior-based rotation advancement flaps. Large, complex, or deep wounds should be reconstructed with distant or free flaps but this may come with the disadvantage of poor skin color and texture match.[18] Finally, the flaps should be designed to place scars at the borders of cosmetic subunits when possible.[2]

## Skin Grafts

Full-thickness and split-thickness skin grafting are feasible modalities in providing external coverage of cheek defects, especially in patients with multiple comorbidities who cannot undergo prolonged anesthesia. A temporary graft is particularly useful while assessing for adequate tumor margins after excision of skin cancer of the cheek. Full-thickness skin grafts harvested from the melolabial fold, postauricular sulcus, and preauricular crease yield the best results in regards to color, character, and texture match whereas skin taken from other areas may produce color and texture mismatch.[2,17] The supraclavicular region provides a larger area for full-thickness grafts; however, the texture and color are often different from cheek skin.[2]

The effect of skin graft contraction should be considered for defects near free margins such as the eyelid, nasal margin, or oral commissure. Skin grafts should be carefully planned near the lower eyelid because primary and secondary contracture results in a high risk of developing ectropion.[19] A Frost suture may be used to suspend the lower lid to improve the survival of the graft and decrease the chance of causing ectropion. Split-thickness skin grafts are more susceptible to contraction and subsequent distortion. Split-thickness grafts offer larger amounts of donor tissue but are less durable and the donor site morbidity is greater than with full-thickness grafts.[2] The scalp is a favorable donor site as it is in close proximity to cheek defects and the donor site is camouflaged by hair.[2]

## Location

For reconstructive planning, multiple classification systems have been proposed which divide the cheek into distinct regions based on similar anatomic considerations or similar skin attributes such as color, texture, and thickness. Classically, the cheek is divided into four cosmetic subunits: medial, zygomatic, buccal, and lateral (Fig. 17.5). For surgical defects in each of these areas, there are common reconstructive considerations.

## Lateral Subunit

The lateral subunit of the cheek represents the preauricular area extending from the zygomaticotemporal region superiorly to the angle of the mandible inferiorly. The skin of the preauricular region is moderately fixed to the SMAS overlying the parotid gland and has less subcutaneous fat.[20] However, the ear has a fixed location and provides no tissue reservoir for local flaps. Because this subunit is the most laterally located subunit of the face, scars in this

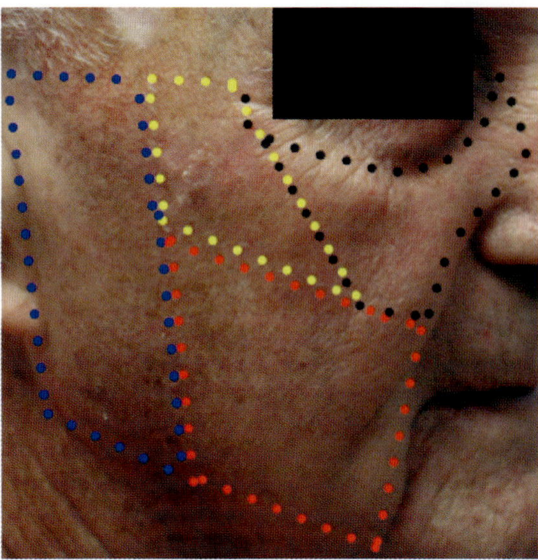

**Fig. 17.5:** Subunits of the cheek. The cheek contains the medial, zygomatic, buccal, and lateral subunits. The cheek is only flat laterally in the buccal and lateral subunits and has a convex surface over the zygomatic bone and medial cheek.

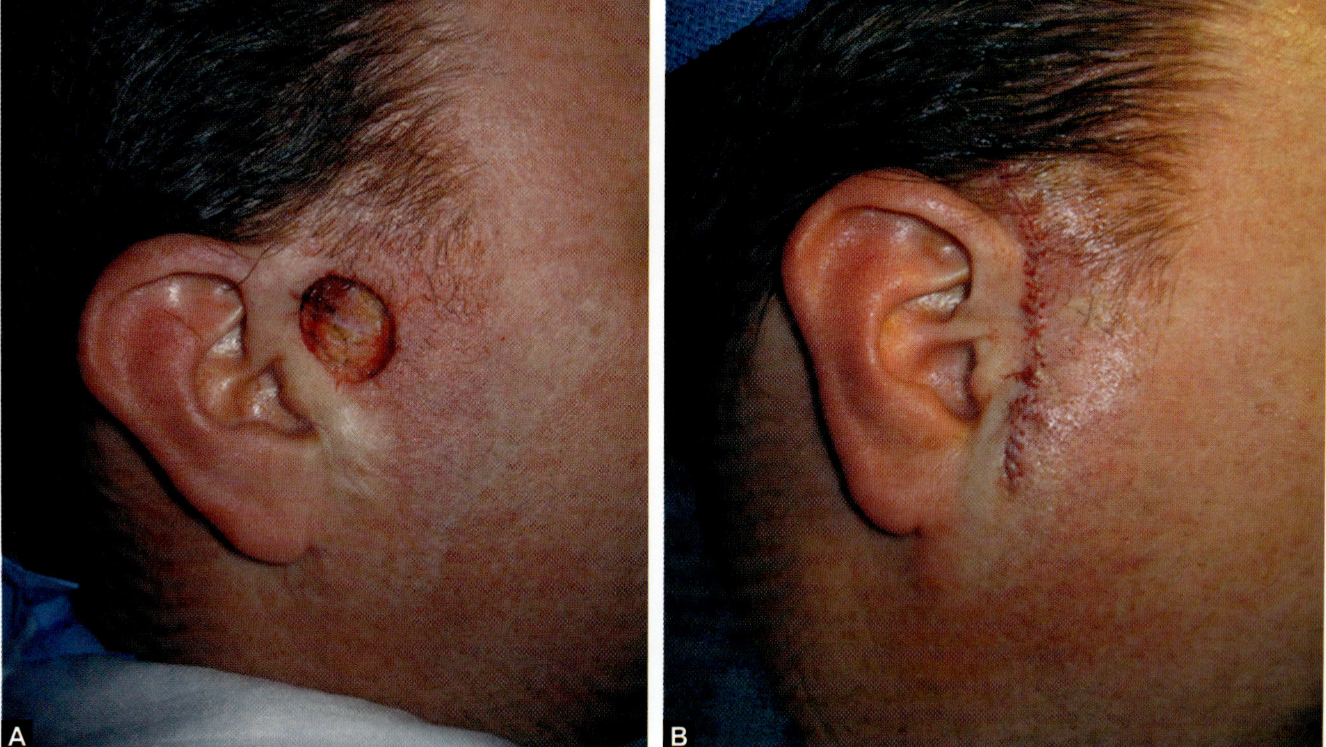

**Figs. 17.6A and B:** Mohs defect of the preauricular cheek. (A) A 41-year-old man underwent Mohs surgery for a nodular basal cell carcinoma (BCC) on the right preauricular area resulting in a 20 × 15 mm surgical defect. (B) Primary closure is placed within the preauricular crease.

area are less noticeable than more centrally located subunits. Caution should be used when dealing with large and deep defects in the preauricular region, as there is inherent risk of injury to multiple branches of the facial nerve and superficial temporal artery.

Small defects in the lateral subunit are best repaired with primary closure (Figs. 17.6A and B). There is typically a small amount of laxity and redundancy of the skin immediately anterior to the ear. When possible, the defect should be closed vertically to place the incision in the preauricular

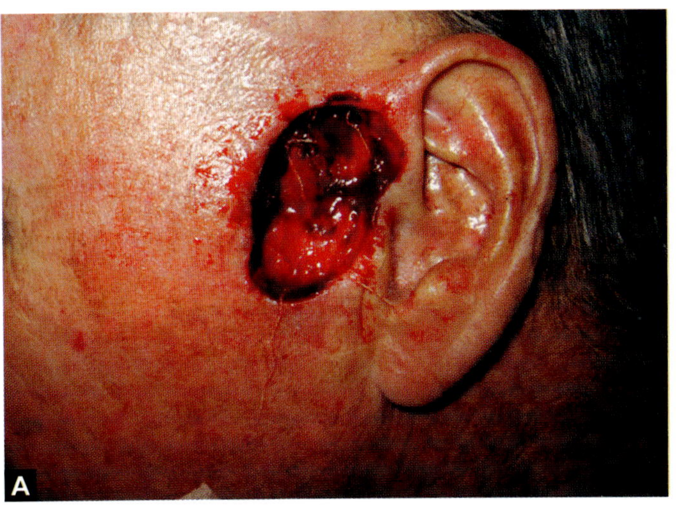

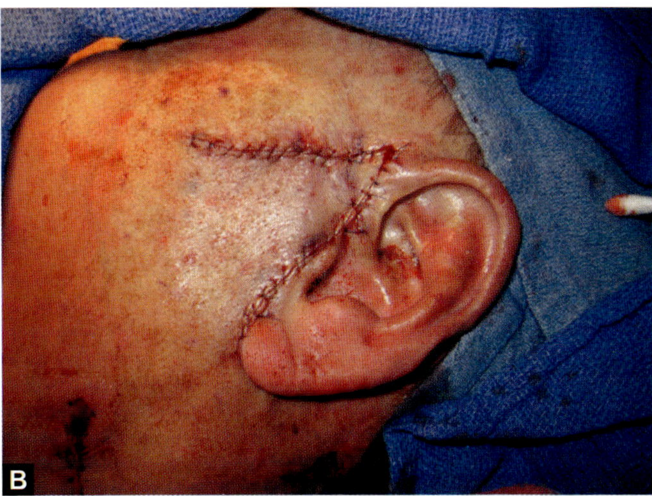

**Figs. 17.7A and B:** Advancement flap for repair of preauricular cheek defect. (A) A 71-year-old man who underwent Mohs surgery for a squamous cell carcinoma (SCC) which cleared in two stages resulting in a 24 × 16 mm defect on the left preauricular area. (B) Repair with a unilateral nonpedicled advancement flap.

sulcus so that the resultant scar is less conspicuous. If the defect is located slightly more anteriorly in men, closure with primary intent with the scar oriented vertically along the anterior border of the sideburn may also be acceptable.

For defects that extend from the lateral subunit onto the tragus (particularly in men), a vertically oriented closure may result in pulling the sideburn onto the tragus. In this situation, it may be preferable to leave the portion of the defect on the tragus to heal via second intention while closing above and below. Because the tragus projects out from the ear, there is concavity just anterior to it that heals well with second intention. In patients with long sideburns, small defects may also be successfully closed horizontally since most of the scar will be hidden in the sideburn. For slightly larger defects that cannot be closed vertically because they exceed the side-to-side tissue laxity of the preauricular area, closing in the horizontal direction should be considered, as there is laxity in the lower cheek and neck to be utilized.

Advancement flaps are suitable for small to medium-sized cheek defects that cannot be closed linearly[17] (Figs. 17.7A and B). Unipedicled flaps are the most commonly employed advancement flap since the neck presents a nearby tissue reservoir. Bipedicle flaps are less commonly used as there is very little laxity from the temple that can be utilized. V-Y advancement flaps are less useful in the lateral subunit where there is very little underlying fat and the overlying skin is more tightly tethered to the underlying SMAS unlike the more mobile medial subunit.[17] For these reasons, V-Y advancement flaps are at increased risk of necrosis from high tension in the lateral subunit.[16]

Rotational flaps work extremely well in the repair of large cheek defects larger than 3–4 cm in diameter within the lower preauricular area by recruiting tissue from the neck.[21] For defects measuring 3–6 cm in diameter, bilobed flaps can be used to transpose adjacent tissue into the lateral cheek defect.[17,22]

Large cervicofacial advancement/rotation flaps are typically used to treat large and deep defects in the lateral subunit (Figs. 17.8A and B). The anterior-based cervicofacial advancement/rotation flap in this region may have a preauricular and postauricular portion designed to transpose over the ear.[16] Anterior-based flaps are useful for posterior and moderate-sized anterior cheek defects. When a greater arc of rotation is needed, a pectoral extension can be used. Large posterior or lower cheek defects up to 10 cm can be repaired with an extended anterior-based cervicofacial flap converting it into a cervicopectoral flap.[18] Lower cheek defects below a line between the tragus and oral commissure are good candidates for the anteriorly based cervicopectoral flap.[18]

In addition to the anteriorly based cervicofacial flap, other regional flaps such as the deltopectoral, platysma myocutaneous, and pectoralis major flaps can also be used. The deltopectoral flap carries many disadvantages, including random vascularization of the distal third, multiple staged nature with a delayed procedure being typically necessary, and a conspicuous skin grafted donor site.[16,18] The platysma myocutaneous flap can be easily

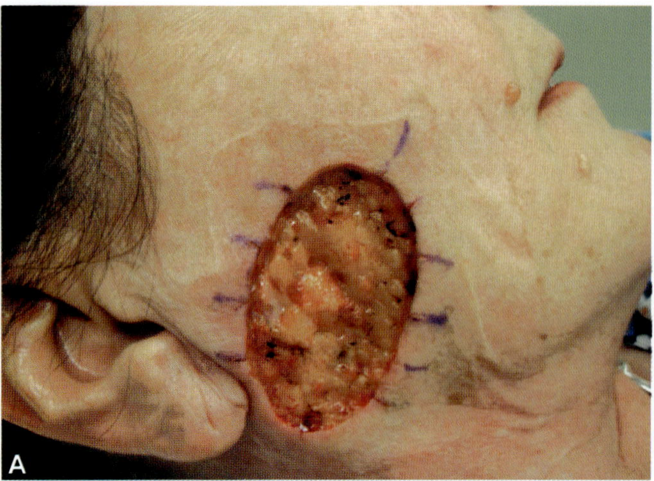


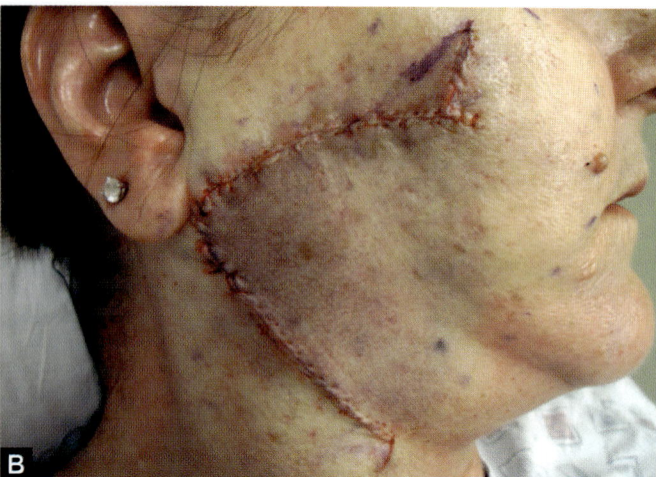


**Figs. 17.8A and B:** Cervicofacial advancement flap utilized for a large lateral cheek defect. (A) A 58-year-old woman who presented for slow Mohs for a lentigo maligna melanoma resulting in a 54 × 33 mm defect. (B) Repair with an anteriorly based cervicofacial advancement flap.

harvested and is a thin, pliable flap.[8] However, it is not a popular choice given its problems with vascularity, and significant rates of partial or total flap necrosis through venous congestion.[18] The pectoralis major flap is unique in that it provides pliable chest skin for both intraoral lining and external coverage (able to cover infraorbital region defect) by folding the flap as a double island technique in full thickness defects.[17]

## Medial Subunit

The superior margin of the medial subunit involves the cheek–eyelid junction where the skin texture becomes finer.[2] Static and dynamic rhytides are common in this region. Underlying the superficial tissues of the cheek-lower eyelid junction are the lower orbital fibers of the orbicularis oculi muscle.[2]

The medial border is defined by the nasofacial sulcus, perialar area, and the melolabial fold. The melolabial bulge is an extension of the buccal fat pad,[1] and descends with age and with increasing tissue laxity.[23] The melolabial crease is indistinct at birth given the abundant layer of subcutaneous fat in the infant face. This fold becomes more pronounced with age, due to changes in the amount and distribution of buccal fat with aging. The architecture of the melolabial crease and bulge should be considered to maintain symmetry during reconstruction planning. In addition, the position and function of the lower eyelid, nose, and mouth must be respected during reconstruction in the medial subunit where ectropion, lateral shifting of the nasal sidewall, alar splaying, and changes in oral commissure position are potential postsurgical complications when repairing the medial cheek.[24]

For small defects of the medial cheek in or near the nasofacial sulcus, primary closure should be considered with the scar placed along the cosmetic junction line where it will not cause ectropion (Figs. 17.9 and 17.10). To avoid tenting, the deep sutures should include a portion of the underlying tissues to tether the skin edges down.

For medium size defects in this area, which are not amenable to primary closure, advancement/rotation flaps are favored due to the ability to hide the scar along cosmetic junction units.[2] Anteriorly based advancement/rotation flaps (Fig. 17.11A) are performed by making an incision along the inferior border of the cutaneous lower eyelid to recruit tissue from the lateral cheek.[2] A standing cone should be removed inferiorly and placed in the melolabial junction if possible. Alternatively, a posteriorly based advancement/rotation flap (Fig. 17.11B) can be used in which tissue is recruited from the portion of the cheek inferior to the defect. The incision is made inferiorly along the nasofacial sulcus and extending into the nasolabial fold. Pexing sutures from just behind the flap tip to the infraorbital rim are placed to reduce the risk of ectropion.[25]

A variant of the posterior-based advancement/rotation flap is the superomedial rotation flap (Fig. 17.12). This flap is a random-pattern, crescentic, sliding cheek rotation

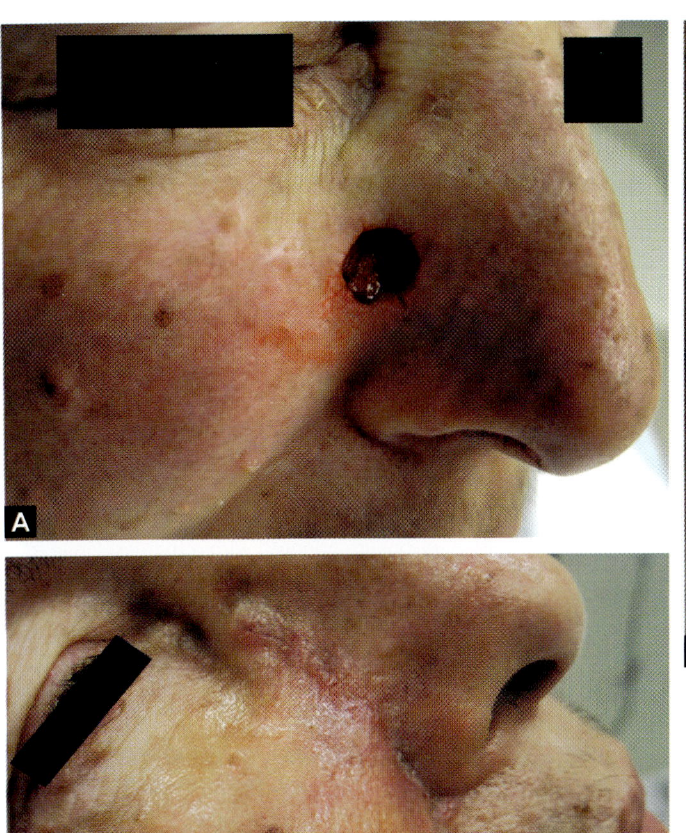


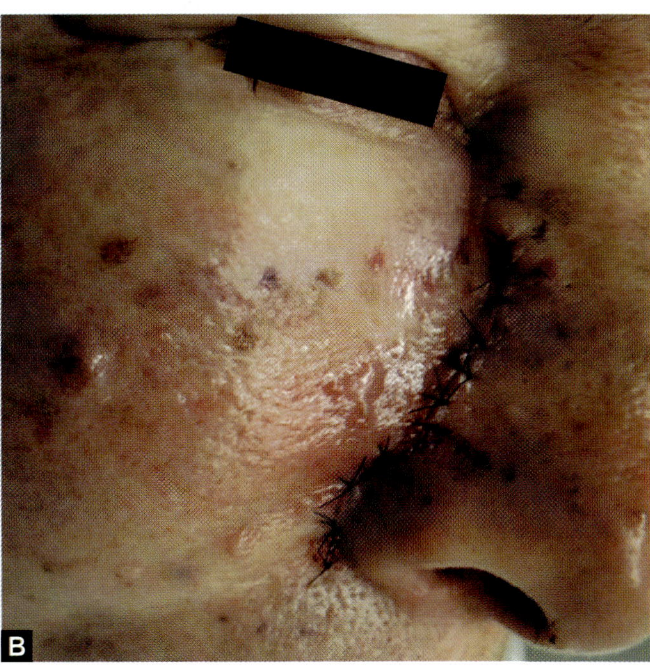


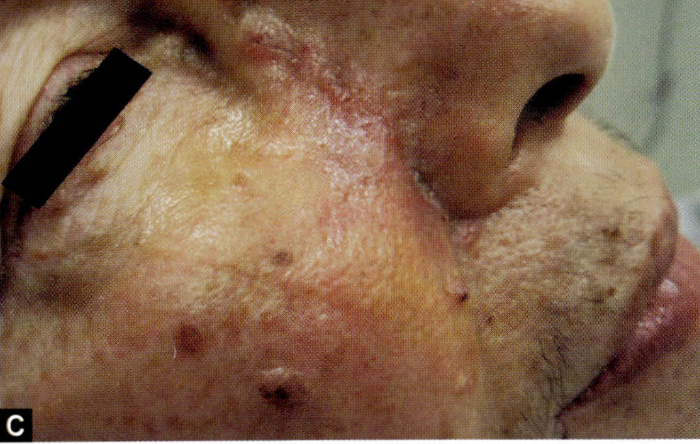


**Figs. 17.9A to C:** Primary repair of medial cheek defect. (A) A 71-year-old woman who underwent Mohs surgery for a nodular basal cell carcinoma (BCC) on the right nasofacial sulcus resulting in a 10 × 8 mm defect. (B) Primary closure with the incision lines placed along cosmetic junction lines. (C) Follow-up 1 week later.

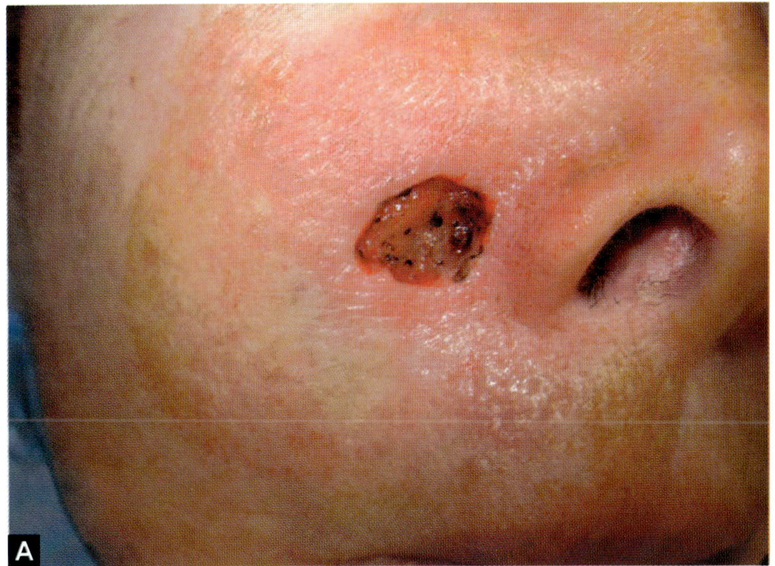


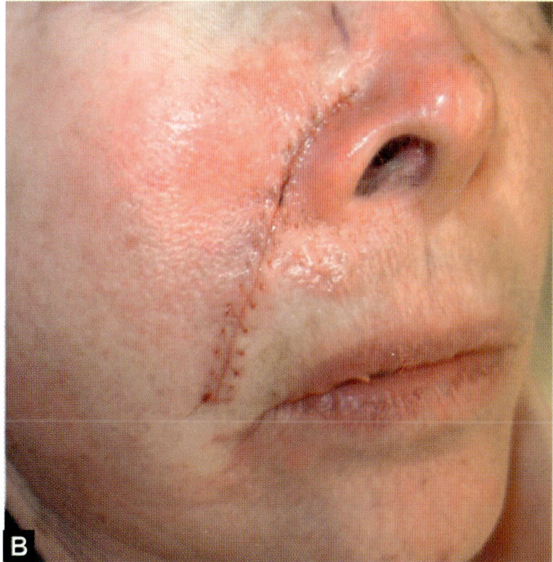


**Figs. 17.10A and B**

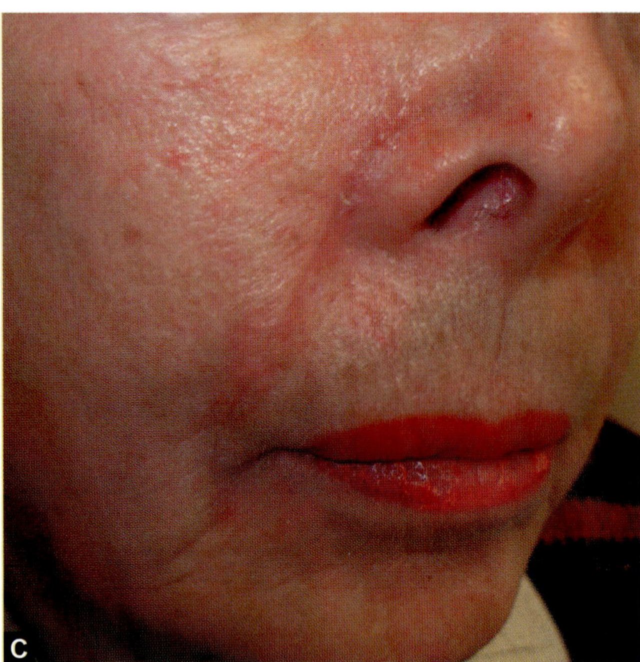


**Figs. 17.10A to C:** Primary closure oriented within the nasolabial fold. (A) A 72-year-old woman who presented for Mohs surgery for a basal cell carcinoma (BCC) on the right medial cheek. She cleared after two layers and was left with a 10 × 14 mm defect. (B) Closed primarily with the scar oriented along the melolabial fold. (C) Follow-up 3 weeks later.

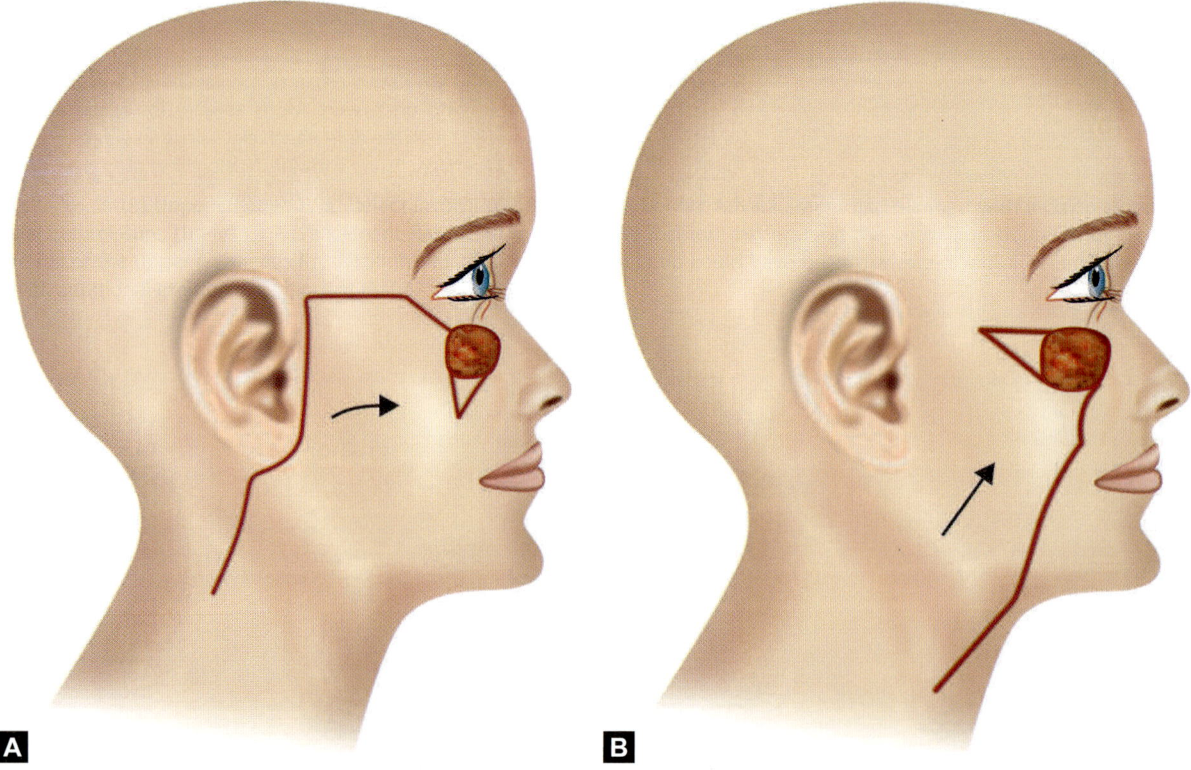


**Figs. 17.11A and B:** Anteriorly and posteriorly based advancement/rotation flaps. (A) Anteriorly based advancement/rotation flaps are performed by making an incision along the inferior border of the cutaneous lower eyelid to recruit tissue from the lateral cheek with standing cone removed inferiorly and placed in the melolabial crease. (B) Posteriorly based advancement/rotation flap involves recruiting tissue inferior to the defect by making an incision along the nasofacial sulcus and extending into the melolabial fold.

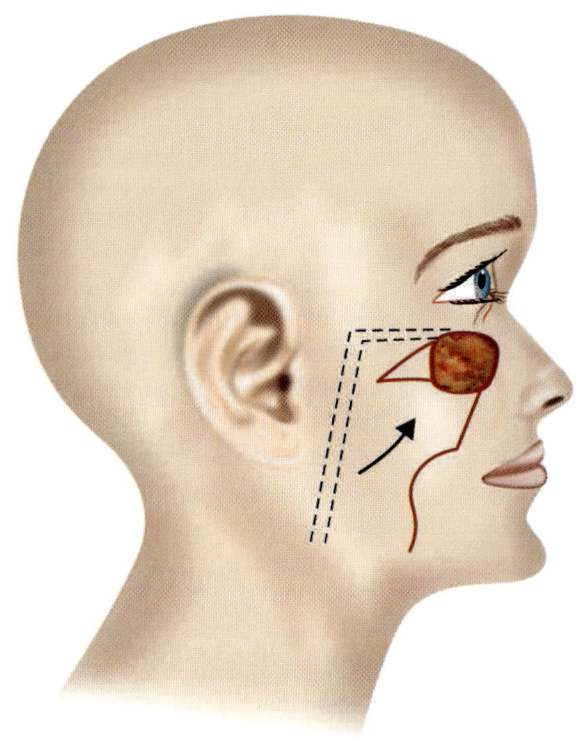

**Fig. 17.12:** Superomedial rotation flap. Similar to the posteriorly based advancement/rotation flap in that an incision is made inferiorly along the melolabial fold. This sliding rotation flap utilizes a crescentic incision to negate the need to remove a standing cone medial to the nasolabial fold. The dotted line signifies that wide undermining should be performed beyond the lateral canthus in the subcutaneous plane.

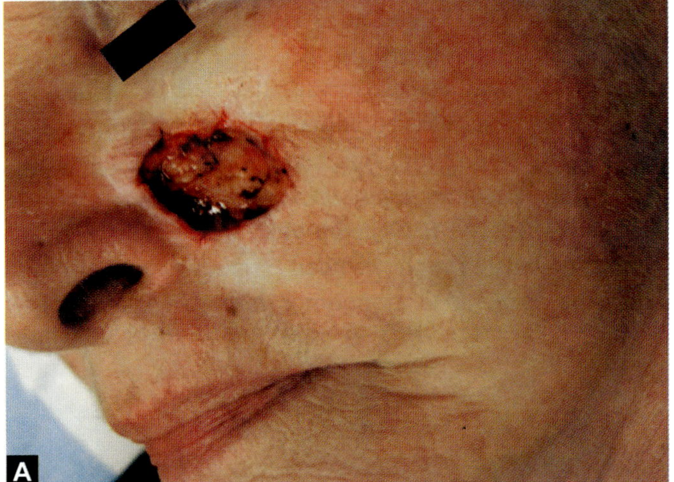


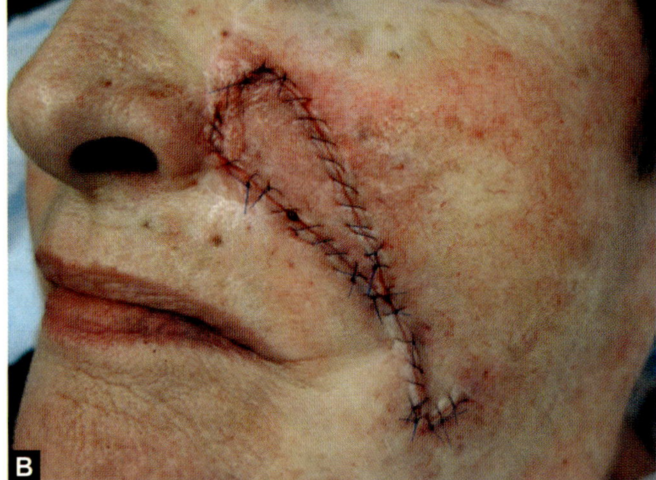


**Figs. 17.13A and B:** V-Y advancement flap for large medial cheek defect. (A) Mohs defect on the medial cheek adjacent to nasolabial fold. (B) Island pedicle flap was effective in repairing defect near nose–cheek junction while being oriented within the melolabial fold.

flap in which a crescent is designed to create extra length on the medial side of the flap[25] rather than removing a standing cone medial to the nasolabial fold. Meticulous care should be taken to conserve melolabial fat to preserve symmetry of the melolabial folds.

For medium-sized defects in this area closer to the ala, V-Y advancement flaps may be considered, especially if one of the limbs of the flap can be oriented in the melolabial fold[2] (Figs. 17.13A and B).

In addition to the advancement flaps, transposition flaps are another option in the medial subunit that yields favorable results. Transposition flaps utilized in this region are designed so that tissue is taken from the jowl where there is the greatest facial skin redundancy.[1]

A disadvantage would be that transposition flaps might not conserve the facial cosmetic units[2,26] as well as V-Y advancement flaps, potentially distorting vulnerable areas like the melolabial fold.

## Zygomatic Subunit

The zygomatic subunit is similar to the lateral subunit as it is also relatively fixed. This is attributed to the zygomatic-retaining ligament extending from the zygoma to the overlying dermis. There are multiple retaining ligaments (zygomatic, orbicularis, upper masseteric, and mandibular) that anchor the overlying soft tissues and dermis to the facial skeleton's intraosseous or interosseous suture lines.[1,2] These lateral retaining ligaments differ in strength: the zygomatic ligament is the strongest followed by orbital, mandibular, and maxillary ligaments.[1,27] In the deep plane hike flap, the zygomatic retaining ligaments need to be transected in order to release and mobilize the cheek flap, allowing for vertical advancement.[18] It is important to remember that the temporal branch of the facial nerve runs in a very superficial plane in the zygomatic region. The malar fat pad adds convexity to the contour of the malar eminence, and the surgeon must respect the fat pad when reconstructing the malar eminence.[2] Reconstruction of this area should involve restoring volume and camouflaging incision lines within relaxed skin tension lines (RSTLs).

Primary closure is feasible for defects that are < 30% of the zygomatic subunit.[18] The closure should be oriented along the relaxed skin tension lines (crow's feet).[2] Due to the convexity of the cheek bone underlying the zygomatic subunit, apical angles of the ellipse should be < 30° to avoid a postoperative standing cone, which may not be obvious intraoperatively due to the volumizing effect of local anesthesia.[2] For small defects close to the lateral canthus, M-plasty may be preferred to avoid extending the ellipse into the canthus.[2]

When the defect is too large, high tension from primary closure can lead to ectropion. Skin from the temporal area and buccal subunit can be used to close larger defects in the zygomatic subunit when primary closure is not possible.[2] Transposition flaps (i.e., rhombic flaps) are typically used to repair medium-sized defects, which comprise 30–70% of the zygomatic subunit, where skin is recruited from the buccal subunit.[2,10,18] This flap is designed to avoid tension on the lower lid or lateral canthus. The surgeon must also be aware of the frontal branch of the facial nerve, which runs superficially in the middle third of the zygoma. Dissection should be carried out superficial to the temporoparietal fascia.

Large defects > 70% of the zygomatic subunit can be reconstructed with a cervicofacial advancement rotation flap.[10] If a large defect involves both the zygomatic and buccal subunits, a large bilobed flap using preauricular skin to cover the defect (primary lobe) and postauricular/cervical skin to cover the secondary defect (secondary lobe).[2]

Advancement-rotation plasties in the medial zygomatic region of the cheek carry a risk of ectropion due to improper flap design. Inferior flap displacement of an advancement-rotation flap can be prevented with the placement of anchoring sutures lateral to the eye and keeping the arc plane above the canthus.[11,19,28,29] Conversely, transposition flaps are associated with the risk of displacement of the lateral canthus.

## Buccal Subunit

The buccal subunit of the cheek is composed of the skin lateral to the inferior melolabial fold and labiomandibular crease. This leaves the skin superior, lateral, or inferior as potential reservoirs for buccal subunit closure but skin medial to the defect should be left alone to avoid deformity of the lip and melolabial fold.[2] Similar to the medial subunit, the mobility of tissues in the buccal subunit allows for primary closure of small- to medium-sized defects, typically up to 30% of the buccal subunit[18] (Figs. 17.14 to 17.16).

Medium-sized defects of the subunit can be closed with transposition flaps (i.e. rhombic flap, bilobed flap, and note flap) or advancement flaps.[2] Transposition flaps involve use of tissue from the lower and lateral cheek along the lines of maximal extensibility in order to achieve less tension and distortion. The rhombic and traditional Limberg flaps are particularly useful in the buccal cheek region.[2,17] Ideally, the rhombic flap should be planned on an area of loose skin to ensure closure of wound edges and should be designed to have scars posterior to the defect, away from the central face where scars can be more noticeable.[2,30]

Large defects of the buccal subunit usually traverse other subunits (lateral or zygomatic) and may be closed with large cheek or cervicofacial advancement rotation flaps (Figs. 17.17A to C). Additionally, these larger defects can also be closed with larger bilobed flaps using pre- and postauricular skin. Given that the buccal region has less underlying bony support, deep defects will need oral lining with free flaps to provide bulky support.[9,31]

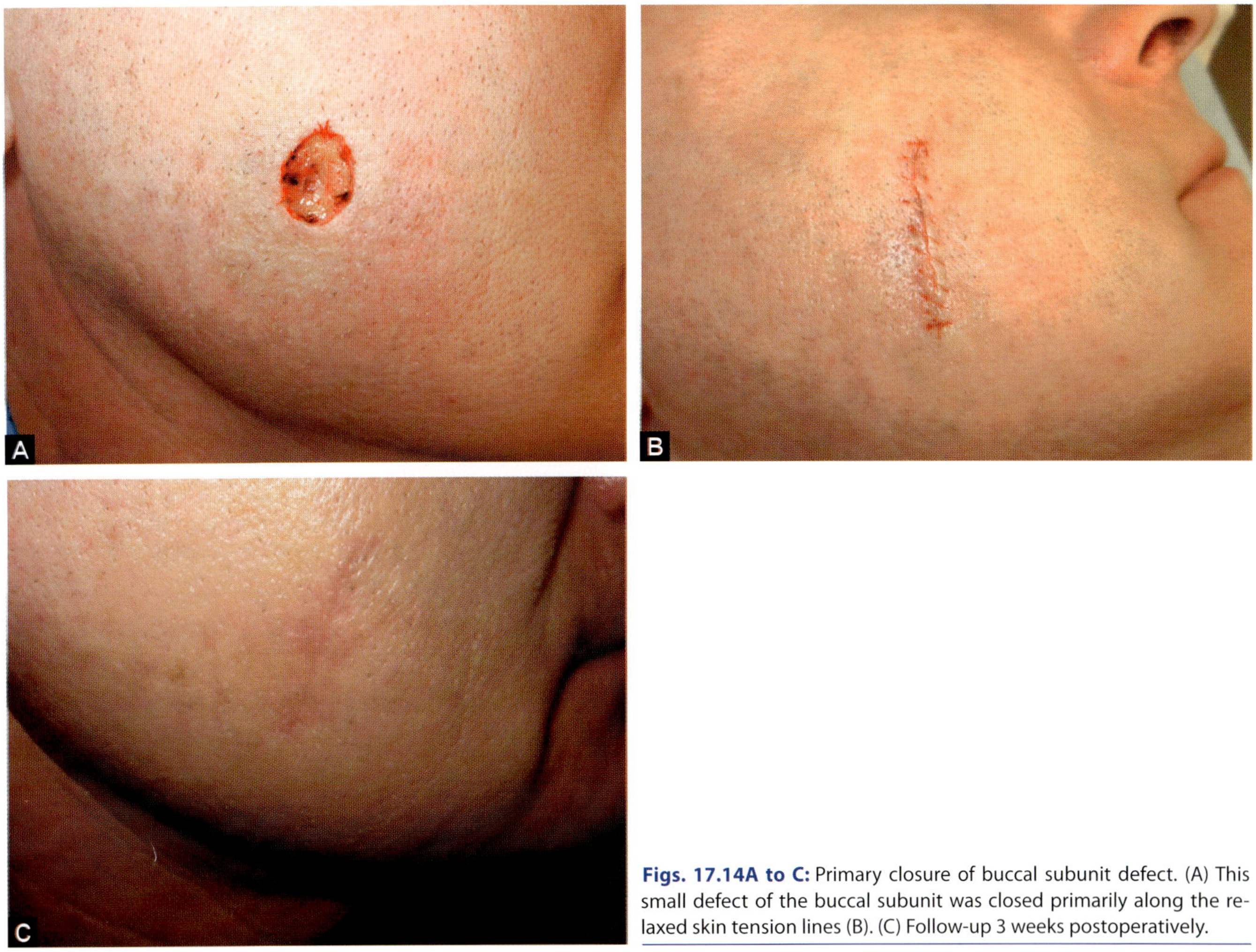

**Figs. 17.14A to C:** Primary closure of buccal subunit defect. (A) This small defect of the buccal subunit was closed primarily along the relaxed skin tension lines (B). (C) Follow-up 3 weeks postoperatively.

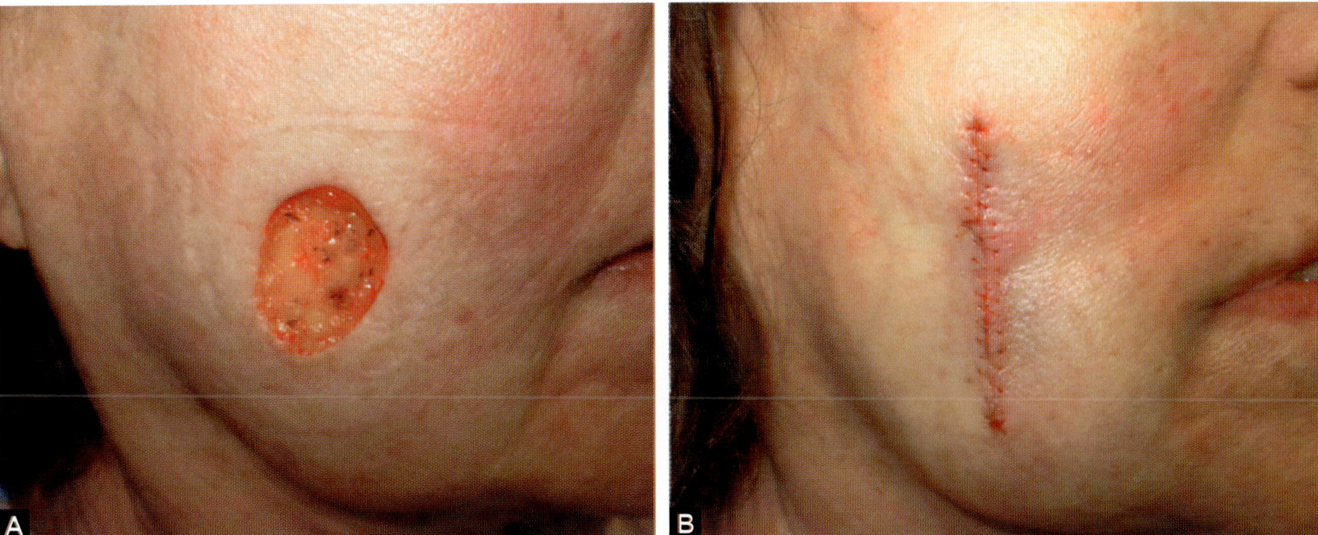

**Figs. 17.15A and B**

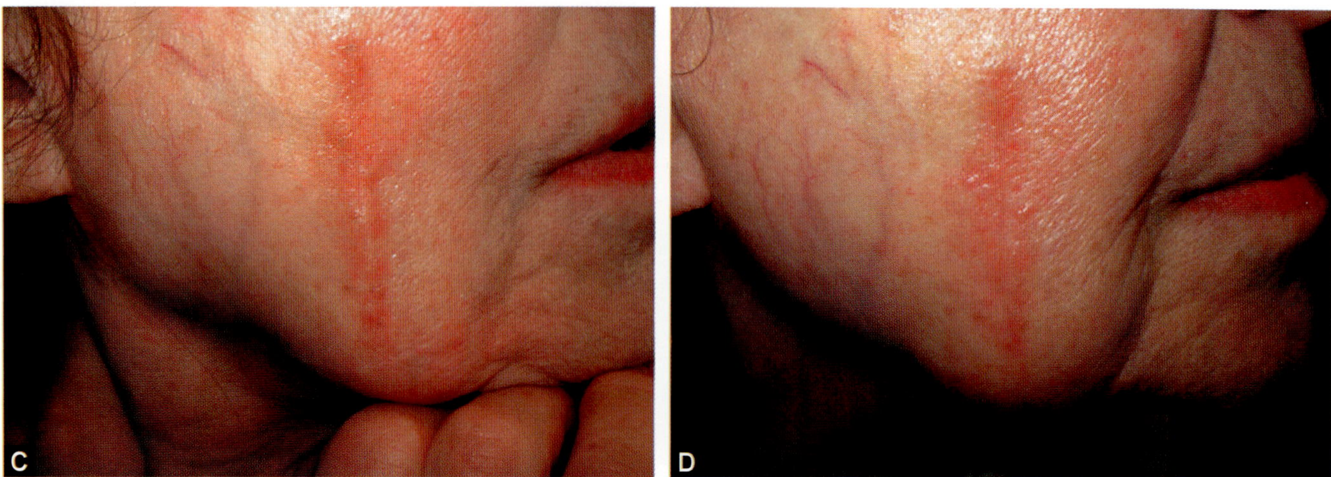

**Figs. 17.15A to D:** Complex layered closure near the jowl on the buccal subunit. (A) Be mindful of the location of the jowl when planning primary closure in this area, especially if the defect is located more inferiorly toward the jowl. (B) Although the jawline is not typically considered a free margin, orienting the linear closure perpendicular to the jawline can result in a pushing displacement that can accentuate the jowl. (C) Temporary postoperative swelling may augment this effect (3 weeks postoperatively). (D) Swelling and accentuation of jowl effect largely resolved by 6 weeks follow-up.

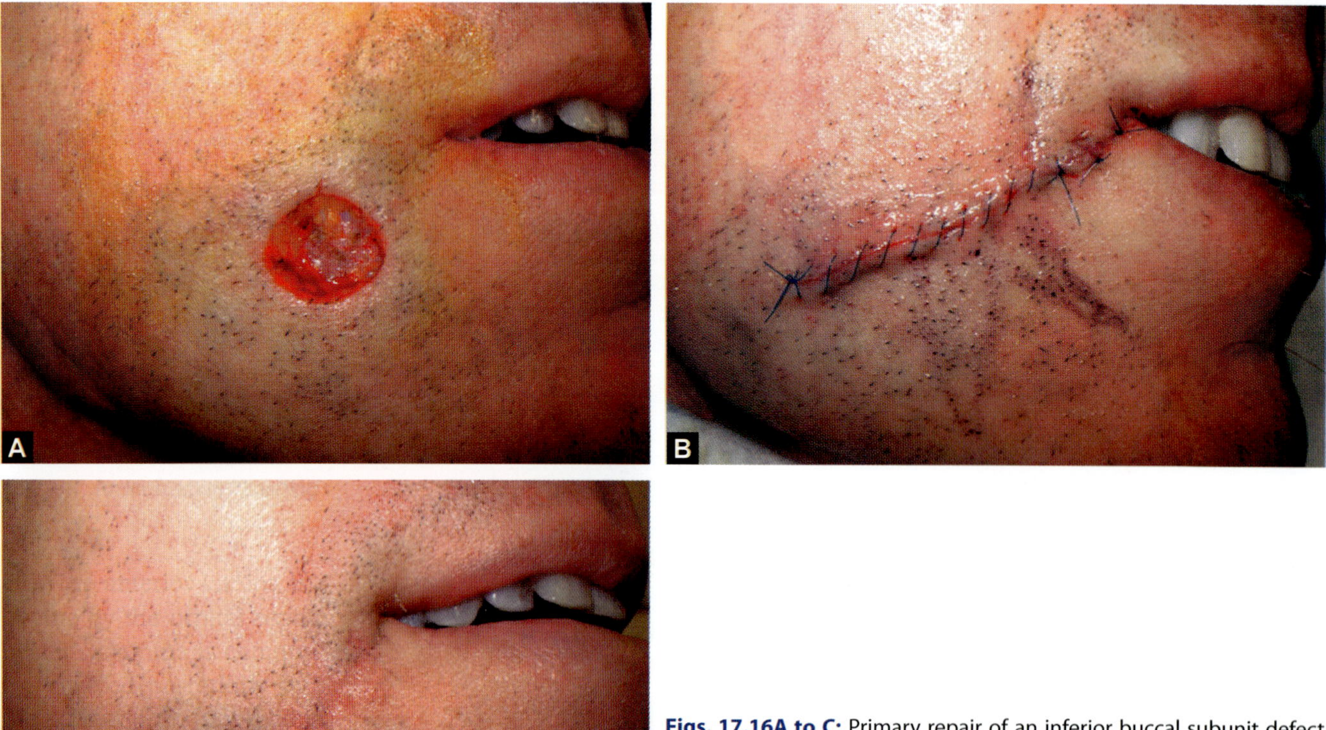

**Figs. 17.16A to C:** Primary repair of an inferior buccal subunit defect near the mouth. (A) Given the inferior location of this buccal defect being near the mouth, this could not be closed vertically without inducing significant distortion of the lip and angle of the mouth. (B) The defect was closed primarily with the scar oriented toward the angle of the mouth to minimize lip distortion. (C) Although the scar is oriented perpendicular to the relaxed skin tension lines, the outcome at one month is acceptable. Note the minor upturned mouth corner as a result of pushing displacement.

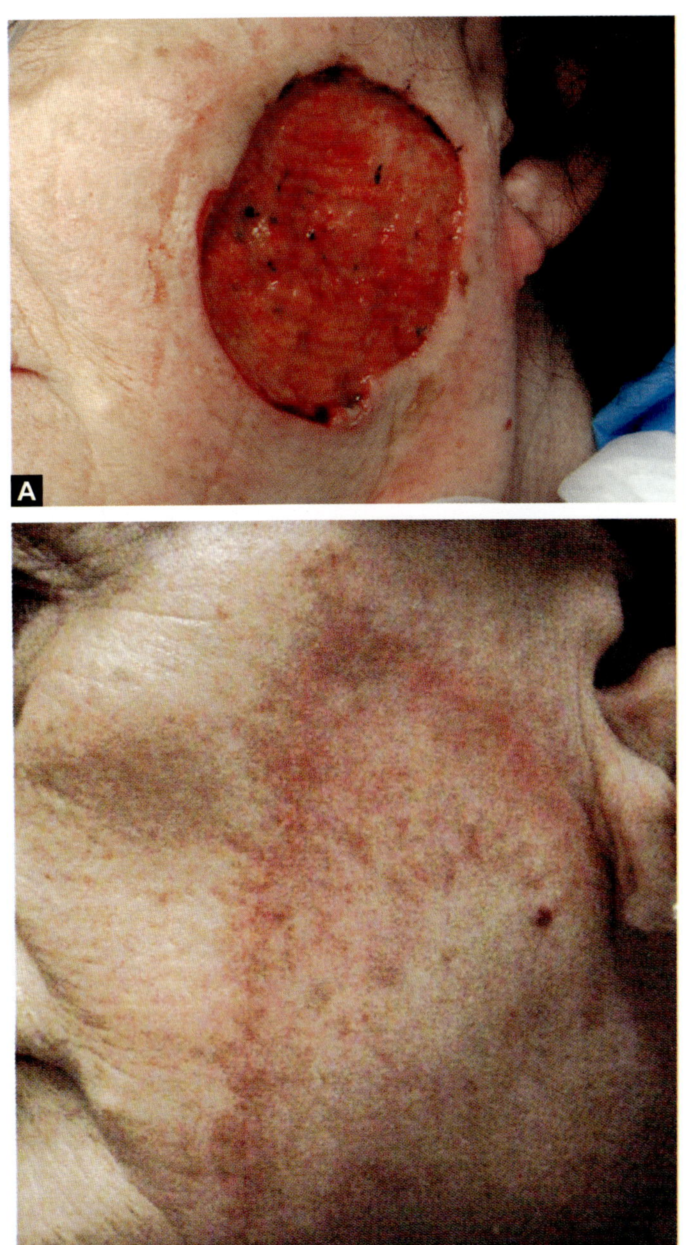

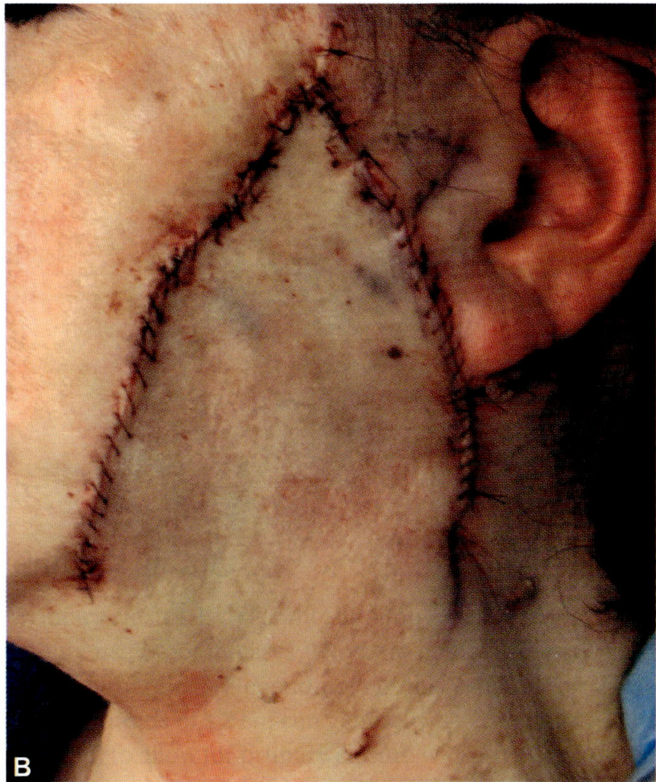

**Figs. 17.17A to C:** Repair of large buccal defect. (A) A 79-year-old woman with a 59 × 49 mm defect following staged excision of a lentigo maligna on the left cheek. Large buccal defect also involving lateral and zygomatic subunits. (B) Cervicofacial advancement flap utilized. (C) Follow-up 3 weeks postoperatively.

## Multi-subunit and Extensive Defects

Defect locations that carry greatest risk for anatomic distortion include the nasal ala, eyelids, and vermillion border. Skin grafting should be avoided in repairing large defects near these free margins given the concern of distortion from skin graft contraction. The following will discuss special reconstructive considerations for defects affecting multiple facial subunits as well as large composite cheek defects with the use of regional and microvascular free flaps.

In general, when defects involve both the cheek and lip, each cosmetic component of the defect should be addressed independently. For smaller defects involving less than half of the lip, primary closure can be considered whereas larger defects involving up to two-thirds of the lip can be addressed with lip switch flaps including Abbe or Estlander flaps.[3,9] When a defect involves the cheek, lip, and nose, the first two cosmetic units should be closed first and then the nasal defect should be repaired subsequently in order to prevent anatomical distortion.[32] In other words, if all three areas are repaired at the same time, wound contraction can cause distortion of the nasal ala.

In medial cheek defects, the melolabial and labiomental creases should be utilized in hiding advancement flap donor site closures.[1] For large medial cheek defects that extend onto the lateral cutaneous lip, the V-Y island pedicle advancement flap is better suited in preserving the boundary between the lip and cheek than the transposition melolabial flap that can distort the melolabial crease.[1] Defects adjacent to the nose or oral commissure can be simply addressed with a perialar crescentic advancement flap.[33] This flap carries the advantage of having the dog-ear excisions follow the melolabial fold after the defect is extended in a crescent shape. Lip retraction can be seen with using this advancement flap and can resolve over several weeks with compensatory movement of the orbicularis oris.[33]

Reconstruction of defects involving both the cheek and lower eyelid poses many aesthetic risks. In the cheek–eyelid region, the infraorbital crease is crucial in distinguishing between the thinner lower eyelid skin from the thicker cheek skin. Reconstruction in this region should ideally preserve this textural transition for combined defects of the cheek and eyelid. Combination defects should ideally be repaired by treating each subunit separately to preserve the transition. For example, a cervicofacial flap can be used to reconstruct the medial cheek, and smaller local flaps, including the nasojugal and Tripier flaps, can be used to address the lower eyelid defect.[10,19]

For defects of the lower cheek near the neck, healthy skin can be advanced from below. Broad horizontally oriented defects along the mandible can be repaired using superior advancement of skin from the neck and chest. Generally, this advancement flap does not include the platysmal muscle in order to maximize mobility and to minimize tissue bulk of the flap[18] although the platysma muscle can be included to provide a reliable blood supply.[4]

Regional flaps involve transfer of tissue from distant sites to cover large cheek defects. These include cervicofacial, cervicopectoral, deltopectoral, platysma musculocutaneous, and pectoralis major flaps.[17,18] Typically, these flaps provide acceptable color and texture match.

The cervicofacial flap is the standard solution for large partial-thickness cheek defects usually 3–4 cm and up to 10 cm.[18] The cervicofacial flap carries many advantages including ease of harvesting, versatility in design, and similar color and texture with the surrounding tissue.[4] Reconstructive planning for cervicofacial flaps must take into account the need for neck incisions or lymph node dissection in melanoma cases, where it may be best to first elevate the flap and then proceed with the sentinel lymph node dissection.[17] In cases of facial nerve tumor involvement requiring nerve resection, nerve grafting from the aural or great auricular nerves can be performed.[3]

Larger complex defects are more routinely addressed in the operating room under general anesthesia with plastic surgery or otolaryngology. Composite cheek defects can be repaired with various flaps, including microvascular free flaps. Pedicle flaps and microvascular free flaps have been used in the repair of full-thickness cheek defects. Pedicle flaps offer multiple advantages over free flaps including providing tissue better in pliability, color, texture, and softness.

Defects measuring 2–5 cm can be repaired with free tissue transfer alone.[9] For very large defects (>10 cm) made from excision of locally advanced primary or recurrent malignant melanoma, free tissue transfer should be considered.[3] These free flaps are the first choice for large through-and-through cheek defects and extensive composite defects with exposed bone, dura, sinuses, or orbit.[18] Examples of free flaps for cheek reconstruction include radial forearm, scapular, latissimus dorsi, and anterolateral thigh.[18,34-36]

## Complications

Complications can be divided into early and late in nature where early complications occur right after surgery to as long as the first couple months after. Early complications most commonly include seroma formation, wound dehiscence, hematoma, and infection. Hematomas compromise the flap's blood supply and require immediate attention. Hematoma and infection are treated with evacuation, drainage, and antibiotic coverage. Flap necrosis usually arises due to errors in design that cause limited blood flow through the flap. Other factors leading to flap necrosis are excessive or linear tension and interruption in normal blood flow (trauma, patient factors, surgical damage). Distal tip necrosis (DTN) is a complication specific to cervicofacial flaps, and may occur from the unreliable random pattern of the flap's vascular supply. History of smoking, radiation therapy, and diabetes are risk factors associated with DTN.[4] Facial nerve injury leading to motor dysfunction is also a potential complication. Use of blunt dissection in a plane perpendicular to the skin and bipolar electrocautery are recommended to minimize the risk for facial nerve injury, especially when working around the anterior margin of the parotid gland.[18]

Late complications typically involve pincushioning deformity, noticeable scars, hypertrophic scars, and keloid formation. Conspicuous scar formation can be limited by proper flap design, proper tissue handling, appropriate postoperative care, and being aware of the RSTLs and cosmetic subunits. Treatment options for hypertrophic scars are excision, Z-plasty, and W-plasty. Pincushioning deformities, particularly seen in V-Y island advancement and transposition flaps, can be revised with defatting the flap or adjacent tissue. These deformities are either caused by an excessively large flap or by scar contraction of bunched up tissue within a curved scar. Avoidance of pincushioning involves adequate undermining for the flap skin to settle into the defect, and ensuring the size of the flap is not too large for the defect.[2,26]

The overall risk of ectropion depends on many variables including pre-existing laxity, the position of the maxilla in relation to the orbit, defect size and depth, and the type of the reconstructive repair performed. In the immediate postoperative period, downward traction on the lower eyelid is mostly due to tension and edema. Scar contracture often worsens this as a late complication and the eyelid is maintained in an everted position.[19]

One method to prevent lower eyelid ectropion in the case of an anterior-based rotation advancement flap is to plan for the lateral superior border of the flap to be above the lateral canthal-helical root plane and thus suspends the flap higher than the eyelid margin. Other methods to prevent ectropion of the lower eyelid include overcorrecting cheek flaps, minimizing tension, and placing permanent sutures into the periosteum at the superior aspect of the flap.3,18 When working in the suborbital region, an incision at the infraorbital rim is associated with less risk of ectropion but may create chronic lymphedema of the lower lid that can take up to one year to resolve.[2]

## SUMMARY

The cheek is the largest aesthetic region of the face that can be further broken down into smaller subunits: lateral, medial, zygomatic, and buccal. Creases and wrinkles of the face can be useful in disguising scars. Design and position of the flap is determined by multiple factors including defect location, size, shape, and depth, as well as regional skin laxity. Depth and size of the defect play important roles in deciding whether to use regional or distant flaps instead of local flap repair. Postoperative complications should be avoided with careful reconstructive planning to prevent structural abnormalities including ectropion, pincushioning, or large noticeable scars.

## REFERENCES


1. Pepper JP, Baker SR. Local flaps: cheek and lip reconstruction. JAMA Facial Plast Surg. 2013;15(5):374-82.
2. Dobratz EJ, Hilger PA. Cheek defects. Facial Plast Surg Clin North Am. 2009;17(3):455-67.
3. Moncrieff MD, Thompson JF, Quinn MJ, et al. Reconstruction after wide excision of primary cutaneous melanomas: part I—the head and neck. Lancet Oncol. 2009;10(7):700-8.
4. Sakellariou A, Salama A. The use of cervicofacial flap in maxillofacial reconstruction. Oral Maxillofac Surg Clin North Am. 2014;26(3):389-400.
5. Bennett RG. Local skin flaps on the cheeks. J Dermatol Surg Oncol. 1991;17(2):161-5.
6. Whetzel TP, Mathes SJ. Arterial anatomy of the face: an analysis of vascular territories and perforating cutaneous vessels. Plast Reconstr Surg. 1992;89(4):591-603.
7. Schaverien MV, Pessa JE, Saint-Cyr M, et al. The arterial and venous anatomies of the lateral face lift flap and the SMAS. Plast Reconstr Surg. 2009;123(5):1581-7.
8. Makkar RM. The faciocervicopectoral flap for non-oncological cases of cheek reconstruction. Ann R Coll Surg Engl. 2013;95(6):397-400.
9. Chinnadurai S, Janus JR, Moore EJ. Algorithm for the repair of cheek defects. Laryngoscope. 2010;121(1):137-41.
10. Eroglu L, Simsek T, Gumus M, et al. Simultaneous cheek and lower eyelid reconstruction with combinations of local flaps. J Craniofac Surg. 2013;24(5):1796-1800.
11. Menick FJ. Reconstruction of the cheek. Plast Reconstr Surg. 2001;108(2):496-505.
12. Khazaeni K, Rajati M, Shahabi A, et al. Use of a sternocleidomastoid myocutaneous flap based on the SCM branch of the superior thyroid artery to reconstruct extensive cheek defects. Aesthetic Plast Surg. 2013;37(6):1167-70.
13. Donaldson MR, Coldiron BM. Scars after secondary intention healing. Facial Plast Surg. 2012;28(5):497-503.
14. Zitelli JA. Wound healing by secondary intention: a cosmetic appraisal. J Am Acad Dermatol. 1983;9(3):407-15.
15. van der Eerden PA, Lohuis PJ, Hart AA, et al. Secondary intention healing after excision of nonmelanoma skin cancer of the head and neck: statistical evaluation of prognostic values of wound characteristics and final cosmetic results. Plast Reconstr Surg. 2008;122(6):1747-55.
16. Sam H. Reconstruction of a large preauricular defect. Dermatol Surg. 2011;37(10):1511-4.

17. Heller L, Cole P, Kaufman Y. Cheek reconstruction: current concepts in managing facial soft tissue loss. Semin Plast Surg. 2008;22(4):294-305.
18. Mureau MA, Hofer SO. Maximizing results in reconstruction of cheek defects. Clin Plastic Surg. 2009;36(3):461-76.
19. Sugg KB, Cederna PS, Brown DL. The V-Y advancement flap is equivalent to the Mustarde flap for ectropion prevention in the recon of moderate-size lid-cheek junction defects. Plast Reconstr Surg. 2013;131(1):28e-36e.
20. Bradley DT, Murakami CS. Reconstruction of the cheek. In: Baker SR (Ed). Local Flaps in Facial Reconstruction. Philadelphia: Mosby/Elsevier; 2007. pp. 525-56.
21. Wells MD, Luce EA, Edwards AL, et al. Sequentially linked free flaps in head and neck reconstruction. Clin Plast Surg. 1994;21:59-67.
22. White CP, Rosen N, Muhn CY. The usefulness of the bilobed flap for lateral cheek defects. Can J Plast Surg. 2012; 20(1):e19-21.
23. Gassner HG, Rafii A, Young A, et al. Surgical anatomy of the face: implications for modern face-lift techniques. Arch Facial Plast Surg. 2008;10(1):9-19.
24. Raklyar E, Zloty DM. Use of a patient and observer scar assessment scale to evaluate the V-Y advancement flap for reconstruction of medial cheek defects. Dermatol Surg. 2012;38(12):1968-74.
25. Hussain W, Tan E, Salmon PJ. Inferiorly based crescentic "sliding" cheek flaps for the reconstruction of paranasal surgical defects. Dermatol Surg. 2012;38(2):249-55.
26. Schultz TA, Cunningham K, Bailey JS. Basic flap design. Oral Maxillofac Surg Clin North Am. 2014;26(3):277-303.
27. Brandt MG, Hassa A, Roth K, et al. Biomechanical properties of the facial retaining ligaments. Arch Facial Plast Surg. 2012;14(4):289-94.
28. Tan ST, MacKinnon CA. Deep plane cervicofacial flap: a useful and versatile technique in head and neck surgery. Head Neck. 2006;28(1):46-55.
29. Austen WG Jr, Parrett BM, Taghinia A, et al. The subcutaneous cervicofacial flap revisited. Ann Plast Surg. 2009;62 (2):149-53.
30. Murillo LM, Fernandez W, Caycedo DJ, et al. Cheek and inferior eyelid reconstruction after skin cancer ablation. Clin Plast Surg. 2004;31(1):49-67.
31. Sun G, Lu M, Hu Q, et al. Reconstruction of extensive through-and-through cheek defects with free anterolateral thigh flap. J Craniofac Surg. 2014;25(1):e31-8.
32. Kawase-Koga Y, Mori Y, Saijo H, et al. Reconstruction of a complex mid face defect from excision of a SCC, according to regional aesthetic units. Oral Surg Oral Med Pathol Oral Radiol. 2014;117(2):e97-101.
33. Rapstine ED, Knaus WJ 2nd, Thornton JF. Simplifying cheek reconstruction: a review of over 400 cases. Plast Reconstr Surg. 2012;129(6):1291-9.
34. Liu ZM, Wu D, Liu XK, et al. Reconstruction of through-and-through cheek defects with folded free anterolateral thigh flaps. J Oral Maxillofac Surg. 2013;71(5):960-4.
35. Kilinc H, Erbatur S, Aytekin AH. A novel flap for the reconstruction of midcheek defects: "rabbit ear flap." J Craniofac Surg. 2013;24(5):e452-5.
36. Camacho-Martínez FM, Rollón A, Salazar C, et al. Free flaps in surgical dermatology. Comparison between fasciocutaneous and myocutaneous free flaps in facial reconstructions. An Bras Dermatol. 2011;86(6):1145-50.

# CHAPTER 18

# Forehead Reconstruction

*Jennifer Herrmann, Consuelo V David, Lisa Chipps*

## INTRODUCTION

The forehead is a slightly convex facial unit that constitutes the upper third of the face. It extends from the anterior hairline superiorly to the glabella and brows inferiorly and zygoma laterally. It can be further divided into four subunits: the medial forehead, lateral forehead, eyebrows, and temples. Depending on gender and ethnicity, its size can vary significantly, and its superior border may become increasingly difficult to define in those with receding hairlines. The convexity of the central forehead becomes flatter more laterally and concave as it transitions into the temporal regions. The skin quality also changes centrally to peripherally. It is relatively thick and inelastic in the middle forehead and becomes increasingly more elastic laterally, especially at the temples where it loosely connects to the underlying temporalis fascia. As such, the temples often serve as tissue reservoirs for more medially located surgical defects.

The major muscles of the forehead include the frontalis, procerus, and corrugator supercilii muscles. The frontalis is located beneath the subcutaneous tissue. It is divided into two vertically oriented bellies, separated by the galeal median raphe, a variably sized, amuscular extension of the scalp. The loose areolar tissue beneath the muscle and galea permits movement of the forehead over the periosteum, which is fixed to the cranial bone. Because this space is devoid of vessels and nerves, it serves as a useful undermining plane. The major function of the frontalis is to elevate the brow, which produces dynamic horizontal rhytids that gradually become static over time. In contrast, the procerus and corrugator muscles depress and furrow the brow creating horizontal and vertical glabellar rhytids, respectively.

The forehead is a highly vascularized anatomic region. Its major vessels from medial to lateral include the dorsal nasal, supratrochlear, and supraorbital arteries, all which are branches of the internal carotid artery. Frontal branches of the superficial temporal artery, a branch of the external carotid artery, supply the temples. These vessels course superiorly as they traverse the forehead.

The main sensory nerves of the forehead include the supratrochlear and supraorbital nerves, which course parallel to their respective arteries. After emerging from their bony foramen, these nerves pierce the frontalis muscle and run vertically in the subcutaneous plane. Along their ascent, they branch laterally and become increasingly superficial as they extend into the scalp. The zygomaticotemporal sensory nerves innervate the temples, and most medially, the infratrochlear nerve partially innervates the glabella.

The most important motor nerve of the forehead is the temporal branch of the facial nerve (CN VII). Its preservation is paramount in forehead reconstruction. Facial countenance critically depends on forehead animation, and brow paralysis produces facial asymmetry. Moreover, in patients who depend on brow elevation to counter dermatochalasis, inability to raise the forehead can result in compromised visual fields.

The temporal branch originates in the parotid gland, travels superomedially and enters the forehead approximately 1.5–2 cm lateral to the orbital rim. It innervates the frontalis, corrugators, and procerus muscles on their deep surfaces. Below the zygomatic arch, the temporal nerve pierces the parotidomassenteric fascia, which is contiguous with the superficial musculoaponeurotic system and travels in the subcutaneous tissue. It then divides into 2–4 rami, which traverse the zygomatic arch and enters the temple in the temporoparietal fascia, an avascular subaponeurotic space. The deep temporal fascia and the temporalis muscle lie beneath this space. The temporal nerve is most prone to damage as it traverses this "danger zone" over the zygomatic arch and temples. Dissection in this region must therefore occur either in the superficial subcutaneous tissue or immediately above the deep temporal fascia to avoid nerve transection.

## RECONSTRUCTIVE PLANNING

### Preoperative Counseling

Reconstructive planning should include preoperative counseling of anticipated surgical sequelae and potential side effects, so as to set postoperative expectations. Swelling and bruising after forehead surgery often migrate inferiorly with gravity. It is not uncommon for patients to develop edema and/or ecchymosis around one or both eyes 2–3 days postoperatively. In addition, because of the vertical orientation of forehead nerves, sensory nerve injury can result in postoperative anesthesia extending from the reconstruction site well into the scalp superiorly. Damaged nerves will often regenerate, but this may take several weeks to months. Finally, for tumors located on the temples, preoperative counseling on possible injury of the temporal nerve is prudent. Local anesthesia on the day of surgery may result in temporary paralysis of the frontalis muscle, while complete transection of the nerve's main trunk can lead to permanent brown ptosis. In some cases, sacrifice of the temporal nerve may be necessary to clear a tumor. Insidious onset forehead palsy may serve as a preoperative clinical clue to peri- or intraneural involvement by an aggressive cancer. Bell's palsy, in contrast, is rapid-onset muscle paralysis, and easily distinguished through a thorough patient history.

### Granulation

Second intention healing of surgical wounds may be an optimal repair option in certain settings. Superficial defects located on concave temporal and glabellar surfaces, especially in patients with fair skin, do well granulating. When such wounds are kept moist with petrolatum to prevent scab formation, they often heal with little to no depression. Moreover, centripetally oriented contractile forces around the wound edges decrease the final size of the scar. Second intention healing might also be considered after excision of aggressive tumors with higher propensity to recur. Early recurrence may be more easily detected when not covered by a local skin flap or full-thickness skin graft. Granulation also reduces intraoperative costs, decreases infection risk, and may best suited for patients with multiple comorbidities who are unable to tolerate prolonged reconstructions.[1] A major disadvantage of this repair is the time required for healing, which depends on both the width and depth of the surgical defect as well as patient fitness. When wounds are large, a purse-string closure may be utilized to reduce defect size and speed healing.

### Linear Closures

Most forehead defects can be closed linearly, with scars placed in glabellar or upper forehead rhytids, in the crow's feet, or along the hairline. Having a patient animate to define natural lines can be helpful when designing a repair. Although horizontal scars hide well in lines on the mid- and upper forehead, horizontally oriented repairs are typically reserved for small defects only (Figs. 18.1A to C). Vertical closures have two distinct advantages. First, they do not asymmetrically pull on one eyebrow, creating a fixed quizzical expression. Second, they minimize sensory nerve damage, given the vertical orientation of nerve fibers (Figs. 18.2A to C).

When performing linear repairs on the forehead, attention to technique can maximize cosmetic outcomes. If a wound is located on the convex portion of the forehead, redundant tissue cones should be lengthened to prevent artificial "squaring off" of the sloped surface. In addition, for closures that reach the subgaleal plane, it is best to repair either the deep fascia or muscular layers before placing dermal and epidermal sutures. Without deeper repair, forehead scars can widen or invert, even if hypereversion of the epidermis is achieved. Finally, if a vertical forehead scar is long, one or more Z-plasties can be designed into the reconstruction to break up the single line scar. A correctly designed Z-plasty reorients a portion of the incision line within the relaxed skin tension lines (RSTLs) of the forehead, making the overall scar less noticeable.[2]

### Grafts

Skin grafts are rarely optimal reconstructive solutions for the forehead. Poorly matched skin thickness and color give them an artificial patch-like appearance. When large defect size precludes primary or local skin flap closure,

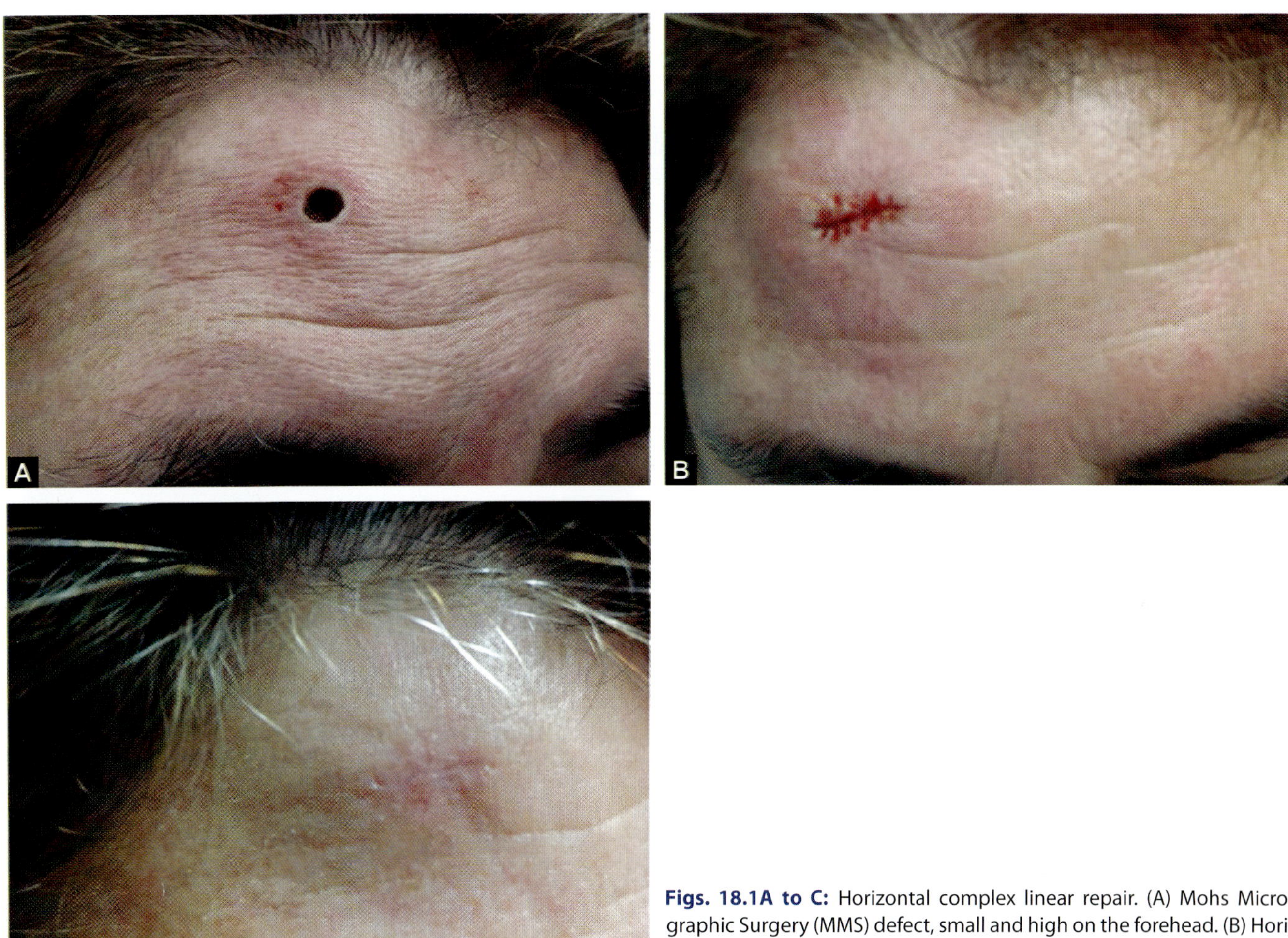


**Figs. 18.1A to C:** Horizontal complex linear repair. (A) Mohs Micrographic Surgery (MMS) defect, small and high on the forehead. (B) Horizontally oriented complex linear repair. (C) Nine months postoperative.

grafts may be acceptable. Local skin is preferred over distant skin as the donor site. Full-thickness skin grafts (FTSG) tend to achieve better color and contour match and may be harvested from adjacent Burow's triangles. Preauricular skin or clavicular skin may serve as donor sites for FTSG (Figs. 18.3A and B). Split-thickness skin grafts (STSG) are often harvested from the anterior thigh, but can also be borrowed from the scalp. A major advantage of the scalp as a STSG donor site is that the scalp heals rapidly because of its rich vascularity and high density of hair follicles and epidermal stem cells.[3] Moreover, pigmentation of the scalp skin is very similar to that of the face, making it a better match than skin harvested from the arm, thigh, or buttock.[4] To improve final skin contour, deeper defects may be allowed to granulate for 2–3 weeks before grafting. This lessens the height difference between the grafted and adjacent skin, minimizing formation of wide depressed graft scars.

## Flaps

Local skin flaps are useful repairs for forehead wounds. They permit replacement of lost with like tissue, yielding cosmetically pleasing results. To optimize skin color and texture match, flap tissue should be recruited from the same cosmetic unit or subunit when possible. Frequent tissue reservoirs include the temples and glabella, but patient age, tissue elasticity, and presence of prior scars all impact the amount of available tissue. Pinching a patient's skin to assess laxity helps determine the best tissue recruitment site or sites for any given defect.

Flap design should include analysis of primary and secondary tissue movement as well as location of anticipated scars. Care should be taken to place surgical incisions in RSTLs and along cosmetic subunit borders. In addition, flaps should be designed so as not to distort free margins, such as the lateral eyelid or eyebrow. Excessive force on

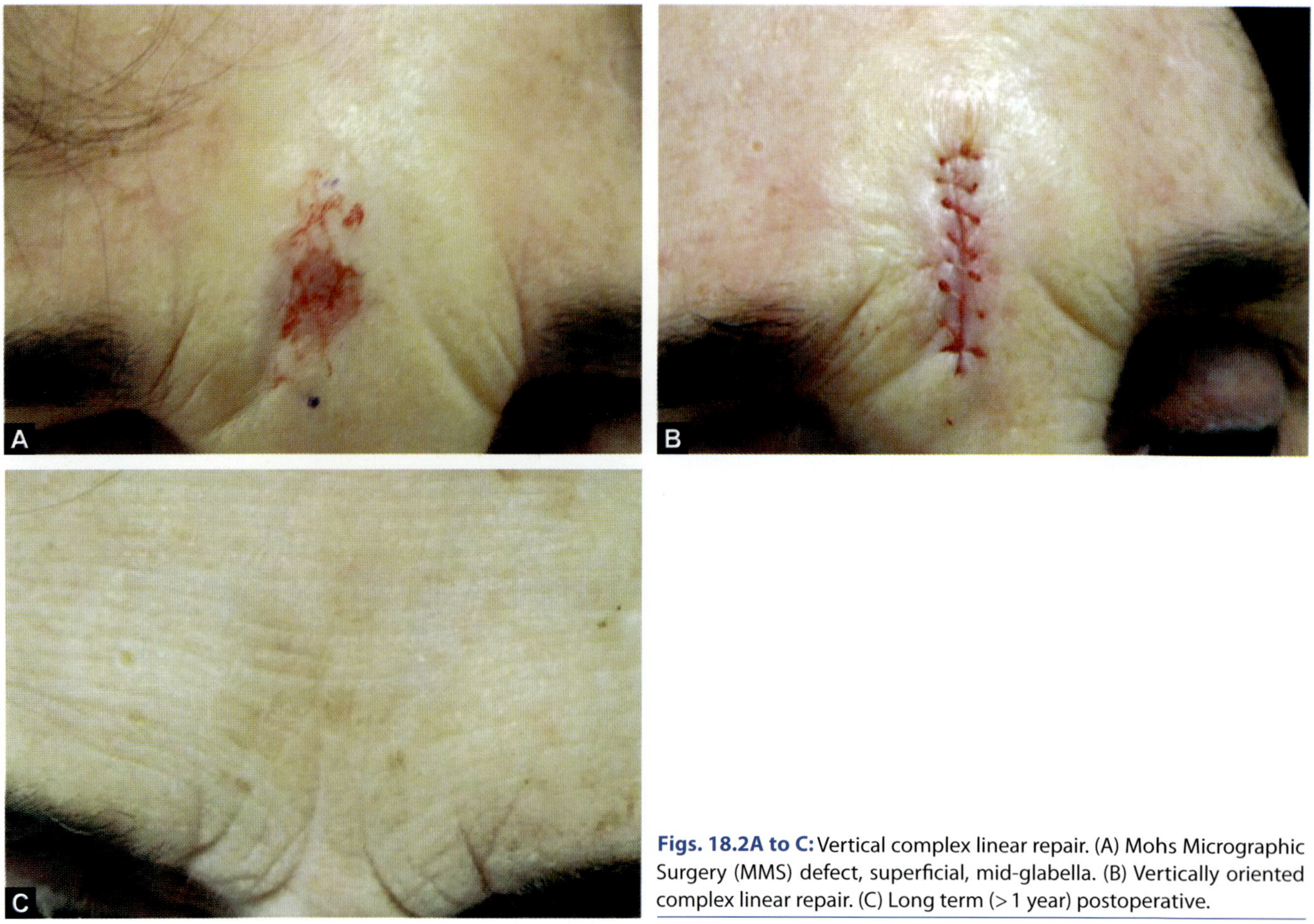

**Figs. 18.2A to C:** Vertical complex linear repair. (A) Mohs Micrographic Surgery (MMS) defect, superficial, mid-glabella. (B) Vertically oriented complex linear repair. (C) Long term (>1 year) postoperative.

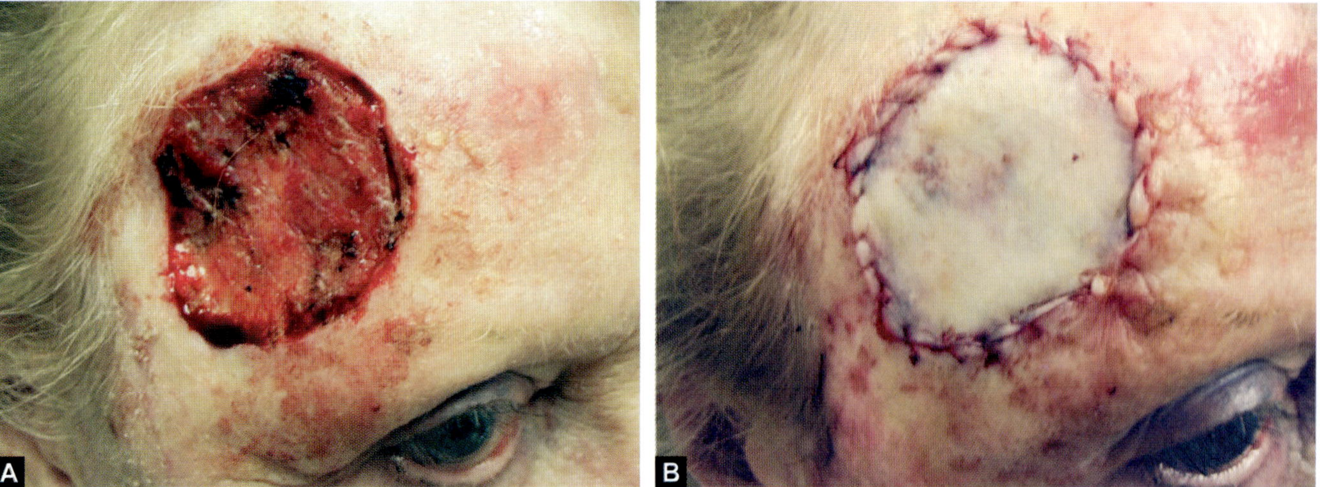


**Figs. 18.3A and B:** Full-thickness skin graft. (A) Mohs Micrographic Surgery (MMS) defect. (B) Full-thickness skin graft (donor site right clavicle).

the eyelid can impair full-lid closure, while asymmetric pull on the eyebrow creates striking facial asymmetry.

Tissue can be moved into surgical defects by advancement, rotation, transposition, or combinations of these

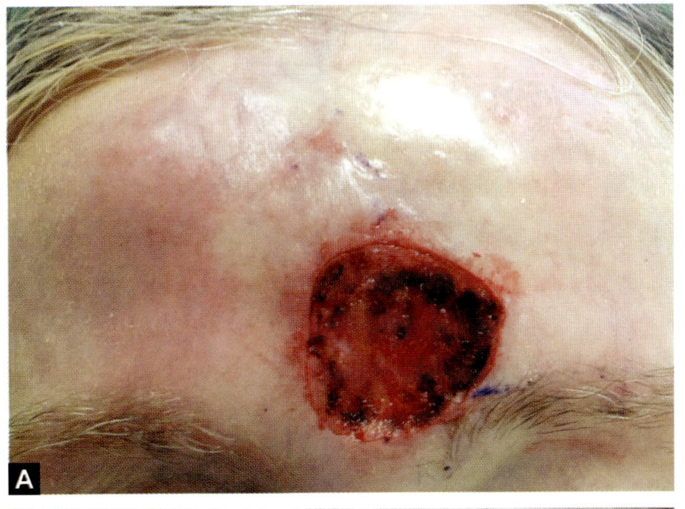


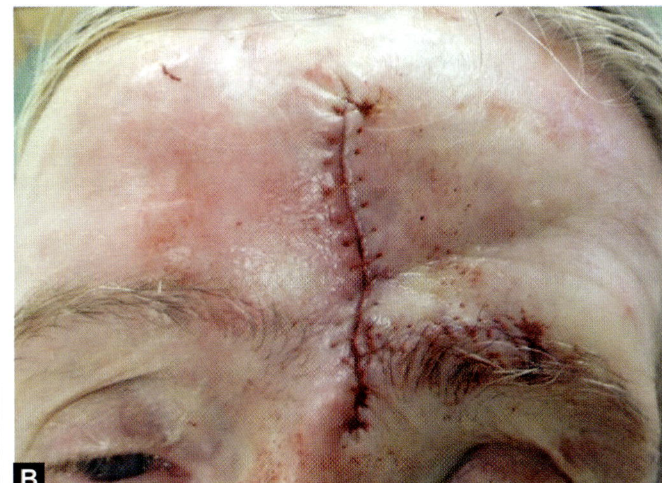


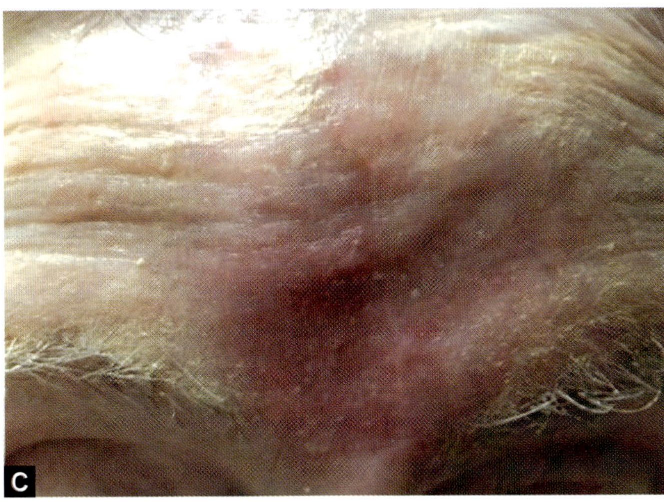


**Figs. 18.4A to C:** Advancement flap, medial forehead. (A) Mohs Micrographic Surgery (MMS) defect. (B) Advancement flap. (C) Long-term follow-up.

motions. Advancement and rotation flaps are "pulling" flaps where maximal tension vectors lie perpendicular to closure of the primary defect. Transposition flaps are "pushing" flaps, where tension is maximized along secondary defect closure. When to choose a particular flap depends on where the defect is located on the forehead, the availability of nearby tissue, the presence of free margins, and the orientation of RSTLs.

## RECONSTRUCTION BY LOCATION

### Medial Forehead

Many surgical wounds located on the medial forehead are successfully closed primarily. In the glabella, small defects can be repaired horizontally or vertically with scars hidden in procerus and corrugator rhytids, respectively. More superiorly over the galeal medial raphe, vertical closures are often preferred as they minimally compromise neurovascular bundles (Figs. 18.2A to C). For defects located adjacent or superior to the eyebrow, linear closures may pull or distort this structure, creating unacceptable brow asymmetry.

Advancement flaps may circumvent this pitfall, leaving eyebrows equally positioned. Flap incisions can be designed along the upper border of the eyebrow with tissue redundancy recruited from the glabella or the lateral forehead (Figs. 18.4A to C). Shallow wounds should be covered with flaps elevated above the muscle to preserve cutaneous nerves and vessels.

Larger defects in this region can also be approached with advancement flaps. Bilateral single-arm ("O-to-T"; "A-to-T") (Figs. 18.5 and 18.6) or double-arm ("H") advancements recruit more tissue than unilateral advancements; however,

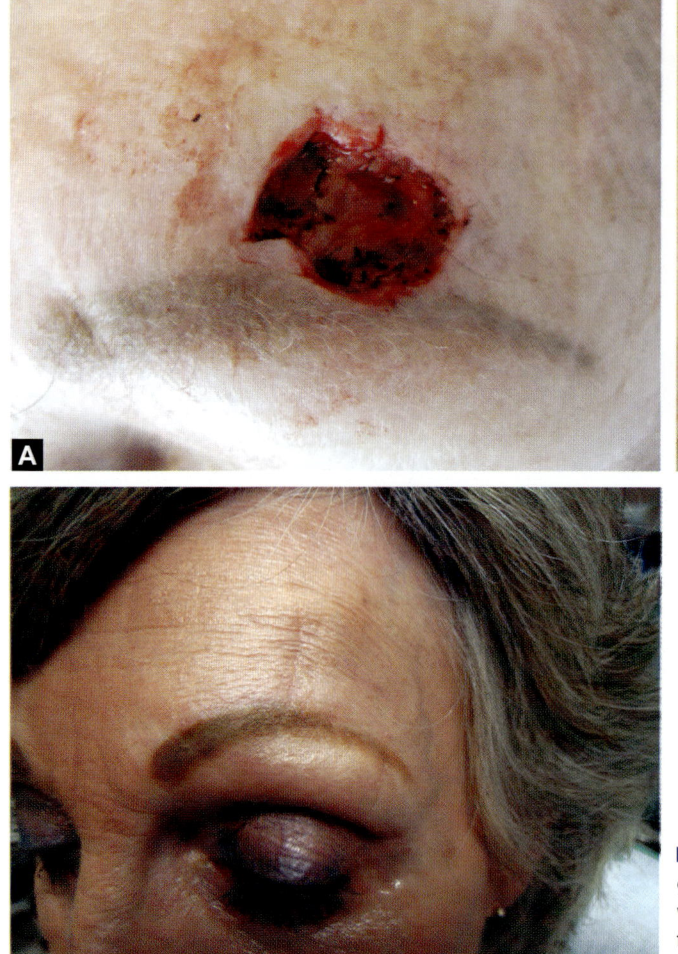


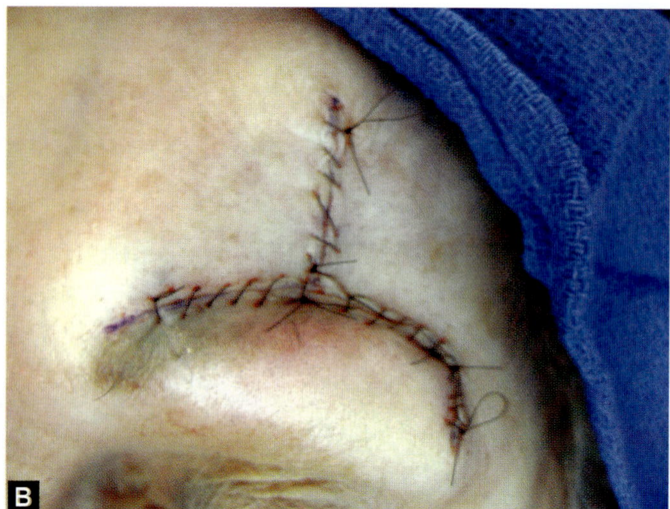


**Figs.18.5A to C:** A-to-T flap on the forehead. (A) Mohs Micrographic Surgery (MMS) defect above the eyebrow. (B) Horizontal incision lines hiding within the suprabrow. (C) Long-term follow-up showing good camouflage of scar within the brow.
*Courtesy*: S Brian Jiang, MD, Sang Diego, California, USA.

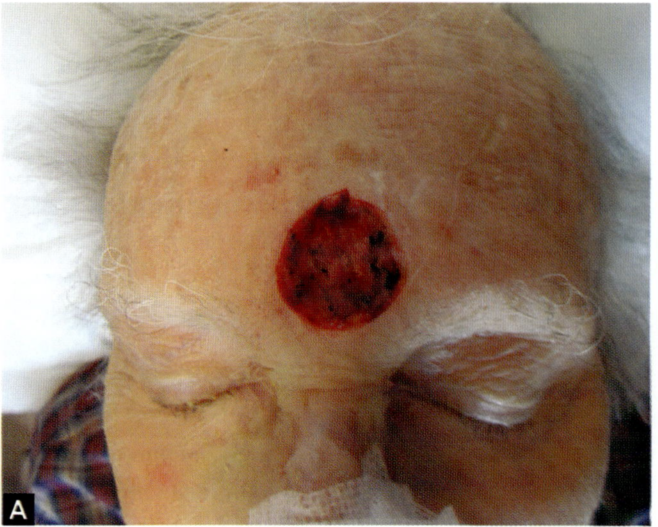


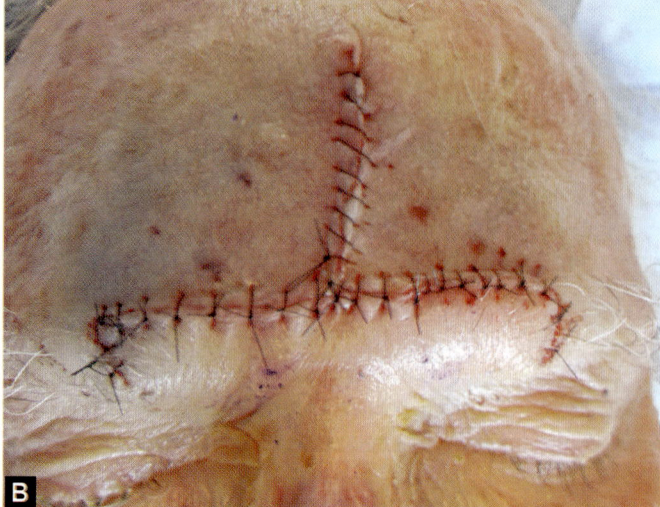


**Figs. 18.6A and B**

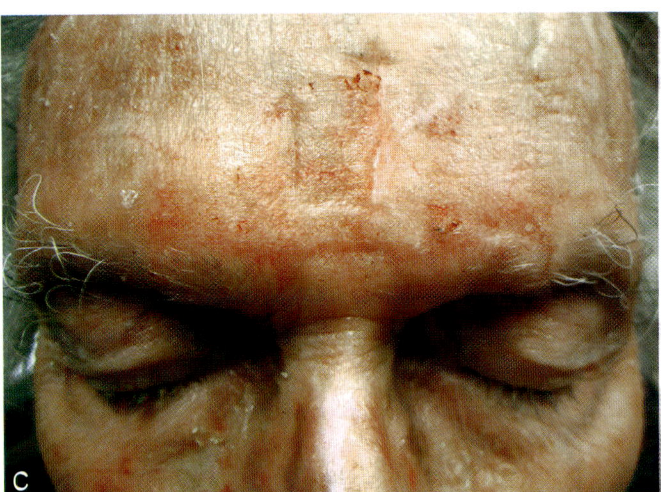


**Figs. 18.6A to C:** A-to-T flap on the mid–forehead. (A) Mohs Micrographic Surgery (MMS) defect on the mid-forehead. (B) A-to-T flap closure. (C) Long-term follow-up.
*Courtesy*: S Brian Jiang, MD, Sang Diego, California, USA.

these repairs can produce geometrically complex lines that may be aesthetically displeasing. Effort should be made to hide scars in RTSLs. For example, a large medial forehead defect can be closed such that removal of Burrow's triangles are aligned superiorly in horizontal forehead creases and inferiorly in glabellar lines.[5] Alternatively, a combination of opposing advancement and rotation flaps may successfully close similarly located, large defects.[6] Both of these reconstructions maintain the forehead's vertical height between the eyebrows and hairline. Undermining is performed beneath the fascia. Although this allows for a bloodless dissection, the long horizontal incisions will disrupt sensory nerves.

Medial forehead defects may also be repaired with muscular sling flaps, which are particularly advantageous in patients who lack lateral tissue laxity. The key to their design is elevating the flap on a muscular pedicle, based on either the frontalis or periocular muscles.[7,8] The muscular pedicle grants significantly more mobility than a traditional island pedicle flap. It also perfuses these flaps with a rich vascularity. One downside to these repairs is that they can appear "graft-like" in shape. However, tissue color and texture match is typically much better than that of grafts harvested from distant sites.

## Lateral Forehead

Closures on the lateral forehead have the potential to raise the ipsilateral eyebrow if not thoughtfully designed. Although minor brow elevation may be tolerated temporarily, significant pull is bothersome to the patient both physically and visually. Linear repairs are frequent reconstructive choices in this region. They are often designed vertically above the eyebrow and become progressively horizontal as defects descend into the temple (Figs. 18.7A to F). With small defects, linear repairs may be oriented horizontally or curvilinearly with respect to the relaxed skin tension lines (Figs. 18.8A to C). If a horizontal repair is designed above the eyebrow, addition of a bipedicled flap may reduce vertical pull. First, a horizontally oriented ellipse encompassing the primary defect is excised. Then, a parallel incision located on the frontal scalp is made through the galea. This second defect is closed with dermal sutures only, allowing the galea beneath to slide inferiorly. This galeotomy results in decreased tension along the primary defect, minimizing vertical pull on the eyebrow.[9]

Advancement flaps are also useful reconstructive options for wounds on the lateral forehead near the eyebrow. Burow's advancement or crescentic advancement flaps allow incision lines to be well disguised (Figs. 18.9 and 18.10). In addition, unilateral or bilateral advancement flaps may be tucked along the hairline for optimal cosmetic results (Figs. 18.11A to D). When redundant tissue cones are removed on the scalp, a bevel-reverse bevel technique may be used to maximally preserve hair follicles. The inferior incision is beveled at 45° as if a Mohs layer was being taken, and the superior incision is reversed beveled at 45°.

For wounds located above the eyebrow that are wider than they are tall, transposition flaps are preferable over advancement flaps. Although transpositions result in slightly more complex geometric lines, they are often aesthetically pleasing if redundant tissue cones are removed along RSTLs (Figs. 18.12 and 18.13).

## Eyebrow

Facial symmetry depends on equally positioned eyebrows, and their movement is fundamental to expressivity. Eyebrows vary tremendously among individuals and may be thick or thin, long or short, arched or flat. Successful reconstruction of defects involving this structure depends on individual eyebrow character as well as the size and location of a surgical defect.

For wounds located centrally in the eyebrow, laterally based V-to-Y advancement flaps can effectively restore eyebrow continuity (Figs. 18.14A to C). These flaps are incised and undermined deep to the hair follicles to insure

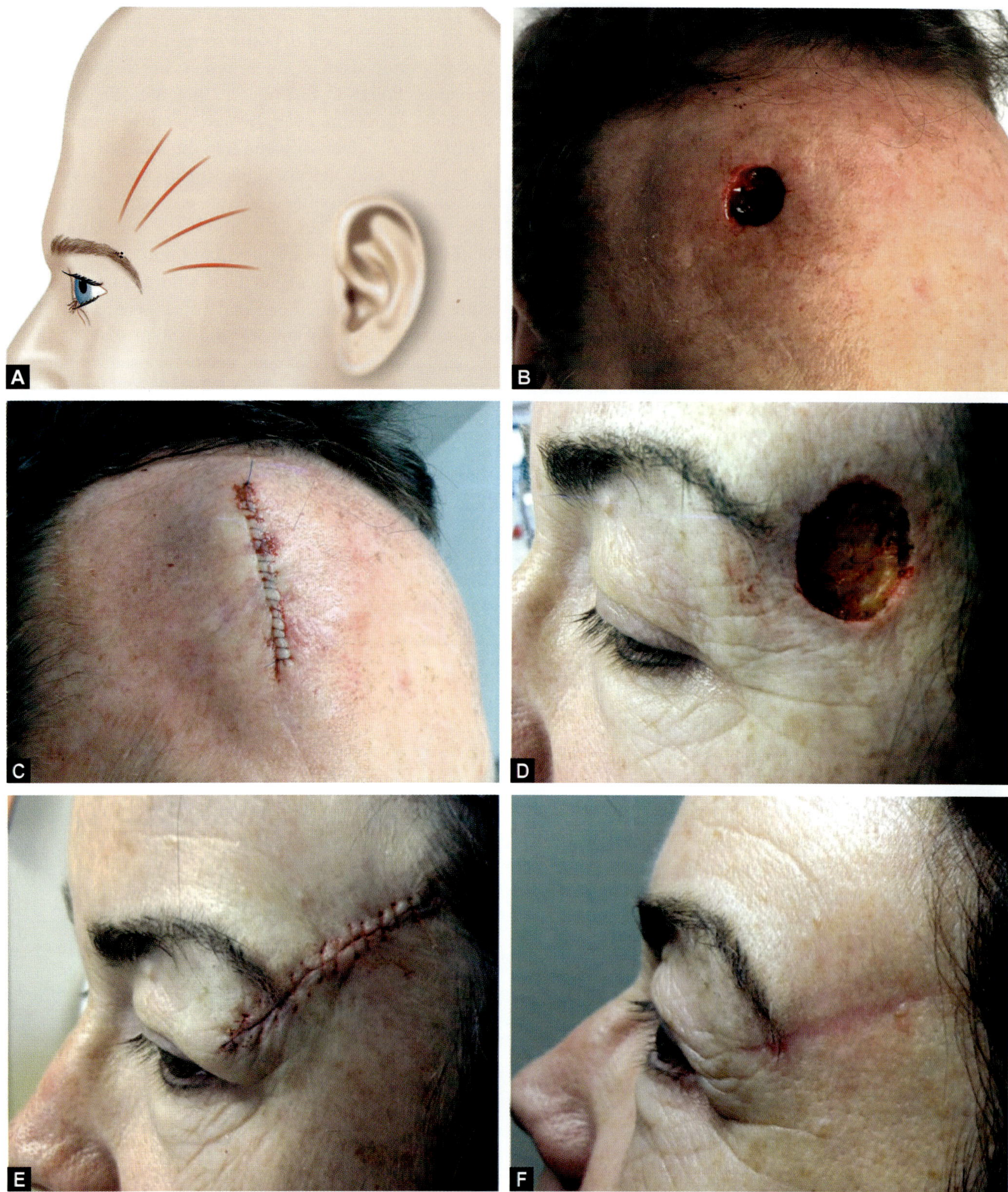


**Figs. 18.7A to F:** Vertical linear repairs, lateral forehead. (A) Diagram of repair designs. (B) Mohs Micrographic Surgery (MMS) defect, right lateral forehead. (C) Vertical linear repair, right lateral forehead. (D) MMS defect, left lateral forehead. (E) Diagonally oriented linear repair, left lateral forehead. (F) Six-week follow-up.

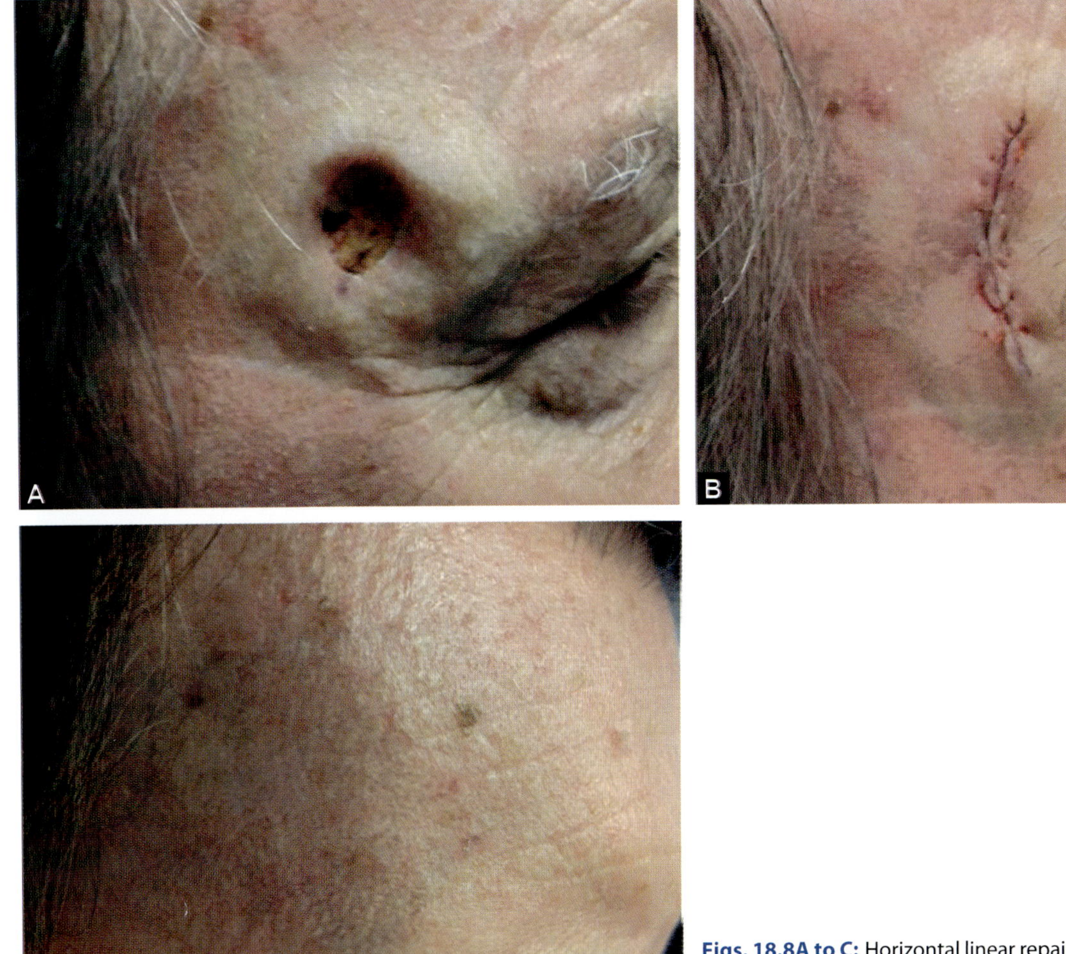


**Figs. 18.8A to C:** Horizontal linear repair, lateral forehead. (A) Mohs Micrographic Surgery (MMS) defect, lateral forehead. (B) Curvilinear repair in relaxed skin tension lines (RSTLs). (C) Long-term follow-up.

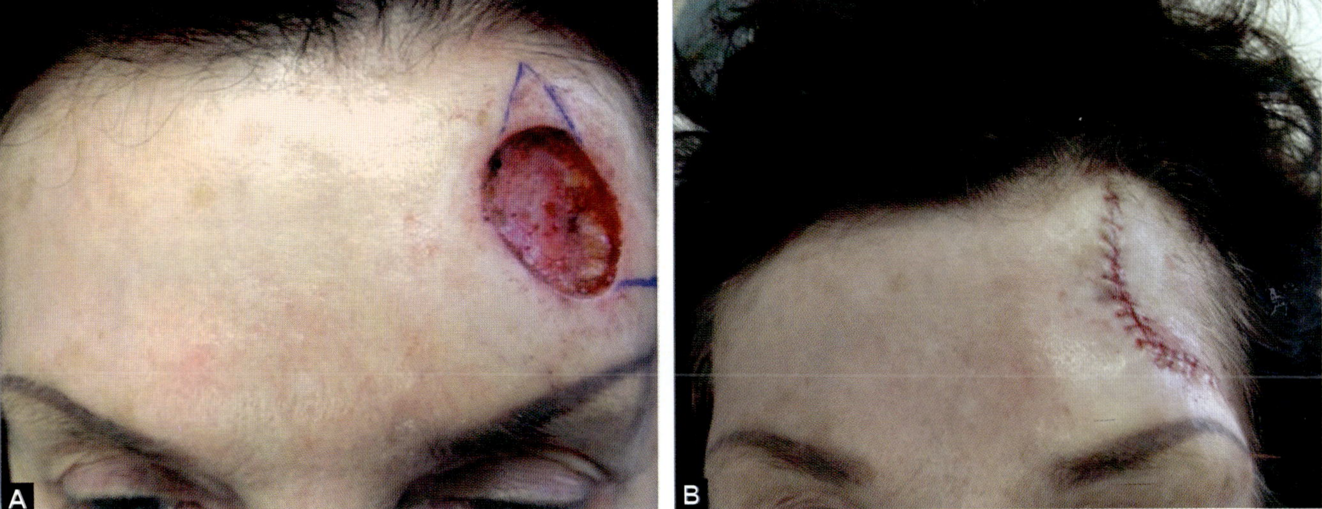


**Figs. 18.9A and B**

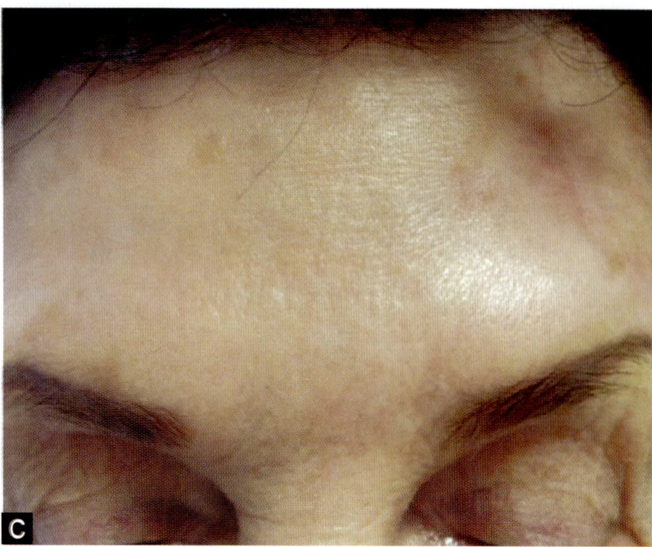

**Figs. 18.9A to C:** Advancement flap on lateral forehead. (A) Mohs Micrographic Surgery (MMS) defect. (B) Advancement flap. (C) Long-term follow-up.

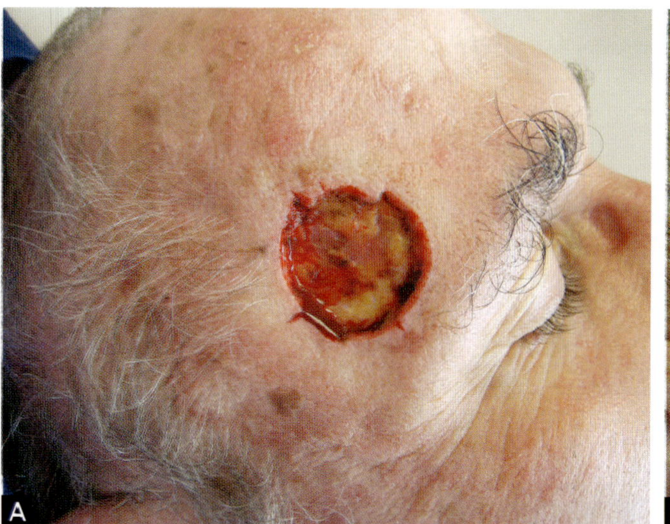

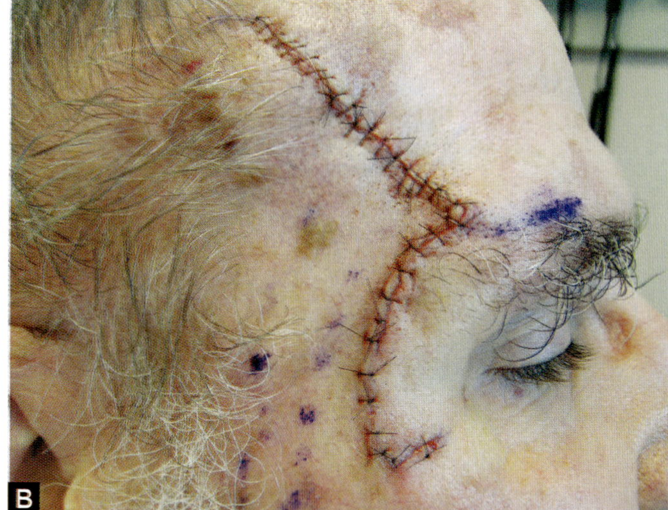

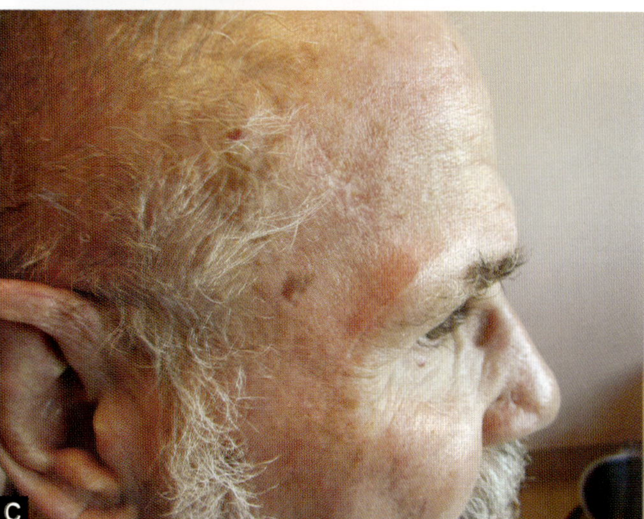

**Figs. 18.10A to C:** Burow's advancement flap on the lateral forehead. (A) Mohs Micrographic Surgery (MMS) defect on lateral forehead. (B) Burow's advancement flap. (C) Long-term follow-up.
*Courtesy*: S Brian Jiang, MD, Sang Diego, California, USA.

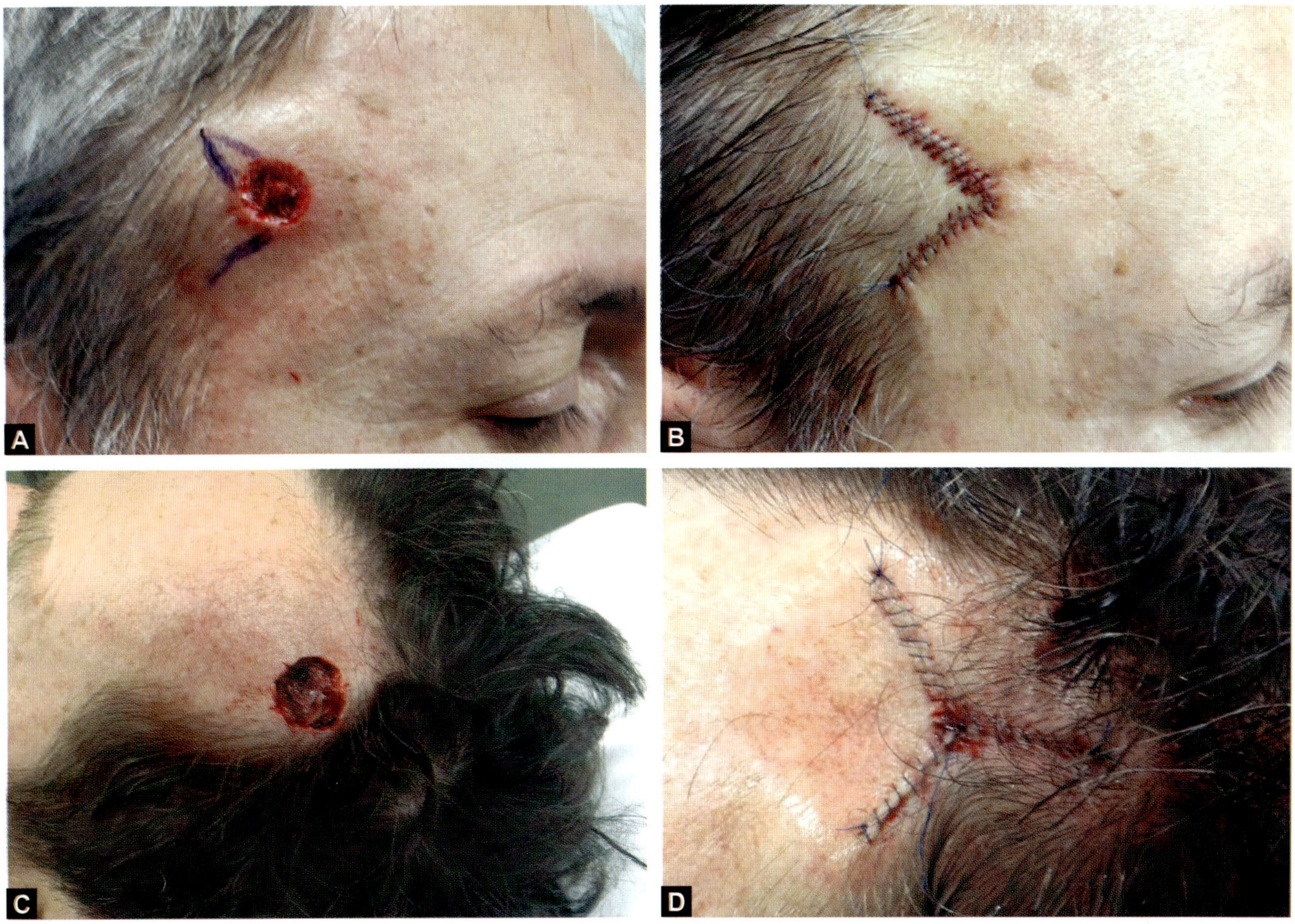

**Figs. 18.11A to D:** Advancement flaps. (A) Mohs Micrographic Surgery (MMS) defect and flap design at lateral forehead near hairline. (B) Unilateral advancement flap. (C) MMS defect at lateral forehead near hairline. (D) Bilateral advancement flap.

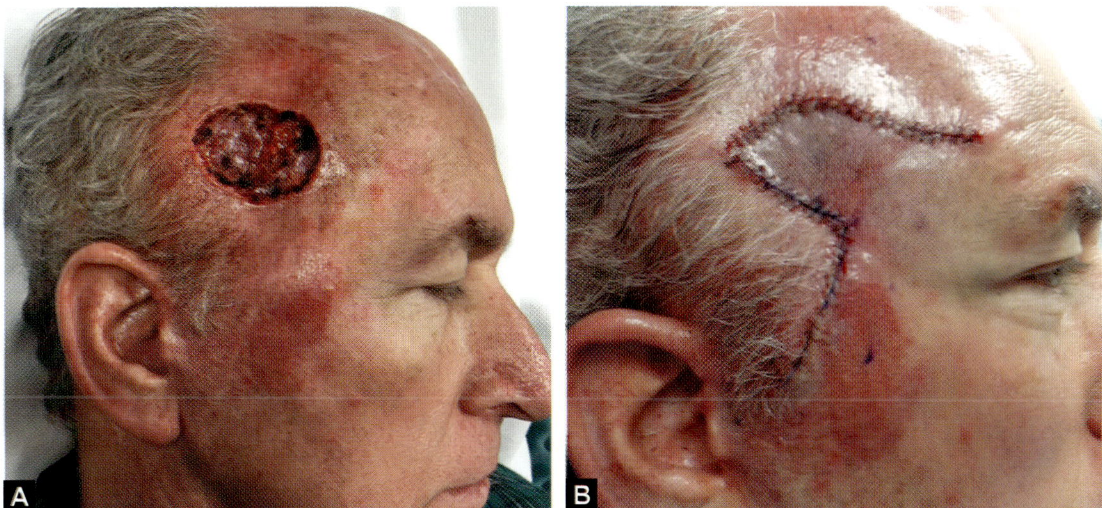

**Figs. 18.12A and B:** Transposition flaps. (A) Mohs Micrographic Surgery (MMS) defect right temple and lateral forehead. (B) Inferiorly based rhombic flap. Temple may serve as a reservoir for redundant tissue for flap design.

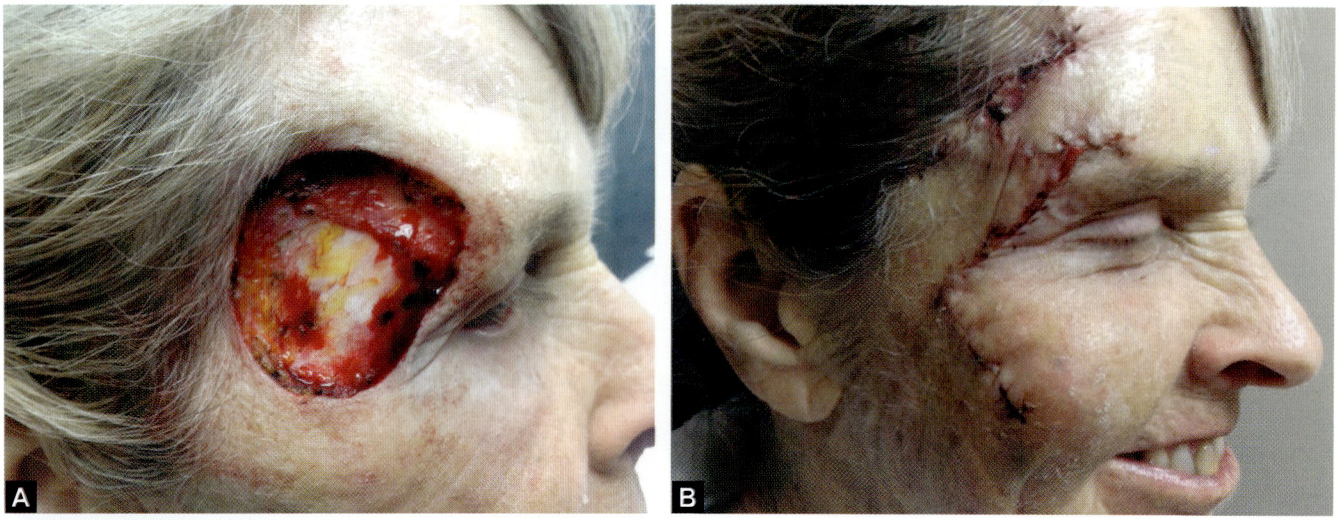

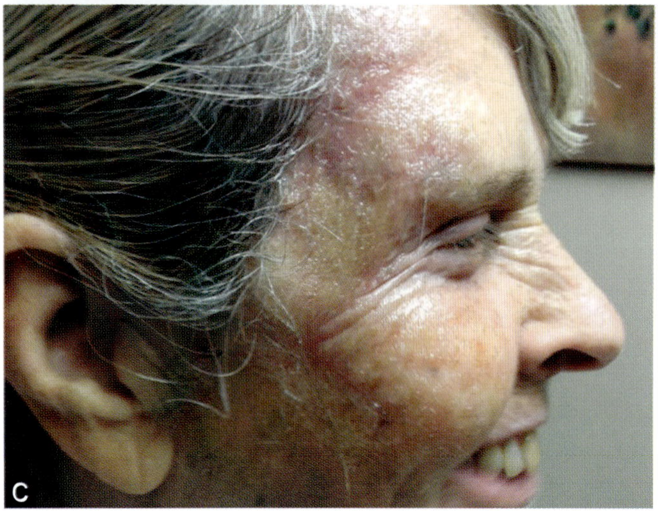

**Figs. 18.13A to C:** Transposition flaps: double rhombic. (A) Mohs Micrographic Surgery (MMS) defect involving lateral forehead and temple. (B) Two rhombic transposition flaps using tissue reservoirs from lateral forehead and from temple and superior cheek. (C) Long-term follow-up.

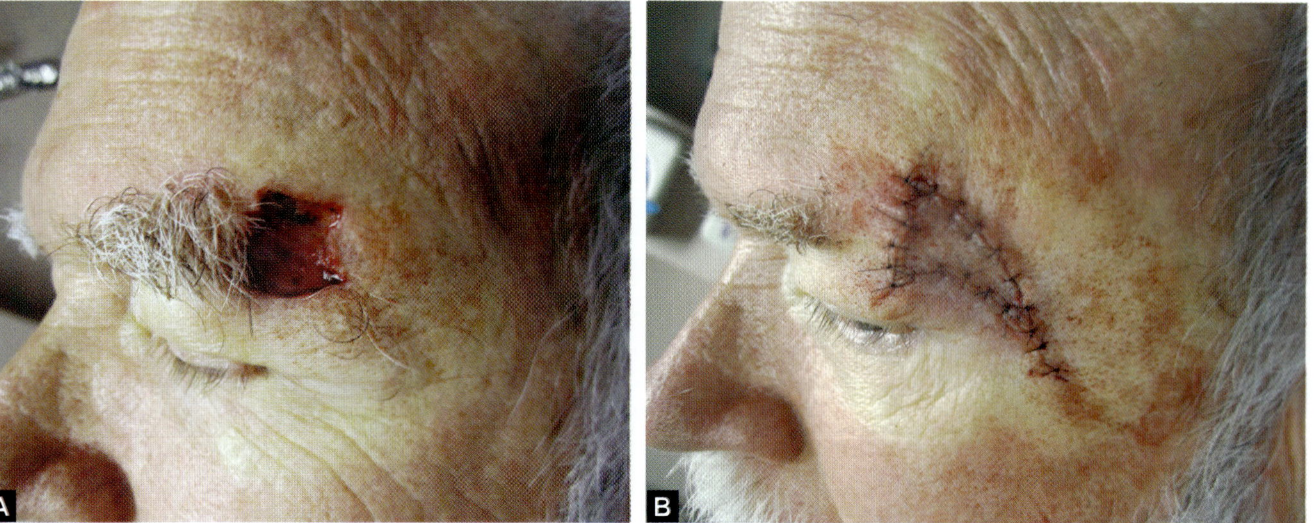

**Figs. 18.14A and B**

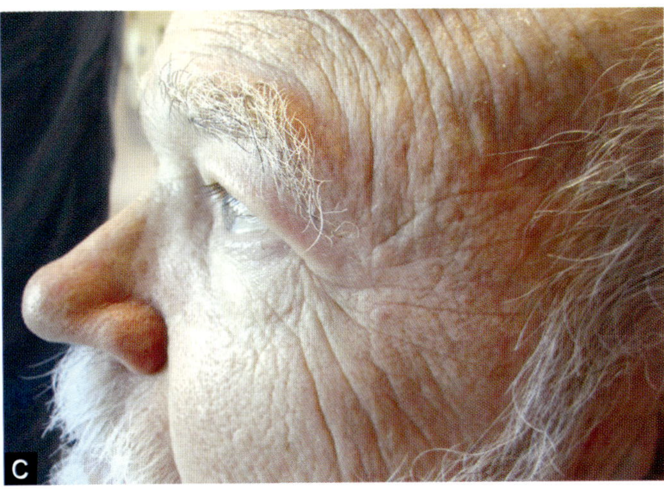

**Figs. 18.14A to C:** V-to-Y advancement flap on the eyebrow. (A) Mohs Micrographic Surgery (MMS) defect on the eyebrow. (B) V-to-Y advancement flap. (C) Long-term follow-up.

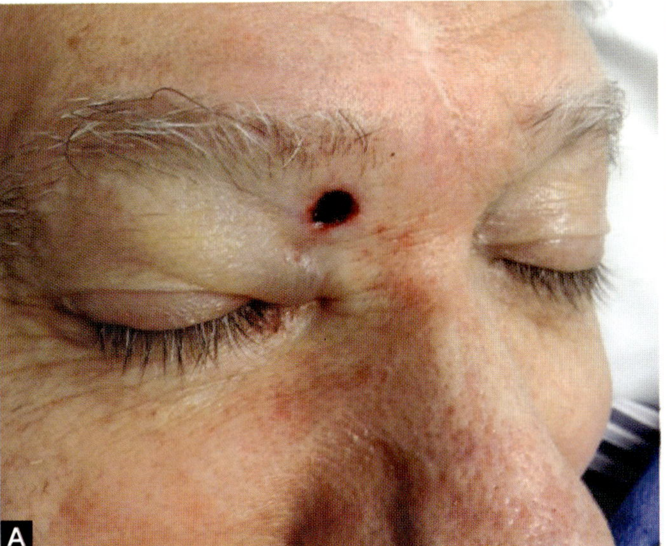

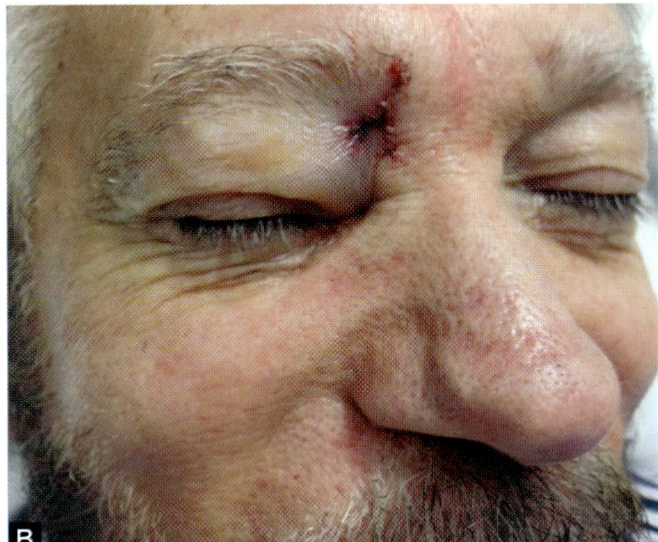

**Figs. 18.15A and B:** Mercedes advancement flap. (A) Mohs Micrographic Surgery (MMS) surgical defect. (B) Mercedes flap.

their preservation. Although this repair necessarily shortens the eyebrow, it restores fullness seen when looking at the patient face-on. For larger more medially based wounds, a subcutaneous island pedicle flap that includes the entire eyebrow can be used.[10] After undermining, the medial edge of the flap should be advanced to a point symmetric to the contralateral eyebrow's medial edge. A releasing incision can be made at the apex or base of the flap to facilitate movement, if necessary. The vascular flap pedicle supports the transferred follicular hair units.

Small defects located at either end of the eyebrow can be closed with a Mercedes advancement flaps. Advancement arms can be angled to avoid extension into the eyebrow (Figs. 18.15A and B). Larger end-defects may be repaired with grafts harvested from the sideburn hair and skin.[11] Although these grafts require a robust host vascular bed, they can offer natural looking results in a one-stage procedure. The preauricular skin offers good color and texture match to the eyebrow region, and the sharp angle between hair shafts and skin in sideburns closely simulates that of the eyebrow. Follicular hair transplantation is an alternate option for restoring local hair; however, this procedure typically requires multiple time consuming procedures.

## Temple

The temple is a concave plane bordered by the lateral canthus and eyebrow medially and scalp hairline laterally.

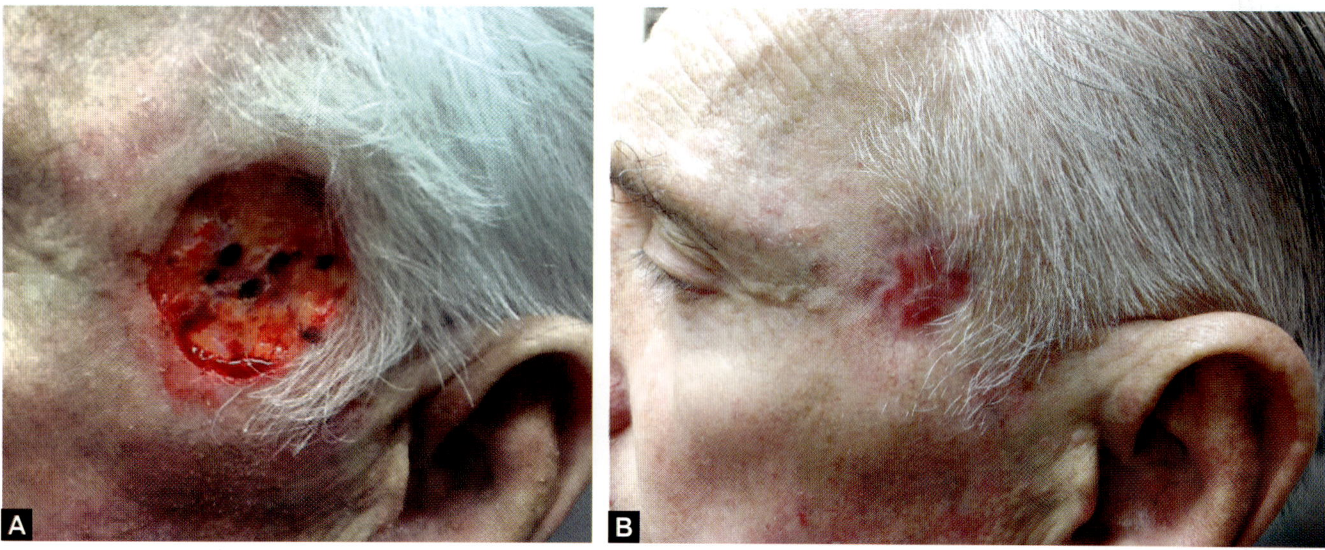


**Figs. 18.16A and B:** Second intention healing. (A) Mohs Micrographic Surgery (MMS) surgical defect. (B) Long-term follow-up.

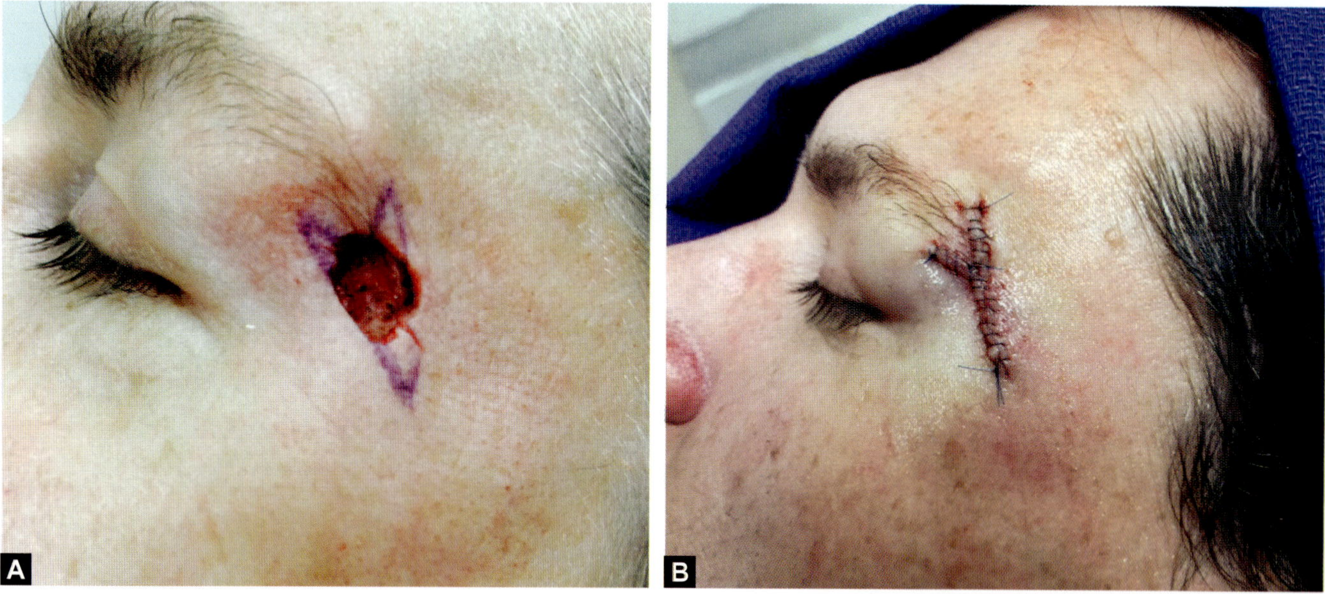


**Figs. 18.17A and B:** M-plasty on temple near lateral canthus. (A) Mohs Micrographic Surgery (MMS) defect and repair design. (B) M-plasty.

The frontal–temporal bone junction marks its superior border, while the zygoma defines it inferiorly. During reconstruction in this region, the temporal branch of the facial nerve is at risk for transection, given its relative superficial location and its minimal protection by thin skin and subcutaneous soft tissues. Keeping closures simple helps avoid unintentional nerve injury.

Because of its general concave shape, temporal wounds often heal well by second intent (Figs. 18.16A and B). When closure is preferred, linear repairs extending radially from the lateral canthus are good choices as incisions can be placed in the crow's feet. To avoid the lateral canthus, an M-plasty can be added to reduce a linear closure's length. M-plasties can be similarly used to avoid the lateral eyebrow (Figs. 18.17A and B). In most patients, the skin and subcutaneous tissues overlying the superficial temporal fascia in the lower temple and upper cheek are meaningfully mobile. Tissue from these regions can thus be recruited for repairing more superiorly located defects. Transposition and advancement flaps tap into this laxity, and large defects are often successfully closed (Figs. 18.18A to E). Advancement flap incisions can be hidden along the hairline and peripheral face with redundant tissue cones removed medially along the RSTLs of the lateral canthus and laterally behind the ear (Figs. 18.19A to C). When large advancement flaps have significant weight, it is helpful to place tacking sutures that anchor the flap to the underlying tightly bound temporalis fascia.

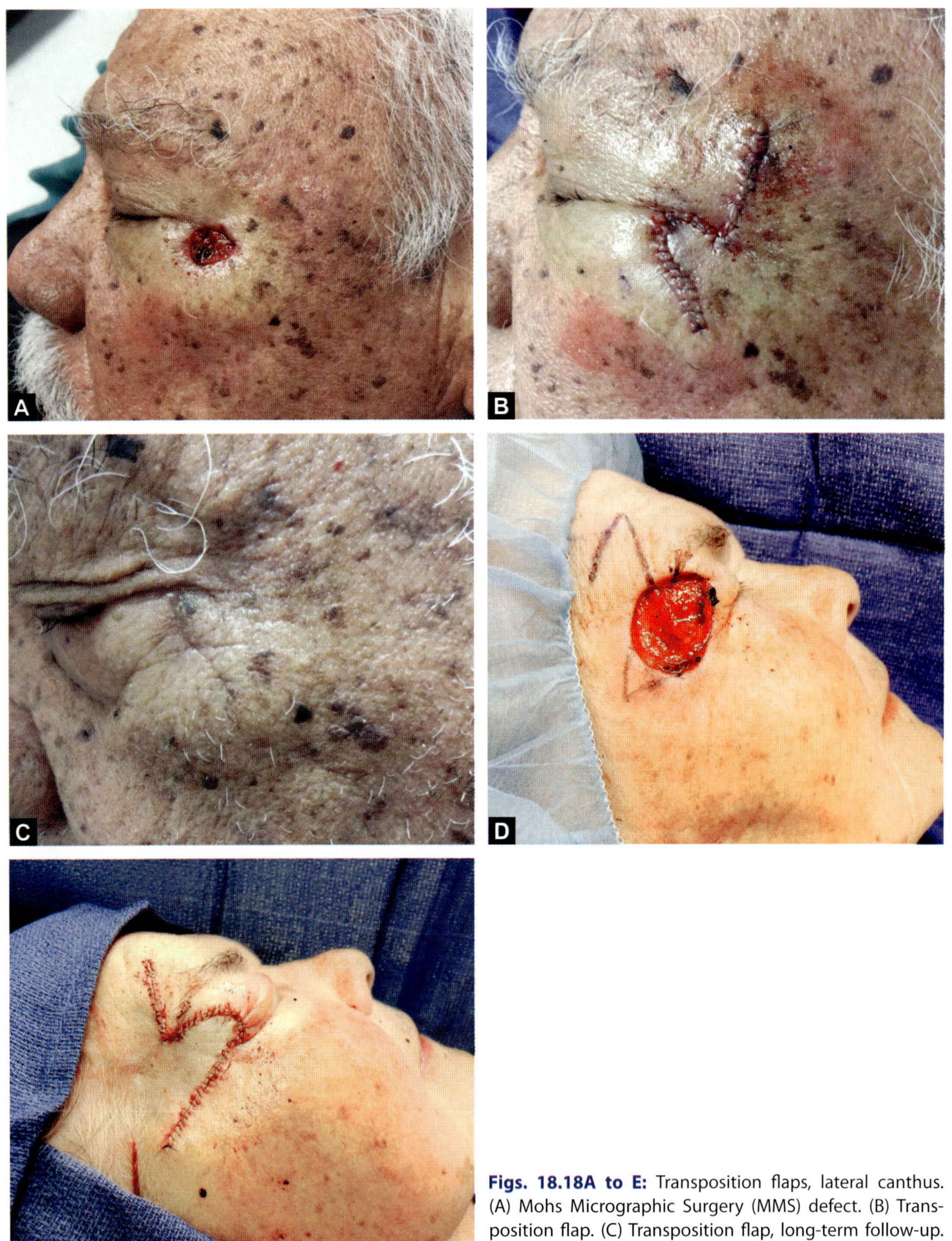

**Figs. 18.18A to E:** Transposition flaps, lateral canthus. (A) Mohs Micrographic Surgery (MMS) defect. (B) Transposition flap. (C) Transposition flap, long-term follow-up. (D) MMS defect. (E) Transposition flap.

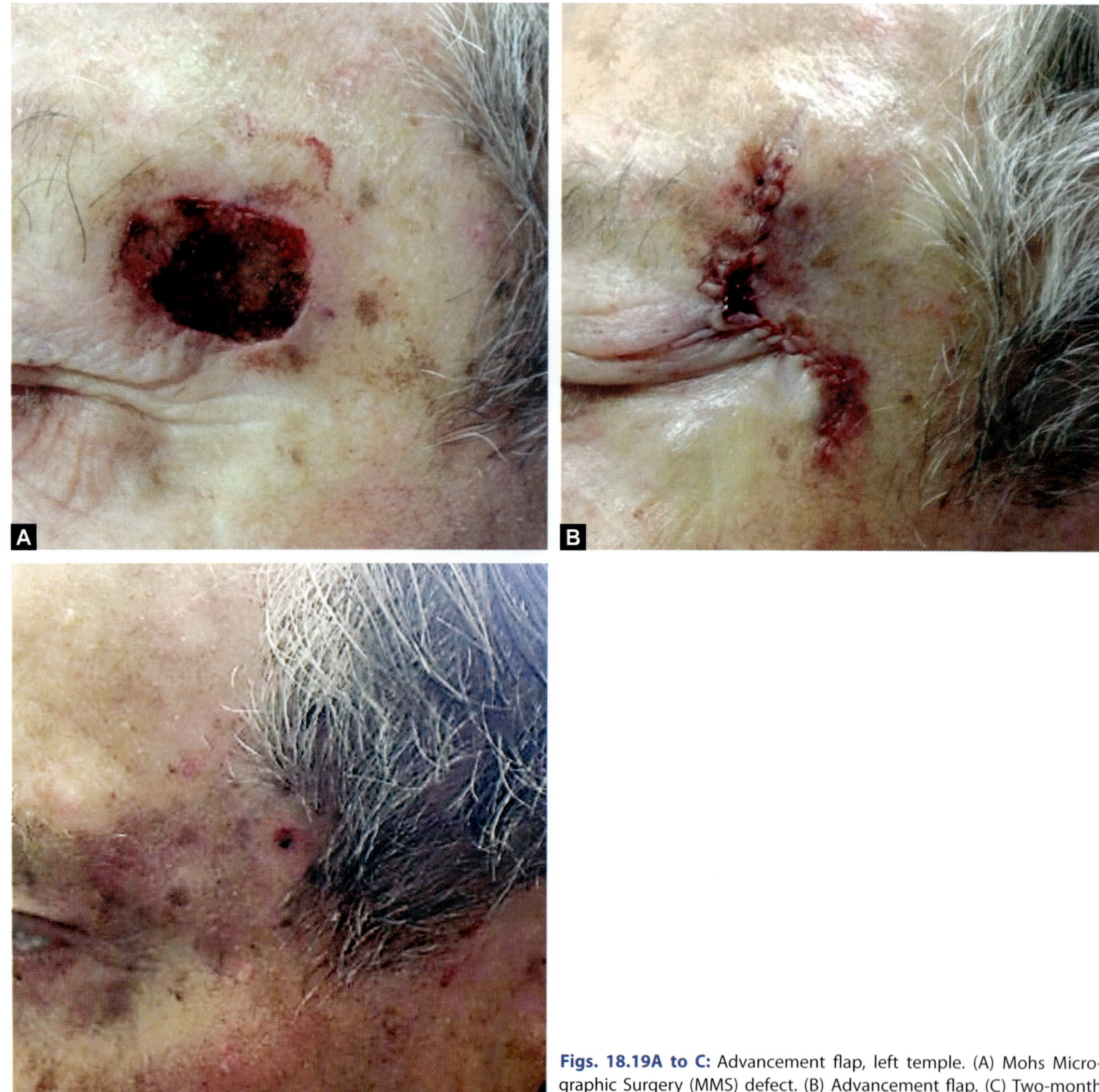


**Figs. 18.19A to C:** Advancement flap, left temple. (A) Mohs Micrographic Surgery (MMS) defect. (B) Advancement flap. (C) Two-month follow-up.

## Combination Closures

For large irregularly shaped defects or for multiple wounds, combination repairs may be necessary. Linear closures combined with Burow's grafts or advancement flaps can cover extensive wounds (Figs. 18.20A to C). Meticulous hemostasis is advisable in large repairs, and temporary drains may be placed in patients at higher bleeding or seroma risk.

In the setting of postoperative temporal nerve injury, a delayed combination repair may also be considered. Temporary paralysis from local anesthesia can be expected on the initial surgery date, and intraoperative nerve manipulation can result in neuropraxia lasting up to 6 months.

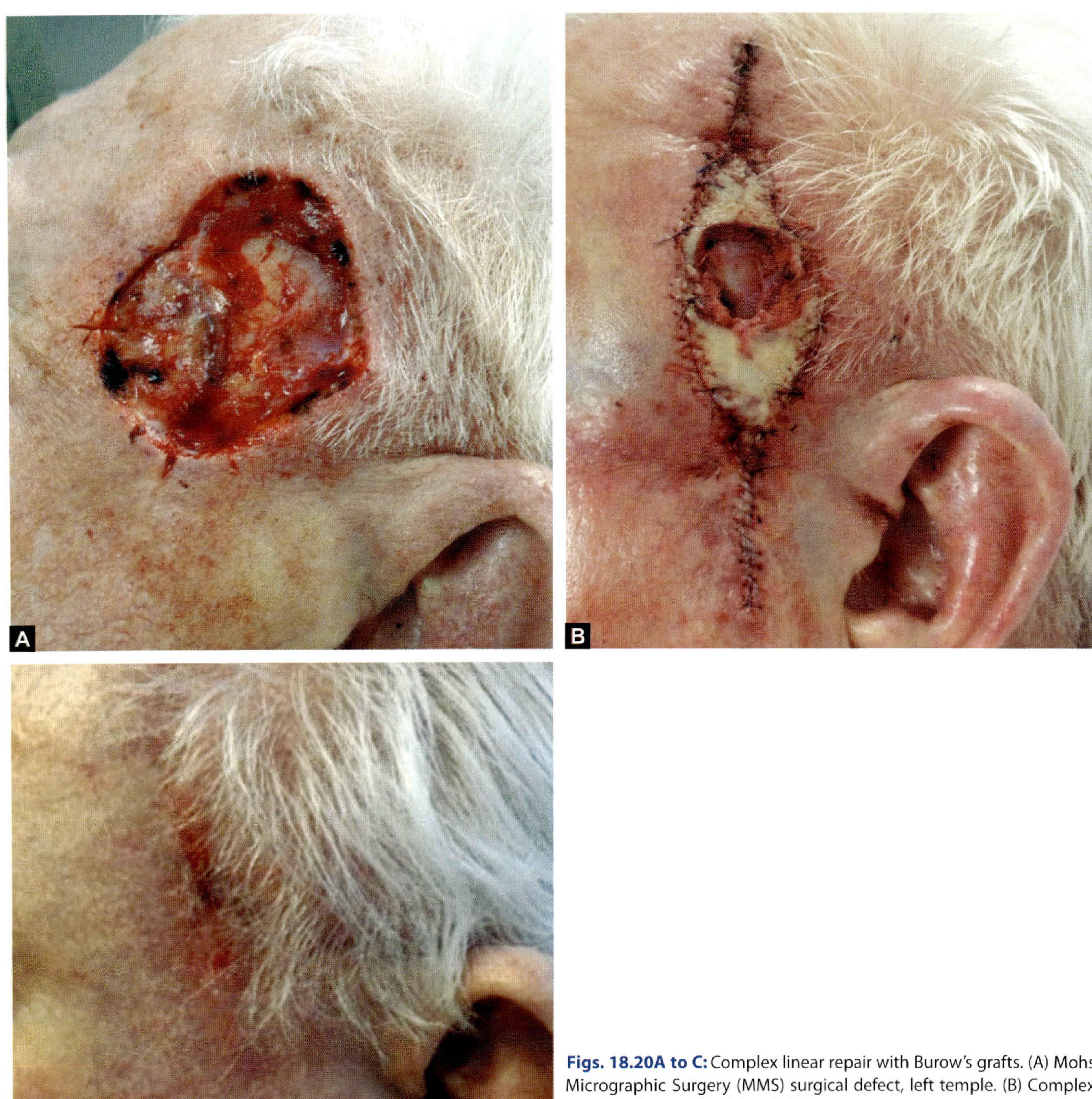

**Figs. 18.20A to C:** Complex linear repair with Burow's grafts. (A) Mohs Micrographic Surgery (MMS) surgical defect, left temple. (B) Complex repair with Burow's grafts. (C) Follow-up.

Although spontaneous return of function may occur through collateral anastomosis, if after 6 months the frontalis muscle remains paralyzed, a direct brow lift can be performed.[12] In this procedure, a tissue ellipse is excised above the ptotic brow. The eyebrow is then elevated and securely tacked to the periosteum at a position slightly above the contralateral eyebrow. Over the next several months, gravity drops the elevated brow to its correct position. Alternatively, if the patient already had loss of function from tumor involvement of the temporal branch of the facial nerve, or if the Mohs Micrographic Surgery sections revealed temporal branch tumor involvement, a direct brow lift may be performed immediately at the time of forehead reconstruction (Figs. 18.21A and B). A direct

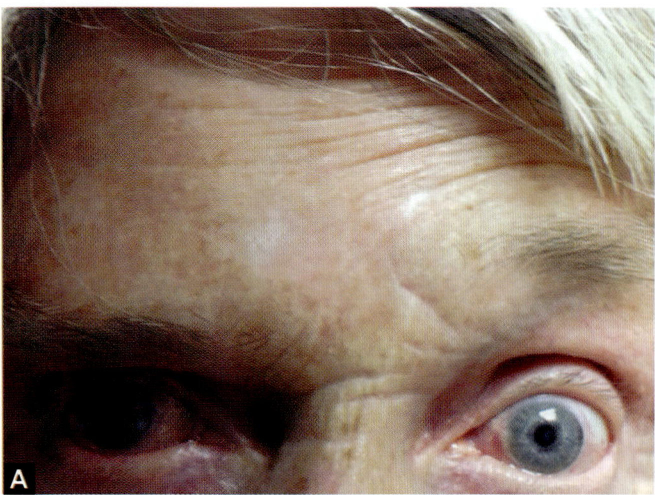
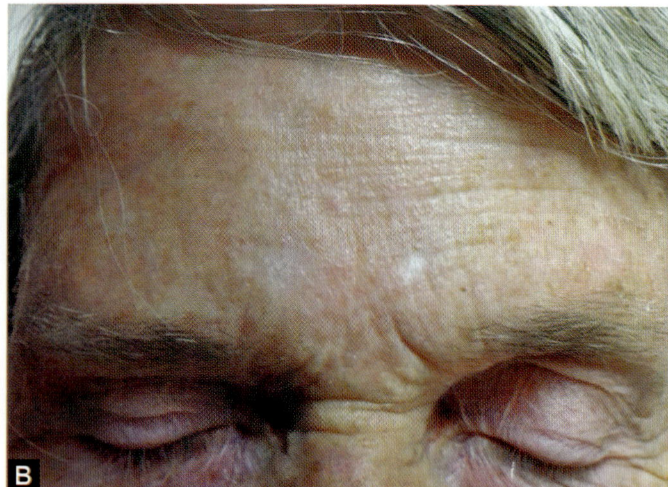

**Figs. 18.21A and B:** Direct brow lift: The patient from Fig. 18.13 had temporal branch involvement from longstanding basal cell carcinoma of right temple. (A) Postoperative loss of right temporal branch function. (B) At rest, right brow remains symmetrical with left brow (no ptosis) because direct brow lift was done at the time of rhombic transposition flap reconstruction.

brow lift can be performed to restore cosmetic symmetry or correct impaired visual fields resulting from the fallen brow.

## CONCLUSION

The forehead is a critical facial region that frames the face. Although most surgical defects can be closed primarily, granulation, skin grafts, and flaps each have their place in the repair armamentarium. Successful reconstructions in this region depend on preservation of facial symmetry and limitation of both sensory and motor nerve injury.

## REFERENCES


1. Donaldson MR, Coldiron BM. Scars after second intention healing. Facial Plast Surg. 2012;28:497-503.
2. Pomaranski MR, Krull EA, Balle MR. Use of the Z-plasty technique for forehead defects. Dermatol Surg. 2005;31:1720-3.
3. Deitch EA, Wheelahan TM, Rose MP, et al. Hypertrophic burn scars: analysis of variables. J Trauma. 1983;23:895-8.
4. Lannon DA, Novak CB, Neligan PC. Resurfacing of colour-mismatched free flaps on the face with split-thickness skin grafts from the scalp. J Plast Reconstr Aesthet Surg. 2009;62:1363-6.
5. Birgfeld CB, Chang B. The periglabellar flap for closure of central forehead defects. Plast Reconstr Surg. 2007;120:130-3.
6. Ransom ER, Jacono AA. Double-opposing rotation-advancement flaps for closure of forehead defects. Arch Facial Plast Surg. 2012;14:342-5.
7. Hussain W, Hafiji J, Salmon P. Frontalis-based island pedicle flaps for the single-stage repair of large defects of the forehead and frontal scalp. Br J Dermatol. 2012;166:771-4.
8. Martinez SA, Masa I, Salinas Velasco V. Nasal root island flap for reconstruction of glabellar defects. Ann Plast Surg. 2015;74:34-6.
9. Stoner JG, Swanson NA. Use of the bipedicled scalp flap for forehead reconstruction. J Dermatol Surg Oncol. 1984;10:213-5.
10. Bakkour W, Ghura V. Medial eyebrow defects: reconstruction with whole eyebrow subcutaneous island pedicle. Ophthal Plast Reconstr Surg. 2013;29:330-2.
11. Matsuda K, Shibata M, Kanazawa S, et al. Eyebrow reconstruction using a composite skin graft from sideburns. Plast Reconstr Surg Glob Open. 2015;3:e290.
12. Kurlander DE, Collins AB, Bordeaux JS. Direct brow lift after Mohs-induced temporal nerve transection. Dermatol Surg. 2013;39:1132-4.

# CHAPTER 19

# Reconstruction of the Ear

*Robert Egbers Jr, Sarah M Sung, Timothy Wang*

## INTRODUCTION

The external ear poses unique and interesting challenges to the reconstructive surgeon due to its composition, shape, and function.

The superior three-quarters of the ear can be thought of as a trilaminate structure of skin, cartilage, and skin. Inferiorly, skin and fibrofatty tissue compose the lobule and its "tail" as it extends up the inferior margin of the helix. The arcuate contour of the ear is familiar and distortion of this free margin is quickly noted. Complex concavities and convexities of the anterior ear add further complication. And any surgery on the ear must preserve its function to collect and channel sound.

The skin of the anterior surface of the ear is relatively inelastic—it moves and stretches little even when separated from the underlying cartilage. In contrast, the skin of the helical rim posterior to its attachment to the free cartilage margin and much of the skin of the posterior surface is relatively mobile. Underlying cartilage possesses shape memory and will exert constant force on repairs that distort it. The ear's "tilted bowl" shape—attached at its side to the scalp—provides opportunities to transpose tissue from the cheek and scalp onto the ear but care must be taken to avoid altering the complex topography of the anterior ear or blunting the posterior auricular sulcus.

## BACKGROUND

The external ear arises embryologically from the first and second branchial arches. The auricle begins its development as six mesenchymal hillocks, which appear during the sixth week of gestation (Figs. 19.1A to F). Each hillock develops into a portion of the auricle, with the anterior hillocks giving rise to the tragus, root (or crus) of the helix, and the superior helix. The posterior hillocks become the triangular fossa, antihelix, antitragus, and lobule. The auricle is completely formed by the 20th week of gestation, including all major topographic landmarks: the helix, antihelix, crura of the antihelix, tragus, antitragus, scaphoid fossa, triangular fossa, concha cymba, concha cavum, and lobule (Fig. 19.2).

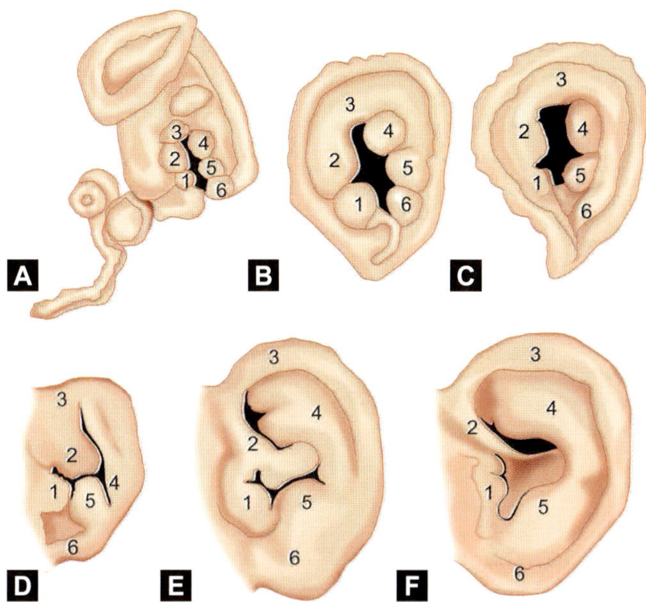


**Figs. 19.1A to F:** Embryology of the ear. Migration of mesenchymal hillocks 1 to 6 through development.

The ear is supported by a single piece of pliable elastic cartilage. Cartilage underlies only the superior three-quarters to two-thirds of the ear (Fig. 19.3). Inferiorly, the lobule is composed of a fibrofatty tissue. Anteriorly, the skin enveloping the cartilage overlies little subcutaneous adipose, and is tightly adherent to the perichondrium. In contrast, the posterior aspect of the ear contains a thick

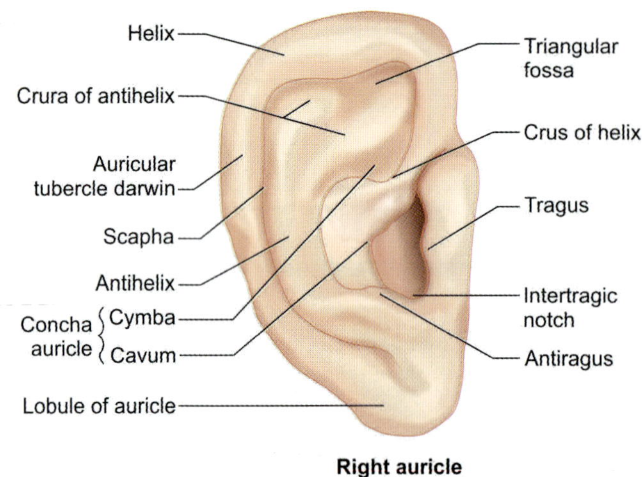


Fig. 19.2: Anatomy of the ear.

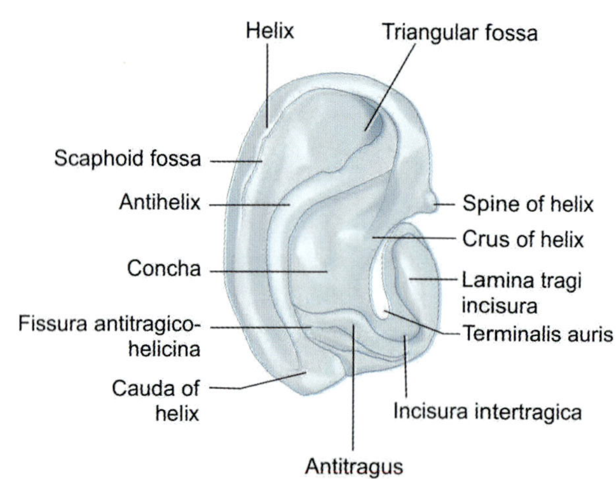


Fig. 19.3: Underlying cartilage of the ear.

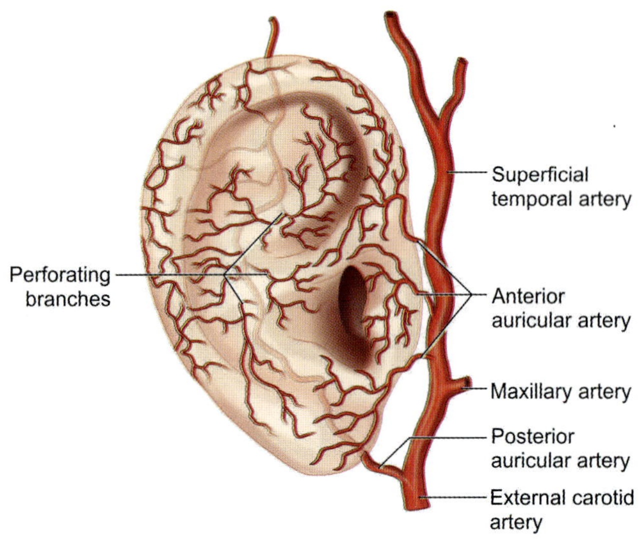


Fig. 19.4: Blood supply of the ear.

layer of adipose between the skin and the perichondrium. The fascial layer between the skin and the perichondrium contains a subdermal plexus of vessels that provides nutrients to the cartilage.

The arterial blood supply to the ear is derived entirely from the external carotid system primarily from branches of the superficial temporal artery (STA) and posterior auricular artery (PAA) (Fig. 19.4). The anterior surface of the ear is supplied by auricular branches of the STA and branches of the PAA that perforate the cartilage from the posterior ear. Three auricular branches of the STA and five perforating branches of the PAA provide a robust and interconnecting blood supply to the anterior ear. The posterior surface of the ear is supplied by branches of the PAA alone. Venous drainage occurs through the superficial temporal, posterior auricular, and to a lesser extent the retromandibular veins, which then drain to the external jugular venous system. Lymphatic drainage is primarily to the preauricular, infra-auricular, and mastoid lymph nodes.

The sensory innervation of the external ear is via nerves derived from the cervical plexus and branches of the cranial nerves (Fig. 19.5). The auriculotemporal nerve, a branch of cranial nerve V3, supplies the helical root and tragus. The superior portion of the auricle is innervated by branches of the lesser occipital nerve (C2, C3). The great auricular nerve (C2, C3) innervates the majority of the external ear. It divides into anterior and posterior branches with the anterior branch supplying the lower half of the anterior ear and the posterior branch supplying the lower half of the posterior ear. The concha is supplied by Arnold's nerve, a branch of the vagus nerve (CN X) and roots of CN VII.

## AURICULAR ARCHITECTURE

The proper orientation and positioning of the ear are critical for the success of auricular reconstruction.[1] There are three measurements critical for the proper positioning of the auricle: axis, level, and distance from the orbit.[2] The axis is defined as the line through the long axis of the ear. Importantly, the vertical axis of the auricle is inclined posteriorly at an angle of 15° to 20°.[3] The superior level of the ear should match the level of the lateral brow or

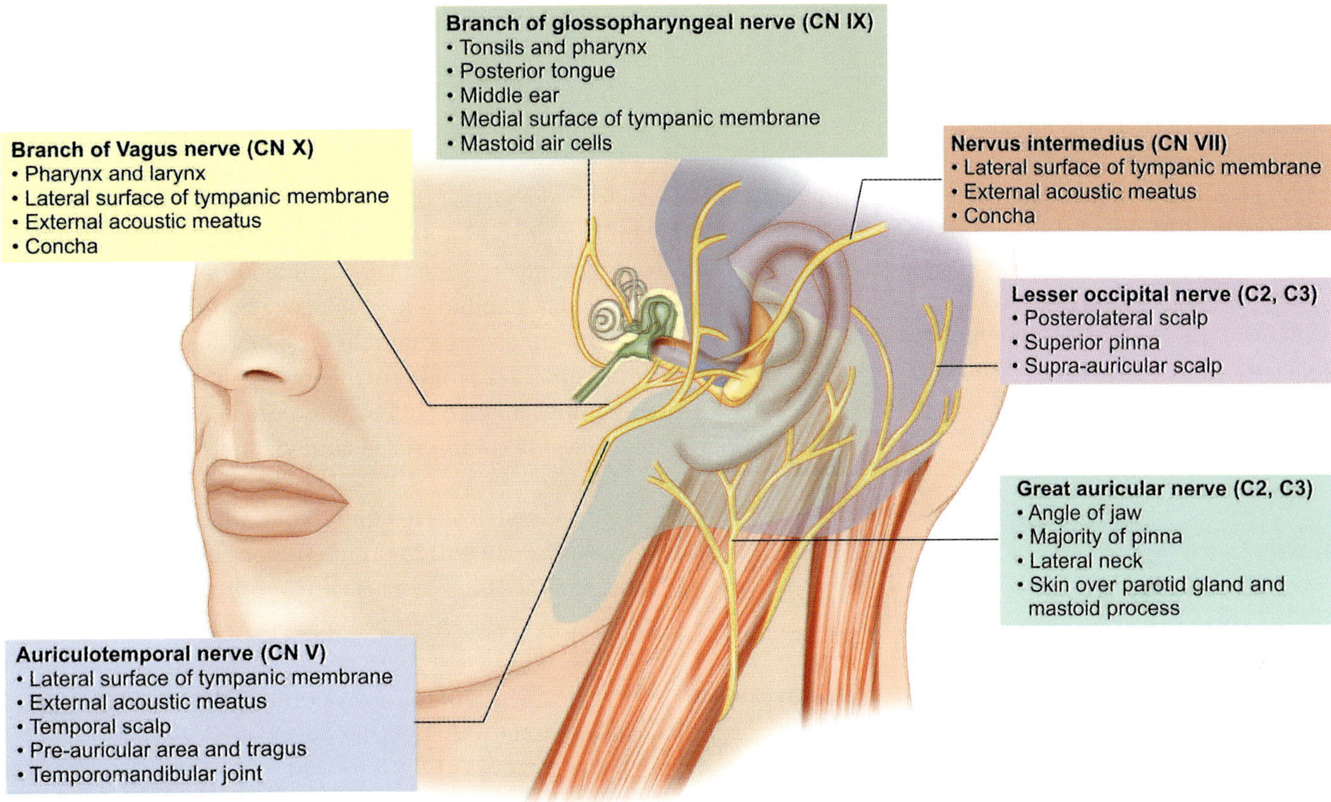


**Fig. 19.5:** Innervation of the ear.

supraorbital rim, while the lobule aligns with the base of the columella.[4] The distance from the root of the helix to the lateral canthus should be 6–7 cm in adults. The horizontal width of the normal adult ear is 3–4 cm, and the vertical height is roughly 6 cm.[5] To account for individual variations in auricular features and positioning, the contralateral ear should always be used as a template in planning reconstruction of the ear. The most important principle of auricular reconstruction is that orientation, location, and size of the reconstructed ear be as similar to the normal ear as possible.

## EAR RECONSTRUCTION

The following largely addresses reconstruction of surgical defects following Mohs extirpation of skin cancer. There are varied approaches to a discussion of ear reconstruction and we have chosen to address defects at specific sites. Although there are often many options, in the majority of cases a few best ones usually exist.

### Conchal Bowl

Reconstructive options in both the conchal cymba and cavum are limited and oftentimes grafting is the best option. In the correct setting, pull-through pedicle flaps based on the retroauricular scalp skin can be successful. Blunting of the posterior auricular sulcus limits these to more anterior, inferior conchal bowl defects. Given its concave contour smaller defects at this site can be allowed to heal by second intention with great success. When larger conchal bowl defects are allowed to heal in this way, it is often helpful to fenestrate the cartilage with 2 or 3 mm punch holes to facilitate granulation from the deep tissues on the other side of the cartilage.

### Triangular Fossa

Transposition flaps utilizing skin from the preauricular cheek or postauricular sulcus can be considered, but as mentioned above, they must take into account crossing the root of the helix. They are most successful when this

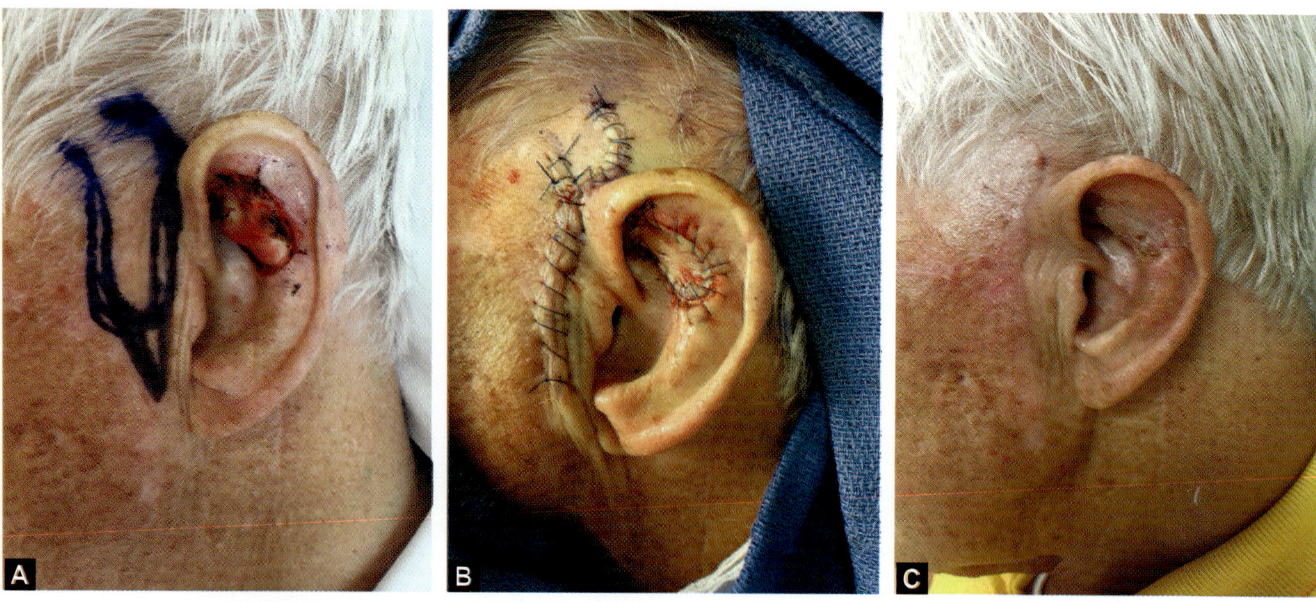

**Figs. 19.6A to C:** Tunneled transposition flap. (A) A post-Mohs defect. (B) Defect repaired with the tunneled transposition immediately post-operative. (C) Well-healed defect, seen in follow-up.

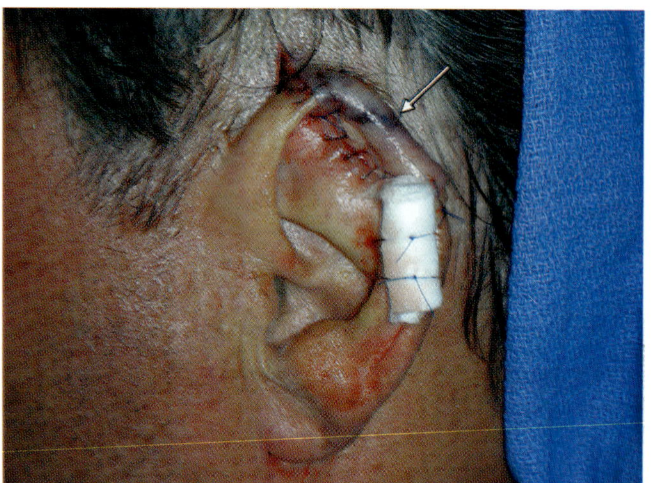

**Fig. 19.7:** Interpolation flap with the helix recreated. Note plicating suture to recreate helical rim (arrow). Also, a bolster (white) was used to tack down the protruding ear, reducing tension on the flap.

margin is removed in the course of tumor extirpation, but when properly designed the margin can be removed prior to repair with relatively little cosmetic impact. Alternatively, transposition flaps can be tunneled beneath the helical root margin as a single-stage repair (Figs. 19.6A to C). This closure requires de-epithelialization of the flap that could compromise flap survival.

As with other partial thickness defects of the ear, both full- and split-thickness grafts can also be utilized, giving an excellent cosmetic result. The editors usually prefer to harvest the graft from the postauricular area.

## Antihelix and Scaphoid Fossa

Interpolated flaps are often the best option for defects in these locations especially those that involve loss of the helical rim. Robust flaps, they allow the surgeon great flexibility in design and are useful in nearly any defect of the anterior ear lateral to the conchal bowl. When the helical rim has been lost, plicating sutures can be used to recreate the helical rim (Fig. 19.7). A pull-through design can be helpful in gaining some anterior extension (Figs. 19.8A and B).

Skin grafting is a good option for defects at these sites especially as a single-stage procedure. Both full- and split-thickness grafts can be used successfully on the ear. Graft survival can be improved by extending defects through cartilage when this does not compromise the structural integrity of the ear or by fenestrating the cartilage. Typical of grafts elsewhere, matching skin tone and quality are sometimes difficult. Due to poorer perfusion and thus graft survival, defects that cross the helical rim but leave intact the free margin of cartilage are best repaired with a flap or wedge rather than a graft. Grafts are good choices for larger defects on the anterior surface of the ear.

The distance of the ear from donor sites on the cheek or scalp make single-stage flaps difficult options for defects on the antihelix and scaphoid fossa.

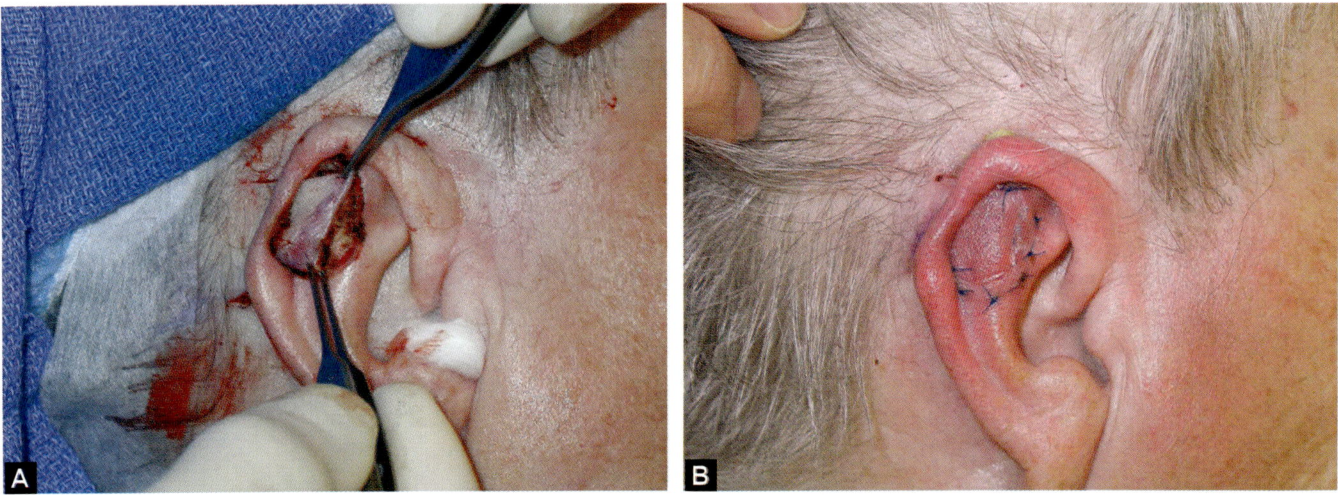


**Figs. 19.8A and B:** Interpolation pull-through. (A) Pull-through interpolation in process. (B) Defect repaired, immediately post-operative.

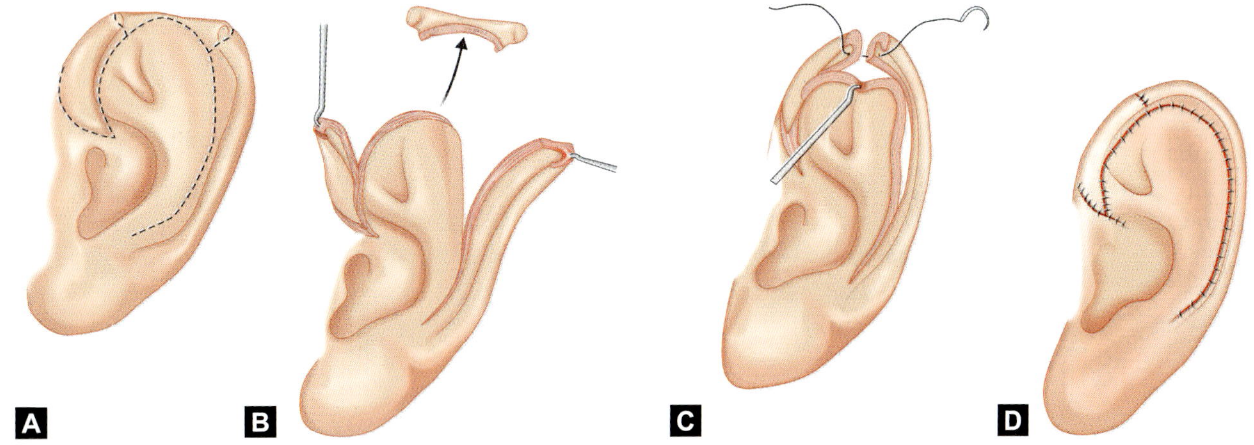


**Figs. 19.9A to D:** Helical advancement flap. (A) Planning incision, with dashed lines. (B) Incision of flap. (C) Placement of key stitch, approximating the helical rim. (D) Repaired defect, immediately post-operative.

## Helical Rim, Helical Root to Helical Apex

For small narrow defects at this site, wedge resection and even composite grafting can be used.

Transposition flaps originating on the preauricular cheek or postauricular sulcus work well here. To avoid blunting of the postauricular sulcus, they must be based near the attachment of the helical root limiting their use much beyond the apex of the helix.

## Helical Rim, Helical Apex to Inferior Margin of Cartilage

Skin covering the helical rim is more elastic with greater mobility when dissected from the underlying cartilage. With undermining posteriorly, smaller helical rim defects can often be closed primarily side to side. But for medium- to large-sized defects, helical advancement flaps are often useful. There are a variety of techniques—unilateral or bilateral (U-plasty and H-plasty) involving skin only or full thickness through cartilage (Figs. 19.9A to D). Most movement comes from inferiorly, utilizing skin from the inferior portion of the helical rim not overlying cartilage. Antia-Buch described advancement closure including skin over the posterior ear (Figs. 19.10A to D). Despite the increased elasticity of helical rim and posterior auricular skin, full thickness removal of auricular cartilage or lobule may be required to allow closure of larger helical rim defects, decreasing the overall height of the ear (Figs. 19.11A and B).

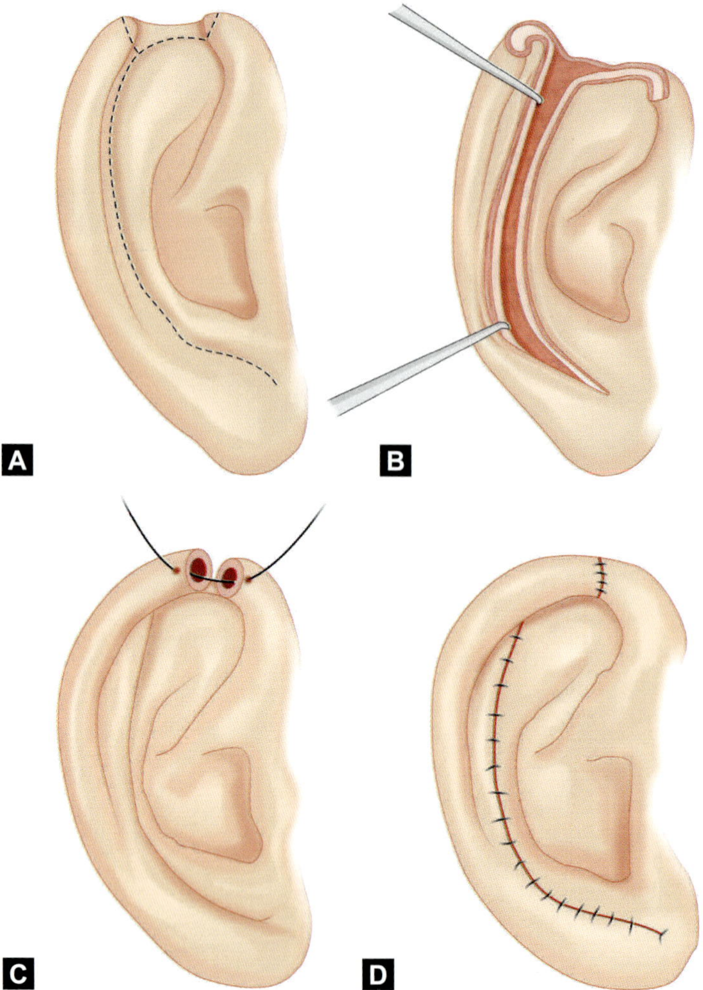


**Figs. 19.10A to D:** Antia-Buch advancement flap. (A) Planning incision, with dashed lines. (B) Incision of flap. (C) Placement of key stitch, approximating the helical rim. (D) Repaired defect, immediately post-operative.

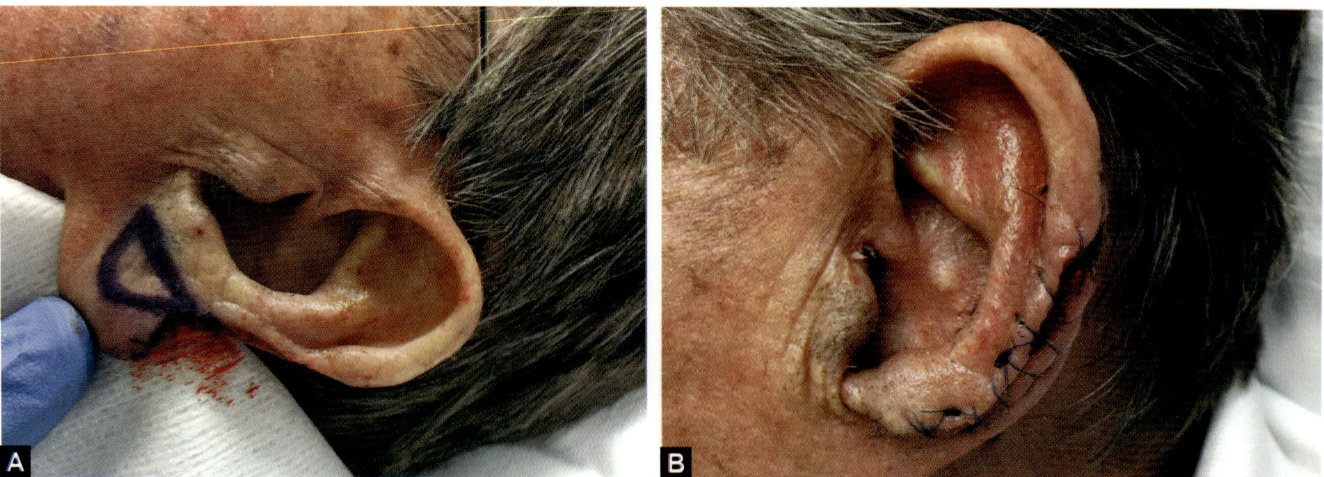


**Figs. 19.11A and B:** Earlobe-based helical advancement with lobule resection. (A) Post-Mohs defect. (B) Repaired defect, 1 week immediately postoperative.

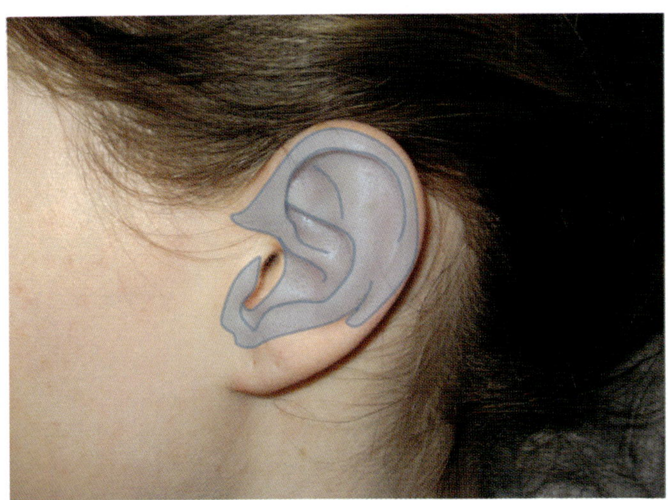

**Fig. 19.12:** Underlying cartilage with demonstration of size of lobule.

Interpolated flaps are extremely useful for medium- to large-sized defects of the helical rim in these locations. As previously mentioned, they are robust and offer great flexibility in design. In contrast to advancement flaps, they do not affect the height of the ear. However, for defects of the helical rim only, a single-stage advancement flap is often preferred over a multistage closure. Interpolated flaps are best when loss along the helical rim is too great to close by advancement.

Wedge resection can be used successfully for small defects of the superior and middle helical rim. However, the inelastic nature of the cartilage must be kept in mind. A helpful analogy is to imagine a triangular wedge removed from the margin of a paper plate. When the cut edges are approximated, the plate does not stretch but instead forms a cone. Coning can be bothersome to the patient and constant pressure on the closure from the distorted cartilage can lead to spreading of the scar over time. In addition, alterations in the smooth radius of the helical rim render wedge resection useful in only relatively smaller defects. Techniques exist to reduce the coning effect of wedge resection, but the authors often prefer alternatives as mentioned above for larger defects at this site.

Defects that involve both the anterior and posterior helical rim where cartilage is left intact are best closed by flap or wedge resection rather than graft due to poor perfusion of exposed cartilage.

## Posterior Ear

The skin on the posterior ear is somewhat more elastic than on the anterior ear. This more easily allows primary closure and adjacent tissue transfer closures. Closure of wounds on the posterior ear exerts force against the free margin of the helical rim and forces that cup the ear. Given this constant force, closures that evert the ear posteriorly will improve with time. As with the anterior ear, transposition flaps can be designed that recruit skin from the postauricular sulcus and scalp. Both split- and full-thickness grafts work well on the posterior ear and as the area is seldom well visualized by the patient, healing by second intention is quite useful for smaller, more superficial defects. Interpolated flaps work especially well for those posterior ear defects closer to the helical rim or those involving both the posterior and anterior ear.

## Lobule

The lobule is the largest reservoir of free tissue on the ear. For purposes of this discussion, we will consider any site on the inferior ear that does not have underlying cartilage as the lobule. The lobule then constitutes a much larger portion of the ear than may be visually apparent and the surgeon is encouraged to palpate the ear when evaluating the lobule's size (Fig. 19.12). Note that nearly the entire lower quarter of the ear has no underlying cartilage. The majority of the lobule lies below the antitragus, but the "tail of the lobule" extends superiorly to approximately the level of the tragus. With age, the lobule grows. Defects of both the anterior and posterior lobule can easily be converted to a wedge by extending the defect through and through. Although simple and easily performed, wedge resection on the lobule poses two unique pitfalls. First, wedge resection on the inferior-most lobule can cause the lobule to taper to a point especially in patients with a hanging lobule. And second, due to tethering of the lobule at its attachment to the cheek, as defects move superiorly along the lobule, wedge resection can result in alteration in the contour of the ear. Therefore, wedge resections in this region of the lobule are best designed with unequal lengths so that the wedge closes with an element of advancement (Figs. 19.13A and B). Z-plasty and other techniques can also be employed to prevent alterations in contour.

Small defects on the anterior and posterior lobule near the attachment to the cheek can be closed with both superiorly and inferiorly based transposition flaps.

Due to its unique composition, shape, and function, the external ear challenges the reconstructive surgeon in interesting and exciting ways. Closure of defects on the ear must always take into consideration the relative inelasticity of the skin of the ear, the helical rim as a free margin, and the underlying cartilage's resistance to distortion.

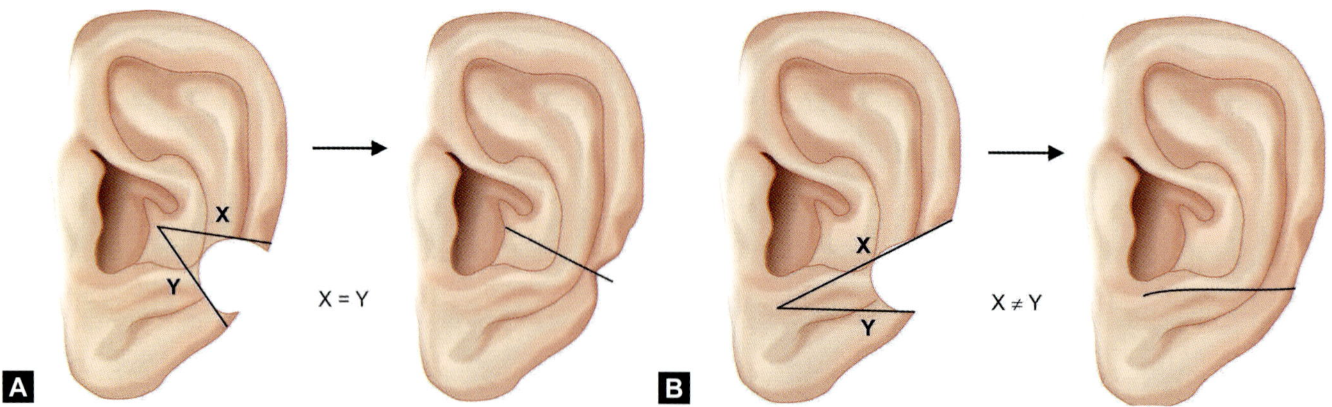


**Figs. 19.13A and B:** Uneven wedge resection. Where X is the length of the superior incising cut of the flap and Y is the length of the inferior incising cut of the flap. This figure depicts that when X = Y, the helical contour is altered, but when X ≠ Y, a component of advancement is introduced along segment Y, maintaining correct helical contour.

## REFERENCES

1. Park SS, Hood RJ. Auricular reconstruction. Otolaryngol Clin North Am. 2001;34:713-38.
2. Tolleth H. Artistic anatomy, dimensions, and proportions of the external ear. Clin Plast Surg. 1978;5:337.
3. Postnick JC, Al-Qatta MM, Whitaker LA. Assessment of the preferred vertical position of the ear. Plast Reconstr Surg. 1993;91:1198.
4. Hadlock TA, Cheney ML, Quatela VC. Reconstruction of the auricle. In: Baker SR (Ed), Local Flaps in Facial Reconstruction. St. Louis, MO: Mosby; 2014.
5. Farkas LG. Anthropometry of the normal and defective ear. Clin Past Surg. 1990;17(2):213-21.

# CHAPTER 20

# Reconstruction of the Scalp

*Brian Hibler, Anthony M Rossi, Kishwer S Nehal*

## INTRODUCTION

Surgery on the scalp is performed for a variety of reasons including incisional or excisional biopsy, removal of benign or malignant lesions, cosmetic purposes, or reconstruction after traumatic injury among many others. When performing an operation on the scalp, there are a number of factors one must account for. In addition to obtaining adequate closure, for many patients it is imperative to obtain acceptable cosmetic outcomes. First and foremost, one needs to contemplate the anatomic and aesthetic elements involved in the surgical site. The physician must assess the depth of injury or excision needed, as well as the quality of the tissue at the surgical site (e.g. history of radiation therapy, presence of infection, or prior surgery). The patient's comorbidities and personal preferences must also be considered. A variety of techniques for reconstruction and wound closure can be utilized depending upon the aforementioned factors. Depending on the surgical defect, the reconstructive treatment ladder includes healing by granulation, and secondary intention, primary closure, local skin flaps, full-thickness or split-thickness skin grafts (FTSG/STSG), as well as tissue expansion. This chapter outlines the essential reconstructive concepts regarding anatomy of the scalp and surgical planning, highlighting potential areas for complications, as well as provide the author's suggestions based on the location and size of the defect.

## ANATOMY

A thorough understanding of the anatomy of the scalp is imperative for successful reconstruction. The scalp is defined as the skin and soft tissue layers extending to the periosteum of the calvaria that encompasses the cranial vault. For the purposes of this chapter, the forehead has been considered as a separate cosmetic unit, with the anterior limit of the scalp ending at the normal frontal hairline. Laterally, the scalp is bordered by the temples and auricles and posteriorly the scalp extends to the superior nuchal line, with the boundaries being demarcated by the lateral and posterior hairlines, respectively.[1] Here we outline the most significant aspects of scalp anatomy that are relevant to reconstruction and surgical planning.

### Anatomic Layers

The scalp has five distinct anatomic layers, commonly remembered by the mnemonic SCALP: skin, subcutaneous tissue, galea aponeurotica, loose areolar (connective) tissue, and pericranium (Fig. 20.1). The skin of the scalp ranges between 3 mm over the vertex and 8 mm over the occiput, and is the thickest skin on the body. This layer contains hair follicles, sebaceous and sweat glands.

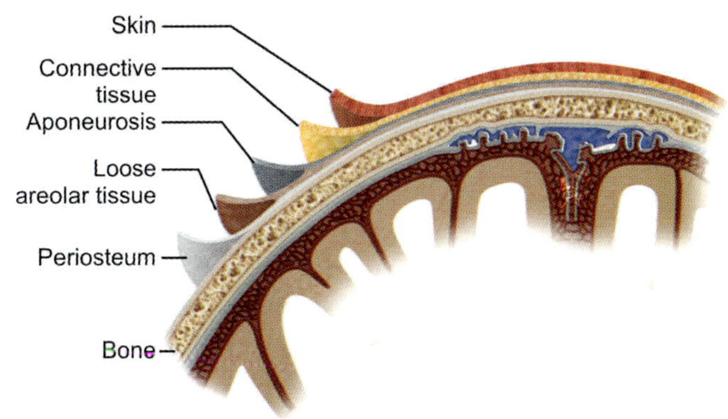


**Fig. 20.1:** Layers of the scalp.

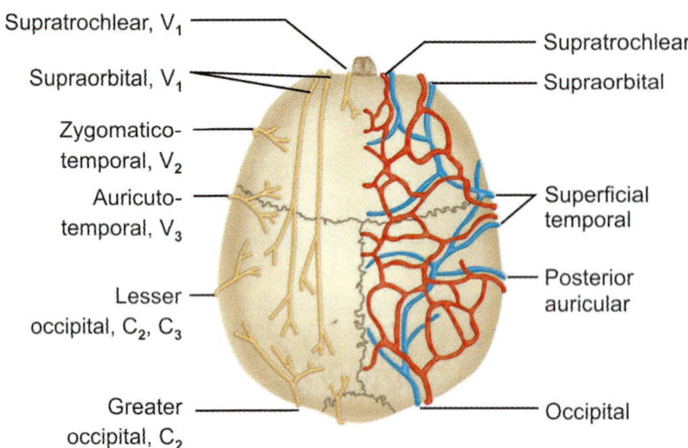


**Fig. 20.2:** Vasculature and innervation of the scalp.

The subcutaneous layer is made of dense connective and fatty tissue. It contains vasculature, lymphatics, and sensory innervation, and is divided into multiple small compartments by fibrous septa. The galea aponeurotica, also called the epicranial aponeurosis, is a fibromuscular layer 1–2 mm thick that lies over the vertex of the scalp, and is contiguous with the frontalis muscle anteriorly, occipitalis muscle posteriorly, and temporoparietal fascia laterally.[2] Dissection in this plane is very difficult, as it is tightly bound to the overlying subcutaneous tissues. Additionally, it is important to limit separation between this layer and the overlying skin to avoid devascularizing the skin. Coronal defects or incisions made through the galea result in antagonistic forces between the frontalis and occipitalis muscles, resulting in widely separating wound edges, leading to increased risk of hemorrhage.[3] Beneath the galea aponeurotica is the loose areolar tissue, a relatively avascular layer. This tissue functions to allow for layers above it to slide as a unit over the cranium.[4] This layer is known as the "danger space" of the scalp, as it readily permits the spread of infections or fluids and is traversed by emissary veins that connect the dural venous sinuses with veins in the scalp. Nevertheless, the ability to surgically dissect this space without significant bleeding is of great importance, and has been discussed later in this chapter. Lastly, the pericranium is the periosteum of the outer surface of the skull and represents the deepest layer of the scalp. It is a dense membranous or fibrous sheet that is loosely attached to the galea aponeurotica and laterally it fuses with deep temporal fascia.[5]

## Vasculature and Lymphatics

The blood supply to the scalp is chiefly cutaneous, with large vessels entering from the periphery and running centrally within the subcutaneous tissues (Fig. 20.2). The paired arterial vessels originate from the carotids. The internal carotid gives rise to the ophthalmic artery whose branches are the supratrochlear and supraorbital arteries that course anteriorly over the forehead. These vessels supply the anterior vascular territory. The external carotid has three branches that supply the scalp. The smallest branch, the posterior auricular artery, leaves the posterior aspect of the external carotid and supplies the area posterior to the ear. The occipital artery also leaves the posterior aspect of the external carotid, and ascends to supply the posterolateral portion of the scalp. Finally, the superficial temporal artery is a terminal branch of the external carotid that supplies the lateral scalp. Each of these arteries is accompanied by veins with similar names. The veins anastomose frequently and ultimately enter the diploic veins of the skull bones and intracranial dural sinuses.[6]

Due to the dense vasculature, high blood flow, and tendency for cut vessels to retract within the subcutaneous fat, transection of vessels in the scalp may lead to excessive bleeding. Furthermore, because the scalp is not supplied by musculocutaneous perforators, transection of subcutaneous vasculature, especially the major vessels at the periphery of the scalp, has consequences for the blood supply of both neighboring and distant tissues from the site of transection,[7] and subsequently reconstructed tissue. As a result, surgical dissection should take place in the relatively avascular subgaleal plane where the overlying blood supply will not be compromised. However, it should be noted that the extensive interconnections between the blood vessels of the scalp can be beneficial, as it allows for the transfer of large scalp flaps, including total scalp replantation, based on a single artery anastomosis without distal necrosis.[8,9] There are minimal contributions of the vessels to the deep pericranial layer; instead, the pericranium receives its blood supply from the middle meningeal and intracranial circulation to the calvarial bone. Therefore, disruption of the superficial vasculature does not result in necrosis of the calvarium.[6]

Like the vasculature of the scalp, the lymphatic system is comprised of a widely anastomotic network of vessels. The exact pattern of drainage is highly variable. Briefly, the lymphatic channels run from superficial to deep, with the frontal and temporal scalp draining to the preauricular and parotid nodes and the posterior scalp draining to the posterior auricular and occipital nodes. Lymph from these nodes eventually drains into the deep cervical chain of lymph nodes.[10]

## Innervation

Sensory innervation of the scalp arises from two primary sources, cranial nerves and cervical nerves. The overall nervous supply of the scalp is similar to the vascular anatomy—the nerves are primarily subcutaneous, originating peripherally and running centrally and are of a similar distribution. All three branches of the trigeminal nerve innervate the scalp (Fig. 20.2): the supraorbital and supratrochlear nerves (V1) innervate the forehead and frontoparietal scalp, the zygomaticotemporal nerve (V2) innervates the lateral brow and temporal scalp, and the auriculotemporal nerve (V3) supplies the lateral scalp. More posterior, the occipital region is innervated by the greater (C2) and lesser (C2, C3) occipital nerves.[11]

Motor innervation to the scalp is derived primarily from the facial nerve. The frontal branch exits the parotid gland and runs to the lateral orbital rim where it supplies the frontalis muscle. The posterior auricular branch innervates the occipitalis muscle.[12]

# RECONSTRUCTION PLANNING: BASIC TENETS

The scalp has both functional and cosmetic roles. There are many elements to consider in order to obtain acceptable aesthetic results and avoid adverse outcomes. Complications from scalp surgery include pain, edema, scarring, distorted hair patterns or alopecia, loss of sensation to the scalp, and stretch-atrophied tissue.[13] Knowledge of the pertinent anatomy covered earlier in this chapter in conjunction with the following principles of reconstruction planning will help anticipate potential complications and improve surgical outcomes. Before commencing with surgery or reconstruction, a thorough cleansing of the hair can be performed with shampoo followed by an antiseptic such as betadine or chlorhexidine. The hair surrounding the area of interest should be parted and clipped short to aid in visualization if necessary. While trimming the hair of the surgical site may be less than ideal for some patients, it allows for a more meticulous reconstruction and less chance for hair to become tangled in the sutures or the closure line. A petrolatum ointment can be used to aid in parting or sectioning of the other areas of the hair. It has been reported that shaving the hair preoperatively may lead to an increased risk of infection postoperatively and consensus is to trim the hair instead.[14]

To anesthetize the surgical site direct injection of lidocaine with epinephrine (barring contraindications) can be suitable to obtain patient comfort. Allowing at least 15–20 minutes for the epinephrine to take effect will aid in vasoconstriction and reduce bleeding. Dilute tumescent anesthesia may be another option to anesthetize larger areas of the scalps if a larger flap or dissection is to be planned. A ring block around the perimeter of the scalp, targeting the supraorbital, supratrochlear, zygomaticotemporal, auriculotemporal, greater and lesser occipital nerves is also another useful tool to provide adequate anesthesia for a larger portion of the scalp.[15]

## Patient Factors

Screening for patients on anticoagulants, nonsteroidal anti-inflammatory drugs, or certain vitamins is important to ascertain potential for intraoperative bleeding and postoperative hematoma formation. Prepping the surgical tray with hemostat clamps and 4–0 absorbable polyglactin 910 sutures should be anticipated to aid in clamping, ligating, and tying off perforating blood vessels. Patients who are smokers are more prone to peripheral vasoconstriction and therefore certain reconstruction techniques such as flaps or grafts may be prone to local necrosis.[16] Patients should be counseled on pre- and postoperative smoking cessation in order to achieve optimal healing. A prior history of radiation, or prior scalp surgeries, may make reconstruction difficult due to inadequate elasticity or lack of tissue reservoir, respectively.

## Incisions/Excisions

When planning for incisions or excisions, it is important to consider both the natural orientation of skin tension and location of the vessels and nerves. Langer's lines, first discovered by Austrian anatomist Karl Langer in 1861, are topographical lines on the human body that correspond to the natural direction of collagen fibers in the dermis.[17] On the scalp, these lines are primarily vertical in orientation, becoming more horizontal as one approaches the occipital scalp (Figs. 20.3A and B). An understanding of the orientation of these lines where tension is minimal is important when performing excisions, as cutting along these lines allows for the greatest width of tissue removal. Furthermore, by cutting along the orientation of collagen, there is less transection of these fibers and subsequent diminution of scarring.[18] As previously described, the vasculature of the scalp is primarily cutaneous and runs centripetally. As such, the ideal scalp incision is at the midline. In doing so, this allows access to the subgaleal

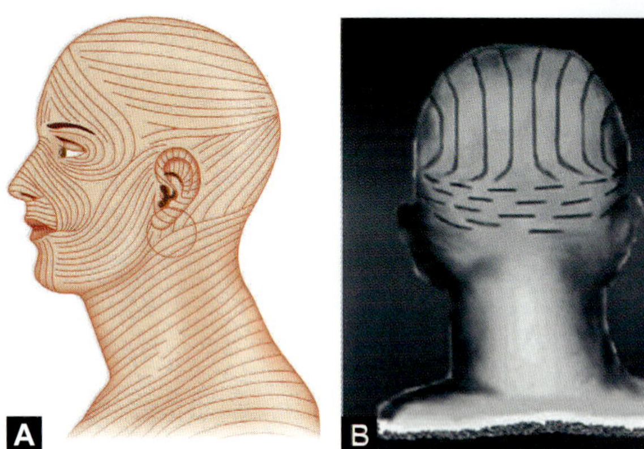

**Figs. 20.3A and B:** (A) Langer's lines (lines of minimum tension) of the scalp. (B) Langer's lines become more horizontal as they approach the base of the scalp.

space while minimizing the risk of trauma to the vasculature or nervous innervation.[7,19]

## Laxity, Galeal Movement, and Undermining

When skin is stretched beyond its resting-length capacity, elastic fibers rupture resulting in irreversible plasticization, also known as stretch atrophy.[7] As a result, fundamental knowledge of the areas of the scalp that are most mobile and techniques to increase movement is essential. The greatest amount of scalp mobility is found at the parietal regions where the temporal fascia overlies the temporalis fascia. The occipital regions have less laxity and are more fixed. The subgaleal loose areolar tissue allows the scalp to slide over the pericranium, enhancing excision in these areas where this layer is present. There is some natural variability among patients, however, as some scalps have relatively poorly developed fibroareolar layers.[7] One can readily assess the extent of laxity allowed by this layer by simply applying pressure with their fingertips on the scalp and sliding the tissues back and forth over the underlying pericranium. Excisions that take advantage of the natural mechanical gliding movement afforded by the loose areolar tissue, rather than utilizing stretching of tissues, can result in fewer complications and negligible topographic distortion. In regions where there is direct adherence of the aponeurotic layers to the pericranium, the mobility can be improved by freeing ligamentous connections between these layers.[20]

Another factor, which may limit the extent of surgical resection, is the relatively inelastic galea aponeurotica. Linear galeal transection, or galeotomy, may be performed to mitigate its restrictive effects.[21] This is achieved by scoring the galea in the direction of desired flap movement in 1-cm intervals. The average actual tissue gain per galeotomy is reportedly 1.67 mm, which results in a 40% reduction of the closing tension.[21] The downside to this maneuver is the additional risk of damaging subcutaneous structures with resultant increased risk of bleeding or infection. One must also be careful with electrocautery, as it may lead to thermal injury of vessels that lie just superficial to the galea.

Finally, undermining of tissues allows for improved closure while minimizing tension at the wound margins. Numerous studies have shown that the effects of undermining are substantial; however, extensive undermining (15 cm as compared to 5 cm) does not result in a significant decrease in tension load required for closure.[22,23] Furthermore, extensive undermining leads to increased risk of traumatic injury to blood vessels or nerves, and risk of infection through disturbed tissue planes with the increased surgical manipulation.

## Towel Clamps and Staples

Towel clamps are often used in scalp reconstruction to help overcome high tensions in wound closure by offering immediate intraoperative tissue expansion (Figs. 20.4A and B). The clamps are placed with adequate margins to prevent tearing through tissue and may be left for 20 minutes. By providing a constant load to help reapproximate wound edges, the towel clamps take advantage of the skin's viscoelastic properties to provide additional cutaneous tissue.[24] This resourceful technique does not require special instrumentation or intense surgical intervention to achieve closure. Similarly the use of pulley sutures during immediate reconstruction can help overcome wound tension. If reconstruction is to be delayed, then use of temporary retention sutures will aid in tissue stretching.

An additional technique that can be used to assist with wound closure is the use of surgical staples. Aside from topical adhesives, stapling offers the method of closure with the least skin ischemia. As a result, surgical staples are particularly useful in hair-bearing areas because they limit the amount of follicular ischemia and resultant alopecia. A randomized study assessing staples versus suture closure of scalp lacerations found that there was no difference in morbidity or the rate of wound infection between the two methods of closure.[25] Furthermore, the use of staples offers the additional benefit of less risk of

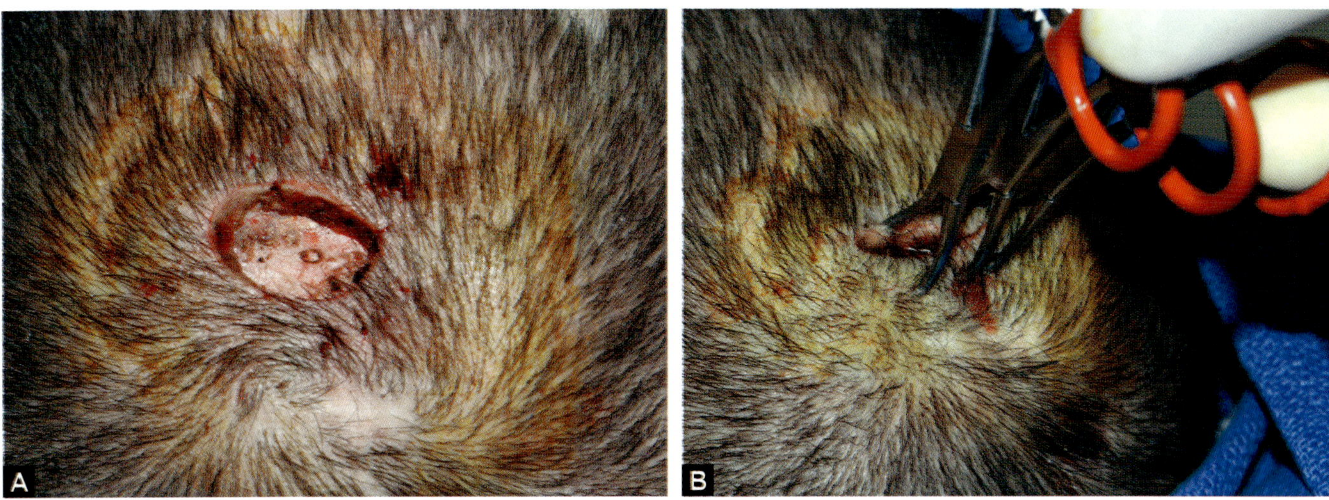


**Figs. 20.4A and B:** Towel clamps. (A) A 2 cm × 3 cm defect over the vertex scalp. (B) Towel clamps in place allowing for local intraoperative tissue expansion.

accidental needle-stick injury to the individual performing the closure as well as the rapid ease of placement.

### Hair-Bearing Areas

In addition to achieving proper coverage of the cranial vault, reconstructive surgeons should strive for a cosmetically pleasing outcome with the least amount of damage to the hair. This requires attention to the hair growth patterns and hairlines to preserve normal anatomy. Hair follicles emerge from the scalp at an angle that varies by region.[26] When making incisions, it is best to plan them parallel to the direction of hair growth so that fewer follicles are disrupted. Conservative use of electrocautery throughout the procedure can help prevent thermal injury to hair follicles, and the use of hemostatic clips on cut edges of scalp should be minimized to prevent additional follicular damage.[27] When closing the wound, the suture used to close the subcutaneous layer should be kept safely beneath the follicles. Finally, excessive tension at wound closure may result in alopecia around the incision site. As the hair density of the scalp is unlike any other area of skin, it is best to close wounds with scalp tissue. Preserving scalp hair not only serves the cosmetic function of hiding the incision, but also functional purposes including prevention of photodamage, protection from blunt trauma or environmental debris, and thermoregulation.[28] Although a more lengthy and drawn-out process, the use of tissue expanders can be employed to recreate normal hair density and patterns.

## RECONSTRUCTION PLANNING: METHODS OF CLOSURE

### Objectives

The primary objective of repairing a scalp defect is to obtain functional closure while minimizing complications. The factors to consider when planning reconstruction are the size, depth, and location of the defect. Whereas smaller defects are more amenable to healing by granulation/secondary intention, or primary closure, larger defects often require local tissue rearrangement or grafting. If the periosteum is damaged and there is extensive exposure of bone, flaps are preferable to grafting due to the lack of a sustainable vascular bed.

The secondary objective of repair is to achieve an aesthetically pleasing result. This may include maintenance of the normal contour of the scalp, similar color and texture of the tissue, and preservation of the natural hairlines. As such, it is best to transpose adjacent hair-bearing tissue into the defect when possible to best conserve the unique characteristics of scalp tissue. In order to obtain a superior cosmetic outcome, it may require a longer, more complicated surgery. It is important to consider the preferences of the patient to assess their desire for good cosmesis at the expense of a potentially more complicated surgical repair. For example, tissue expansion can result in excellent aesthetic outcome with preservation of normal cosmetic aspects of the scalp, but the patient must be willing to undergo a prolonged procedure with an inconvenient and significant cosmetic deformity until the final operation.

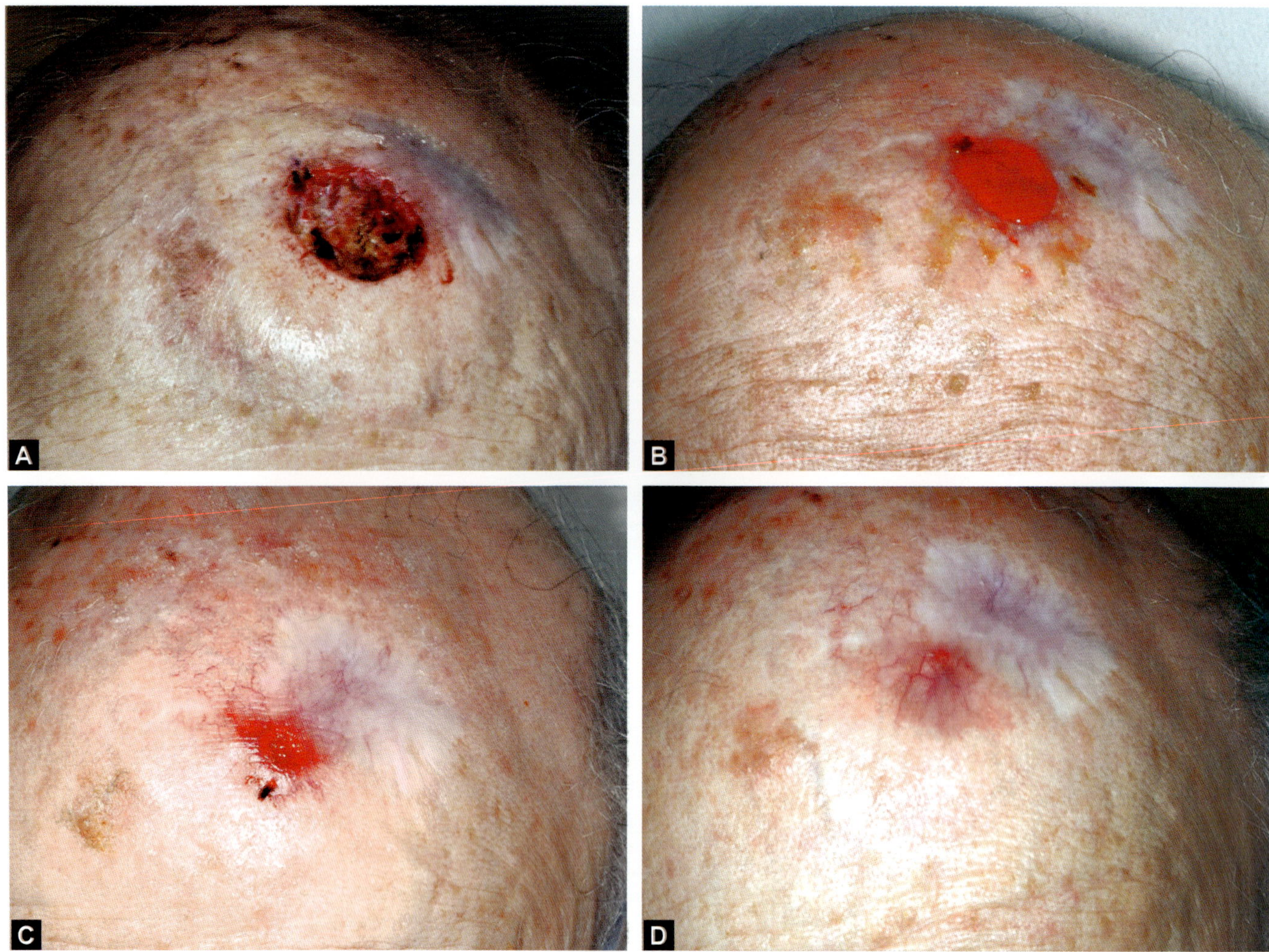


**Figs. 20.5A to D:** Secondary intention. (A) Patient treated for recurrent squamous cell carcinoma leaving a 4 cm × 6 cm defect. (B) One-month postsecondary intention. Field cancerization effect precluded the use of flaps for reconstruction. Secondary intention was opted for improved monitoring. (C) Two-months postsurgery. (D) Five months postoperative showing fully healed surgical site.

## Secondary Intention

Healing by granulation is often preferred by patients who wish to undergo the minimal amount of surgery possible. It can be performed on any location of the scalp, but is dependent on the depth of the surgical defect.[29] It is beneficial in patients with superficial defects, a history of radiation therapy, or wounds with potential residual tumor (Figs. 20.5A to D).[30] However, patients must be able to perform proper wound care that entails keeping the wound moist with a nonirritating emollient to prevent desiccation. In addition to the prolonged wound healing, granulation may result in an area of alopecia depending on the depth of the defect. If there is bone exposed, burr holes should be created in the outer table of the cranium to expose the vascularized diploic space.[31] Other techniques to improve healing by granulation include porcine xenograft-assisted granulation and purse-string suture-assisted granulation. Porcine xenografts provide temporary coverage of the wound and help facilitate granulation formation and limit loss of protein and fluid (Figs. 20.6A to D).[32] The use of a purse-string suture may allow for the surface area of the defect to be decreased for larger defects (Figs. 20.7A and B).

## Primary Closures

Primary closure is performed for full-thickness scalp defects, most often <3 cm, where wound edges can be reapproximated without significant tension. Due to the

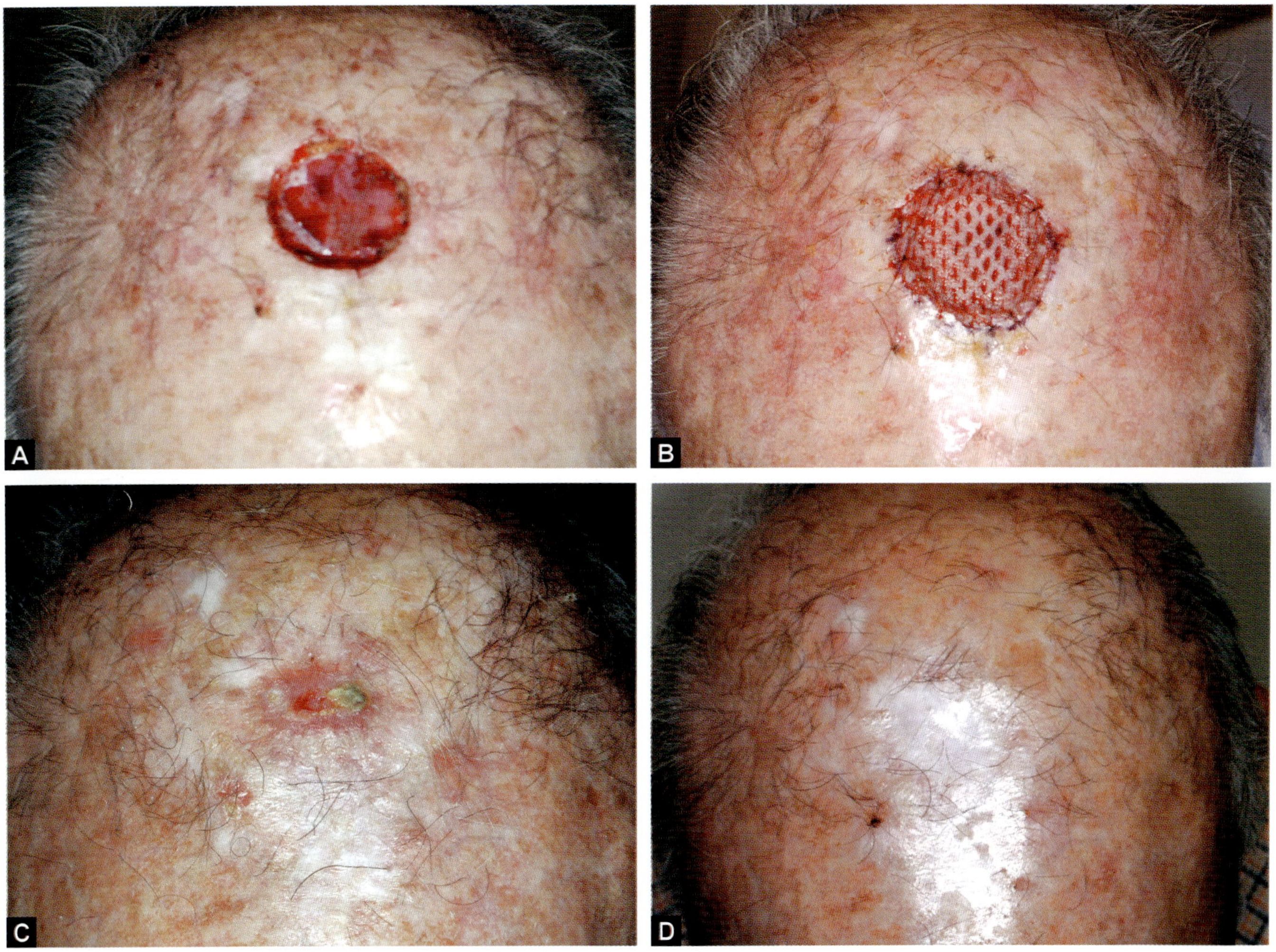

**Figs. 20.6A to D:** Porcine xenograft. (A) A 3.3 cm × 3.3 cm defect down to periosteum in the mid-frontal scalp. (B) Porcine xenograft was used due to patient preference and field cancerization. (C) Result at 6-week follow-up. (D) Result at one-year follow-up.

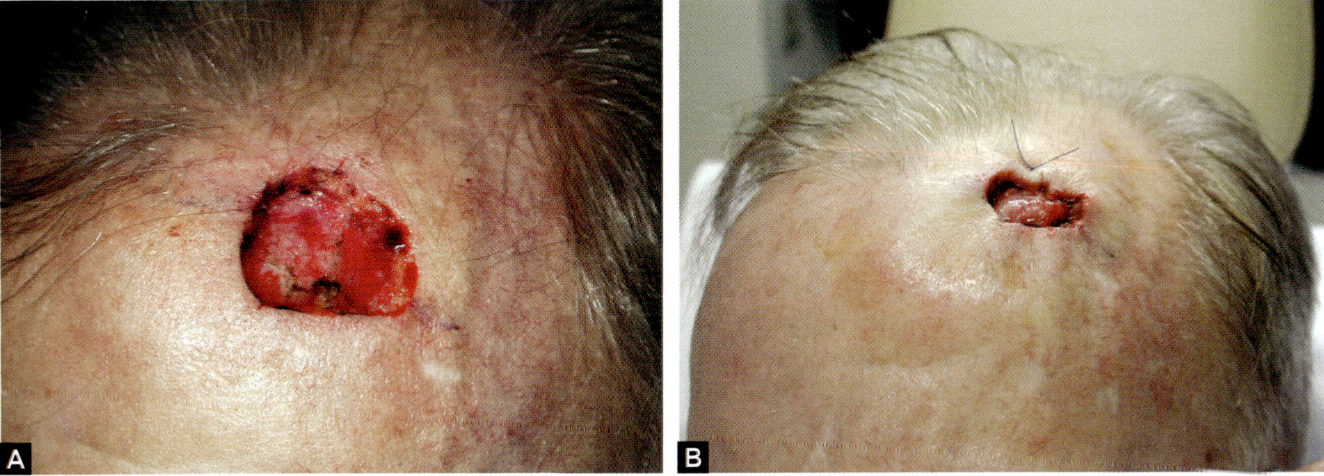


**Figs. 20.7A and B:** Purse-string suture. (A) A 2.5 cm × 2.5 cm defect on the left frontal scalp. (B) Purse-string suture in place decreasing defect size to 1 cm × 1.5 cm.

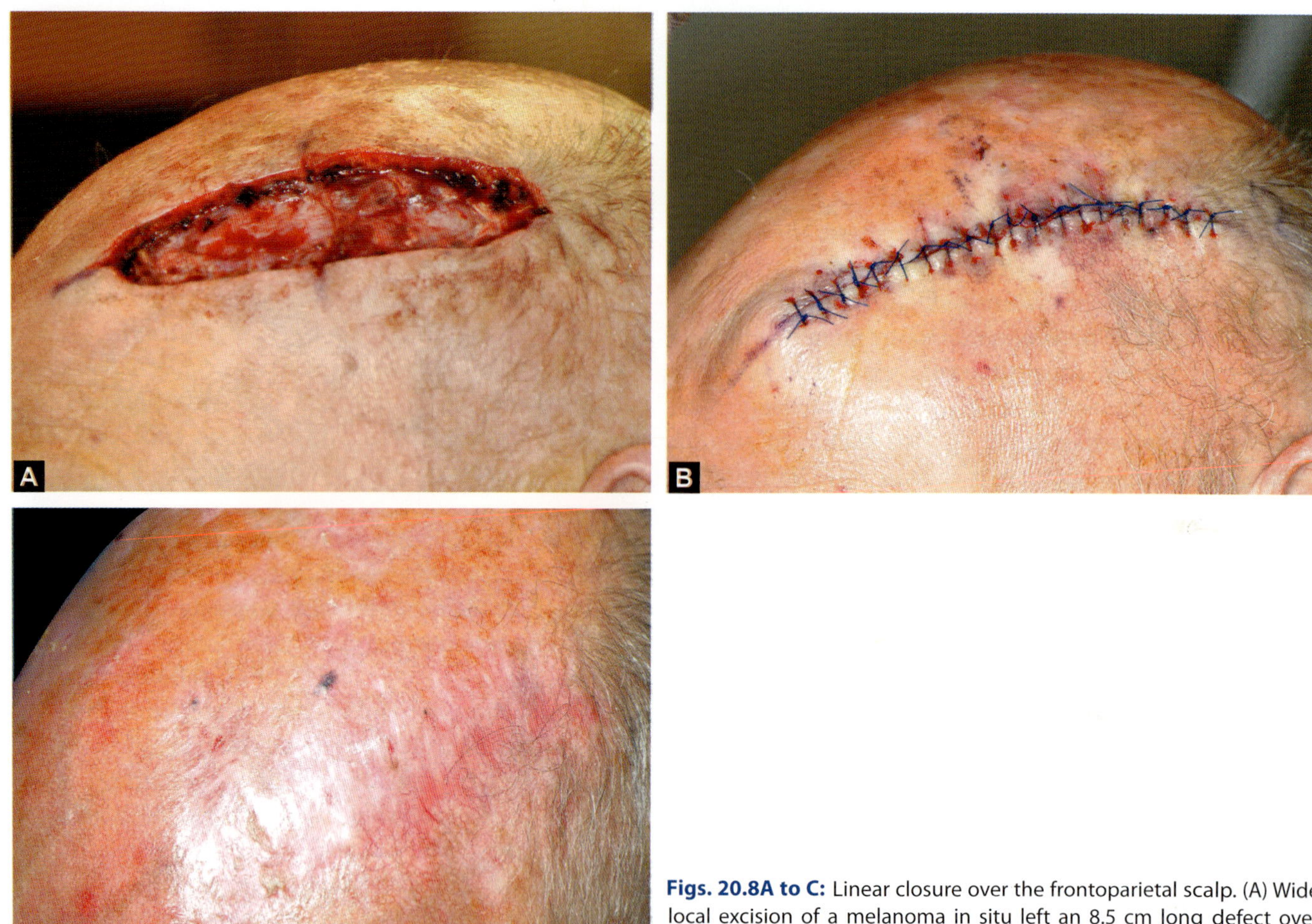

**Figs. 20.8A to C:** Linear closure over the frontoparietal scalp. (A) Wide local excision of a melanoma in situ left an 8.5 cm long defect over the left frontoparietal scalp. (B) The elliptical lesion was primarily closed in a linear fashion. (C) Follow-up 10 months later showing a linear scar.

convex shape of the scalp and differing levels of elasticity depending on the location, primary closure of larger defects is not always possible without subjecting the wound site to excessive tension. It is important to assess tissue laxity before closing, as the elasticity of scalp tissue varies with age and between individuals. This closure may be performed rapidly with the least amount of additional surgery compared to flaps and grafting. Primary closure on the scalp is assisted by undermining in the avascular subgaleal plane. The defect should be elliptical, following the standard 3:1 length:width ratio with ~30° end angles. As is true for linear closure of other sites, the wound ellipse should be oriented among relaxed skin-tension lines to minimize closure tension and reduce the risk of dehiscence or depressed appearance (Figs. 20.8A to C). Surgical sites on the hair-bearing scalp areas can be closed in a trichophytic manner to aid in improving the final appearance. This is accomplished by removing ~1 mm of skin from the lower margin of the incision at an oblique angle, allowing the opposing edge to overlap. This allows the hair to grow through a thinner scar, thereby improving the appearance.[33]

## Local Tissue Rearrangement

A variety of flaps are often performed for closing scalp defects when the size of the wound and the relative inelasticity of scalp tissue prevent primary closure. The type of flap depends largely on the location of the defect, and suggestions for specific flaps by location has been covered later in the chapter. On the scalp, subcutaneous flaps run the risk of poor protection, compromised vascularity, and interruption of hair follicles.[26] As a result, large flaps are dissected in the subgaleal plane where they can be easily elevated with preservation of the vasculature and adnexal structures. Furthermore, the presence of the

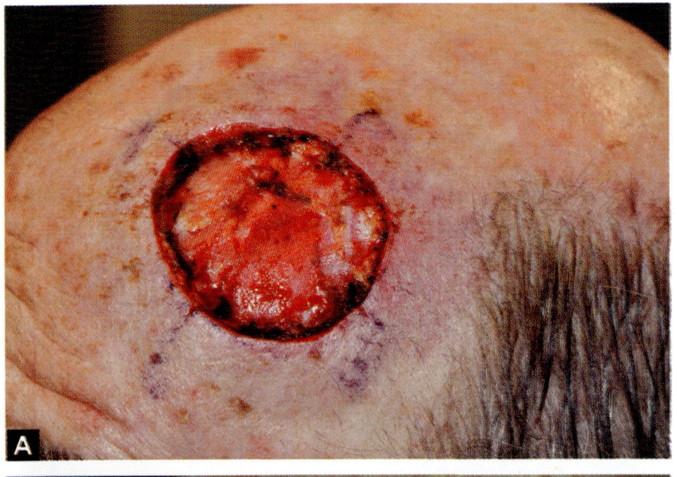


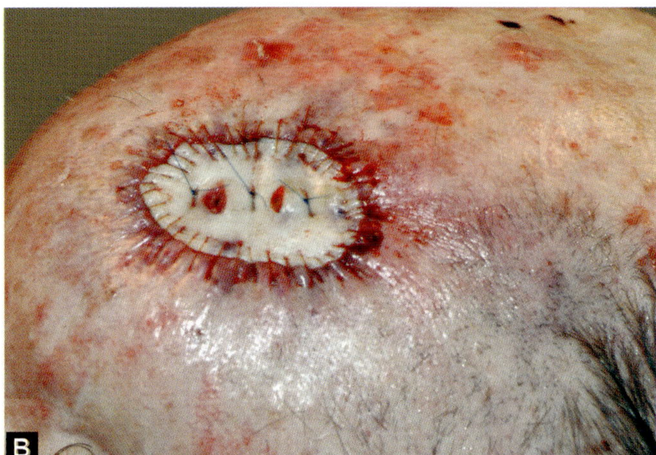


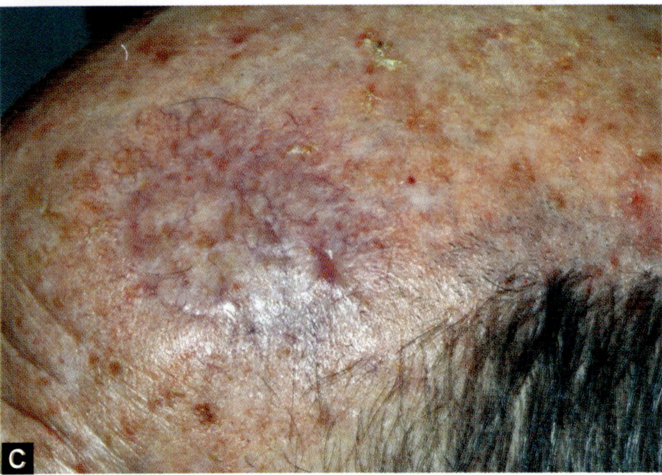


**Figs. 20.9A to C:** Full-thickness skin graft. (A) Patient treated for a lentigo maligna arising in a seborrheic keratosis leaving a 4.5 cm × 5 cm defect down to the periosteum. (B) Wound was closed with a full-thickness skin graft. (C) Follow-up 4 months later showing take of the graft with good cosmetic match.

rigid galea in flaps dissected in the loose areolar tissue helps prevent excessive stretching or torsion of vessels.[34] When planning for scalp repair with flaps, it is important to place incisions in skin with the greatest laxity and to align them with adjacent cosmetic subunits for camouflage. As such, it is preferred to use the minimum number of flaps to minimize surgical manipulation and trauma. However, using multiple flaps is beneficial in locations, such as the vertex, where the recruitment of additional tissue aids in disseminating the tension over a greater surface area. Since the flap created is larger relative to the size of the defect, closure may result in a standing cone of tissue.[35] This redundancy normally flattens over the course of months, and it may be desirable to wait to remove it in standard fashion after complete healing of the original wound, although the Burow's technique can be used for large standing cones.[26] The use of flaps on the scalp can provide immediate closure with good cosmesis by preserving normal scalp tissue characteristics, and hair swirl pattern.

## Skin Grafts

Skin grafts are the preferred method of closure for patients who are poor candidates for flap reconstruction and who are willing to accept an inferior aesthetic result. In general, STSGs have a higher take rate than FTSGs and may be used for closure of secondary defects after flap closure.[36] In cases where bone is exposed, the bone may be ground down and Integra (LifeSciences, Plainsboro, New Jersey), a porous scaffold for regenerating skin, may be placed on the wound.[37] Upon granulation, the wound can then be covered with an STSG. However, STSGs do not accurately reflect the color, normal hair-bearing qualities, or contour of the scalp, thus making them a more functional than cosmetic option.

Full-thickness skin grafts provide a better cosmetic match than STSGs and offer a better thickness match for full-thickness defects (Figs. 20.9A to C). Compared to STSGs, these grafts are less susceptible to contraction and more capable of resisting trauma.[36] Donor sites may

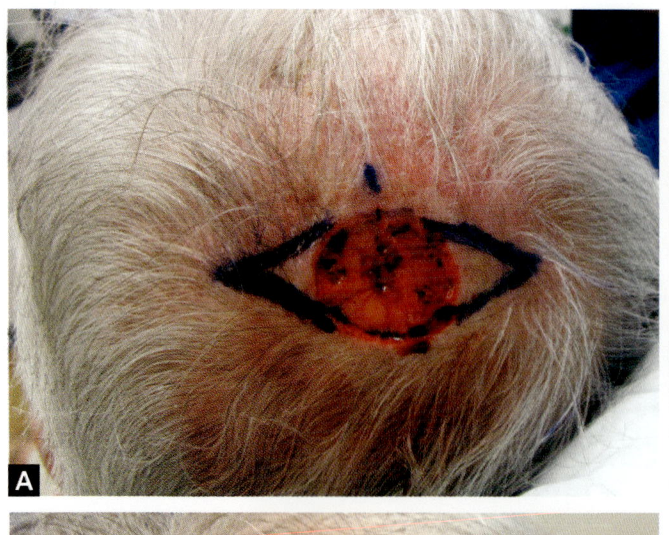


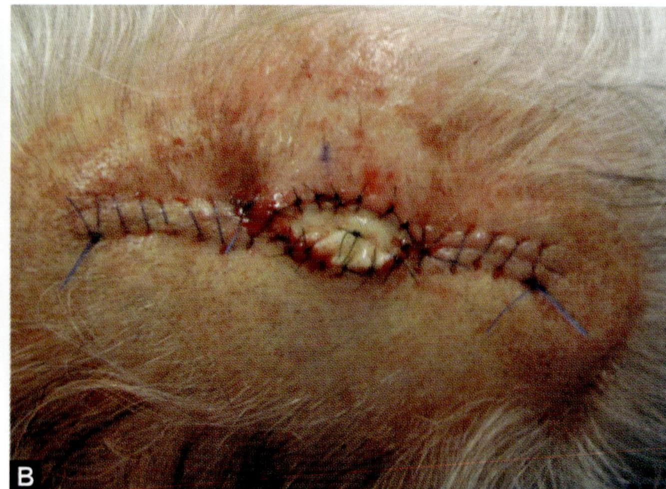


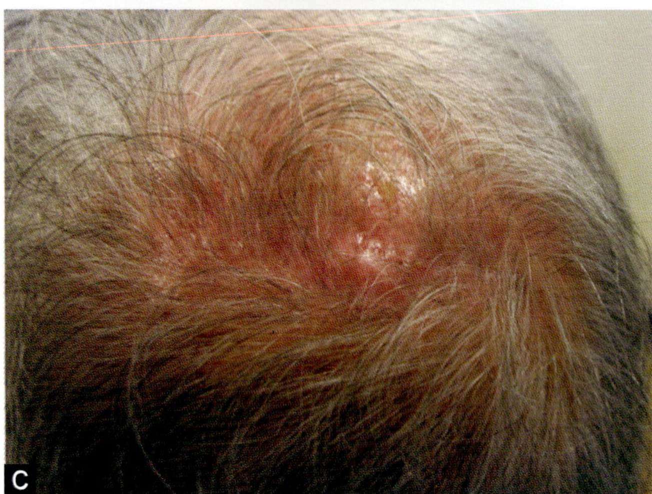


**Figs. 20.10A to C:** (A) Medium depth wound on the scalp. (B) Combination of linear closure and Burow's graft. (C) Long-term follow-up showing good cosmesis.
*Courtesy*: S Brian Jiang, MD, Sang Diego, California, USA.

include the supraclavicular region, lateral neck, or upper arm.[38] The editors also utilize adjacent tissue as a donor site for medium depth and size defects that can be repaired with a combination of linear closure and Burow's graft (graft harvested from the Burow's triangle removed during closure) (Figs. 20.10A to C). In order to maintain the convexity of the scalp, the editors preserve a small dermal island during the linear closure as a base for the FTSG (Figs. 20.11A to D).[39] Bolster dressings should be placed to allow for important apposition of the graft to the wound bed to aid in the three phases of graft take, imbibition, inosculation, and revascularization.

## Free Tissue Transfer

Microvascular free tissue transfer allows for reconstruction of larger scalp defects where primary closure is not obtainable and local tissue is inadequate. This strategy allows for closure to be completed in a single surgery while maintaining both the functional and aesthetic outcome.[40] The most commonly used free tissue transfer for scalp reconstruction is the latissimus dorsi flap that may be taken with the serratus anterior to provide better coverage.[41] The latissimus dorsi flap may be covered by an STSG, and upon atrophy of the muscle the volume of the transferred tissue closely approximates that of the native scalp.[40] Other examples of free tissue flaps that have been used for reconstructing large scalp defects include the anterolateral thigh flap and the radial forearm free flap.[42,43] The main disadvantages to these types of flaps are donor site morbidity, lack of similar hair-bearing quality, and a prolonged surgery.[44] These procedures are performed in an operating room setting but are important to keep in mind when reconstruction of the scalp is planned.

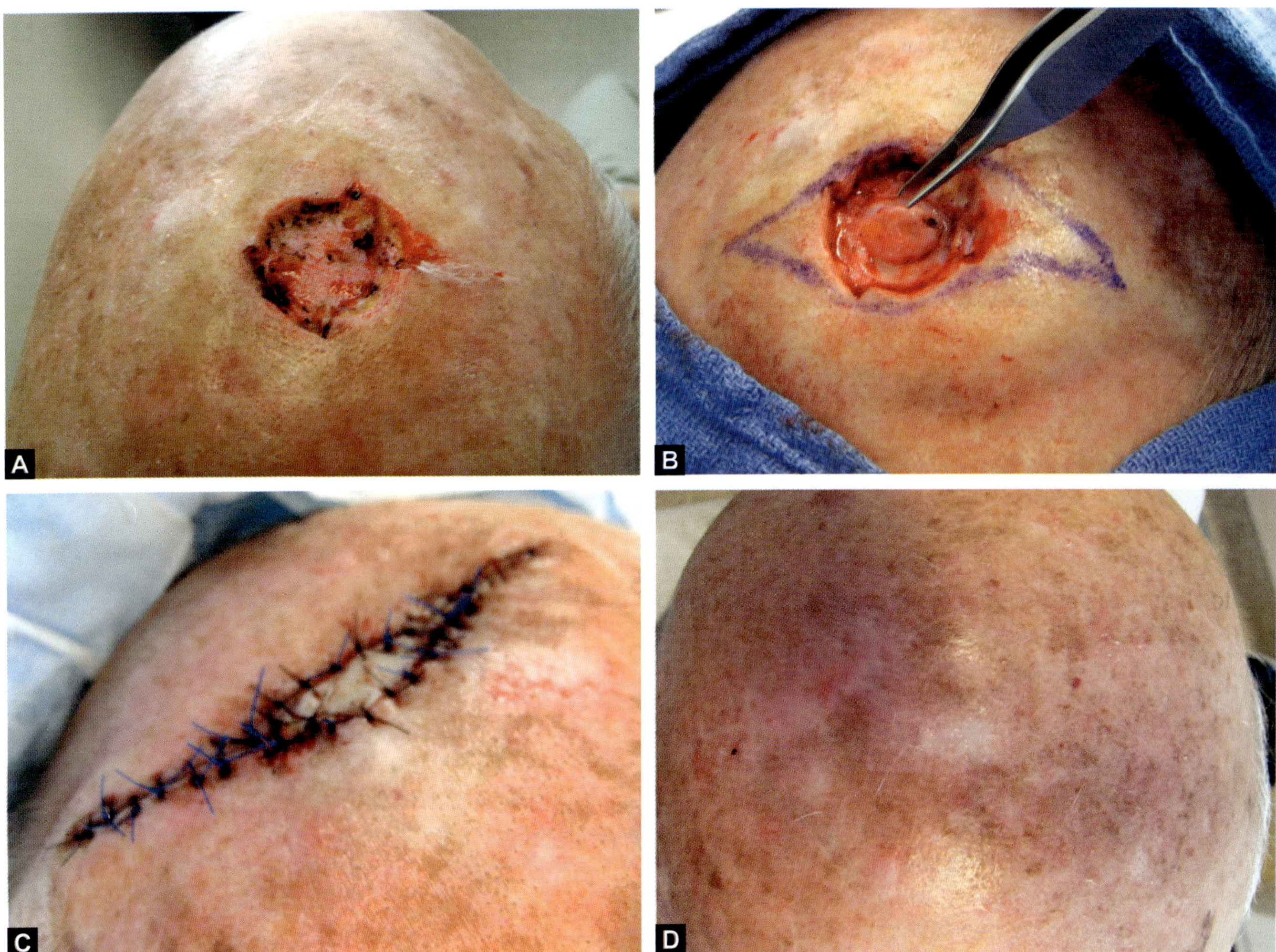


**Figs. 20.11A to D:** (A) Scalp wound prior to repair. (B) Preserved dermal island used as a base for the full-thickness skin graft (FTSG). (C) FTSG placed above dermal island. (D) Long-term follow-up showing preservation of scalp convexity.
*Courtesy*: S Brian Jiang, MD, Sang Diego, California, USA.

Tissue expansion should be considered when the size of the defect is too large for local tissue transfer or the quality of surrounding tissue is poor. The benefits of this technique on the scalp are preservation of the texture, color, sensation, and thickness of the normal scalp tissue along with matching hair-bearing qualities. This technique also avoids donor site morbidity associated with skin grafting. However, not all patients are candidates for the multiple surgeries and prolonged course required for this method of reconstruction.

## Location

The scalp is commonly divided into sections based upon different characteristics of the anatomy in these locations. This section reinforces key anatomic differences among the sites with suggestions for wound closure based on the size of the defect to provide the best functional and cosmetic outcome.

### *Frontal Scalp*

The major consideration when repairing defects on the frontal scalp is preservation of the anterior hairline. Incisions should be confined and hidden within hair-bearing areas or placed such that scars may be camouflaged within horizontal forehead rhytids. When cutting over hair-bearing regions, the scalpel blade should be oriented parallel to hair follicles to minimize transection.

For small defects along the anterior hairline where there is sufficient tissue laxity, primary closure is preferred. This can be achieved using redundant forehead

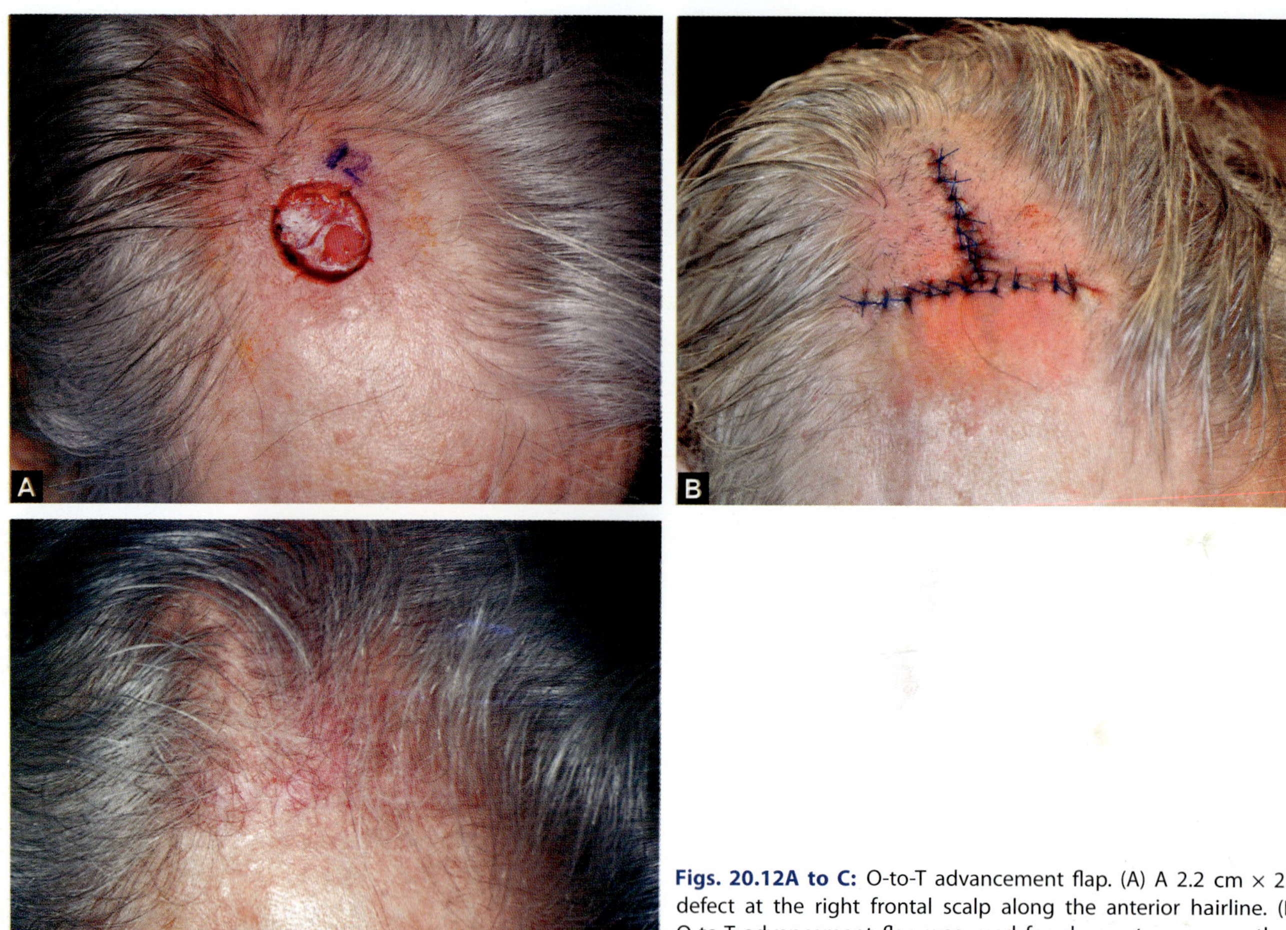


**Figs. 20.12A to C:** O-to-T advancement flap. (A) A 2.2 cm × 2.5 cm defect at the right frontal scalp along the anterior hairline. (B) An O-to-T advancement flap was used for closure to preserve the hairline and hide the scar within hair-bearing tissue. (C) Result at 6-month follow-up.

skin or preferential undermining toward the vertex scalp to prevent backward migration of the hairline.[45] When utilizing these techniques, care should be taken to prevent formation of an asymmetric outcome.

When primary closure is not feasible with defects in the frontal region, an O-to-T flap is an excellent option. By aligning the cross of the "T" with the frontal hairline and the edges of the advance flap within the scalp, the incision lines can be effectively concealed (Figs. 20.12A to C).

Medium or larger defects of the frontal scalp may be amenable to a variety of local skin flaps, including rotation (Figs. 20.13A to C), transposition (Figs. 20.14A to C), and bilateral advancement flaps.[46] For balding patients or elderly who are poor candidates for large flap reconstruction, skin grafting is an acceptable alternative that affords a good functional outcome (Figs. 20.15A to C). For larger defects, an Orticochea flap[47] or the use of tissue expanders can result in good cosmesis, but both require extensive surgical manipulation. When repairing the frontal scalp, it is important to inform the patient of the possibility of significant postoperative edema and ecchymosis that may travel down the forehead and settle periorbitally. Sleeping propped up or upright will help facilitate gravitational drainage of the postoperative edema.

## *Parietal Scalp*

The parietal scalp is unique in that it has more mobility than other regions of the scalp due to the temporoparietal fascia overlying the deep temporal fascia. As a result, this region is more compliant with local tissue rearrangement and tissue advancement flaps. Small defects can also be readily repaired with primary closure (Figs. 20.16A to C). Alternatively, a variety of flaps including V to Y (subcutaneous pedicled flaps), rotation (Figs. 20.17A to C), and transposition flaps can be used with great cosmetic outcome.

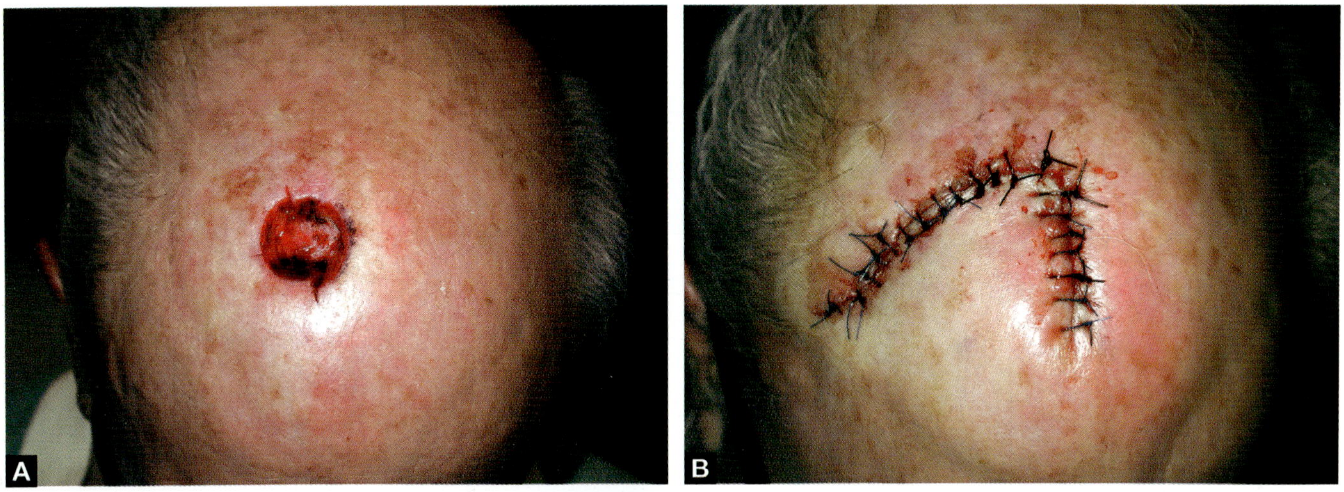

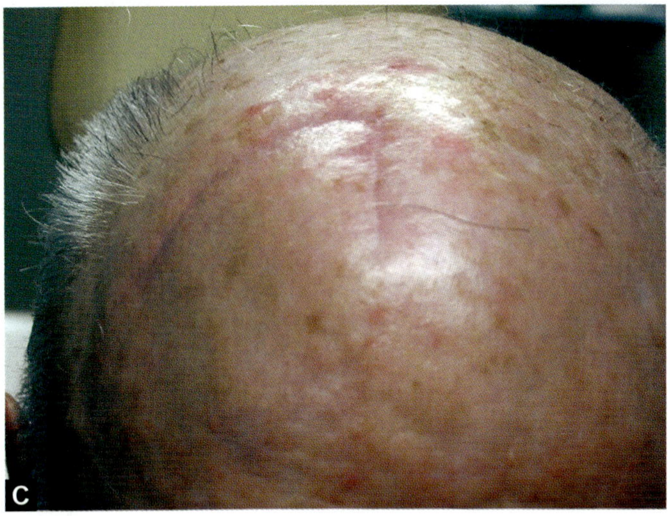

**Figs. 20.13A to C:** Rotation flap. (A) A 2.5 cm × 2.0 cm defect down to the galea layer on the frontal scalp. (B) Because the defect was not amenable to primary closure, a rotation flap was used. (C) Follow-up at 3.5 months.

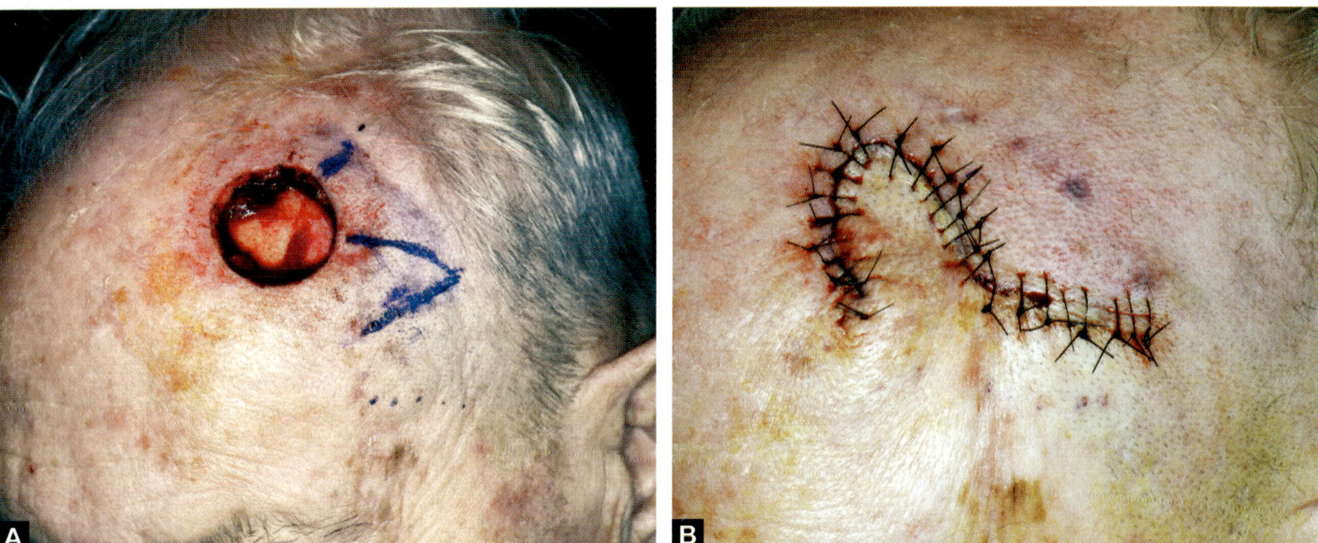


**Figs. 20.14A and B**

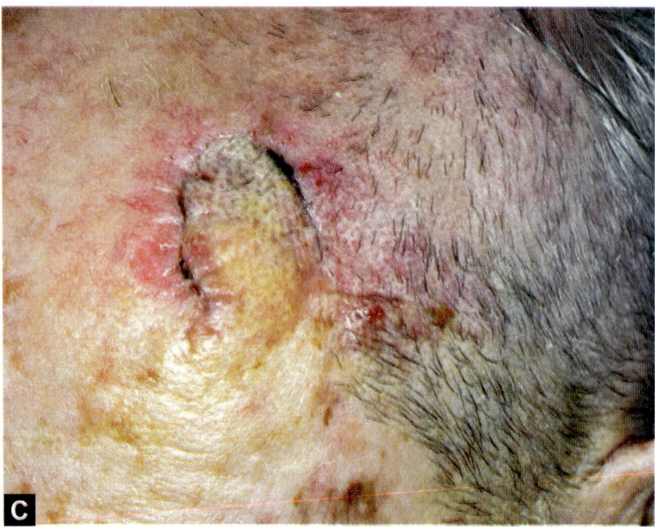

**Figs. 20.14A to C:** Transposition flap. (A) A 3.1 cm × 3.3 cm defect down to periosteum. (B) A transposition flap was used to cover the wound. (C) 2-week follow-up showing wound healing with resultant scar.
*Courtesy*: Erica Lee, New York, New York.

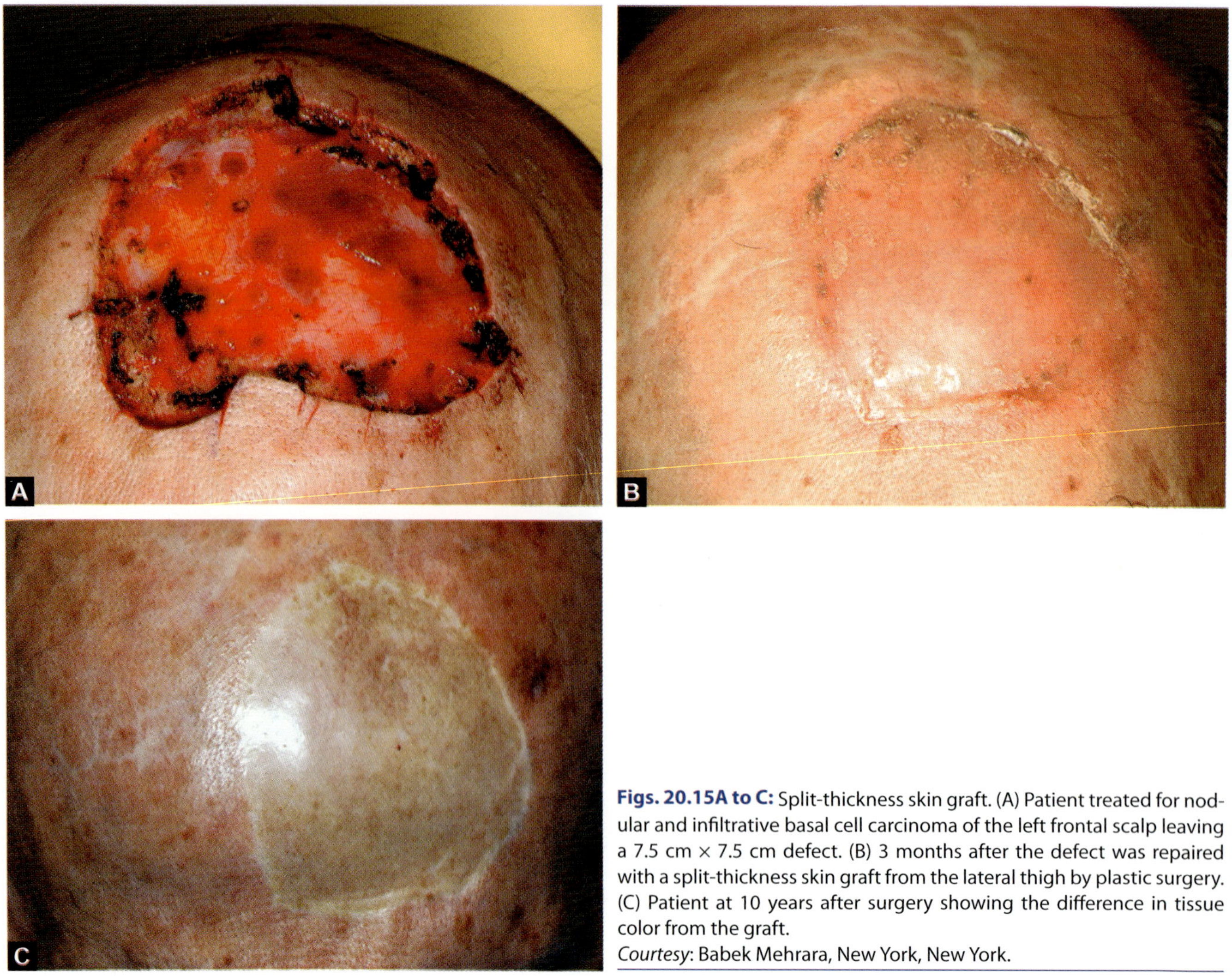

**Figs. 20.15A to C:** Split-thickness skin graft. (A) Patient treated for nodular and infiltrative basal cell carcinoma of the left frontal scalp leaving a 7.5 cm × 7.5 cm defect. (B) 3 months after the defect was repaired with a split-thickness skin graft from the lateral thigh by plastic surgery. (C) Patient at 10 years after surgery showing the difference in tissue color from the graft.
*Courtesy*: Babek Mehrara, New York, New York.

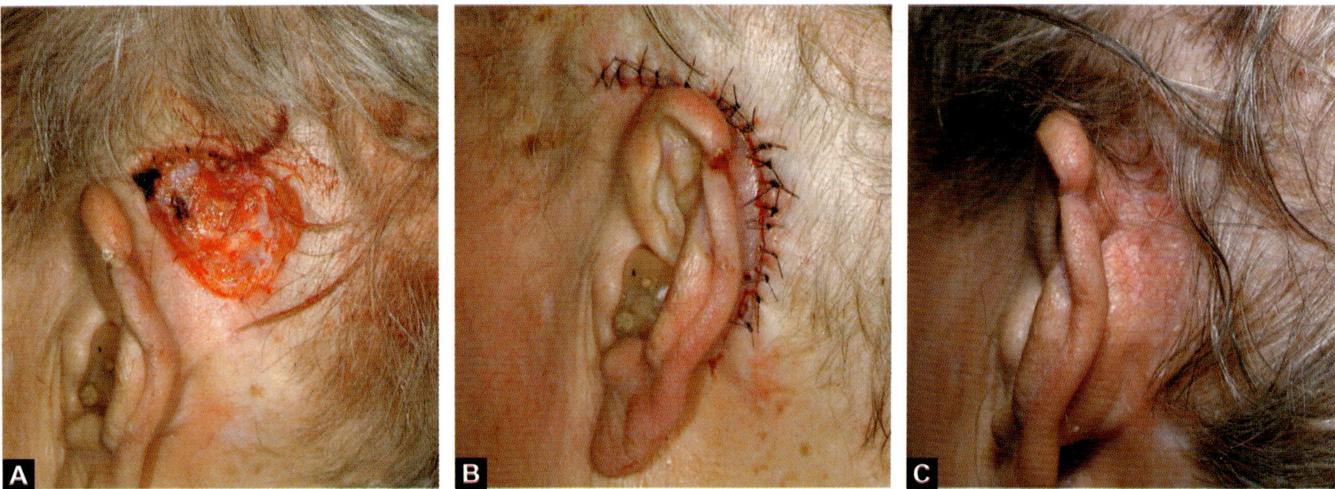


**Figs. 20.16A to C:** Postauricular closure. (A) A 3.5 cm × 2.0 cm postauricular defect down to temporoparietal fascia. (B) Laxity of the tissue in the parietal scalp allowed for the defect to be closed with a curvilinear approach. (C) 6-month follow-up showing the scar concealed behind the ear along the lateral hairline.

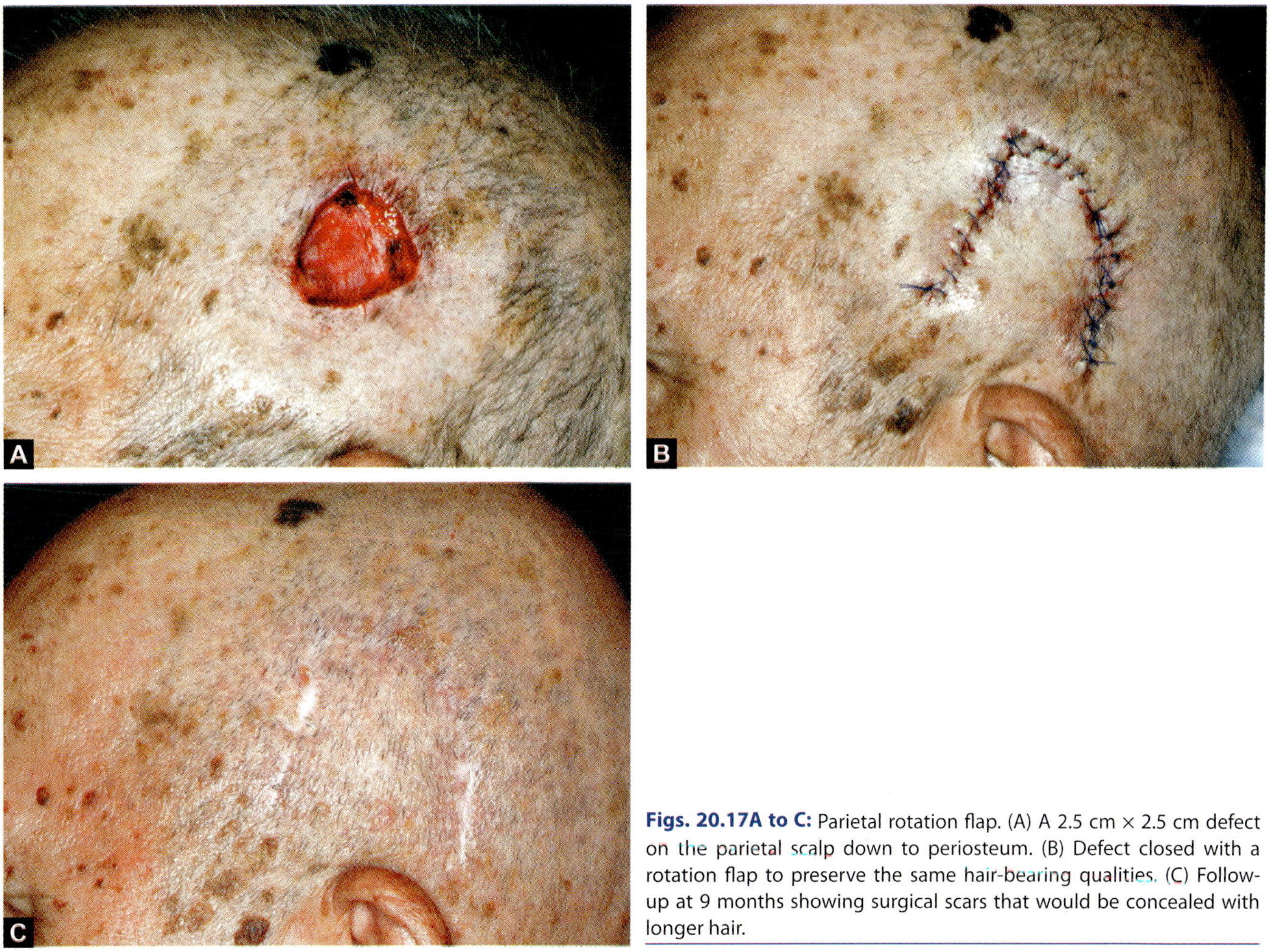

**Figs. 20.17A to C:** Parietal rotation flap. (A) A 2.5 cm × 2.5 cm defect on the parietal scalp down to periosteum. (B) Defect closed with a rotation flap to preserve the same hair-bearing qualities. (C) Follow-up at 9 months showing surgical scars that would be concealed with longer hair.

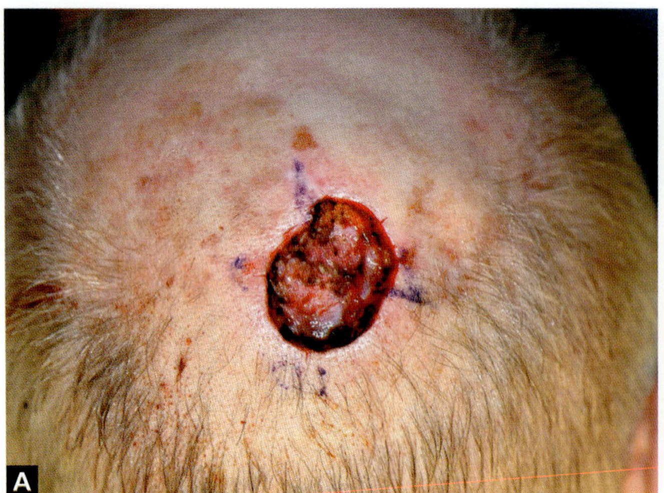


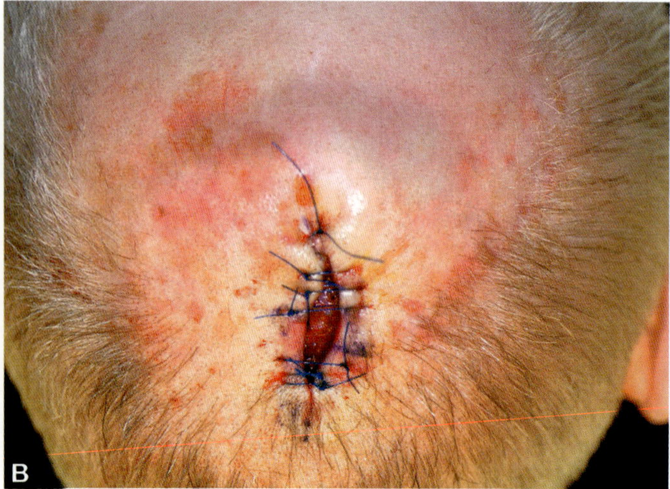


**Figs. 20.18A and B:** Partial closure with secondary intention. (A) A 2.9 cm × 2.8 cm defect located over the vertex scalp. (B) The inelastic tissue precluded primary closure, so the wound was partially closed and allowed to heal via secondary intention.

When repairing defects at the temporoparietal scalp junction, flaps should be inferiorly based and widely undermined. More laterally, the temporoparietal fascia can be pedicled or used as a free flap, and is useful for reconstruction of full-thickness postauricular defects.[48] Flaps in the parietal region are generally based on the posterior branch of the superficial temporal artery, thus avoiding potential injury to the frontal branch of the facial nerve and preservation of the anterior hairline, but may be based on the anterior branch or both branches simultaneously.[49]

Rhomboid or subcutaneous pedicle is often preferred for reconstruction of the temporal area. The rhomboid flap allows for the scar to be hidden behind the ear. Care must be taken in the case of larger flaps to avoid a significant shift in the natural hairline. Tissue expanders may also be used for significant wounds to preserve a normal contour and hair-bearing quality.

## Vertex Scalp

Surgical reconstruction over the vertex scalp requires extensive undermining due to the limited mobility of tissue. The relative lack of mobility is due to the dense galeal layer, no underlying muscle, and poor tissue distensibility. Cosmetically, it is important to attempt to preserve the natural whorled hair pattern.

Small defects can be closed directly with expansive subgaleal dissection.[50] Alternatively, the use of a purse-string suture or partial closure and retention sutures can be used to decrease the surface area of the lesion and allow for healing by secondary intention (Figs. 20.18A and B). In general, larger flaps are required to repair defects over this region than are required for other areas of the scalp, as there is less redundant tissue to mobilize for closure (Figs. 20.19A to C).[51] For large scalp defects, transposition flaps with FTSG/STSG or a xenograft for the secondary defect may be used (Figs. 20.20A and B).[52] Multiple rotation flaps, such as an O-to-Z flap can be used to disperse the tension over a greater surface area at the expense of additional surgical manipulation (Figs. 20.21A to C). Alternatively, large rotation flaps with near-complete scalp undermining and galeal scoring can be used. In balding patients with a defect over the vertex, skin grafting should be considered to produce a reasonable appearance. As is true for the other regions of the scalp, tissue expanders may be used for large defects.

## Occipital Scalp

The occipital scalp contains the thickest skin on the scalp and is an area of moderate mobility. The back of the scalp, including the posterior hairline, is not as cosmetically sensitive as it may be covered by long hair in some individuals. Although the tissue of the occipital scalp is not as loose as that of the parietal scalp, small defects are amenable to linear closure (Figs. 20.22A to C), or may be reduced in surface area with a purse-string suture and allowed to heal by granulation (Figs. 20.23A to C).[53] Again trichophytic closures in this area can help camouflage resultant scars and cut down on obvious alopecia associated with this area.

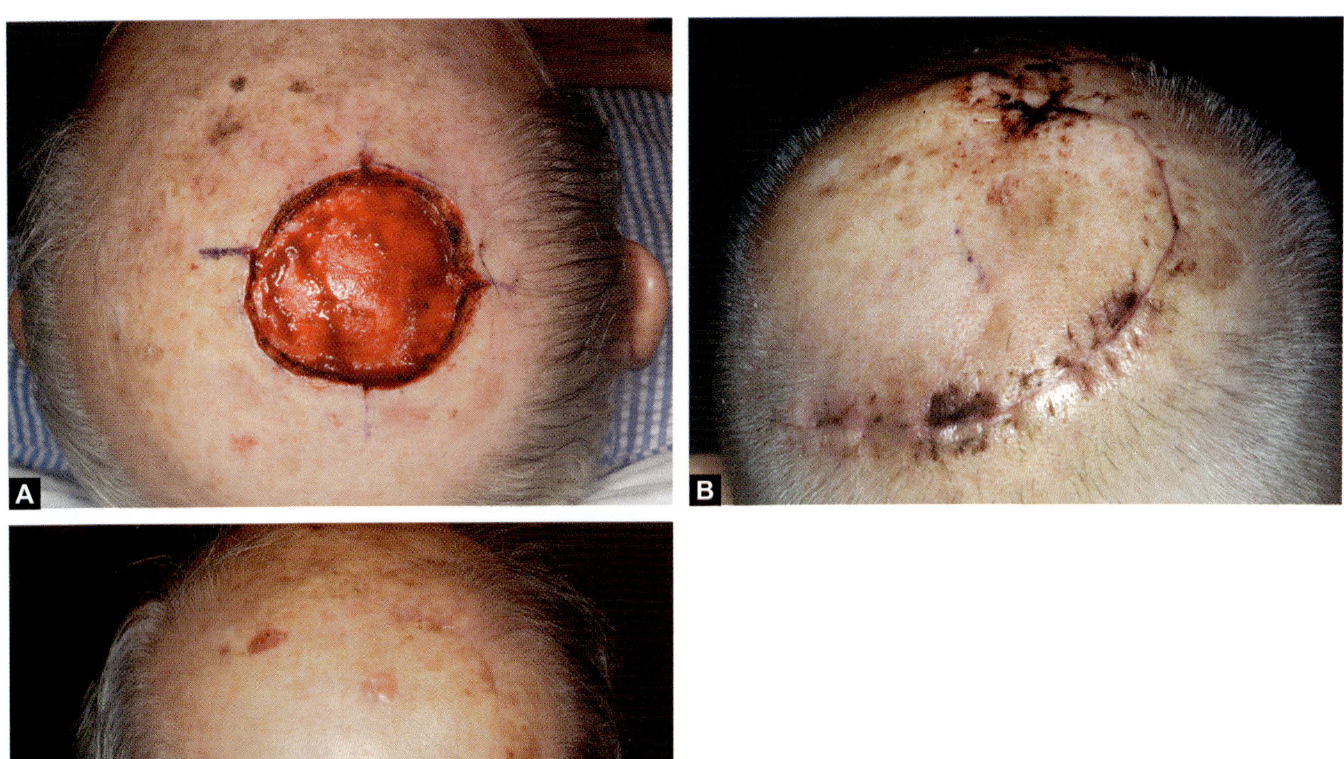

**Figs. 20.19A to C:** Bilateral rotation flap. (A) A 6.5 cm × 6.5 cm defect over the vertex scalp in a patient treated for a well-differentiated, invasive squamous cell carcinoma. (B) A large bilateral rotation flap was designed necessitating wide undermining due to vertex scalp's lack of laxity. (C) Follow-up at 7 months shows preservation of normal appearing scalp tissue with a scar.
*Courtesy*: Colleen McCarthy and Erica Lee, New York, New York.

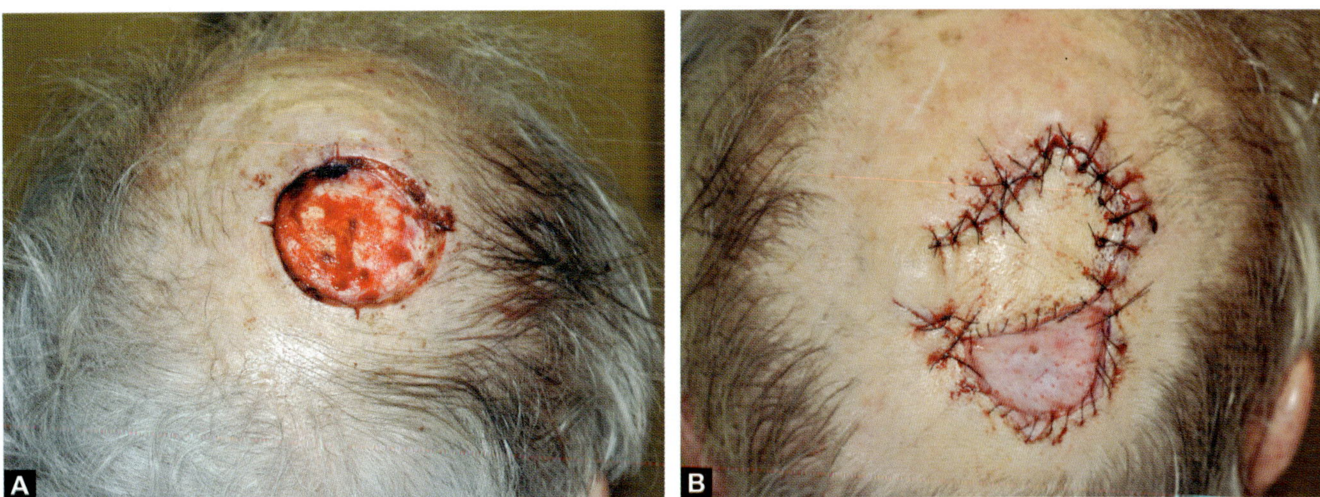

**Figs. 20.20A and B:** Combined local flap with xenograft repair. (A) A 7 cm × 6 cm defect over the vertex scalp down to periosteum. (B) The wound was closed with a rotation flap and the secondary defect was covered with a xenograft.
*Courtesy*: Erica Lee, New York, New York.

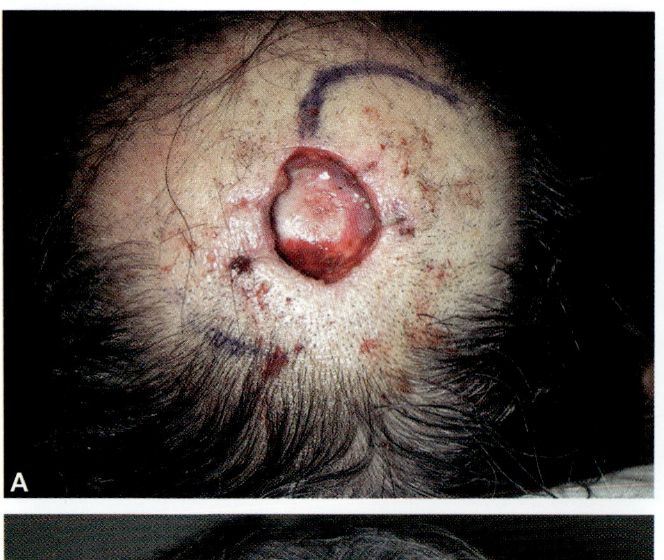


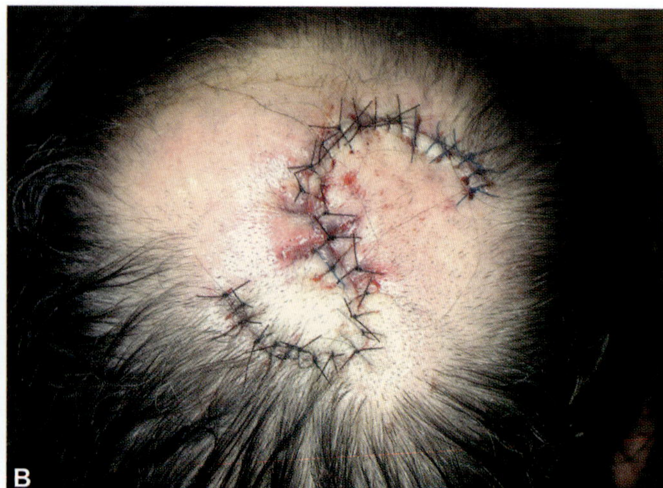


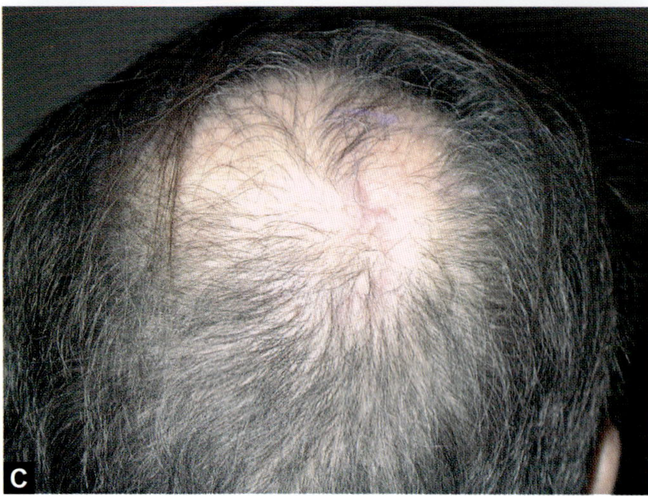


**Figs. 20.21A to C:** Bilateral rotation flap (O-to-Z). (A) A 2.5 cm × 2.5 cm defect over the vertex scalp down to periosteum in a patient treated with wide local excision for a lentigo maligna. (B) The defect was closed with a bilateral rotation (O-to-Z) flap to distribute the tension over a greater surface area. (C) Follow-up 6 months later.

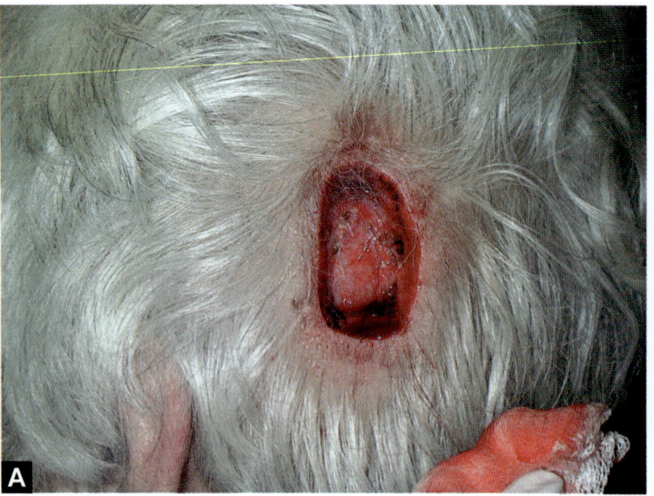


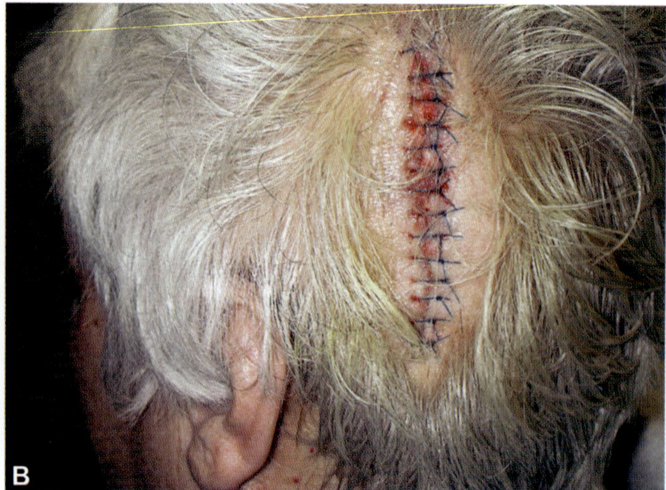


**Figs. 20.22A and B**

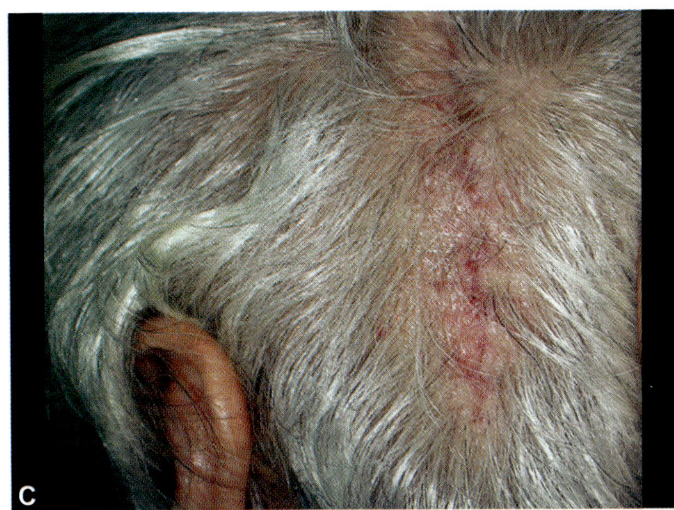

**Figs. 20.22A to C:** Linear closure on the occipital scalp. (A) A 4 cm × 2.5 cm defect over the occipital scalp. (B) The wound edges were reapproximated in a linear fashion. (C) 2-month follow-up showing a linear scar concealed by normal hair growth.

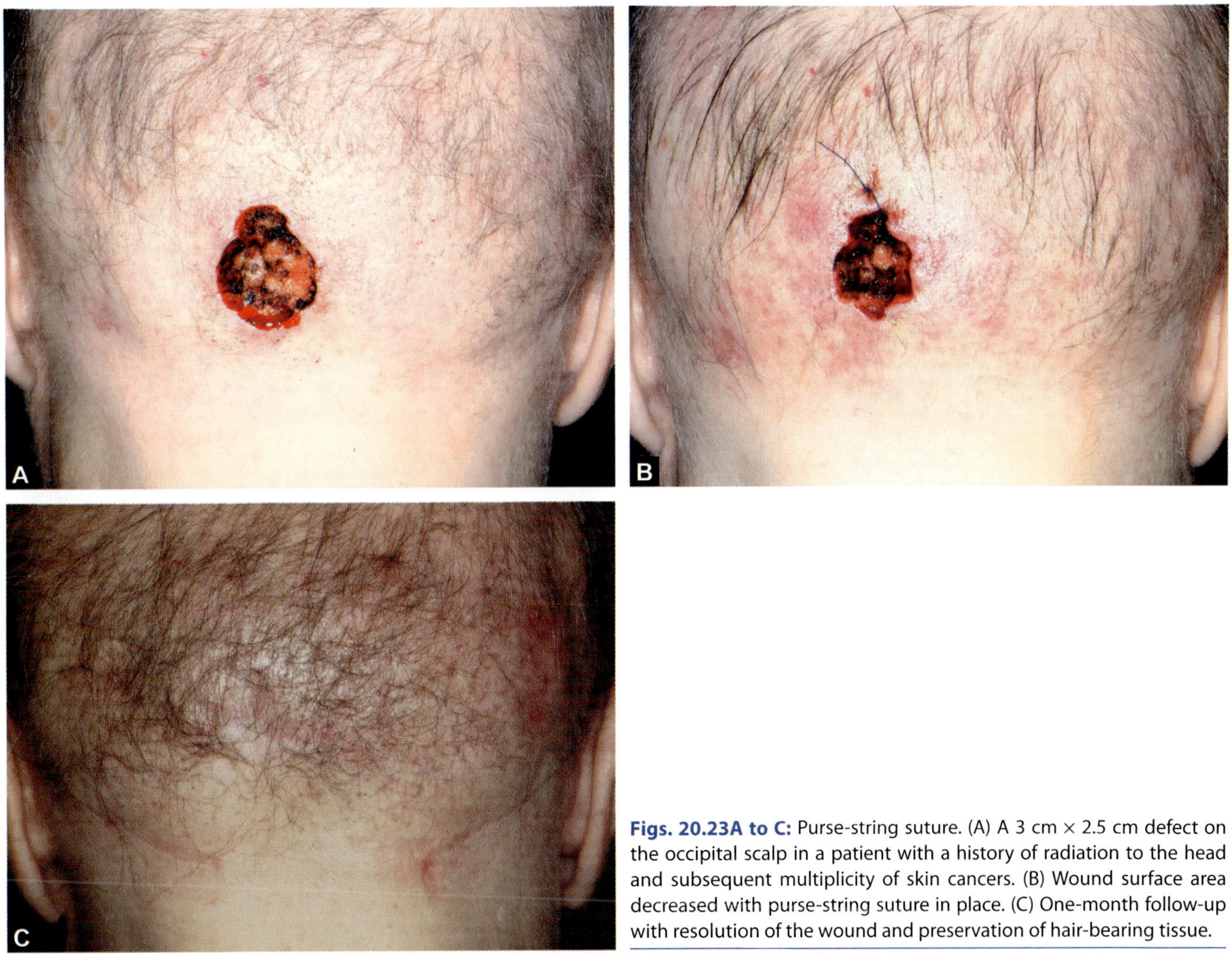

**Figs. 20.23A to C:** Purse-string suture. (A) A 3 cm × 2.5 cm defect on the occipital scalp in a patient with a history of radiation to the head and subsequent multiplicity of skin cancers. (B) Wound surface area decreased with purse-string suture in place. (C) One-month follow-up with resolution of the wound and preservation of hair-bearing tissue.

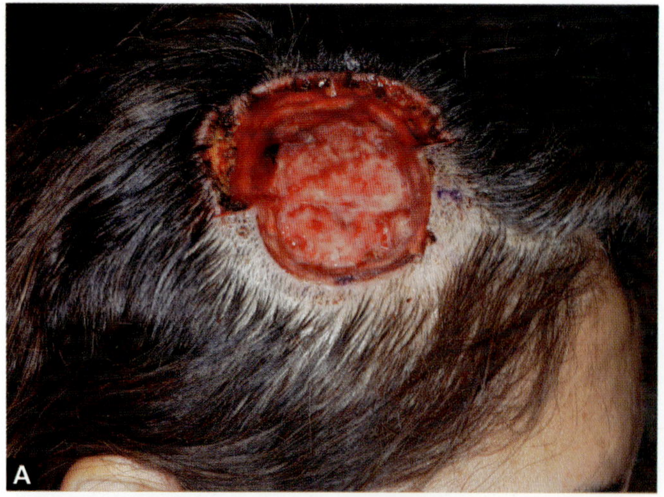

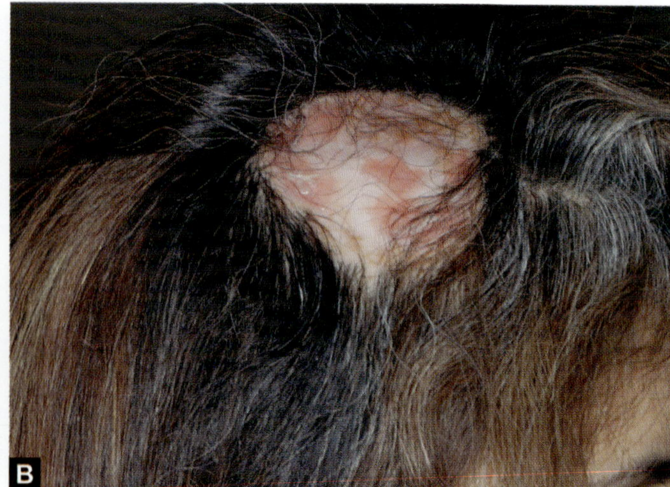

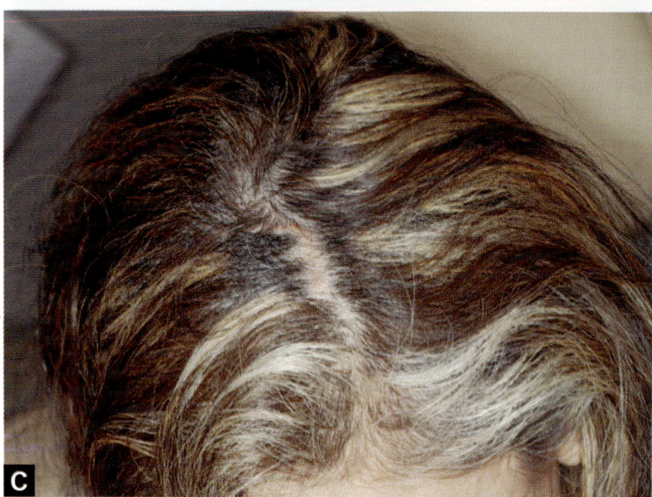

**Figs. 20.24A to C:** Split-thickness skin graft and tissue expansion. (A) Patient treated for microcystic adnexal carcinoma with perineural invasion resulting in a 6.5 cm × 6.5 cm defect over the right parietal scalp down to periosteum and galea. (B) A split-thickness skin graft from the thigh was used due to potential for recurrence, leaving a functional but poor cosmetic match. (C) Patient after undergoing tissue expansion and rotation flap to restore normal hair-bearing tissue. *Courtesy*: Evan Matros and Joseph Disa, New York, New York.

## COMPLICATIONS AND POSTOPERATIVE CARE

Postoperative bandaging serves a multitude of purposes. It provides pressure hemostasis, which can be imperative for patients on anticoagulants. It stabilizes wounds and protects the area from outside shearing forces or environmental pathogens. Depending on the amount of hair surrounding the closure, the use of an adhesive bandage may not be practical. Therefore, one can use a combination of nonadherent padding and a traditional postoperative garment for the head. This will provide necessary pressure and protection without the use of adhesive. Alternatively one can create a similar compression bandage using an elastic wrap. Bandages can be left in place for 48 hours before commencing with wound care. Afterward washing with gentle soap and water or even a baby-formulated shampoo may help keep the area cleansed. Telling the patient to not let the shower directly hit the wound will help from avoiding excessive water pressure on the area. Afterward, the area can be pat dry and a layer of petrolatum can be placed over the incision. Again, bandage placement will depend on the amount of hair surrounding the wound. Sutures or staples are traditionally left in for 2 weeks; however, if on follow-up the wound is not fully healed these can be left in for additional time.

Complications of scalp reconstruction include standard complications of surgery such as infection, postoperative bleeding, hematoma formation, ecchymosis, wound dehiscence, and flap or graft necrosis. Maintaining sterile or clean technique is essential to any surgery but postoperative care by the patient is also paramount. Deeper and larger defects, as well as patient factors such as immunosuppression or radiation, can all affect wound healing and increase the risk for complications.[54] Additionally, informing the patient to sleep with their head at an upright angle will allow for gravitational forces to assist with post-operative edema. Postoperative ice packs can also help with edema and local pain control. Avoiding strenuous exercise or bending of the head below the heart will prevent increases in blood pressure that could compromise healing. Alopecic scars or areas of skin grafts can be treated with local hair transplantation[55] or delayed tissue expansion and revision (*see* Figs. 20.24A to C).

## SUMMARY

Surgical reconstruction of the scalp is a highly individualized procedure where a thorough understanding of the anatomy and meticulous presurgical planning is of utmost importance. Although the major factors that determine the options for closure are the size, depth, and location of the defect, it is equally important to consider the patient's comorbidities and ability to tolerate further surgery, quality of surrounding tissue, and desire for a good cosmetic result. The suggestions provided in this chapter are not meant to function as an all-inclusive list, but rather a collection of options to serve as a foundation when planning reconstruction. Comprehensive knowledge of the broad spectrum of techniques available for closure along with understanding the patient's wishes and expectations will help create a superior end result.

## REFERENCES

1. Ioannides C, Fossion E, McGrouther AD. Reconstruction for large defects of the scalp and cranium. J Craniomaxillofac Surg. 1999;27:145-52.
2. Kirolles S, Haikal FA, Saadeh FA, et al. Fascial layers of the scalp. A study of 48 cadaveric dissections. Surg Radiol Anat. 1992;14:331-3.
3. Singh V. Textbook of Anatomy (Regional and Clinical) Head, Neck, and Brain. Elsevier Health Sciences APAC; New Delhi, India. 2014.
4. Hayman LA, Shukla V, Ly C, et al. Clinical and imaging anatomy of the scalp. J Comput Assist Tomogr. 2003;27:454-9.
5. Tolhurst DE, Carstens MH, Greco RJ, et al. The surgical anatomy of the scalp. Plast Reconstr Surg. 1991;87:603-12; discussion 13-4.
6. Cutting CB, McCarthy JG, Berenstein A. Blood supply of the upper craniofacial skeleton: the search for composite calvarial bone flaps. Plast Reconstr Surg. 1984;74:603-10.
7. Seery GE. Surgical anatomy of the scalp. Dermatol Surg. 2002;28:581-7.
8. Mehrara BJ, Disa JJ, Pusic A. Scalp reconstruction. J Surg Oncol. 2006;94:504-8.
9. Nguyen HH. The microsurgical replantation of seven complete scalp avulsions: is one artery sufficient? J Plast Reconstr Aesthet Surg. 2012;65:1639-44.
10. Pan WR, Le Roux CM, Briggs CA. Variations in the lymphatic drainage pattern of the head and neck: further anatomic studies and clinical implications. Plast Reconstr Surg. 2011;127:611-20.
11. Mosser SW, Guyuron B, Janis JE, et al. The anatomy of the greater occipital nerve: implications for the etiology of migraine headaches. Plast Reconstr Surg. 2004;113:693-7; discussion 98-700.
12. Stuzin JM, Wagstrom L, Kawamoto HK, et al. Anatomy of the frontal branch of the facial nerve: the significance of the temporal fat pad. Plast Reconstr Surg. 1989;83:265-71.
13. Seery GE. Galea fixation in alopecia reduction surgery. Dermatol Surg. 2001;27:931-6.
14. Sebastian S. Does preoperative scalp shaving result in fewer postoperative wound infections when compared with no scalp shaving? A systematic review. J Neurosci Nurs. 2012;44:149-56.
15. Davies T, Karanovic S, Shergill B. Essential regional nerve blocks for the dermatologist: Part 1. Clin Exp Dermatol. 2014;39:777-84.
16. Egemen O, Bingol D, Ozkaya O, et al. Use of scalp flaps as a salvage procedure in reconstruction of the large defects of head and neck region. Turkish Neurosurg. 2012;22:712-7.
17. Wilhelmi BJ, Blackwell SJ, Phillips LG. Langer's lines: to use or not to use. Plast Reconstr Surg. 1999;104:208-14.
18. Son D, Harijan A. Overview of surgical scar prevention and management. J Korean Med Sci. 2014;29:751-7.
19. Sattur SS. A review of surgical methods (excluding hair transplantation) and their role in hair loss management today. J Cutan Aesthet Surg. 2011;4:89-97.
20. Raposio E, Nordstrom RE, Santi PL. Undermining of the scalp: quantitative effects. Plast Reconstr Surg. 1998;101:1218-22.
21. Raposio E, Santi P, Nordstrom RE. Effects of galeotomies on scalp flaps. Ann Plast Surg. 1998;41:17-21.
22. Raposio E, Santi PL, Nordstrom RE. Serial scalp reductions: a biomechanical approach. Dermatol Surg. 1999;25:210-4.
23. Seery GE. Improved scalp surgery results by controlling tension vector forces in the tissues by galea to pericranium fixation sutures. Dermatol Surg. 2001;27:569-74.
24. Liu CM, McKenna J, Griess A. Surgical pearl: the use of towel clamps to reapproximate wound edges under tension. J Am Acad Dermatol. 2004;50:273-4.
25. Ritchie AJ, Rocke LG. Staples versus sutures in the closure of scalp wounds: a prospective, double-blind, randomized trial. Injury. 1989;20:217-8.
26. Sherris DA, Larrabee WF. Principles of Facial Reconstruction: A Subunit Approach to Cutaneous Repair. Thieme; New York, New York, 2011.
27. Frodel JL, Mabrie D. Optimal elective scalp incision design. Otolaryngol Head Neck Surg. 1999;121:374-7.

28. Yesudian P. Human hair—an evolutionary relic? Int J Trichol. 2011;3:69.
29. Becker GD, Adams LA, Levin BC. Secondary intention healing of exposed scalp and forehead bone after Mohs surgery. Otolaryngol Head Neck Surg. 1999;121:751-4.
30. Payne WG, Naidu DK, Wheeler CK, et al. Wound healing in patients with cancer. Eplasty. 2008;8:e9.
31. Drosou A, Trieu D, Goldberg LH. Scalpel-made holes on exposed scalp bone to promote second intention healing. J Am Acad Dermatol. 2014;71:387-8.
32. Ersek RA, Hachen HJ. Porcine xenografts in the treatment of pressure ulcers. Ann Plast Surg. 1980;5:464-70.
33. Kim CK, Kim DY, Kim JY. Asymmetric dermal-subdermal suture in trichophytic closure for wide hair transplantation donor wound. Dermatol Surg. 2013;39:1124-7.
34. Gottlieb LJ, Krieger LM. From the reconstructive ladder to the reconstructive elevator. Plast Reconstr Surg. 1994;93: 1503-4.
35. Weber PJ, Moody BR, Dryden RM, et al. Electrosurgical standing cutaneous cone modification. Dermatol Surg. 2001;27:960-2.
36. Thornton J. Skin grafts and skin substitutes. In: Selected Readings in Plastic Surgery, Vol 10, No 1; 2004. Pp. 1-23.
37. Komorowska-Timek E, Gabriel A, Bennett DC, et al. Artificial dermis as an alternative for coverage of complex scalp defects following excision of malignant tumors. Plast Reconstr Surg. 2005;115:1010-7.
38. Stephenson AJ, Griffiths RW, La Hausse-Brown TP. Patterns of contraction in human full thickness skin grafts. Br J Plast Surg. 2000;53:397-402.
39. Tran HT, Gladsjo JA, Jiang SB. Two simple ways to maintain contour on convex surfaces: the lateral nasal ala and scalp. Cutis. 2013:26(2)16-20.
40. Fowler NM, Futran ND. Achievements in scalp reconstruction. Curr Opin Otolaryngol Head Neck Surg. 2014;22: 127-30.
41. Kalra GS, Goil P, Chakotiya PS. Microsurgical reconstruction of major scalp defects following scalp avulsion. Ind J Plast Surg. 2013;46:486-92.
42. Sweeny L, Eby B, Magnuson JS, et al. Reconstruction of scalp defects with the radial forearm free flap. Head Neck Oncol. 2012;4:21.
43. Choi MS, Kim EJ, Lee JH, et al. Scalp reconstruction after resection of a large recurred proliferating trichilemmal tumor using an anterolateral thigh free flap. Arch Plast Surg. 2013; 40:458-60.
44. O'Reilly AG, Schmitt WR, Roenigk RK, et al. Closure of scalp and forehead defects using external tissue expander. Arch Facial Plast Surg. 2012;14:419-22.
45. Schaefer SD, Byrd HS, Holmes RE. Forehead and scalp reconstruction after wide-field resection of skin carcinoma. Arch Otolaryngol 1980;106:680-4.
46. Gundeslioglu AO, Selimoglu MN, Doldurucu T, et al. Reconstruction of large anterior scalp defects using advancement flaps. J Craniofac Surg. 2012;23:1766-9.
47. Orticochea M. Four flap scalp reconstruction technique. Br J Plast Surg. 1967;20:159-71.
48. Mavropoulos JC, Bordeaux JS. The temporoparietal fascia flap: a versatile tool for the dermatologic surgeon. Dermatol Surg. 2014;40 Suppl 9:S113-9.
49. Yap LH, Langstein HN. Reconstruction of the scalp, calvarium, and forehead. In: Thorne C, Grabb WC, Smith JW, et al. (Eds). Grabb and Smith's Plastic Surgery. Wolters Kluwer Health/Lippincott Williams & Wilkins; Philadelphia, PA; 2007.
50. Raposio E, Nordstrom RE, Santi P. Aesthetic reconstruction of the vertex area of the scalp. Case report. Scand J Plast Reconstr Surg Hand Surg. 1998;32:358-66.
51. Ahuja RB. Geometric considerations in the design of rotation flaps in the scalp and forehead region. Plast Reconstr Surg. 1988;81:900-6.
52. Aldabagh B, Cook JL. Reconstruction of scalp wounds with exposed calvarium using a local flap and a split-thickness skin graft: case series of 20 patients. Dermatol Surg. 2014;40:257-65.
53. Earnest LM, Byrne PJ. Scalp reconstruction. Facial Plast Surg Clin North Am. 2005;13:345-53, vii.
54. Janus JR, Peck BW, Tombers NM, et al. Complications after oncologic scalp reconstruction: a 139-patient series and treatment algorithm. Laryngoscope. 2014;125(3):582-8.
55. Jung S, Oh SJ, Hoon Koh S. Hair follicle transplantation on scar tissue. J Craniofac Surg. 2013;24:1239-41.

# CHAPTER 21

# Reconstruction of the Hand/Nail

*Joseph F Sobanko, Christopher J Miller*

## INTRODUCTION

Although the hand accounts for <2% of the total body surface area, ~10–15% of all skin cancers occur on the hands.[1,2] The most common cutaneous malignancy of the hand is squamous cell carcinoma, and other cutaneous neoplasms such as basal cell carcinoma and melanoma occur less frequently.[2,3] Reconstructive surgery may be necessary to preserve or restore function after excision or Mohs micrographic surgery of cutaneous neoplasms.[4] This chapter will focus specifically on reconstruction of soft tissue defects of the dorsal surface, where the hand, digits, and nail unit are particularly vulnerable to skin cancer from chronic ultraviolet exposure.

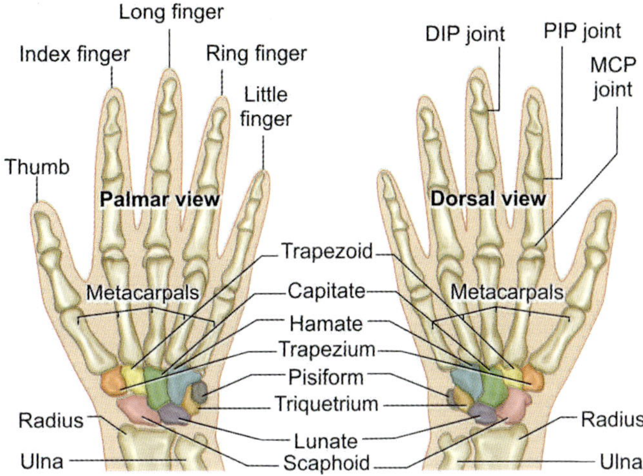


**Fig. 21.1:** Hand skeletal anatomy.
(MCP: Metacarpophalangeal; PIP: Proximal interphalangeal; DIP: Distal interphalangeal).

## ANATOMY OVERVIEW

### Skeletal Anatomy

The skeleton of the hand includes eight carpal bones in the wrist, five metacarpals in the hand proper, and phalanges in each of the five digits (thumb and four fingers). The digits are numbered and named as follows: digit 1, thumb; digit 2, index finger; digit 3, long finger ("middle finger"); digit 4, ring finger; digit 5, small finger ("little finger"). Each finger (digits 2–5) has three joints: the distal interphalangeal (DIP) joint between the distal and middle phalanges, the proximal interphalangeal (PIP) joint between the middle and proximal phalanges, and the metacarpophalangeal (MCP) between the proximal phalanx and metacarpals and corresponding to the distal palmar crease (Fig. 21.1). The thumb has an MCP joint and only one interphalangeal (IP) joint.

An intricate musculotendinous system controls the motions of the skeleton. A detailed discussion of the muscles and tendons of the hand and digits is beyond the scope of this chapter, and readers are referred to other sources for more comprehensive information.[5] Briefly, the tendons on the dorsal hand insert on the phalanges to control motion of the digits. The tendons lie immediately superficial to the deep dorsal fascia investing the dorsal interosseous muscles and periosteum of the metacarpals. On the proximal two-thirds of the dorsal hand, the extensor tendons are linked by a connective tissue network called the junctura tendinae.[6] The distal aspect of the junctura tendinae is an important landmark to identify perforating arteries from the palmar to dorsal hand. This chapter addresses more detailed anatomy of the muscles and tendons when applicable to a specific reconstruction or critical anatomic relationship.

### Vascular Anatomy

The radial and ulnar arteries supply all of the blood to the hand and digits (Fig. 21.2). The ulnar artery enters the

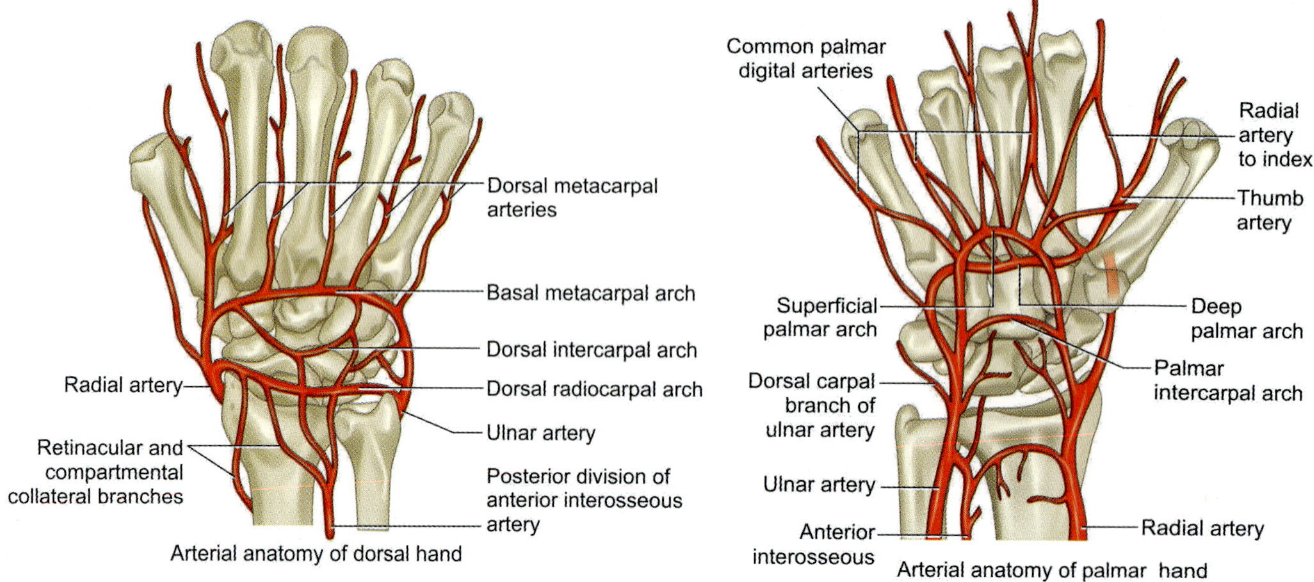


**Fig. 21.2:** Hand arterial anatomy.

hand anterior to the flexor retinaculum via the ulnar canal located between the pisiform and the hook of the hamate. The radial artery enters the hand as it crosses the floor1 of the anatomic snuffbox between the easily palpated tendons of the extensor pollicis longus and extensor pollicis brevis muscles. The palmar aspect of the hand and fingers receives the bulk of its blood supply from the ulnar artery, while the dorsal aspect is supplied primarily from the radial artery. However, each side benefits from a series of anastomoses, which are critical contributors to some flaps on the hand and fingers.

The palmar blood supply comes from two arterial arches. The superficial palmar arch is a direct continuation of the ulnar artery and is completed laterally by the superficial branch of the radial artery. Kaplan's cardinal line (drawn across the palm parallel to a fully abducted thumb) overlies the superficial palmar arch. The superficial palmar arch gives rise to the common palmar digital arteries, which further divide into the proper palmar digital arteries that run along the palmar aspect of the midaxial line of the second through fifth digits. The proper palmar digital arteries give rise to consistent dorsal cutaneous branches in the proximal and middle phalanges of digits 2–5 and near the MCP joint and IP joint of the thumb.[7] These dorsal cutaneous branches can be utilized to provide the blood supply for digital flaps.

The deep palmar arch is a direct continuation of the radial artery and is completed medially by the deep palmar branch of the ulnar artery. The deep palmar arch lies across the metacarpals just distal to their bases and is located ~1 cm proximal to the superficial palmar arch. The deep palmar arch gives rise to the princeps pollicis artery of the thumb and three palmar metacarpal arteries. The palmar metacarpal arteries from the deep palmar arch have rich anastomoses with the common palmar digital arteries from the superficial palmar arch. The palmar metacarpal arteries give rise to dorsal perforating arteries 1 cm proximal to the metacarpal head and immediately distal to the junctura tendinae. These perforating arteries anastomose with the dorsal metacarpal arteries and are the basis for single-stage perforating flaps to reconstruct dorsal defects of the proximal digits.

The blood supply to the proximal two-thirds of the dorsal hand arises primarily from the dorsal metacarpal arteries.[8] The first dorsal metacarpal artery arises from the radial artery.[9] The second through fifth dorsal metacarpal arteries arise from the dorsal carpal arterial arch, which is formed by branches of both the radial and ulnar arteries. The third and fourth metacarpal arteries may also arise from a perforating artery from the palmar arterial system at the level of the metacarpal base.[10] The dorsal metacarpal arteries run parallel to the metacarpal bones within the fascia of the dorsal interosseous muscles and deep to the extensor tendons.[10,11] Each of the dorsal metacarpal arteries supplies blood to the dorsal skin of the hand via four to eight cutaneous perforator vessels that arise along its length.[10] The number and diameter of perforators are larger at the level of the distal third of the metacarpal compared

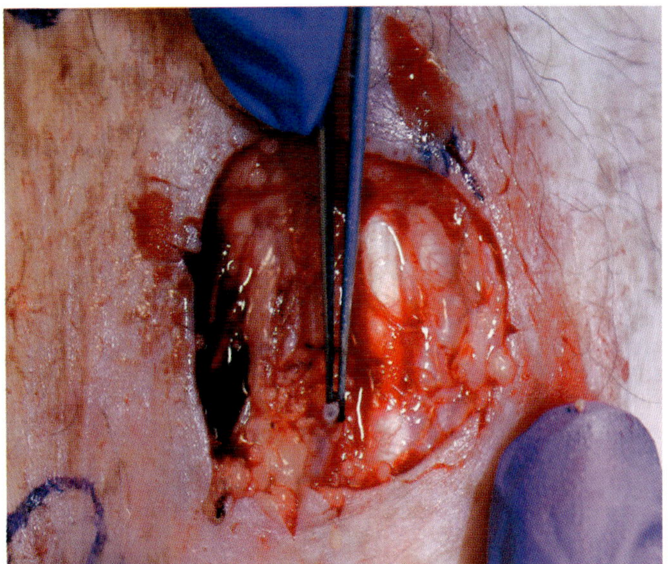

**Fig. 21.3:** Dorsal metacarpal artery cutaneous perforator.

to the proximal and central thirds because of perforating arteries from the palmar arterial system (Fig. 21.3).[10] The dorsal metacarpal arteries give rise to dorsal digital branches that supply the dorsal aspect of the digits.

Skin perforators from the palmar metacarpal arteries constantly arise at the level of the second to fifth metacarpal head and help supply blood to the distal dorsal hand and digits.[10] The deep palmar arch also sends one to two dorsal perforating branches at the level of the metacarpal neck.[8] Perforators from the palmar system have distal branches that anastomose with the dorsal cutaneous branches of the palmar digital arteries, proximal branches that anastomose with the dorsal metacarpal arteries, and lateral branches that anastomose with adjacent dorsal metacarpal perforating branches.[8] The first through third dorsal metacarpal arteries consistently communicate with perforators from the palmar arterial system at the metacarpal head, whereas connections between the fourth and fifth dorsal metacarpal arteries and the palmar system are more variable.[10]

The dorsal surface of the digits derives much of its blood supply from dorsal cutaneous branches of the proper palmar digital arteries. These branches communicate with the dorsal digital branches of the dorsal metacarpal arteries, which help supply blood to the dorsal surface of the proximal and middle phalanges.[7] These anastomoses between the palmar and dorsal circulation on the hand and digits are the anatomic basis for several intrinsic flaps that are discussed in the following text.[8]

## Fascial Anatomy

The fascial system of the dorsal hand, detailed by Kanavel in 1938, was initially discussed because of its importance as a conduit for hand infections.[12] A recent comprehensive analysis[13] of the distinct dorsal hand laminae and their relation to the neurovascular and tendinous structures proves useful for reconstruction of dorsal hand defects.[14] The soft tissue of the dorsal hand consists of three distinct fascial layers separated by fatty-areolar laminae: the dorsal superficial lamina (DSL) separates the dorsal superficial fascia (DSF) from the overlying dermis; the dorsal intermediate lamina (DIL) separates the DSF from the dorsal intermediate fascia (DIF); and dorsal deep lamina (DDL) separates the DIF from the dorsal deep fascia (DDF) (Fig. 21.4). The dorsal venous system and sensory nerves lie between the DSF and DIF, the latter of which is contiguous with the antebrachial fascia in the forearm. Extensor tendons lie beneath the DIF in the DDL. Deep to the extensor tendons, the DDF forms a contiguous layer over the dorsal interosseous muscles and periosteum of the metacarpals.[13] Running between all of these fascial layers are loose connective tissue adhesions that can be separated by blunt dissection (Fig. 21.5). Within the adhesions are perforating vessels that originate from the dorsal metacarpal arteries and progress superficially to supply the dermal plexus.

The digits have a complex soft tissue network called Cleland's ligaments, which maintain the digital skin in a fixed relationship to the underlying skeleton during motion and functional tasks (Fig. 21.6). These ligaments extend from fascial structures enveloping the bone, IP joints, and tendons to insert on the lateral and palmar skin of the digits. They also create a gliding path for the lateral slips of the extensor tendon and protect the neurovascular bundle, which lies closer to the volar aspect of the lateral digits, an important relationship to understand for nerve blocks and reconstructions that utilize the proper palmar digital artery or digital nerves.[15]

## Hand Innervation

Three terminal branches of the brachial plexus that have motor, sensory, and sympathetic capabilities innervate the hand: the median, ulnar, and radial nerves. The radial nerve (C5–8, T1) allows for supination of the forearm and extension of the wrist and digital joints. The median (C6–8, T1) and ulnar (C8, T1) nerves allow for pronation of the forearm, flexion of the wrist, digital joints, and movement of the intrinsic hand muscles.

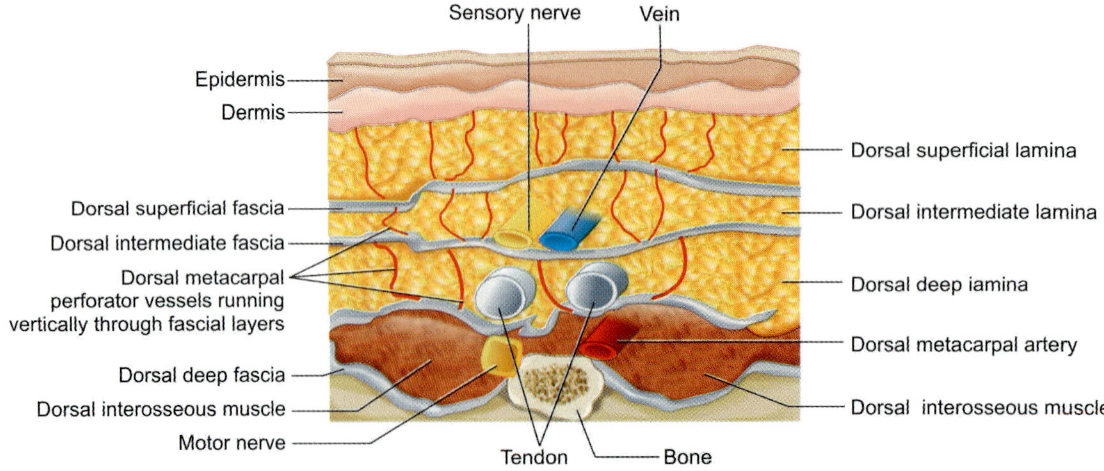


**Fig. 21.4:** Dorsal hand fascial anatomy.

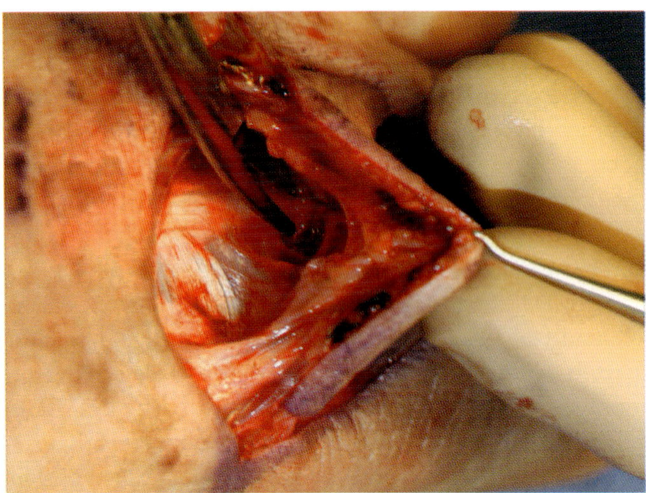

**Fig. 21.5:** Connective tissue adhesions between fascial layers

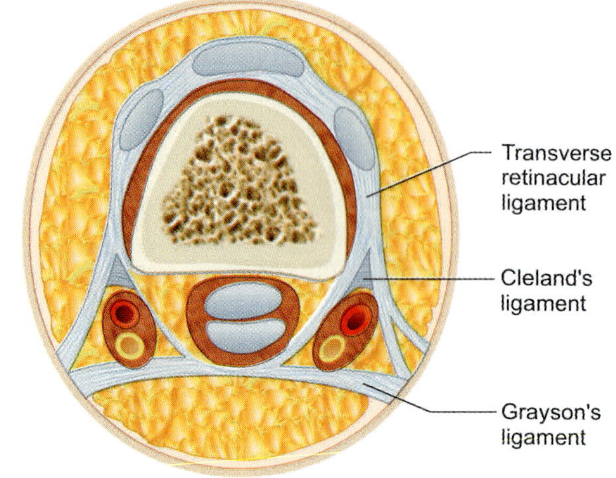


**Fig. 21.6:** Digit ligaments.

While the depth of the motor nerves often precludes injury from tumor resection and reconstruction in dermatologic surgery, the superficial branch of the radial nerve and the dorsal branch of the ulnar nerve are vulnerable to resection in the fatty-areolar lamina between the DSF and DIF. Both nerves flank the hand and turn medially as they move distally. In order to plan reconstructions on the dorsal hand and avoid nerve injury, it is helpful to use the carpometacarpal (CMC) joint of the third ray as a landmark. A safety zone for incisions can be found proximal and 1.5 cm ulnar to the third CMC joint (Fig. 21.7).[16]

Knowledge of sensory nerve distribution also permits effective nerve blocks to maximize patient comfort during hand and nail procedures. The radial aspect of the dorsal hand skin is innervated by the radial nerve. Its branches can be blocked by injecting 4–5 cc of anesthetic over the distal radius where the nerve can be felt to roll under a palpating fingertip. The remainder of the dorsal hand skin can be anesthetized with a dorsal ulnar nerve block by injecting anesthetic on the side of the wrist in the subcutaneous plane alongside and distal to the styloid process.[16] The ulnar aspect of palmar skin is blocked by placement of 4–5 cc of anesthetic just deep to the flexor carpi ulnaris tendon, ensuring not to injure the ulnar artery. The palm of the hand can be further blocked by inserting the needle between the palmaris longus and flexor carpi radialis and injecting into the carpal tunnel without eliciting paresthesia of the median nerve.

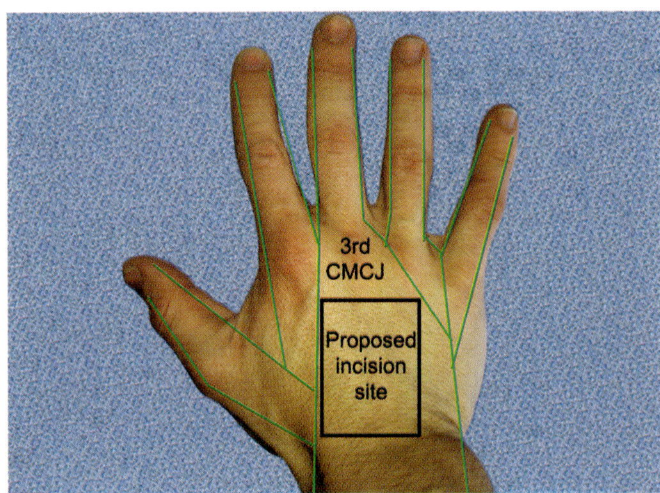


**Fig. 21.7:** Safety zone for dorsal hand incisions through dorsal superficial fascia. The area over the skin of the dorsal wrist where no major nerve passes. CMCJ: Carpometacarpal joint.

Superficial injection at this location also anesthetizes the palmar cutaneous branch of the median nerve.

Digital nerve blocks ensure patient comfort for digit and nail procedures. The surgeon may approach the nerve through an interdigital web or on the side of the digit, recognizing that the nerves of the digit lie palmar to the arteries. About 1 cc of solution injected on each side of the digit should be sufficient to gain anesthesia. Alternatively, a single volar injection just distal to the distal palmar crease can achieve anesthesia of the entire digit except for the dorsal proximal aspect. Anesthesia with epinephrine is safe in the digits.[17,18]

## Distal Phalanx and Nail Anatomy

This section will give a brief description of distal phalanx and nail anatomy. Readers are referred to excellent sources for more comprehensive nail anatomy.[19]

The function of the nail unit and pathways of vessels and nerves are closely interrelated to the bony topography and fibrous framework of the distal phalanx. The distal phalanx has an hourglass shape with a broad proximal base, a tapered waist, and a broader head with a horseshoe-shaped ungual process. A strong fibrous network of ligaments, tendons, and connective tissue lends strength to the distal digit, protects neurovascular structures, and provides stability to the nail unit. Most prominently, the lateral interosseous ligament adds strength to the more delicate waist of the phalanx as it extends from the lateral tuberosities and the base of the distal phalanx to the spines of the ungual process. The extensor tendon attaches to the base of the dorsal distal phalanx ~ 1.2 mm proximal to the germinal matrix, controls extension of the distal phalanx, and provides support to the DIP joint.[20]

The bone and fibrous network are covered by the nail unit and its skin frame dorsally and by a more generous soft tissue at the distal tip and pulp on the palmar aspect (Fig. 21.8). The nail plate is framed by invaginations of skin at the lateral and proximal nail folds. The proximal and lateral nail grooves are the cul-de-sacs between the nail frame and nail plate where the skin of the proximal and lateral nail folds merges with the nail matrix and nail bed. Distally, the hyponychium marks the convergence of the skin of the terminal phalanx with the distal nail bed epithelium. The nail frame seals the nail unit and prevents infection and penetration of foreign bodies.

The majority of the nail plate is formed from the nail matrix. The lunula is the topographic landmark for the distal matrix, and the proximal matrix extends on average 55% of the distance from the proximal nail fold to the DIP joint.[21] Put simply, the proximal matrix forms the dorsal nail plate and the distal matrix forms the ventral nail plate. Therefore, injury to the proximal matrix is more likely to cause dystrophy of the dorsal nail plate. The nail plate lifts easily from the nail matrix but is firmly adherent to the nail bed epithelium. In cross section of the digit, the matrix and nail bed epithelium form a near semicircle that curls around to the midaxial line of the distal phalanx.

The paired proper palmar digital arteries give rise to branches that supply both the palmar and dorsal aspects of the distal digit. As with the proximal digits and hand, anastomoses between the dorsal and palmar vessels ensure adequate blood supply after damage to either the dorsal or palmar vascular systems.

The blood supply to the palmar surface is comprised of middle and distal transverse arches that arise from the paired proper palmar digital arteries. The middle transverse arch occurs near the head of the middle phalanx and runs deep to the flexor tendon. The distal transverse arch arises immediately distal to the insertion of the flexor tendon on the distal phalanx and is protected by the digital pulp. The distal transverse arch gives rise to a cruciate anastomosis, which supplies blood to the distal palmar tips of the fingers.

The blood supply to the dorsal distal digit is comprised of three arcades that arise from the palmar vessels. The superficial arcade traverses the dorsal digit at the base of the distal phalanx immediately proximal to the nail matrix

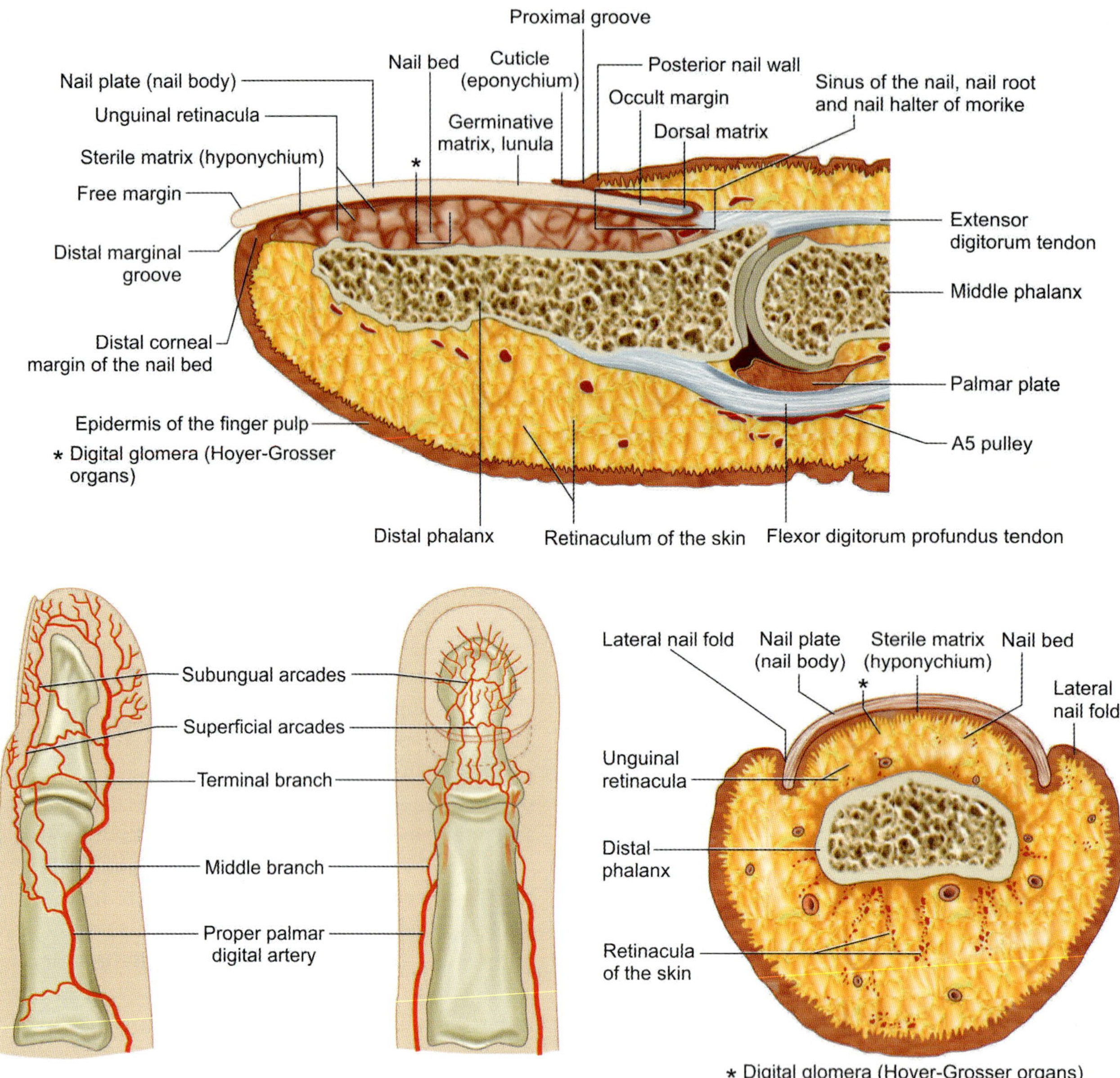


**Fig. 21.8:** Nail anatomy schematics.

and superficial to the insertion of the extensor tendon. The superficial arcade is formed from dorsal branches arising both directly from proper palmar digital arteries and from the middle transverse palmar arch.

Two additional dorsal arcades arise from the cruciate anastomosis in the pulp of the distal digit. The proximal subungual arcade passes transversely across the waist of the dorsal distal digit deep to the nail matrix and the distal subungual arcade passes transversely over the ungual process deep to the nail bed epithelium. Distal branches arising from the distal subungual arcade anastomose with palmar vessels that pass over the distal phalanx. The venous drainage of the finger occurs through deep and superficial systems. The nail bed corium deep to the nail bed epithelium contains numerous glomus bodies and neurovascular structures that serve as arteriovenous anastomoses for regulating blood supply amidst temperature changes.[22]

The nerve supply to the distal digits varies.[23] The second through fourth digits are innervated by the volar proper digital nerves, which divide distally into three branches that provide sensation to the proximal nail fold, matrix, and nail bed. The dorsum of the thumb and fifth dorsal digits may be innervated by the dorsal proper digital nerves,

| Table 21.1: Principles to guide reconstruction of soft tissue hand defects. |
|---|
| Exposed joints, bone, and tendon should be covered with a vascularized surface whenever possible |
| Vascularized flaps are preferred over grafts when paratenon has been removed |
| Repair design should be based on the size of the defect when the hand and fingers are in full flexion |

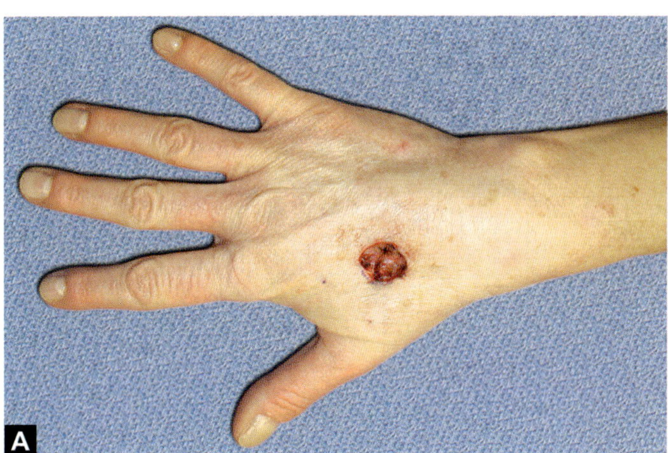
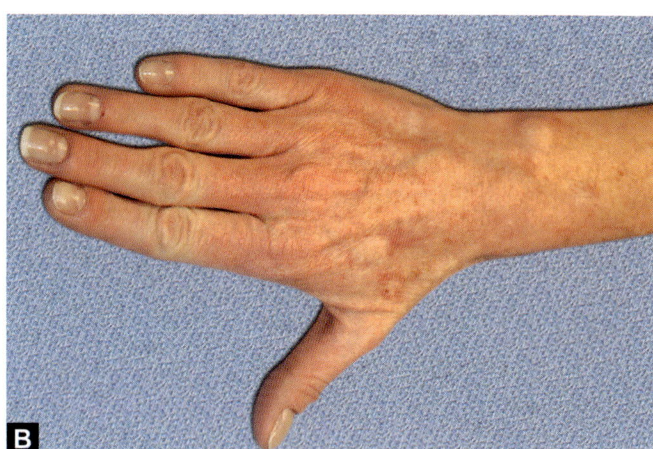

**Figs. 21.9A and B:** (A) Defect amenable for second intention healing. (B) Three months postoperative after second intention healing.

while the palmar aspect of these digits is supplied by the palmar proper digital nerves.

## PLANNING RECONSTRUCTION

Before initiating surgery, the surgeon must account for the patient's hand dominance, occupation, and history of upper-extremity problems. The optimal surgical plan considers the ability of a patient to tolerate postoperative restrictions and prepares the patient for any anticipated hand therapy.

Reconstruction options are diverse and vary depending on the size, depth, and specific location of the defect. A few general principles help guide selection for repair (Table 21.1). Exposed joints, bone, and tendon should be covered with a vascularized surface whenever possible. Vascularized flaps are preferred over grafts when paratenon has been removed. Finally, reconstruction design should be based on the size of the dorsal defect when the hand and fingers are in full flexion (i.e., a fist), as this position places the wound and reconstruction under maximum tension.

### Second Intention Healing

Second intention healing is a useful option for a subset of dorsal defects of the hand and digit (Figs. 21.9A and B).[24] A prospective study of 28 defects on the dorsum of the hand with a size ranging between 1.5 and 4.6 cm (median 2.4 cm) revealed a median healing time of 44 days with no episodes of postoperative bleeding or infection.[25] The appearances of the resultant scars were acceptable for patients, although almost half of the cases were complicated by hypergranulation tissue that required topical steroid treatment and discontinuation of a hydrocolloid dressing. The ideal defect for granulation has intact DSF and is not located over a joint. Purse-string or guiding sutures can reduce the wound surface and speed healing. Second intention healing of defects overlying joints risks contracture and restriction of motion; and exposed tendon without paratenon may desiccate and restrict motion without a vascularized cover. The extensor tendon of the distal digits is especially vulnerable to desiccation with resultant mallet deformities as possible sequelae (Figs. 21.10A to C).

### Linear Repair and Variations (S-Plasty, M-Plasty)

The linear repair is a workhorse for smaller defects, particularly those of the mid and proximal dorsal hand. A fusiform repair should be designed with the skin under maximal tension in the fist position, since the dorsal skin

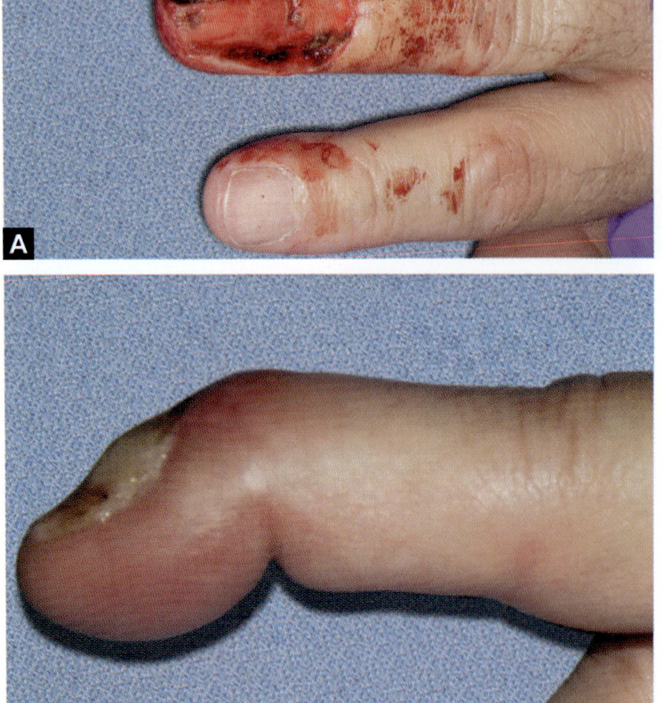

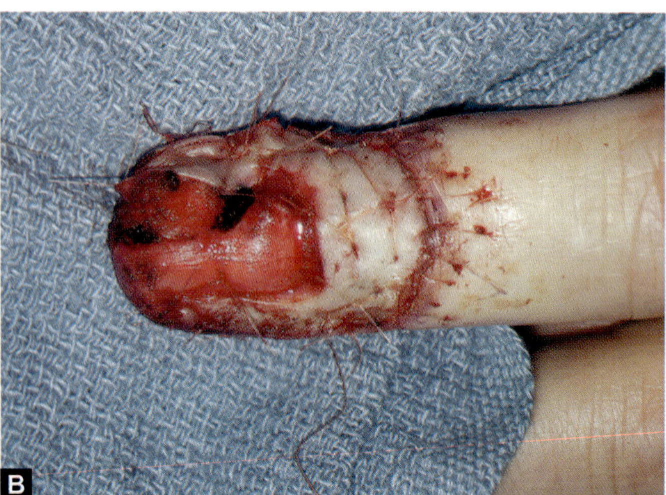

**Figs. 21.10A to C:** (A) Distal digit defect. (B) Full-thickness skin graft coverage of proximal portion of defect with distal area left to granulate. (C) Resultant mallet deformity.

lengthens by ~3 cm when the hand moves from full extension to full flexion.[5] Ideally, the two limbs of the fusiform design can be pinched together with the patient's hand in full flexion, an undertaking almost always easier in elderly patients with thin, photodamaged skin. Orientation of the closure may vary but will usually run from proximal to distal rather than transversely. Whereas traditional fusiform design typically has a length to width ratio of 4:1 or 5:1 with apical angles of 15°–20°, the intrinsic elasticity of the dorsal hand skin reduces the risk of redundant tissue cones and the length to width ratio in design may approach 3:1 with apical angles of 30°.[26] Incisions that are close and parallel to the webs, especially the first web space, should be avoided because of limitations in digital abduction.[27] Curvilinear or S-plasty modifications may displace tension away from the surrounding joints and may be preferred to simple linear repairs (Figs. 21.11A and B).

Incisions are typically carried through the skin into the DSL in order to avoid sensory disturbances. Blunt undermining is performed in this plane by scissors tips spreading and lifting the overlying dermis off the DSF. Wide undermining is not necessary in most instances because of the skin's mobility. Most surgeons opt for a layered repair on the dorsum, though some use only a single layer of epidermal sutures, especially in thin, photoaged skin that is prone to shearing. Small to moderate tissue protuberances in this location do not need to be "chased" as they almost certainly resolve with time because of the skin's elasticity.

While palmar defects are uncommon in dermatologic surgery, when closing small defects in this location it is also essential to ensure incisions occur in appropriate orientations. Damaging incisions include (1) Longitudinal incisions across a flexural crease; (2) incisions that parallel

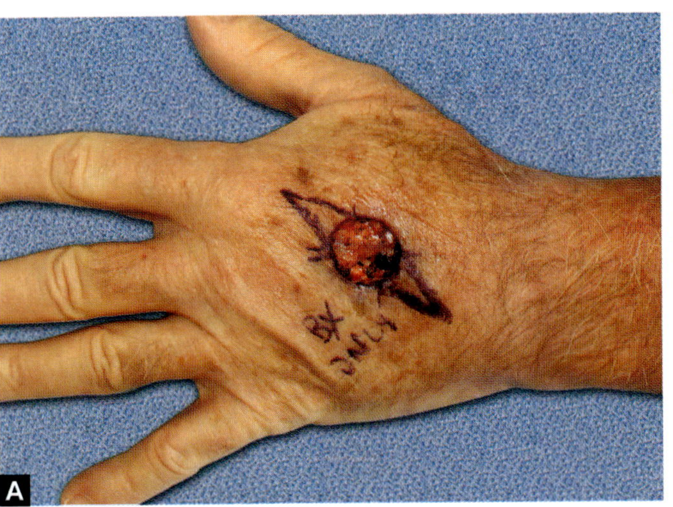

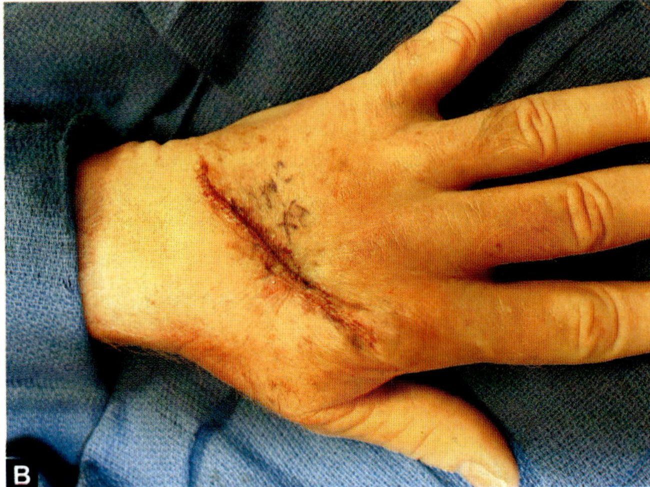

**Figs. 21.11A and B:** (A) Defect amenable to linear repair. (B) Immediately postoperative linear repair obliquely oriented.

**Table 21.2:** Potentially harmful incisions to avoid on the hand and digits.

- Longitudinal incisions across a flexural crease
- Incisions that parallel the web spaces
- Longitudinal incisions on the anterolateral aspects of the fingers
- Incisions crossing the thenar crease in the hollow of the palm
- Incisions on the palmar pulp
- Circumferential spiral incisions around a digit

the web spaces; (3) longitudinal incisions on the anterolateral aspects of the fingers; (4) incisions crossing the thenar crease in the hollow of the palm; (5) incisions on the palmar pulp; (6) circumferential spiral incisions around a digit (Table 21.2).[5] Scar lines in any of these locations can tether the hand and restrict its functional activities.

## Grafts

A skin graft may be the preferred method of repair when primary closure with a linear repair or flap is not possible. The ideal wound for immediate grafting has preserved DSF, since the extensor tendons are not exposed and the base of the wound does not shift with hand motion. The decision to select a full-thickness skin graft (FTSG) or split-thickness skin graft (STSG) depends on the size, depth, and location of the primary defect as well as the reservoir size and morbidity of the secondary defect at the donor site. Full-thickness skin graft are more metabolically demanding than STSGs but preserve adnexal structures and offer better cosmesis (Figs. 21.12A to C). Split-thickness skin grafts allow for coverage of a wider area and are more likely to survive compared to FTSG but may have inferior cosmetic results (Figs. 21.13A to D).

The graft template should be based on the maximal size of the wound when the hand is in full flexion. Full-thickness skin grafts may be harvested from any number of locations, though the most frequently utilized sites are the clavicle, inner arm, and abdomen. Split-thickness skin grafts are typically taken with a dermatome from the thigh or buttock. An intermediate (0.4 mm or 16/1,000 inch) STSG may be preferred to a thin STSG (0.2 mm or 8/1,000 inch) because of the reduced likelihood of postoperative contraction (Figs. 21.13A to D).[28]

Defects that extend deeper than the DSF into the DIF are also amenable to skin grafting; however, graft survival may be threatened if hand motion shifts the wound base, or if vascularity is compromised from removal of paratenon or periosteum. Skin grafts have less reliable survival compared to flaps and fail to provide a gliding surface for the underlying mobile structures.[29] Adhesions and fibrosis may ensue, potentially compromising tendon motion.[30] If paratenon has been removed or the base of the wound shifts with hand motion, it may be preferable to initially cover the defect with a dermal substitute to avoid desiccation of the tendons and to create a well-vascularized buffer of granulation tissue before placing a skin graft. The authors prefer to suture a bilayer dermal regeneration template (Integra, Plainsboro Township, NJ) into these deeper defects and immobilize the hand for the 1st week in order to maximize the "take" of the product. Three weeks after placement, the silicone layer is removed and a skin graft (STSG or FTSG) may be sutured to the new, shallower recipient area (Figs. 21.14A to D).

Graft survival is the result of a three-step process. The first 48 hours are marked by plasmatic imbibition followed by 7–10 days of inosculation or revascularization.

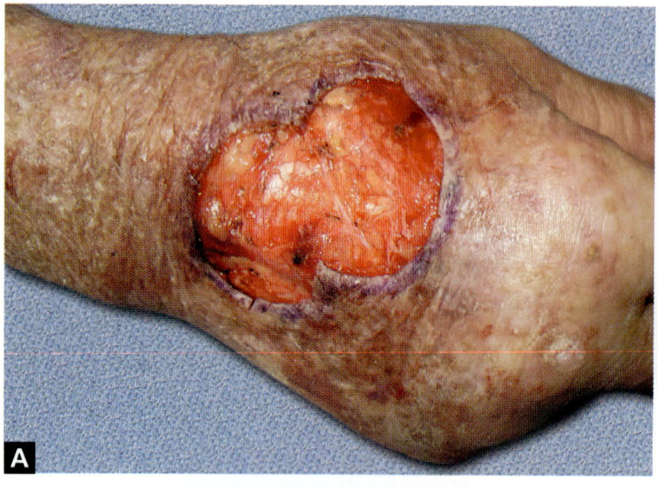

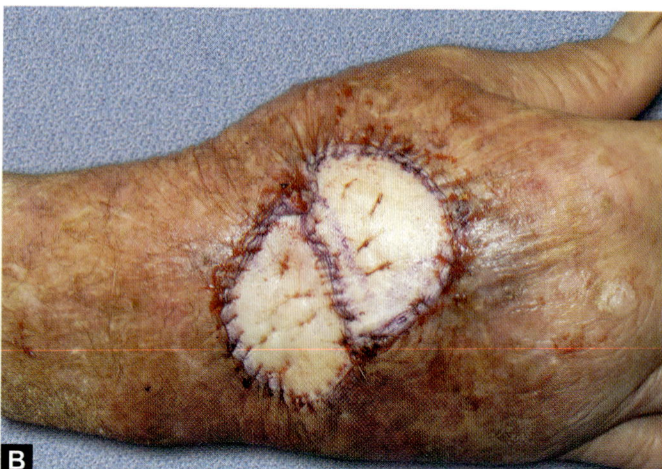

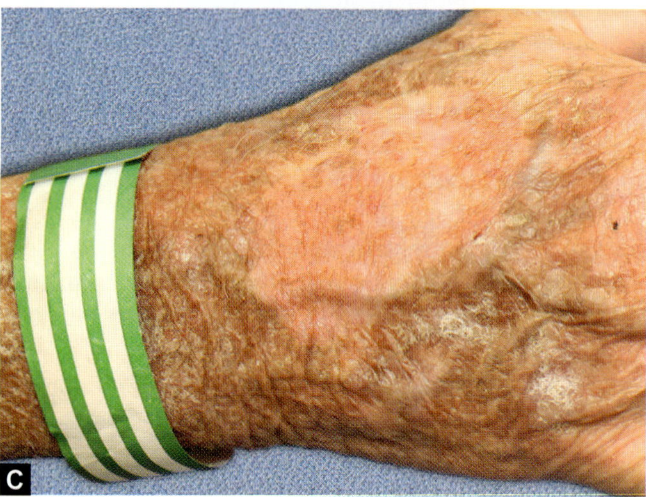

**Figs. 21.12A to C:** (A) Defect amenable to full-thickness skin graft (FTSG) reconstruction. (B) FTSG immediately postoperative. (C) Three-month follow-up after FTSG placement.

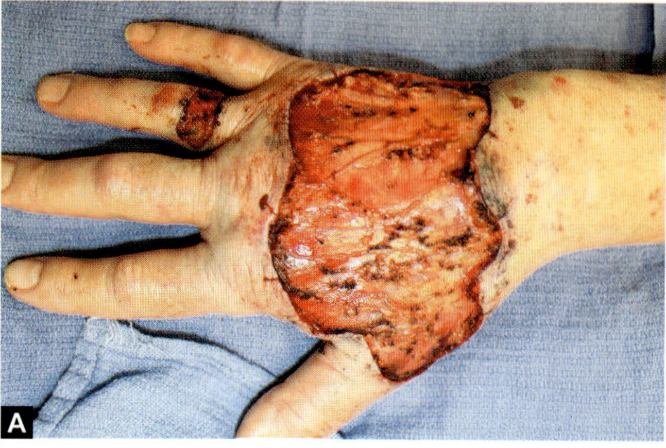

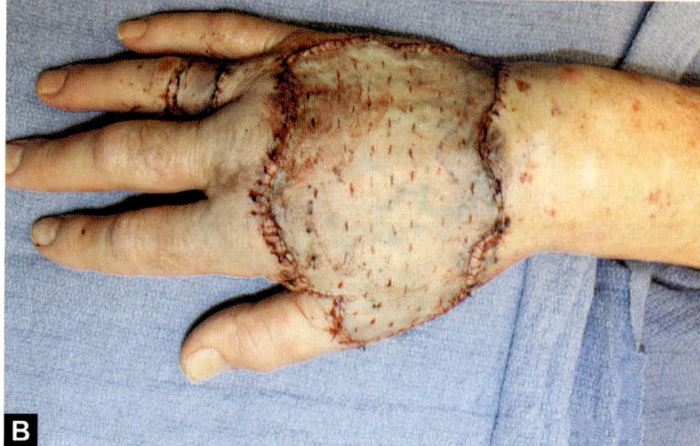

**Figs. 21.13A and B:** (A) Defect amenable to split-thickness skin graft (STSG) repair. (B) Immediately postoperative STSG.

Neovascularization parallels inosculation and grafts often become stable by the 3rd or 4th week.[31] Enhancement of graft viability can be achieved in a number of ways. Transferring the graft to the wound bed immediately after harvesting limits the time the graft is devoid of blood. When suturing grafts into place, "basting" sutures throughout the surface

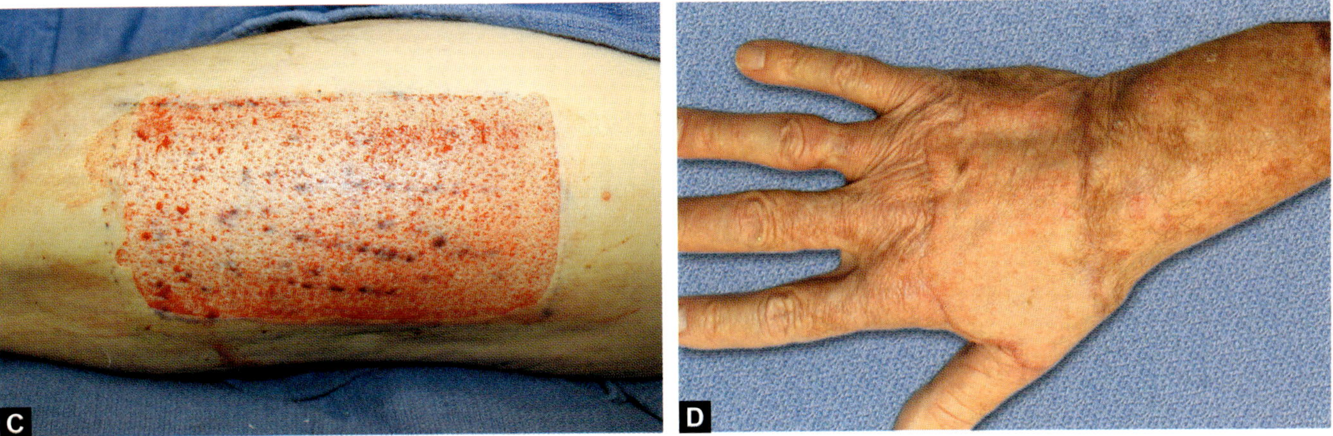

**Figs. 21.13C and D:** (C) STSG donor site. (D) Four-month follow-up after STSG.

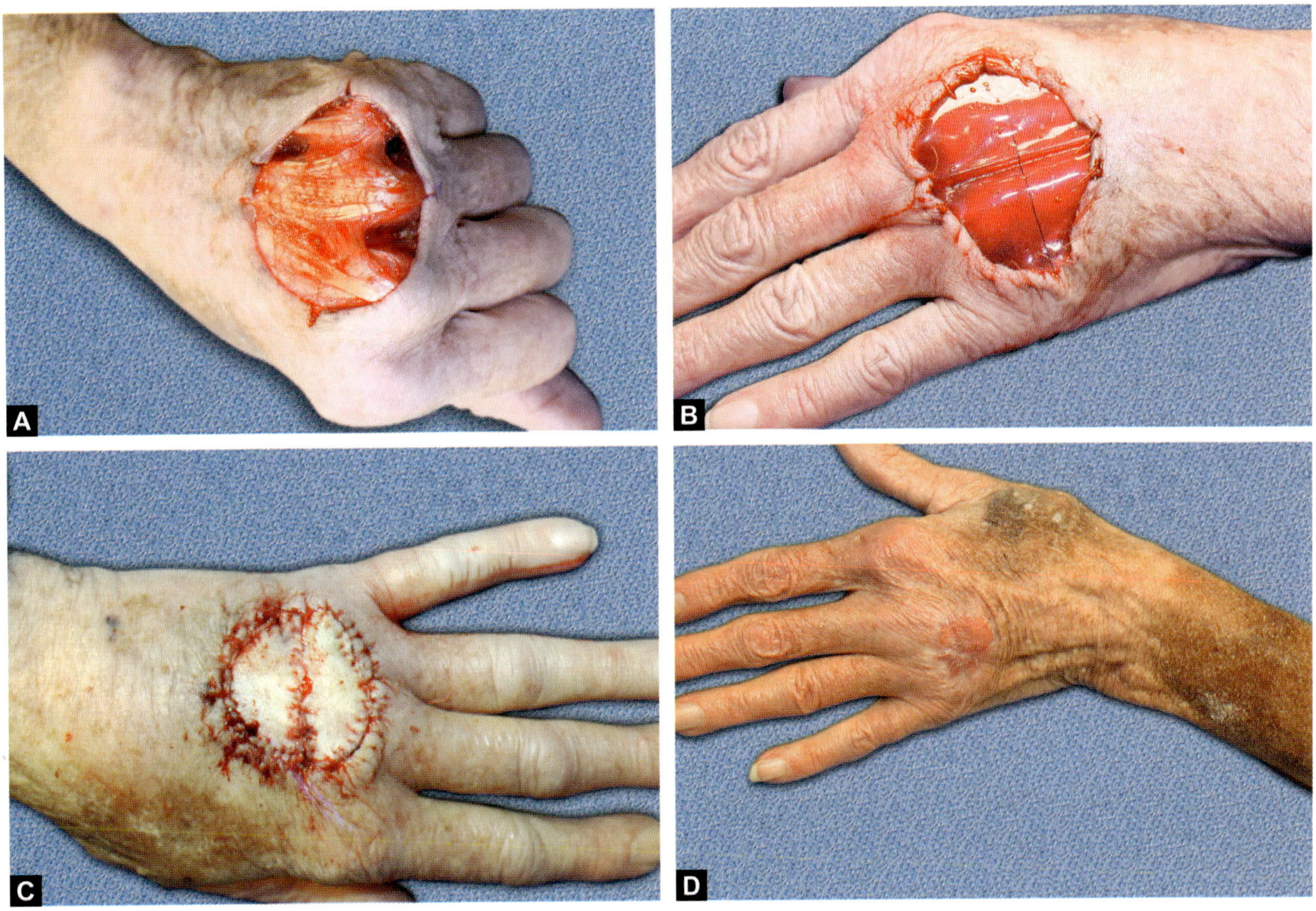

**Figs. 21.14A to D:** (A) Defect with exposed paratenon. (B) Immediately after Integra placement. (C) Silicone layer pulled, full-thickness skin graft (FTSG) placed on wound bed. (D) Early postoperative appearance after FTSG placement.

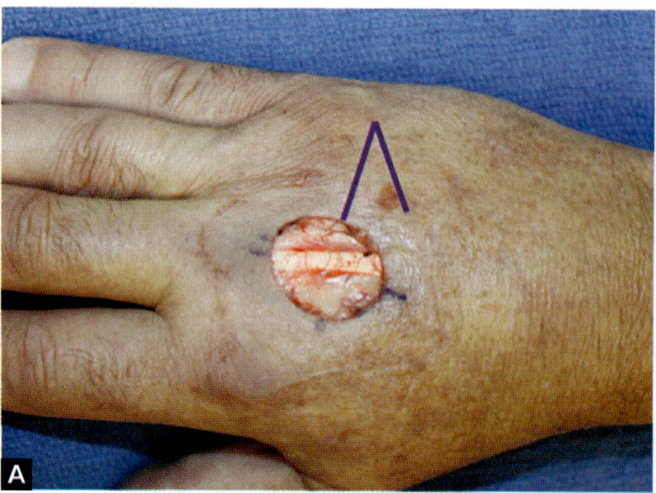


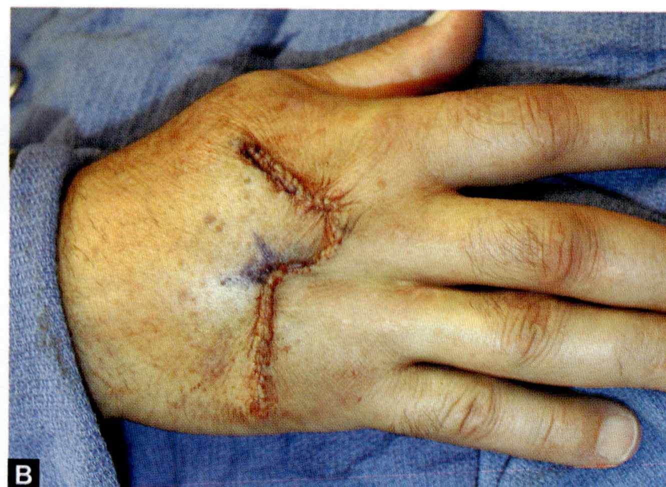


**Figs. 21.15A and B:** (A) Defect with rhombic flap design. (B) Immediately postoperative rhombic flap.

area of the graft maximizes contact between the graft and bed. Finally, bolstering the graft and splinting the patient's hand (discussed below) in the early postoperative period will reduce the likelihood of graft shearing and separating from the bed below.

Volar surface defects that require grafting pose a unique challenge since the aforementioned donor sites fail to provide the thickness necessary to resist environmental forces. Furthermore, nonglabrous donor sites lack the dermal mechanoreceptors to provide sensation to the palmar aspect of the hand and digits. Donor sites such as the nonweight-bearing region of the instep of the foot and the hypothenar eminence are locations with a limited reservoir of specialized skin that may act as an ideal replacement for smaller, volar surface wounds.[28]

## Flaps

Reconstruction with vascularized random-pattern, fasciocutaneous, and axial-pattern flaps is ideal for defects with exposed bone or tendon. Since the dorsal hand has a finite reservoir of skin, careful planning is necessary to minimize donor site morbidity, prolonged rehabilitation, or ischemia.[29,32]

### *Random Pattern Flaps (Advancement, Rotation, and Transposition)*

Since sliding flaps such as advancement or rotation flaps principally displace scar lines but do not recruit large amounts of tissue to the reconstruction site they possess limited utility on the hand. Transposition flaps such as the rhombic and bilobed flaps, however, offer multiple benefits in this location. First, they transfer key tension vectors away from the primary defect to avoid undue tension on joints. Second, they recruit skin from more ample reservoirs of skin such as the wrist or forearm.[33]

Rhombic flaps can be implemented when the skin immediately adjacent to the defect has a sufficient reservoir. Pinching this reservoir between two fingers allows the surgeon to determine whether it can provide sufficient volume to cover the defect. In order to reduce the risk of postoperative dysfunction, skin from the webs should not be used as a donor site. The rhombic flap's first limb is designed from the midline of the defect and the second limb points toward the preferred donor site (Figs. 21.15A and B).[33] Incisions for the flap are carried into the DSL or DIL and the flap's undersurface and the recipient area are bluntly undermined with scissors. The key suture closes the secondary defect and the remainder of the flap is closed in a layered manner.

If the skin immediately adjacent to the defect is insufficient then a bilobed or trilobed flap may be considered to access a more generous reservoir near the proximal hand and wrist. The design of the bilobed flap is analogous to that used on other anatomic sites such as the nose—the primary lobe surface area should match the size of the defect and the secondary lobe may be undersized by 10–15%.[34,35] As with the rhombic flap, the bilobed flap is lifted in the DSL or DIL and undermined in a way to preserve as many fasciocutaneous perforating vessels as possible (Figs. 21.16A to C). After the random pattern flaps are completed, splinting of the hand for 1 week may help in avoiding wound dehiscence.

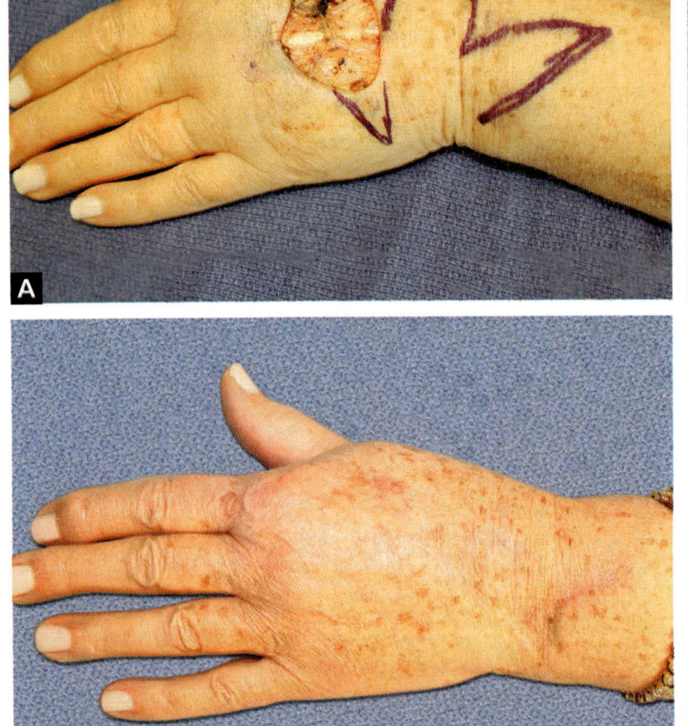

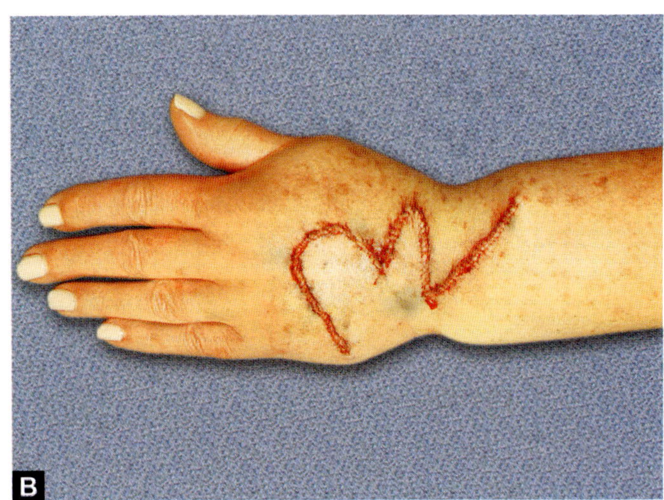

**Figs. 21.16A to C:** (A) Bilobed flap design. (B) Immediately postoperative bilobed flap. (C) Four-month follow-up after bilobed flap repair.

One modification to aforementioned transposition flaps that can be utilized for larger defects with exposed bone or tendon sans paratenon is the "jump flap" where skin immediately adjacent to the defect is lifted and sutured over the defect. If the secondary defect from lifting the flap is too large to close or would result in postoperative hand dysfunction then this donor site may be grafted (Figs. 21.17A to D). Since the flap is elevated in the DSL, the DIF is preserved and may be covered with an FTSG/STSG from another site or a redundant tissue cone.

## *Fasciocutaneous Flaps*

Because of the hand's finite reservoir of skin and thin dermis and subcutaneous fat, random pattern flaps have increased risk for necrosis or dehiscence from excessive tension. For moderately sized defects of the dorsal hand and proximal digits not amenable to random-pattern flaps or grafting, a "sliding fasciocutaneous flap" may be used, whose blood supply derives from dorsal perforating arteries and that uses bilevel undermining for improved mobility. The flap may be used to repair defects situated on the dorsal surface of the hand between the MCP joint/proximal digit and the extensor crease of the wrist. The defect may extend down to tendon and bone, but more superficial defects may also be repaired with this flap.

The defect should be measured with the hand in full flexion and the lateral borders of the flap may then be designed proximally off the defect as two lateral limbs that arise from the widest portions of the defect. A third limb should connect the two lateral flap limbs. The length of the lateral limbs should be at least 1.5–2.0 times the defect diameter to incorporate a sufficient number of dorsal perforating arteries. These lateral flap limbs may parallel one another to create a rectangular flap or they may gently diverge from one another so that an arciform or keystone-

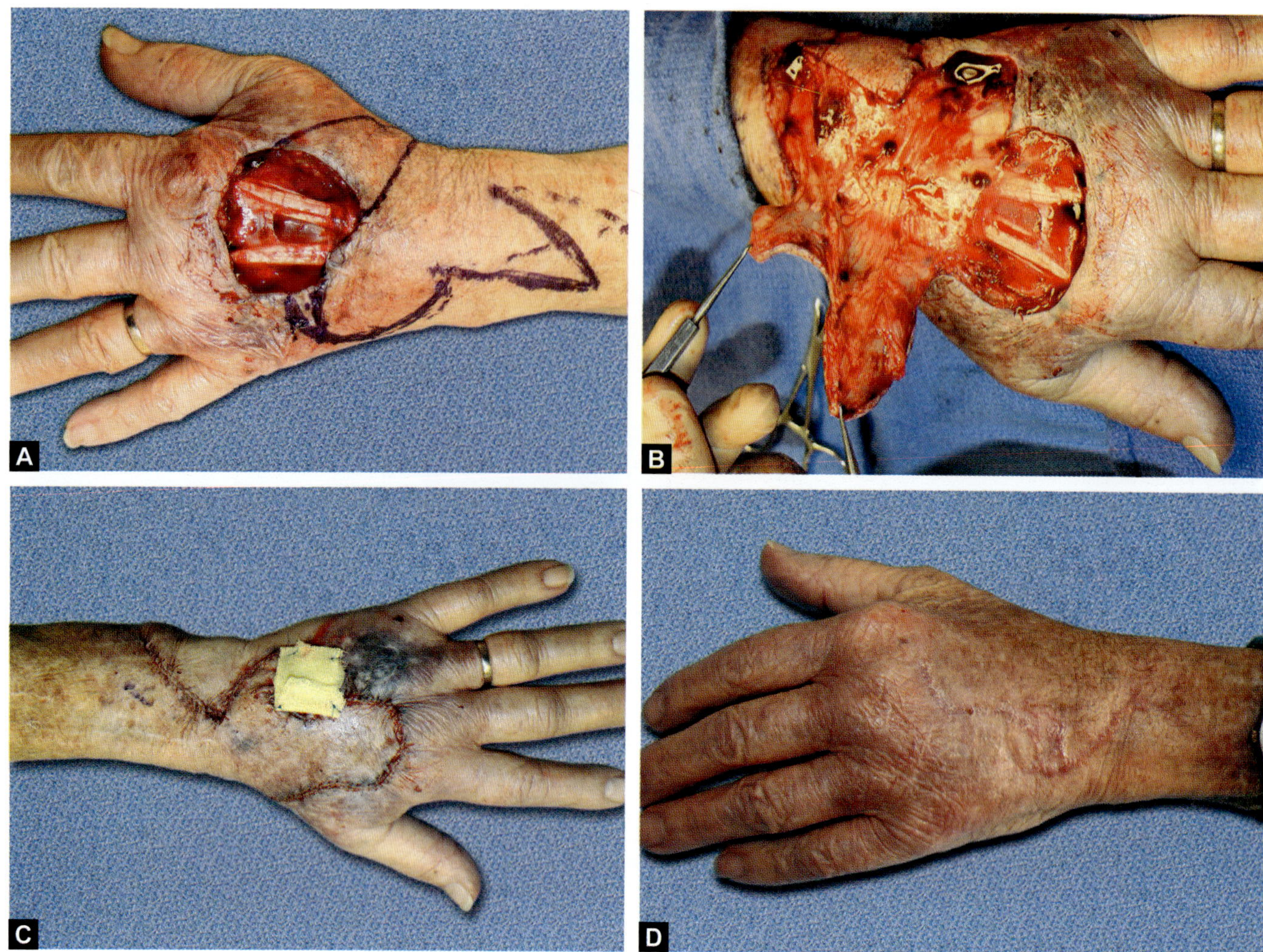

**Figs. 21.17A to D:** (A) Defect with exposed tendon. (B) Lifting bilobed flap for tendon coverage and preserving fascia over anticipated graft site. (C) Jump bilobed flap and full-thickness skin graft (FTSG) immediately postoperative. (D) Three-month follow-up after jump bilobed flap and FTSG.

shape is created. For defects that will be under tension, the keystone design allows for easier recruitment of skin with the V-Y closure at the proximal corners. Ideally, the flap is centered over the intercarpal space or second through fourth web spaces, where perforating arteries abound (Fig. 21.18A).

Once the flap is designed, it may be gently incised through the dermis of all three limbs into the DSL (Fig. 21.18B). The ideal flap pedicle depends on the mobility of the skin. To gain mobility, one, two, or three limbs of the flap must be released through the dorsal superficial and intermediate fascia to the level of the DDL immediately superficial to the paratenon and DDF (Fig. 21.18C). As more limbs of the flap are released, more mobility may be gained, but flap vascularity grows more tenuous, especially if the flap is not centered over a generous supply of perforating arteries.

The undermining that occurs in the plane above the paratenon and DDF should be done bluntly to preserve perforator arteries. The perforating arteries have a small diameter of 0.1–0.3 mm, so they are not readily visible. For flaps on the dorsal hand, the midpoint between the carpal bones should be preserved whenever possible, since the underlying dorsal metacarpal artery and its perforators emerge along this line. For flaps based on the second through fourth web spaces, the area immediately distal to the junctura tendinae, which is ~ 1 cm proximal to the metacarpal heads, should be preserved to protect Quaba's perforators. Doppler ultrasound is not used in our clinic, but may be helpful to locate perforators

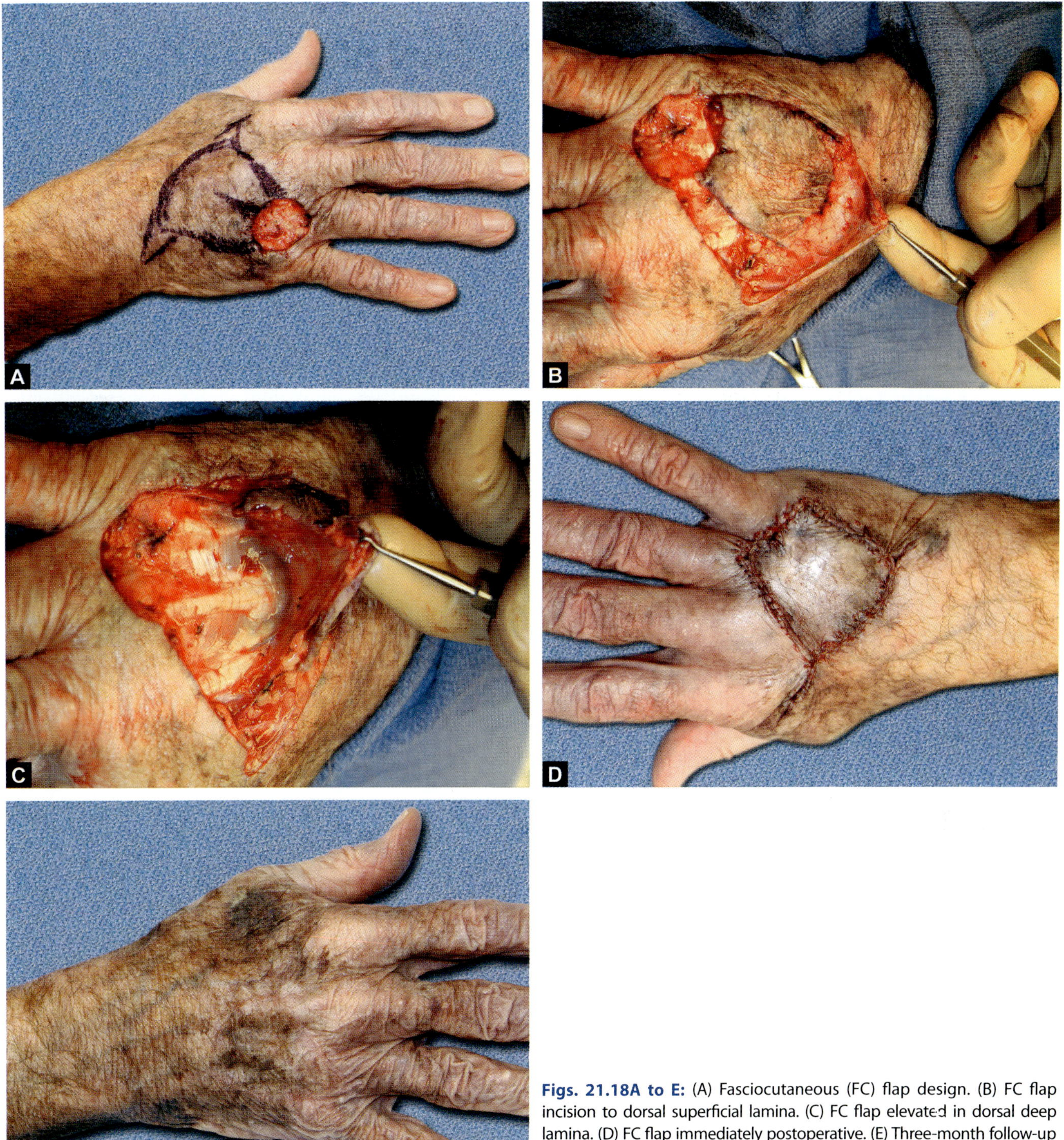

**Figs. 21.18A to E:** (A) Fasciocutaneous (FC) flap design. (B) FC flap incision to dorsal superficial lamina. (C) FC flap elevated in dorsal deep lamina. (D) FC flap immediately postoperative. (E) Three-month follow-up after FC flap repair.

preoperatively. The fascial pedicles of the bipedicled and sling variations of this flap may provide sufficient random blood supply, even if the perforators under the flap have been severed.

Once the flap has been adequately released to the paratenon on the desired limb(s), the remaining attached limbs are undermined in the DSL to mobilize the fascial pedicle. Once the flap has been sufficiently released and undermined, it should easily move into the defect without undue tension (Figs. 21.18D and E). A layered repair should be able to secure the flap in a tension- free manner with preserved function and range of motion just after closure.

The sliding fasciocutaneous flaps are not truly axial but their blood supply is robust. Consistent cutaneous perforator vessels from the parallel arrangement of the dorsal arterial network permit these sliding flaps to be raised and mobilized with a reduced risk of ischemia when compared to random pattern flaps based on the dermal plexus (Figs. 21.19A to F). Often, there is a communication between the palmar and dorsal systems, which may further reinforce blood flow to these flaps.[8,36,37]

## DIGITAL RECONSTRUCTION

Reconstruction options with local flaps are limited on the digit due to scant tissue reservoirs. Consequently, defects on the digits frequently require second intention healing, skin grafting, axial flaps, perforator flaps, or staged reconstruction. This section will address flaps specific to reconstruction of the digits.

### Adipofascial Turnover Flaps

Homo- or heterodigital adipofascial turnover flaps can cover deep defects of the dorsal aspect of the digits with vascularized tissue and allow for immediate grafting. The pedicles of these turnover flaps are based on the dorsal cutaneous branches of the proper palmar digital arteries.[7,38] The advantages of these flaps are their ease and reliability. The disadvantages are the long scar at the donor site and the need for immobilization to protect the graft.

Homodigital adipofascial turnover flaps are reliable to cover defects of the middle and distal phalanges of the long digits and the proximal and distal phalanges of the thumb (Figs. 21.20A to C).[7] The midline dorsal skin of the digit is incised from the proximal aspect of the defect to the MCP or further proximally. Transverse incisions are made at the proximal and distal ends of the longitudinal incision, and the skin flaps on each side are elevated in the immediate subdermal plane, taking care to leave the adipofascia intact. The proximal and lateral aspects of the newly exposed adipofascia are incised to the level of the paratenon, taking care to preserve the dorsal communicating arteries in the pedicle, which is usually based near the PIP of the long digits and MCP or IP of the thumb. The adipofascial flap is undermined at the level of the paratenon from its proximal aspect to the pedicle. The flap is elevated and turned toward the defect like a page in a book and sutured to the defect with dissolving sutures. The skin flaps at the donor site are closed primarily and the primary defect, which is now covered with the turnover flap, is repaired with an STSG or FTSG. A bolster is placed and the digit is splinted for 5–7 days to protect the graft.

A heterodigital adipofascial flap, also called a reverse cross-finger flap, may cover deep dorsal defects of the adjacent digit, most commonly located on the proximal or middle phalanges (Figs. 21.21A to E).[39] A rectangular dorsal skin flap is elevated with its pedicle facing away from the injured digit. The skin flap is elevated in the immediate subdermal plane to preserve the underlying adipofascia. A rectangular flap of the adipofascia is then incised with its pedicle on the same side of the injured digit. The adipofascial flap is elevated immediately superficial to extensor tendon paratenon to preserve the dorsal communicating arteries from the proper palmar digital arteries in its pedicle. The adipofascial flap is turned over like a page in a book and secured with dissolving sutures to the primary defect on the adjacent digit. The secondary defect at the donor site is closed primarily with the initial skin flap, and the primary defect, which is now covered with the turnover adipofascial flap, is repaired with an STSG or FTSG. A bolster is placed to protect the graft for 5–7 days. Two to three weeks later, the pedicle of the adipofascial flap is divided and inset. The heterodigital flap has the disadvantage of requiring prolonged immobilization of both digits and a secondary procedure to divide and inset the flap pedicle.

### Perforator Flaps

The reverse dorsal metacarpal arterial perforator flap is a one-staged procedure useful for reconstruction of dorsal defects of the proximal thumb and fingers (Figs. 21.22A to E).[10,37,40] This flap has the advantage of a reliable blood supply, simple execution, and quick return to mobility.

As reviewed in the anatomy section at the start of the chapter, the dorsal metacarpal arteries run in the intercarpal spaces immediately superficial to the dorsal interosseous muscles. They have dorsal perforators that supply blood to the skin of the proximal two-thirds of the dorsal hand. Approximately 1 cm proximal to the metacarpal head and immediately distal to the junctura tendinae, the palmar metacarpal arteries from the deep palmar arch give rise to a dorsal perforating artery.[10] This perforating artery consistently anastomoses with the first through third metacarpal arteries and variably communicates

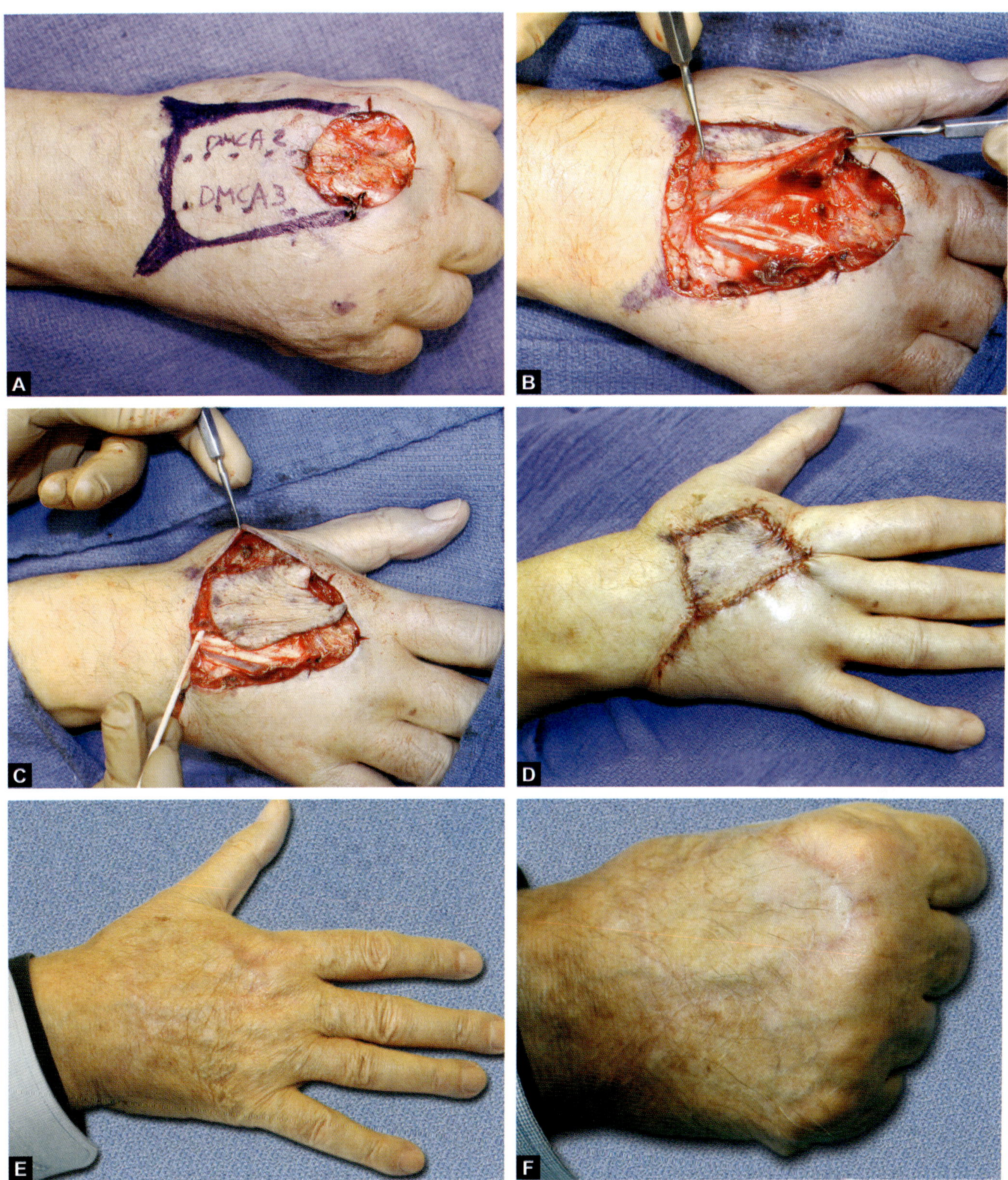


**Figs. 21.19A to F:** (A) Fasciocutaneous (FC) flap design. (B) FC flap bilevel undermining. (C) FC flap mobilized and advanced with robust pedicle. (D) FC flap immediately postoperative. (E) Three-month follow-up after FC flap repair. (F) Three-month follow-up after FC flap repair in flexion. (DMCA: dorsal metacarpal artery).

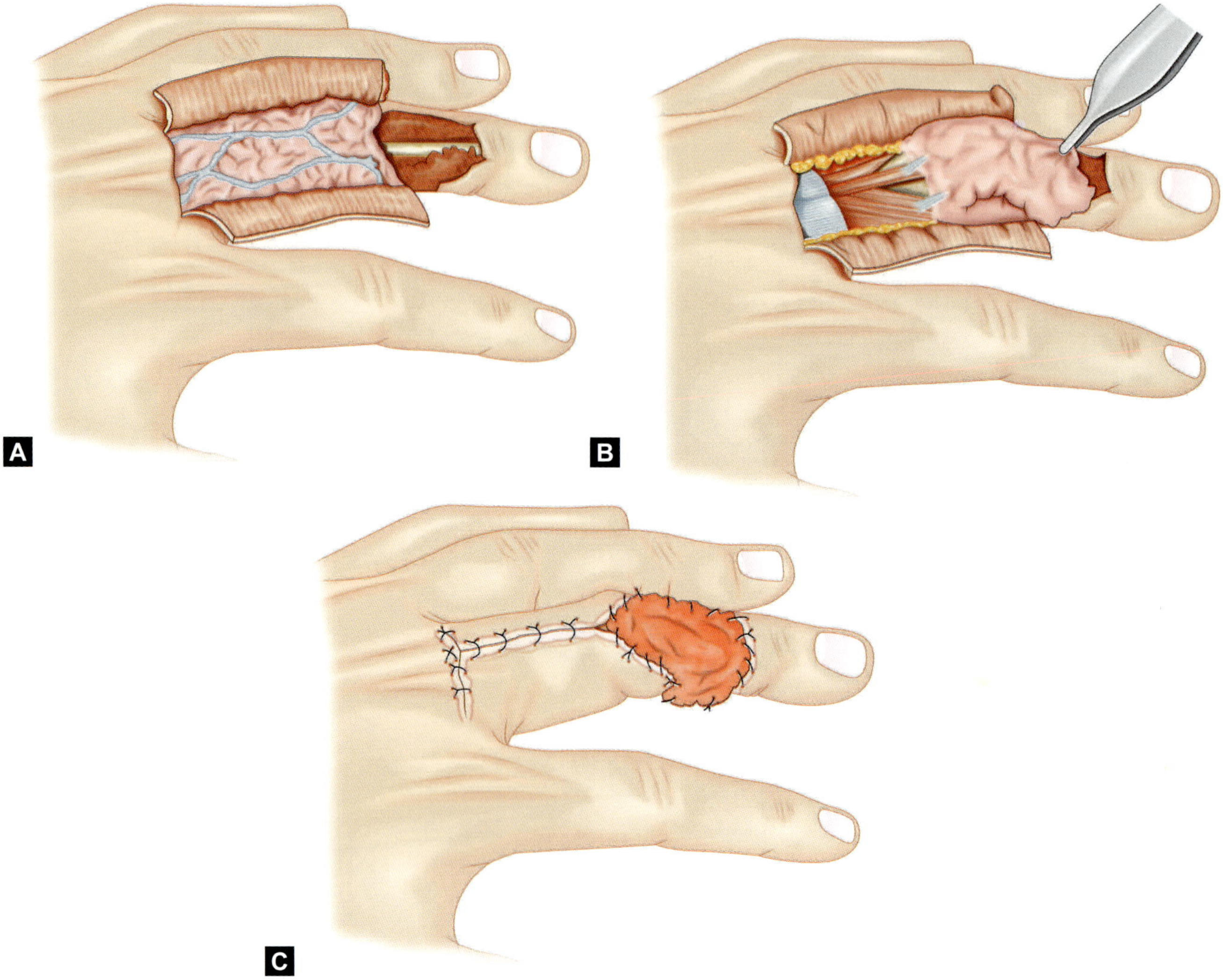

**Figs. 21.20A to C:** Homodigital adipofascial turnover flap.

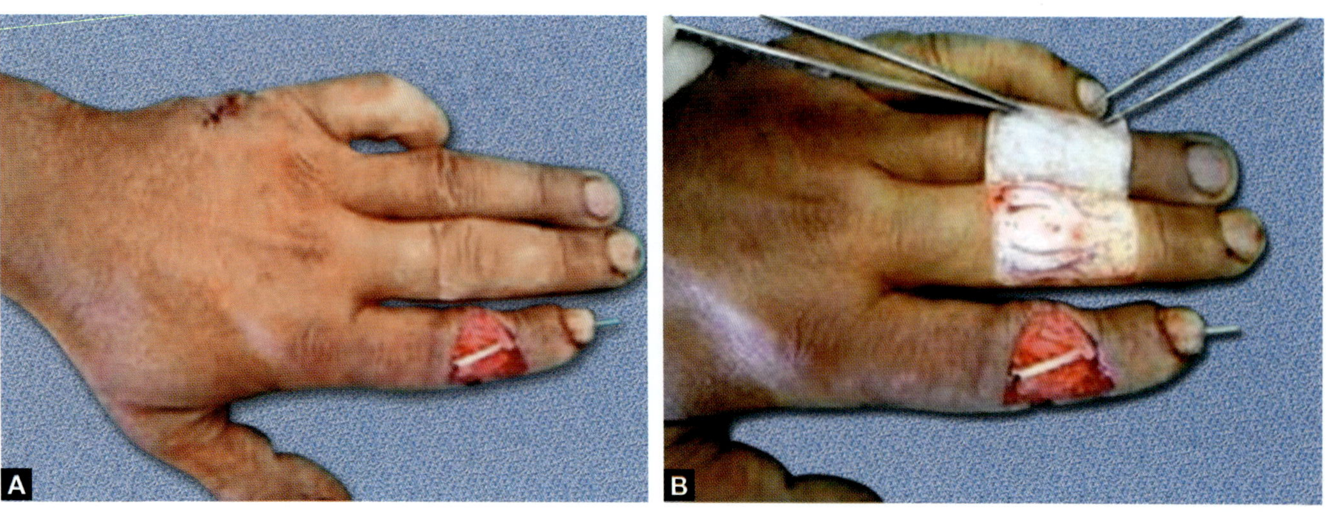


**Figs. 21.21A and B**

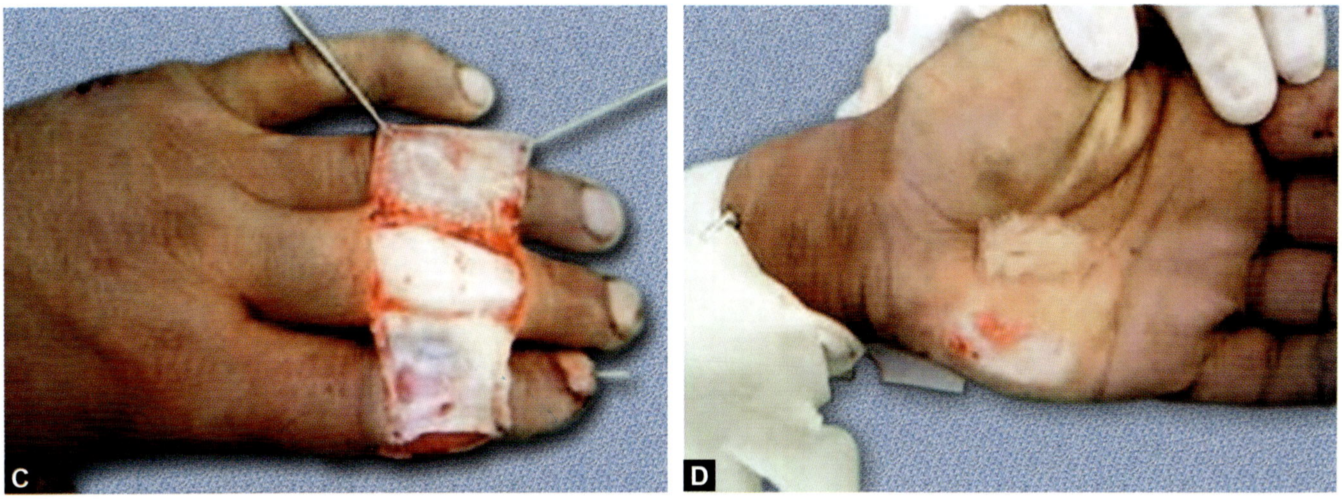

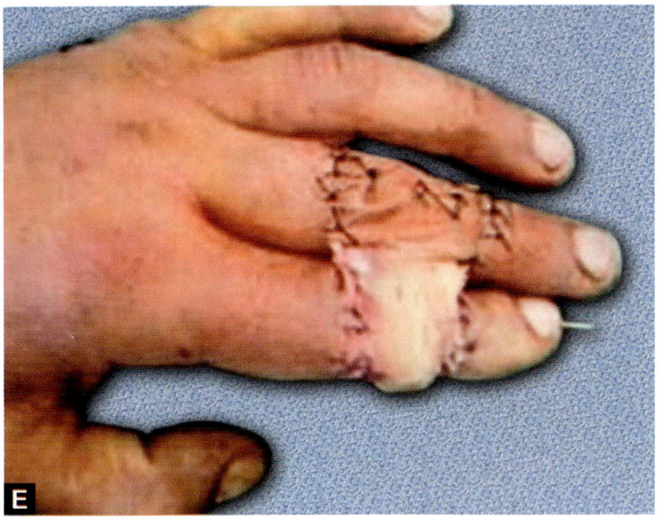

**Figs. 21.21A to E:** Reverse cross-finger flap.

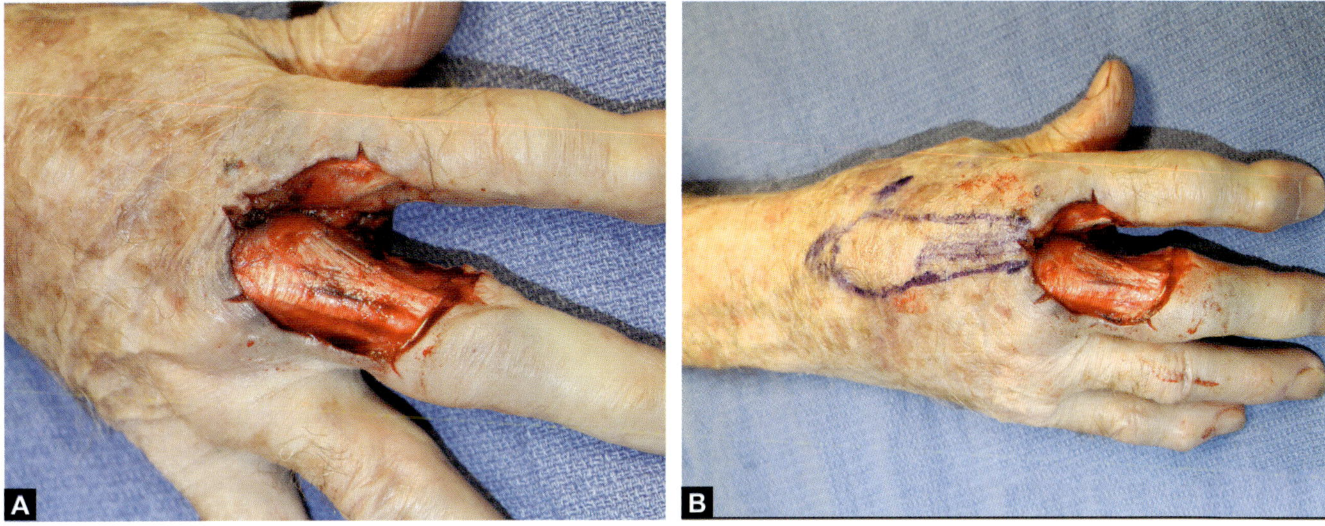


**Figs. 21.22A and B:** (A) Challenging digit and intercarpal web space defect. (B) Reverse dorsal metacarpal artery (RDMCA) flap design.

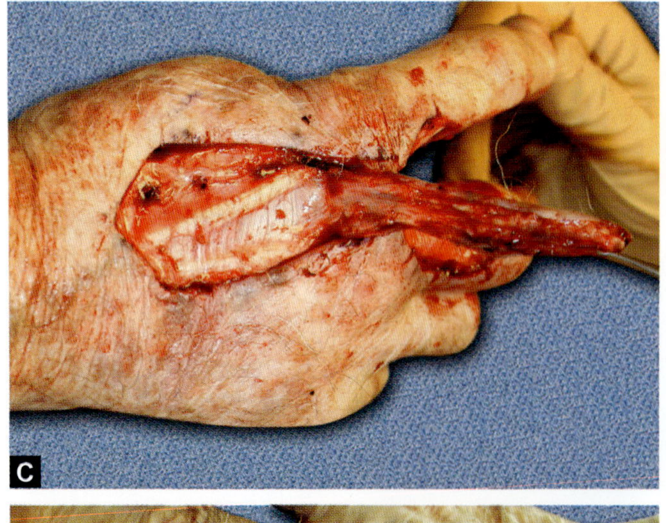
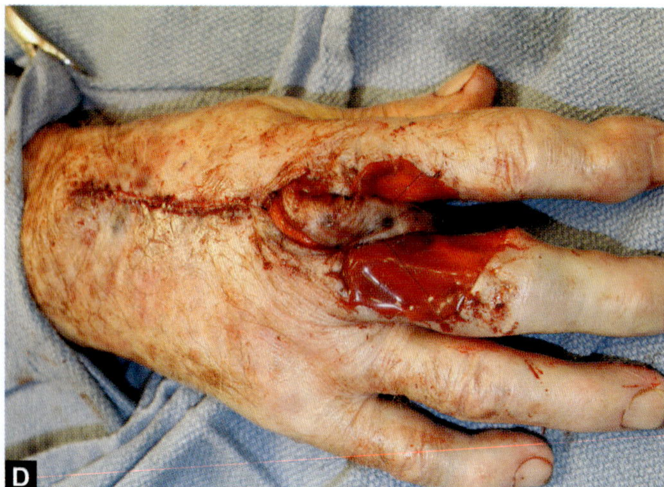
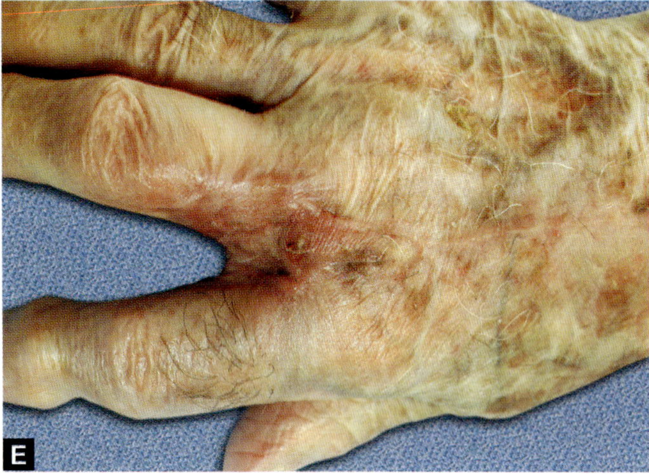

**Figs. 21.22C to E:** (C) RDMCA flap elevation. (D) RDMCA rotated into web space and Integra coverage of remainder. (E) Early postoperative appearance after full-thickness skin graft coverage on Integra. Note suture granuloma in center.

with the fourth and fifth dorsal metacarpal arteries. This anastomosis between the palmar and dorsal blood supplies forms the basis for the reverse dorsal metacarpal artery perforator flaps.

A Doppler probe can be used to verify the precise location of the perforator artery, although this may not be necessary since the artery can be reliably located distal to the junctura tendinae. A template of the digital defect is rotated 180° proximally and transferred to the intercarpal space of the dorsal hand so that its base lies over the perforating artery 1 cm proximal to the metacarpal head. The flap may be lengthened to account for shortening from pivotal restraint during rotation of the flap.

The flap borders are incised to the fascia of the dorsal interosseous muscle. Note that when the dorsal metacarpal artery is cut and ligated at the proximal portion of the secondary defect, flap survival depends on retrograde blood flow from the source dorsal perforating artery at the metacarpal head. The flap is elevated from proximally to distally and includes the fascia of the dorsal interosseous muscle to ensure that the dorsal metacarpal artery is contained in the flap. As the dissection approaches the metacarpal heads, caution is taken to preserve the primary blood supply from the dorsal perforating artery and a generous cuff of adipofascial tissue can help protect the artery.

The flap is rotated 180° to the digital defect and inset with sutures. For distal digital defects, there may be an isthmus of skin between the flap's pedicle and the proximal defect. This intervening skin can be removed to facilitate inset of the flap. The donor site on the dorsal hand is closed primarily. If it is anticipated that the donor site on the dorsal hand will be too large to close primarily, it is possible to raise an adipofascial flap without the overlying dorsal hand skin so that the donor site can be closed primarily.[39] The adipofascial flap requires a graft for coverage

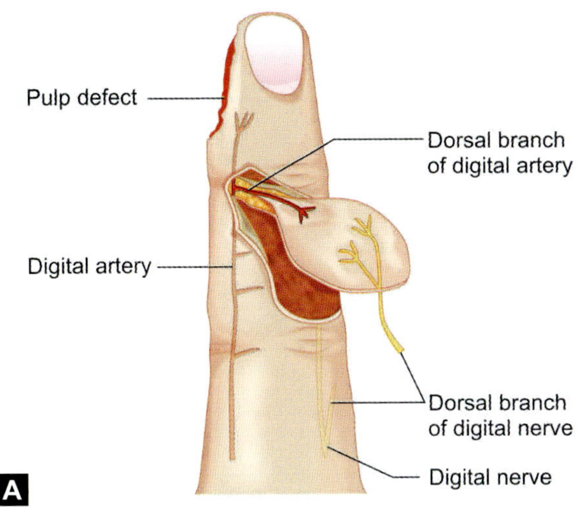


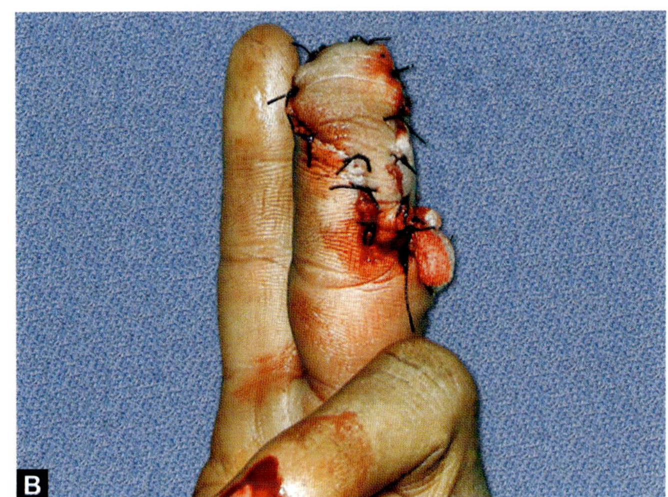


**Figs. 21.23A and B:** Dorsal digital island flap.

of the digit. For smaller defects, skin flaps based entirely on the perforator between the metacarpal heads without inclusion of the dorsal metacarpal artery may be useful.[36,37]

## Homodigital Dorsal Cutaneous Axial Flaps

Homodigital axial flaps based on the dorsal branches of the proper palmar digital artery can be used as a one-staged procedure to reconstruct deep defects of the fingertip and proximal and middle phalanges.[41,42] As reviewed in the anatomy section, the proper palmar digital arteries have dorsal cutaneous branches that communicate with the dorsal digital branches of the dorsal metacarpal arteries and help supply blood to the dorsal surface of the digits.[43] There are two or three dorsal cutaneous branches arising from the proper palmar digital arteries on the proximal phalanx. While the most proximal branch is variable, the two branches closest to the PIP are consistent, reliable, and arise 10 and 4 mm from the PIP.[43] Two dorsal cutaneous branches also occur reliably and consistently in the middle phalanx, occurring within 6–8 mm and 9–12 mm from the PIP. The most distal dorsal cutaneous branch arises near the DIP.[42]

A template of the defect is transferred to the dorsal skin of the middle and/or proximal phalanges. The flap is oversized by 10–15%.[42] The pedicle of the flap is centered on the first intact dorsal cutaneous branch nearest to the defect. For distal defects, the pedicle is centered on the DIP or the midportion of the midlateral line of either the ulnar or radial aspect of the digit, depending on which side will allow the flap to reach the defect (Figs. 21.23A and B). For defects of the middle or proximal phalanges, the flap pedicle is based on the dorsal cutaneous arteries in the proximal phalanx.

The distal and lateral edges of the flap are incised to the extensor paratenon. The flap is elevated from distal to proximal immediately superficial to the paratenon, leaving a minimum of a 0.5–0.8 cm cuff of soft tissue to preserve the dorsal cutaneous branch at the pedicle. Some authors leave the skin intact over the pedicle,[41] whereas other authors incise the flap as an island and have a pedicle based entirely on the subcutaneous tissue.[42] Leaving the skin intact over the pedicle may decrease venous congestion, which is a common complication of this flap.[42] The flap is rotated to the defect and secured under minimal tension with interrupted cutaneous sutures. The secondary defect at the donor site is covered with an STSG or FTSG. Wound care consists of a bolster dressing for the graft for 5–7 days. Immobilization of the finger may be necessary if the secondary defect spans a joint.

Compared to other flaps that will not be covered in this chapter, such as the homo- and heterodigital reverse digital artery flaps,[44,45] the homodigital dorsal cutaneous artery axial flap does not require sacrifice of the proper palmar digital artery, protects the digital nerve, and leaves a secondary defect easily amenable to skin grafting. Sensation of the flap is diminished, so some authors advocate for flaps that contain the dorsal branches of the proper digital nerve and neurorrhaphies to the cut nerves at the primary defect to improve sensation.[42]

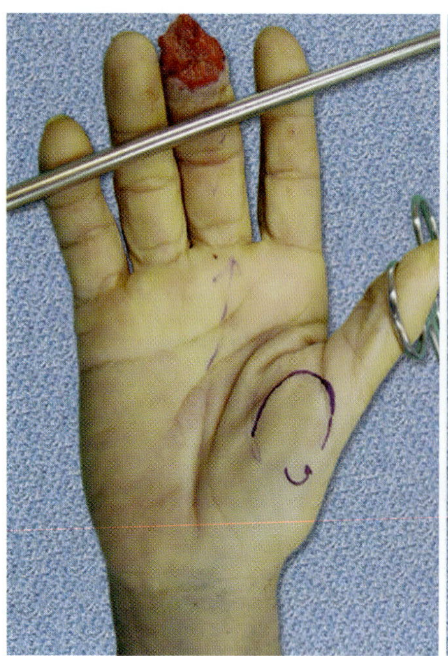
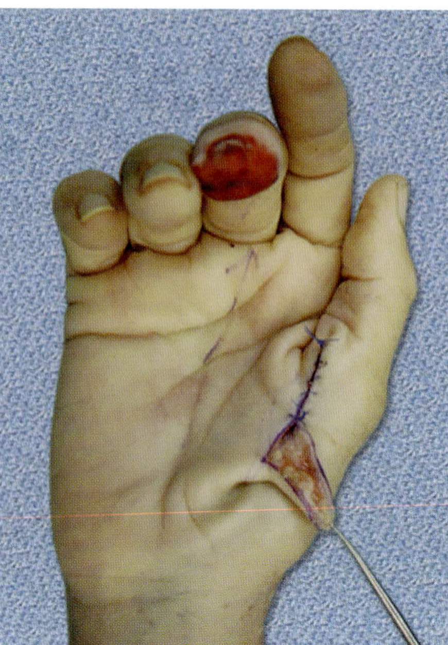
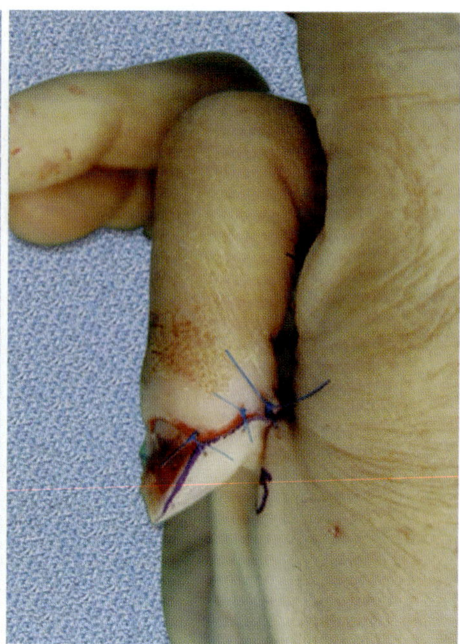

**Fig. 21.24:** Thenar flap.

## Staged Heterodigital Flaps

### *Thenar Flap*

The staged thenar flap is useful to repair defects of the fingertips, particularly the volar aspects of the second and third digits (Fig. 21.24).[39] A template of the defect is transferred to the thenar aspect of the palm proximal to the MCP crease of the thumb, where the injured digit should easily reach. The flap should be slightly oversized to avoid tension. Three sides of the template are incised, and the flap is elevated superficial to the thenar fascia, taking care to preserve the radial digital nerve of the thumb. The injured digit is flexed to reach the thenar hand and the flap is sutured to the wound. The pedicle is divided and the flap is inset 2–3 weeks later. The disadvantages of this flap are the two stages and the risk for contracture of the PIP due to immobilization in the flexed position between the first and second stages.

### *Cross-Finger Flap*

The cross-finger flap is useful for reconstruction of the palmar aspect of the middle and distal phalanges (Fig. 21.25). A template of the defect is transferred to the dorsal surface, usually over the middle phalanx, of an adjacent digit. The flap should be slightly oversized to avoid tension. A three-sided rectangular flap is elevated immediately superficial to the extensor paratenon with the broad pedicle on the same side of the injured digit. The distal flap is flipped like a page of a book and sutured primarily to the defect. The secondary defect at the donor site is repaired with an FTSG or STSG. A bolster is placed over the skin graft, and both digits are immobilized until division and inset of the pedicle is performed ~3 weeks later. Like the thenar flap, the cross-finger flap has the risk of PIP contracture from prolonged immobilization.

The traditional cross-finger flap has limited mobility due to the broad base of its pedicle. To improve flap mobility and allow for coverage of completely degloved fingertips, Feng et al. have successfully utilized a cross-finger flap that narrows the pedicle to a 0.5-cm cuff based on the dorsal cutaneous branch of the proper palmar digital artery at the middle phalanx.[46] To improve static two-point sensory discrimination, the authors performed neurorrhaphies. Note that for dorsal digital defects, the reverse cross-finger flap (also called the heterodigital adipofascial flap), which is described above, is more useful.

### *V–Y Advancement Flaps and Moberg Flap for Distal Tip Defects*

For small (<1.5 cm) defects of the distal fingertip with exposed bone and sufficient nail bed length, a V–Y advancement flap may be used. In the classic Kutler V–Y advance-

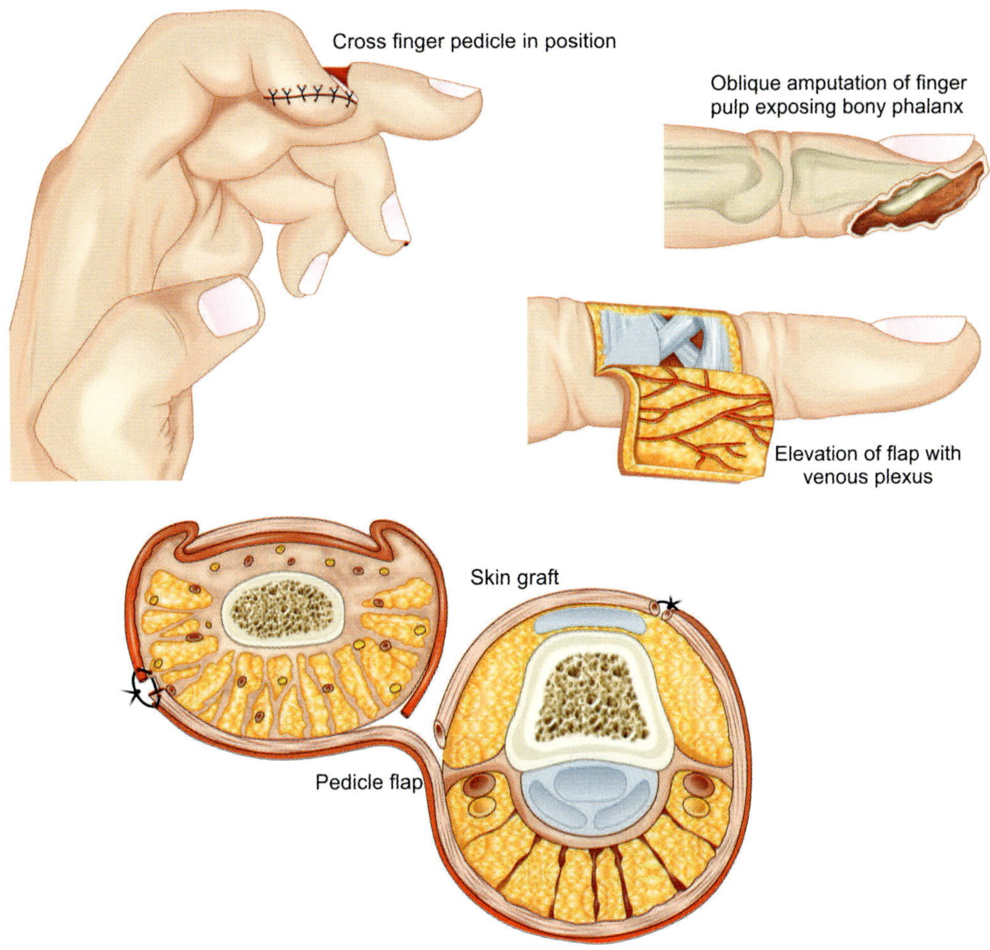


**Fig. 21.25:** Cross-finger flap.

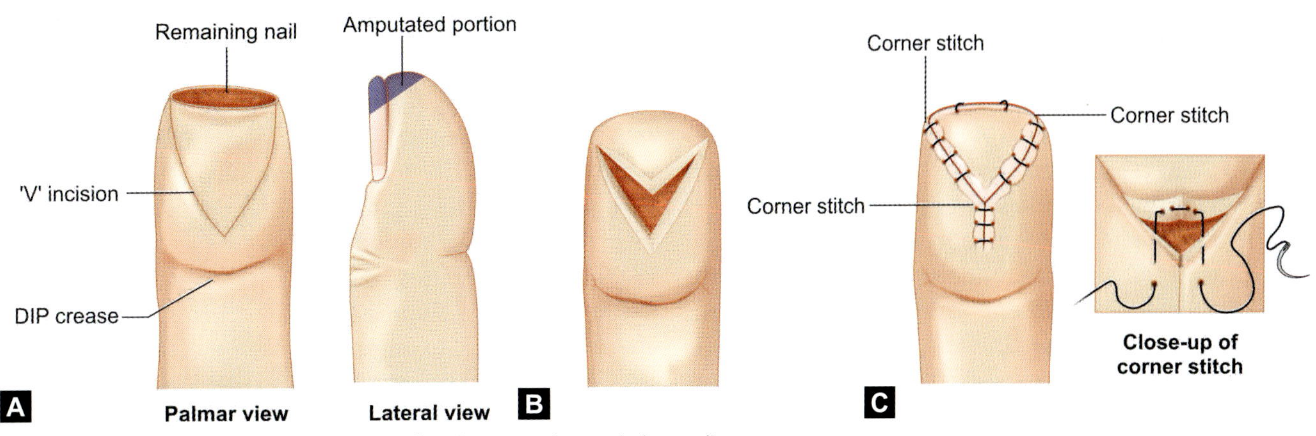


**Figs. 21.26A to C:** Kutler V–Y advancement flap. (DIP: Distal interphalangeal).

ment flap, V-shaped incisions are made to the subcutaneous tissue on the lateral aspects of the defect with the point of each V extending proximally to the level of the DIP joint crease (Figs. 21.26A to C).[47] The incision of the dorsal limb of the flap may be extended to the periosteum, but the volar limb should remain at the depth of the subcutaneous tissue to preserve the neurovascular supply. The fibrous adhesions are released with sharp-pointed scis-

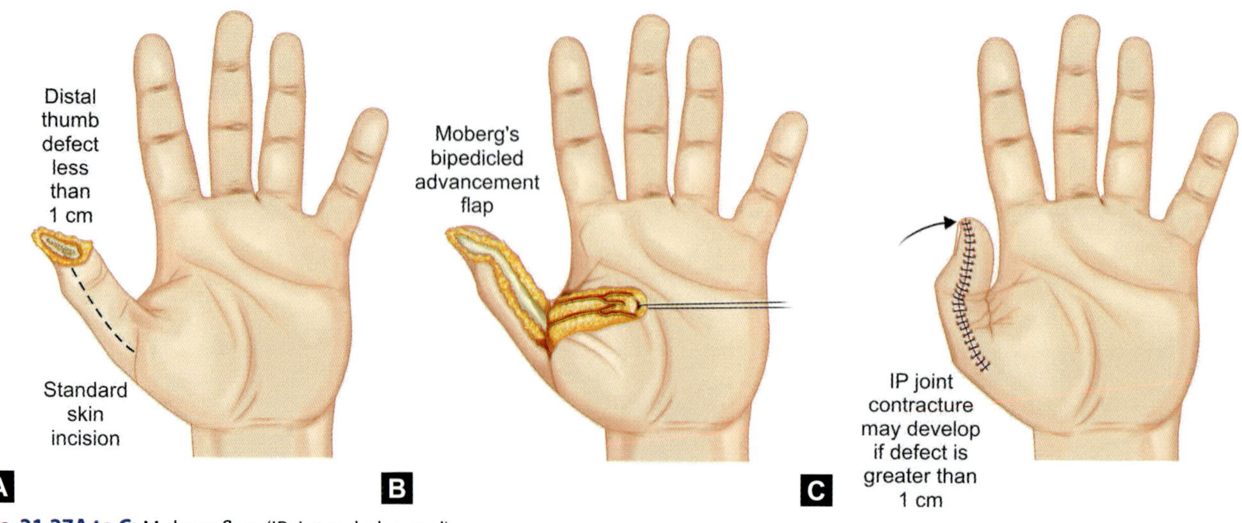


**Figs. 21.27A to C:** Moberg flap. (IP: Interphalangeal).

sors until the flaps can be advanced distally. Note that the flap will advance only 0.5–1.0 cm.[48] The distal edges of the flap are sutured together, and the secondary defects at the proximal flaps are closed in a V to Y fashion. This flap has the advantage of transferring sensate skin and the disadvantage of limited mobility. Variations of the traditional V-Y advancement flap design may improve mobility.[49] For smaller defects, a single V-Y advancement flap based on the pulp of the distal digit may be sufficient.[39] Undermining at the leading edge of the flap should be minimal, but should be done at the level of the periosteum or flexural tendon sheath, if necessary, in order to preserve the neural and blood supplies. The lateral incisions should remain at the depth of the subcutaneous fat.

The Moberg flap utilizes a similar principle for reconstruction of defects of the pulp of the thumb with a size of up to 1.5 cm (Figs. 21.27A to C).[32,39] The palmar skin of the thumb can be elevated more aggressively than that of the skin of the digits due to an independent blood supply to the dorsum of the thumb. Incisions are made at the mediolateral axis of the thumb from the proximal defect to the MCP flexion crease. The flap is raised from distal to proximal immediately superficial to the flexor tendon and the neurovascular bundles on both sides of the flap are incorporated to retain sensation. The flap is advanced distally and sutured into place.

### *First Dorsal Metacarpal Artery Flap (Kite Flap)*

The first dorsal metacarpal artery flap, also knows as a kite flap, can repair dorsal defects of the thumb (Figs. 21.28A to C).[32] In contrast to the retrograde blood flow in the reverse dorsal metacarpal artery flaps discussed elsewhere, the first dorsal metacarpal artery flap has anterograde blood flow. A template of the defect is transferred to the dorsal surface of the proximal phalanx of the second digit. A curved linear incision is made over the second metacarpal to harvest the pedicle, whose pivot point lies at the radial border of the second metacarpal base. One of the large dorsal veins is identified and the pedicle is harvested from the proximal template to the pivot point by elevating the fascia and a minimum 0.5 cm width of connective tissue around the vein. The pedicle includes the first dorsal digital nerve from the superficial branch of the radial nerve. A strip of skin can be harvested over the pedicle to avoid compression during flap transfer. Next, the templated portion of the flap is incised and elevated immediately superficial to the extensor tendon of the second digit. The flap and pedicle are rotated to the thumb and sutured through an open or closed tunnel. The secondary defect on the second digit is grafted and the curvilinear incision over the flap pedicle is sutured primarily. Microsurgical neurorrhaphy is possible to improve sensation of the flap.[50]

## Nail Reconstruction

Several of the reconstruction strategies described above are useful for defects of the distal digit, including larger defects involving the nail unit. Smaller defects of the nail unit may be amenable to reconstruction strategies that restore the nail matrix and frame to minimize dystrophy of the nail plate. Readers are referred to excellent and

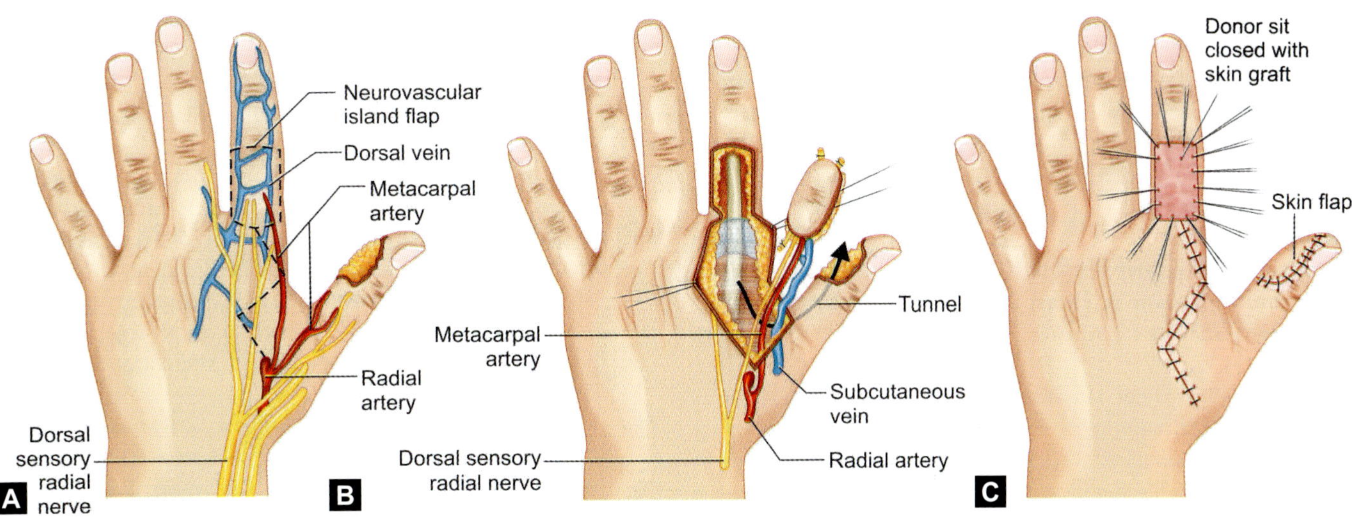


**Figs. 21.28A to C:** First dorsal metacarpal artery flap.

**Table 21.3:** Preferred method of postoperative hand immobilization.

- Wrist in moderate (30°–45°) extension
- MCP joints in 50°–75° of flexion
- PIP joints nearly full extension
- Uniform pressure applied lightly

(MCP: Metacarpophalangeal; PIP: Proximal interphalangeal).

more comprehensive references for discussion of reconstruction specific to the nail unit.[51-53]

## POSTOPERATIVE WOUND CARE

Bandaging, wound care, and sometimes immobilization after reconstruction are critical steps to ensuring a successful postoperative outcome. Patients should be educated that it is common to have hand swelling that develops a few days after suturing and can persist up to a few weeks after surgery. Elevation of the hand above the level of the elbow may limit or reduce the amount of edema. If a good deal of swelling is anticipated or if hand motion is likely to compromise the outcome via dehiscence then use of a prolonged compression bandage that immobilizes the hand is preferred (Table 21.3). The ideal position for hand immobilization is moderate wrist extension (30°–45°) with moderate MCP joint flexion (50°–75°), thumb abduction, and full PIP extension.[28] Fluffed gauze may be used between the fingers to prevent maceration. It is important to apply a uniform degree of light pressure that does not result in ischemia or nerve compression. Hand pain postoperatively should be vetted carefully with removal of the bandage to eliminate the risk of nerve damage.

## CONCLUSION

Dermatologic surgeons frequently encounter defects on the hand that require reconstruction after tumor extirpation. A comprehensive knowledge of hand anatomy, with specific attention to the hand's unique fasciocutaneous and vascular makeup, allows the surgeon to approach reconstructing these defects with confidence.

## REFERENCES


1. Martinez JC, Otley CC. The management of melanoma and nonmelanoma skin cancer: a review for the primary care physician. Mayo Clin Proc. 2001;76(12):1253-65.
2. Maciburko SJ, Townley WA, Hollowood K, et al. Skin cancers of the hand: a series of 541 malignancies. Plast Reconstr Surg. 2012;129(6):1329-36.
3. Hsu CS, Hentz VR, Yao J. Tumours of the hand. Lancet Oncol. 2007;8(2):157-66.
4. Sobanko JF, Dagum AB, Davis IC, et al. Soft tissue tumors of the hand. 2. Malignant. Dermatol Surg. 2007;33(7):771-85.
5. Yu H, Chase RA, Strausch B. Atlas of Hand Anatomy and Clinical Implications. St Louis, MO: Mosby; 2004.
6. von Schroeder HP, Botte MJ. Anatomy of the extensor tendons of the fingers: variations and multiplicity. J Hand Surg Am. 1995;20(1):27-34.
7. Braga-Silva J. Anatomic basis of dorsal finger skin cover. Tech Hand Up Extrem Surg. 2005;9(3):134-41.

8. Yang D, Morris SF. Vascular basis of dorsal digital and metacarpal skin flaps. J Hand Surg Am. 2001;26(1):142-6.
9. Pistre V, Pelissier P, Martin D, et al. Vascular blood supply of the dorsal side of the thumb, first web and index finger: anatomical study. J Hand Surg Br. 2001;26(2):98-104.
10. Omokawa S, Tanaka Y, Ryu J, et al., The anatomical basis for reverse first to fifth dorsal metacarpal arterial flaps. J Hand Surg Br. 2005;30(1):40-4.
11. Vuppalapati G, Oberlin C, Balakrishnan G. "Distally based dorsal hand flaps": clinical experience, cadaveric studies and an update. Br J Plast Surg. 2004;57(7):653-67.
12. Koch SL, Allen B. Kanavel (1874–1938). Clin Orthop. 1959; 15:1-4.
13. Bidic SM, Hatef DA, Rohrich RJ. Dorsal hand anatomy relevant to volumetric rejuvenation. Plast Reconstr Surg. 2010;126(1):163-8.
14. Sobanko JF, Fischer J, Etzkorn JR, et al. Local fasciocutaneous sliding flaps for soft-tissue defects of the dorsum of the hand. JAMA Dermatol. 2014;150(11):1187-91.
15. Zwanenburg RL, Werker PM, McGrouther DA. The anatomy and function of Cleland's ligaments. J Hand Surg Eur Vol. 2013;39(5):482-90.
16. Mok D, Nikolis A, Harris PG. The cutaneous innervation of the dorsal hand: detailed anatomy with clinical implications. J Hand Surg Am. 2006;31(4):565-74.
17. Thomson CJ, Lalonde DH, Denkler KA, et al. A critical look at the evidence for and against elective epinephrine use in the finger. Plast Reconstr Surg. 2007;119(1):260-6.
18. Lalonde D, Martin A. Tumescent local anesthesia for hand surgery: improved results, cost effectiveness, and wide-awake patient satisfaction. Arch Plast Surg. 2014;41(4): 312-6.
19. Morgan AM, Baran R, Haneke E. Anatomy of the nail unit in relation to the distal digit. In: Zook EG, Krull EA, Baran R, et al. (Eds). Nail Surgery: A Text and Atlas. Philadelphia, PA: Lippincott, Williams, & Wilkins; 2001. Pp. 1-28.
20. Shum C, Bruno RJ, Ristic S, et al. Examination of the anatomic relationship of the proximal germinal nail matrix to the extensor tendon insertion. J Hand Surg Am. 2000;25(6): 1114-7.
21. Reardon CM, McArthur PA, Survana SK, et al. The surface anatomy of the germinal matrix of the nail bed in the finger. J Hand Surg Br. 1999;24(5):531-3.
22. de Berker D. Nail anatomy. Clin Dermatol. 2013;31(5):509-15.
23. Haneke E. Surgical anatomy of the nail apparatus. Dermatol Clin. 2006;24(3):291-6.
24. Bosley R, Leithauser L, Turner M, et al. The efficacy of second-intention healing in the management of defects on the dorsal surface of the hands and fingers after Mohs micrographic surgery. Dermatol Surg. 2012;38(4):647-53.
25. Lateo SA, Langtry JA. A prospective case series of secondary intention healing for surgical wounds on the dorsum of the hand. Clin Exp Dermatol. 2013;38(6):606-11.
26. Sobanko JF, Miller CJ. Fusiform excisions. In: Avram M, Avram M, Ratner D (Eds). Procedural Dermatology. New York: McGraw-Hill; 2015;177-92.
27. Moran S, Cooney WP. Master Techniques in Orthopaedic Surgery: Soft Tissue Surgery, 1st edition. Lippincott Williams & Wilkins; Philadelphia 2009.
28. Wolfe S, Hotchkiss RN, Pederson WC, et al. Green's Operative Hand Surgery. Philadelphia, PA: Elsevier; 2010.
29. Davami B, Porkhamene G. Versatility of local fasciocutaneous flaps for coverage of soft tissue defects in upper extremity. J Hand Microsurg. 2011;3(2):58-62.
30. Rahoma AH. Use of local sliding flaps to manage deep localized burns of the hand. J Hand Microsurg. 2011;3(2): 45-50.
31. MacNeal R, Messingham MJ, Arpey J. Surgery of the skin. In: Robinson J, Hanke CW, Siegal DM, et al. (Eds). Procedural Dermatology. Philadelphia, PA: Elsevier; 2010; 306-23.
32. Germann G, Biedermann N, Levin SL. Intrinsic flaps in the hand. Clin Plast Surg. 2011;38(4):729-38.
33. Miller CJ. Design principles for transposition flaps: the rhombic (single-lobed), bilobed, and trilobed flaps. Dermatol Surg. 2014;40 (Suppl 9):S43-52.
34. Cook JL. Reconstructive utility of the bilobed flap: lessons from flap successes and failures. Dermatol Surg. 2005;31 (8 Pt 2):1024-33.
35. Cook JL. A review of the bilobed flap's design with particular emphasis on the minimization of alar displacement. Dermatol Surg. 2000;26(4):354-62.
36. Quaba AA, Davison PM. The distally-based dorsal hand flap. Br J Plast Surg. 1990;43(1):28-39.
37. Bailey SH, Andry D, Saint-Cyr M, The dorsal metacarpal artery perforator flap: a case report utilizing a quaba flap harvested from a previously skin-grafted area for dorsal 5th digit coverage. Hand (N Y). 2010;5(3):322-5.
38. Braga-Silva J, Gehlen D, Bervian F, et al. Randomized prospective study comparing reverse and direct flow island flaps in digital pulp reconstruction of the fingers. Plast Reconstr Surg. 2009;124(6): 2012-8.
39. Biswas D, Wysocki RW, Fernandez JJ, et al. Local and regional flaps for hand coverage. J Hand Surg Am. 2014;39 (5):992-1004.
40. Appleton SE, Morris SF. Anatomy and physiology of perforator flaps of the upper limb. Hand Clin. 2014;30(2): 123-35, v.
41. Qin JZ, Wang PJ. Fingertip reconstruction with a flap based on the dorsal branch of the digital artery at the middle phalanx: a simple and reliable flap. Ann Plast Surg. 2012;69 (5):526-8.
42. Chen C, Tang P, Zhang X. A comparison of the dorsal digital island flap with the dorsal branch of the digital nerve versus the dorsal digital nerve for fingertip and finger pulp reconstruction. Plast Reconstr Surg. 2014;133(2):165e-73e.
43. Braga-Silva J, Kuyven CR, Fallopa F, et al. An anatomical study of the dorsal cutaneous branches of the digital arteries. J Hand Surg Br. 2002;27(6):577-9.

44. Henry M, Stutz C. Homodigital antegrade-flow neurovascular pedicle flaps for sensate reconstruction of fingertip amputation injuries. J Hand Surg Am. 2006;31(7):1220-5.
45. Adani R, Busa R, Scagni R, et al. The heterodigital reversed flow neurovascular island flap for fingertip injuries. J Hand Surg Br. 1999;24(4):431-6.
46. Feng SM, Gu JX, Liu HJ, et al. Treatment of distal fingertip degloving injuries using a cross-finger flap based on the dorsal branch of the proper digital artery at the middle phalanx. J Reconstr Microsurg. 2013;29(9):623-30.
47. Gaber M. Kutler repair for the amputated fingertip. Ann R Coll Surg Engl. 1979;61(4):298-300.
48. Rehim SA, Chung KC. Local flaps of the hand. Hand Clin. 2014;30(2):137-51, v.
49. Sungur N, Kankaya Y, Yildiz K, et al. Bilateral V-Y rotation advancement flap for fingertip amputations. Hand (N Y). 2012;7(1):79-85.
50. Zhang X, Shao X, Ren C, et al., Reconstruction of thumb pulp defects using a modified kite flap. J Hand Surg Am. 2011;36(10):1597-603.
51. Haneke E. Advanced nail surgery. J Cutan Aesthet Surg. 2011;4(3):167-75.
52. Haneke E. Nail surgery. Clin Dermatol. 2013;31(5):516-25.
53. Jellinek NJ. Flaps in nail surgery. Dermatol Ther. 2012;25(6):535-44.

# CHAPTER 22

# Scar Revision

**Steven Chow, Richard G Bennett**

## INTRODUCTION

Scar revision is the surgical approach to make a scar less conspicuous and more functional than it was prior to revision. This chapter focuses on the operative techniques for scar revision. Other revision techniques that may be important in scar revision, such as laser or dermabrasion, will be addressed in other chapters.

## SCAR ASSESSMENT

The ability to analyze how to revise a scar is an important skill. The patient is essentially trading a visually unacceptable scar for one that is cosmetically acceptable. Knowledge of the advantages and limitations of each scar revision technique will help the surgeon decide the appropriate technique to implement. For instance, if the patient is bothered by the long appearance of a linear incision line from a prior surgery, then converting the linear incision line into a series of crooked lines may make it less conspicuous. Techniques based on this concept include the running W-plasty, "geometric" broken lines closure and the Z-plasty. Other surgical techniques may be utilized to change certain characteristics of an existing scar. The Z-plasty and V-to-Y advancement flap can lengthen a contracted scar. Conversely, a Y-to-V advancement flap can shorten a scar. Scars may have their orientation changed; transposition of the triangular flaps in a Z-plasty reorients the overall tension vector of a revised scar. Another problem one may face with scars is contour issues: elevations or depressions. These can be dealt with in any number of ways that are discussed in the following text.

## TIME TO REVISE A SCAR

The best time to revise a scar is when the scar itself has matured, which occurs months after the initial surgery is performed. Scar revisions are typically not performed prior to 3 months, and usually occur between 6 months to a year after surgery. If the revision surgery is performed prematurely, disruption of collagen, capillary and lymphatic maturation can adversely affect the final result. Revision surgery may not even be necessary for some elevated scars that are massaged with pressure over a few months.

## FUSIFORM EXCISION

The fusiform or curvilinear excision is a common technique used in scar revision surgery. This technique is often used to change the shape or remove a spread or atrophic scar. When a flap has been utilized as a repair, the fusiform excision may be used as the subsequent surgical procedure to correct the deformity created by the initial flap. For example, performing a bilobe flap on the nose can result in a cutaneous cone deformity that occurs from transposing the primary and secondary lobes into their appropriate defects. Patients who undergo a bilobe flap may need a subsequent excision to remove the standing cone deformity.

### Case Example: Standing Cone Excision

A 92-year-old woman had a bilobe flap repair after undergoing Mohs surgery for a basal cell carcinoma on her left nose tip. At the time of the repair, a standing cone (dog-ear) was not removed at the flap base to ensure an adequate blood supply to the distal lobe. The patient returned 2 months later at which time the standing cone was still present and produced an obvious contour deformity of the dorsal nose (Fig. 22.1A). The standing cone was removed by a fusiform excision (Fig. 22.1B) and the subsequent wound closed side to side. The healed result (Fig. 22.1C) showed a flat dorsal nose without the contour deformity.

When planning the fusiform excision, the tissue to be removed is initially outlined with a surgical skin marker.

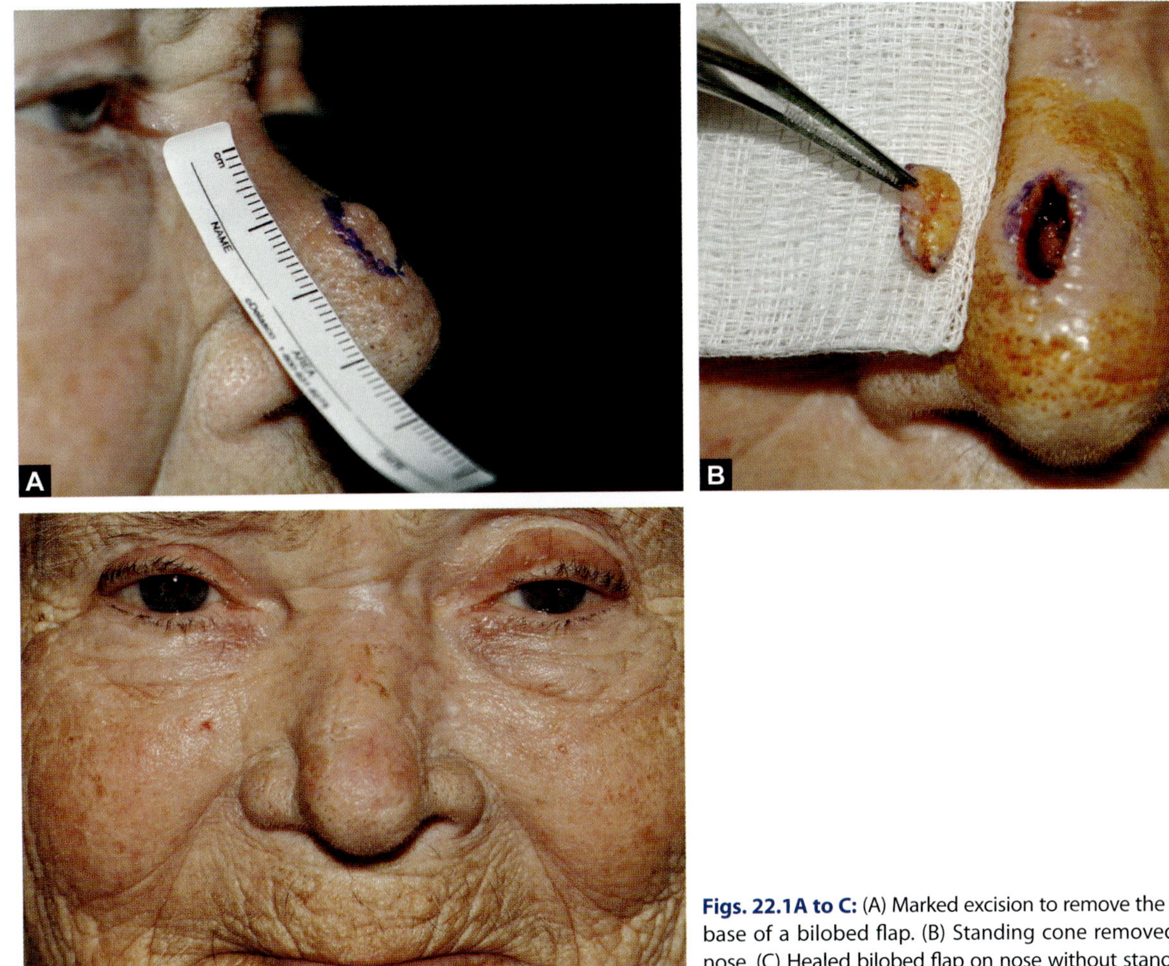

**Figs. 22.1A to C:** (A) Marked excision to remove the standing cone at the base of a bilobed flap. (B) Standing cone removed leaving wound on nose. (C) Healed bilobed flap on nose without standing cone 15 months after standing cone removal.

This planned excision should ideally run parallel to the relaxed skin tension lines (RSTL) to minimize overall wound tension. Classical conventions of having apical angles about 30° and a length to width ratio of approximately 3:1 should be followed. Undermining the surrounding skin reduces its tensile forces on the sutured wound and the subsequent scar. Dermal-subdermal sutures help eliminate dead space and evert tissue, while the percutaneous sutures align the wound edges both vertically and horizontally. When a fusiform excision is used as a scar revision technique, it is important to realize that the new incision line may be longer than the previous one. If the length of the new incision line is of concern, then an M-plasty may be used to shorten the overall incision length.

For large spread scars, the fusiform excision may be performed in stages to gradually decrease the overall tension on the wound as it heals. By serially excising a wound, the final scar length may also be shorter compared to excising the entire initial scar in one stage. To perform the serial excision technique, the fusiform excision is initially placed within the spread scar. Each subsequent excision removes a portion of the scarred tissue until the entire scar is removed[1] (Fig. 22.2).

## TRAPDOOR DEFORMITY REPAIR

Trapdoor, or pincushion deformity, is a complication that can occur following the utilization of round or U-shaped flaps. After a flap is placed onto a wound bed, curved contraction of the flap and the wound base during the healing process can cause the flap to buckle and protrude above the surrounding tissue. This process occurs more frequently when a thick flap is placed into a shallow wound bed, if the flap size is larger than the wound size, or if the recipient wound edges are not undermined adequately. Trapdoor deformity may be corrected through various

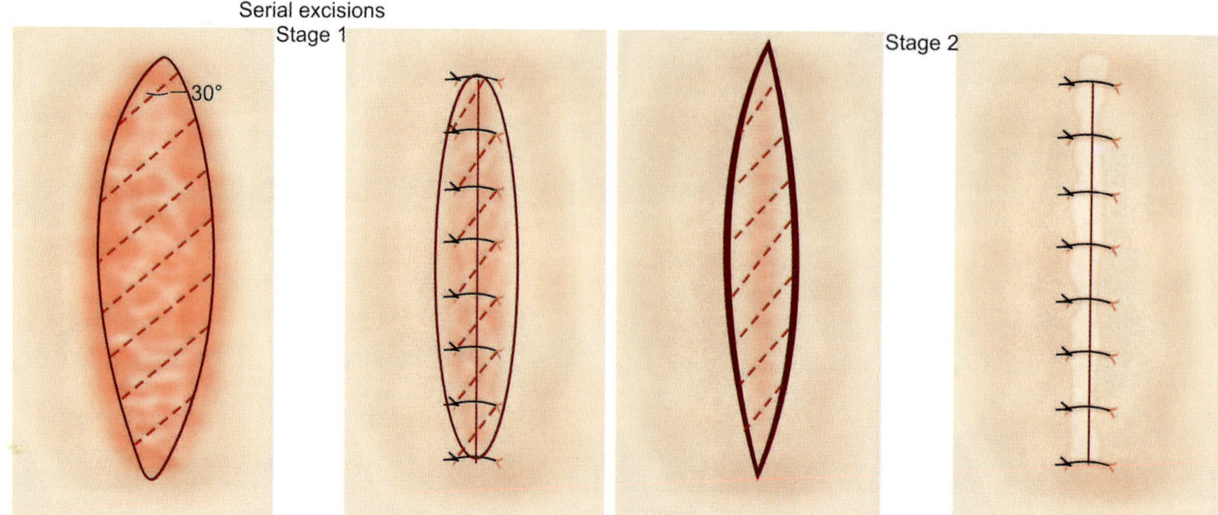


**Fig. 22.2:** Scar removed with serial excisions. Stage 1: Central portion of scar removed with first excision. Stage 2: Remaining scar removed with second excision.

means. If the amount of elevation is minimal, intralesional triamcinolone acetonide 10 mg/mL (Kenalog®-10) may be injected during the postoperative period, usually beginning 1 month after suture removal. If the trapdoor decreases in response to Kenalog®-10 injection, subsequent injections may be performed. When a large section of a flap has elevated, or is unresponsive to multiple Kenalog®-10 injections, then a surgical revision may be considered.

When surgically revising the trapdoor deformity, an incision should ideally be made along the prior incision line adjacent to the bulkiest portion of the flap to minimize additional scars. Assuming that the scar is mature and its blood supply robust, the bulky portion of the flap is reflected back, and its undersurface is thinned using tenotomy scissors or a scalpel. When excising the fibrofatty scar tissue causing the trapdoor, one needs to judge the amount of tissue to excise. One should start by excising only a small amount, then lay the flap onto the wound bed to gauge if any additional fibrofatty tissue need be removed. This repetitive fine tuning process allows one to remove the appropriate amount of tissue. Aggressive defatting should be minimized so that flap vascularity is not compromised and one does not trade an elevated flap for a depressed flap.

### Case Example: Defatting a Flap

A 66-year-old man had a cheek transposition flap to repair a wound on his left nose subsequent to the removal of a basal cell carcinoma. Two months after the sutures were removed, the patient returned with an elevated trapdoor deformity (Fig. 22.3A). The main portion of the flap to be thinned was marked with gentian violet so that blanching with local anesthetic does not obscure the scar lines (Fig. 22.3B). The fibrofatty tissue excised is shown on the grid (Fig. 22.3C). Note the blue color of the flap due to "sympathetic shock" to the vascular blood supply. The bleeding was stopped with biterminal electrocoagulation and the wound sutured (Fig. 22.3D). A tacking suture was placed from the underside of the flap to the underlying wound bed to help contour the flap to the underlying wound surface. The distal portion of the flap was subsequently injected with Kenalog®-10 to which it responded by flattening down.

## Z-PLASTY

The Z-plasty is an important surgical technique utilized for scar revision. Its ability to alter numerous aspects of a previously existing scar results in extensive use of the Z-plasty in our practice. The Z-plasty performs three important tasks: it changes the orientation of a scar, elongates a contracted scar, and disrupts its linearity. The fundamental concept of this technique is that two adjacent triangular flaps are made with a "Z"-shaped incision and are transposed with each other. The classic Z-plasty has equal triangular flaps drawn at angles 60° from the central limb of the "Z". If the angles of the triangles are ≤60°, the limbs of the Z-plasty should follow the RSTL with the central limb of the "Z" placed along the contracted scar to be elongated. The angles should not be >60° because of the difficulty associated with flap transposition.[2] In practice, the

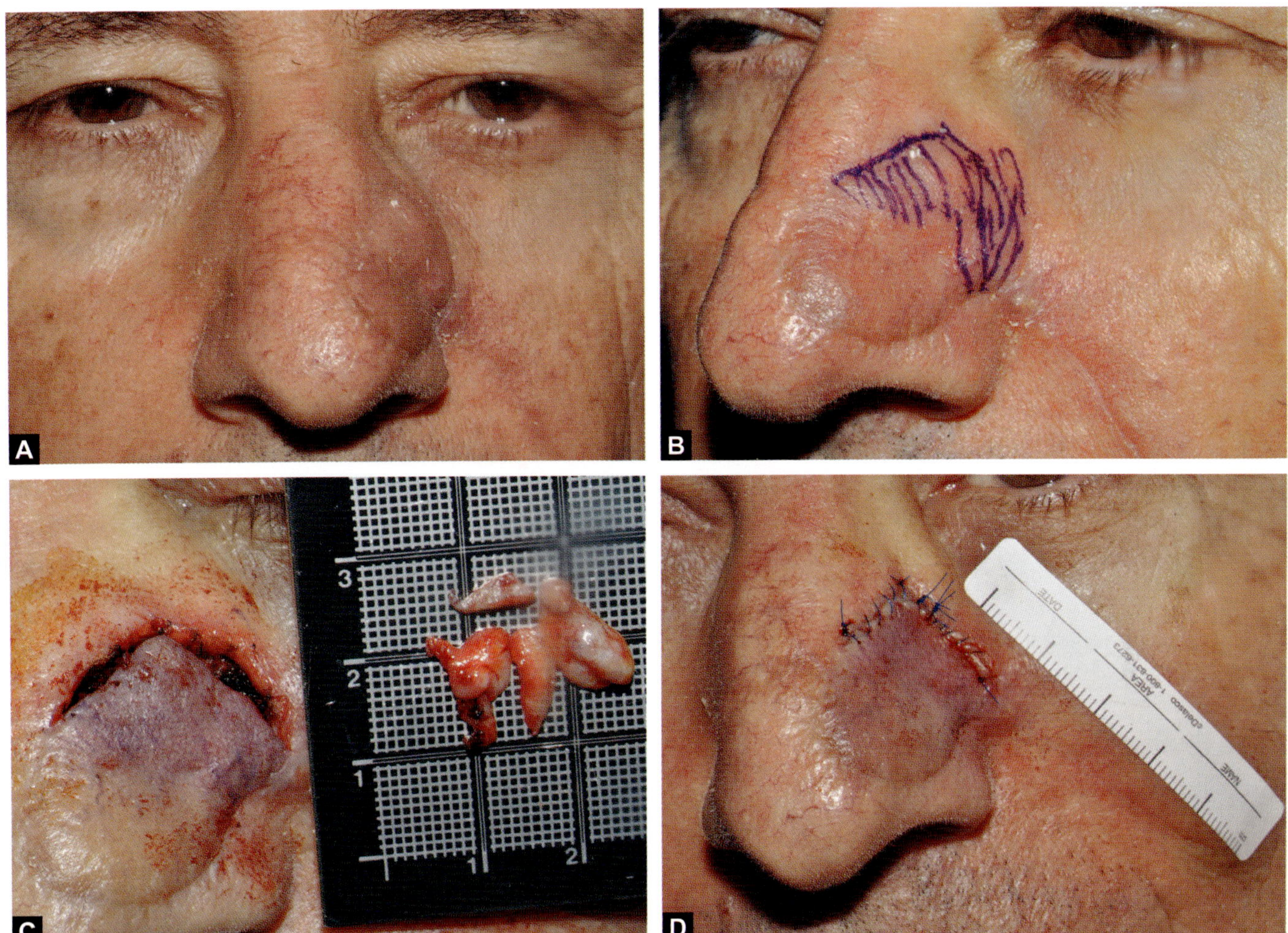


**Figs. 22.3A to D:** (A) Trapdoor flap deformity on the nose 2 months after a melolabial transposition flap repair. (B) Marked region is the location where the flap undersurface is to be thinned. (C) Excision of fibrofatty tissue. (D) Sutured flap after trapdoor correction.

size and the angles of the flap may vary to accommodate a particular feature or facial area. When this occurs, the flaps may be somewhat dissimilar. Multiple smaller Z-plasties may also be used instead of a single large Z-plasty. One benefit of using a series of multiple Z-plasties is that the revised scar is more irregular and thus less noticeable.[3]

Important concepts to understand with the Z-plasty are that relationships exist between both the angles used for the Z-plasty and the Z-plasty limb length in association with overall scar lengthening. When the triangular flaps are transposed in the classic 60° Z-plasty, the overall scar length theoretically increases by 75%. Smaller Z-plasty angles with the same size limbs result in a smaller gain in overall scar length (Figs. 22.4A and B).[4] Longer limbs with the same angles used in a Z-plasty result in a larger gain in overall scar length (Fig. 22.4B).[5]

## Case Example: Z-Plasty to Correct Medial Canthal Position

A 51-year-old woman had a basal cell carcinoma that involved her medial canthus and left nose. A glabella transposition flap repair was successfully performed and left the patient with a good cosmetic result. However, the patient's left medial canthus was slightly displaced inferiorly compared to that on the right (Fig. 22.5A). To elevate the inferiorly displaced canthus, a Z-plasty was designed with the superior triangle medially based, and the inferior triangle laterally based (Fig. 22.5B). The Z-plasty was positioned this way so that after transposition, the patient's left medial canthus would be reoriented superiorly and match the patient's opposite medial canthus. The two triangles were incised, undermined, transposed, and sutured (Fig. 22.5C).

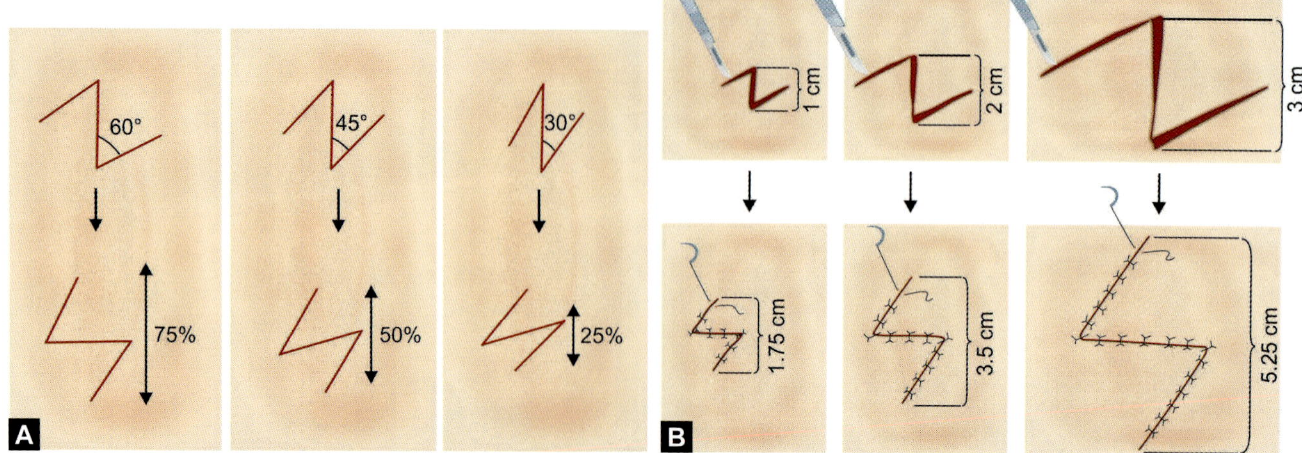


**Figs. 22.4A and B:** (A) Relationship between Z-plasty angles and gain in overall tissue length. The smaller the Z-plasty angles the less gain in tissue length. (B) Relationship between Z-plasty limb length and gain in overall tissue length. The longer the limb length, the greater gain in tissue length.

Two months after suture removal, the patient had appropriate elevation of her left medial canthus (Fig. 22.5D).

### Case Example: Correction of Saddle Nose Deformity

A 59-year-old man presented with a contour ("saddle nose") deformity of his dorsal nose (Fig. 22.6A). The patient had a basal cell carcinoma removed from his dorsal nose, and a vertical side-to-side linear repair was performed at another physician's office. This repair shortened the tissue across the patient's dorsal nose. A rhombic flap with a double Z-plasty (essentially a triple Z-plasty as the rhombic flap is really a Z-plasty) was designed on the patient's right nose (Fig. 22.6B). Note that the horizontal arm of the rhombic is oriented almost horizontally like the middle arm of a Z-plasty. Thus, lengthening will occur in this horizontal direction. The rhombic flap with a double Z-plasty flap was cut, undermined, electrocoagulated (Fig. 22.6C), transposed (Fig. 22.6D), and sutured into place (Fig. 22.6E). Note the recipient wound edges were squared inferiorly to precisely receive the flap corners to prevent trapdoor formation. Not shown is the incision and transposition of the Z-plasty from the left nose. After the rhombic flap with a double Z-plasty was sutured into place it became apparent that further loosening was necessary across the dorsal nose. Therefore, a separate Z-plasty on the left nose was cut as drawn in Figure 22.6B. The Z-plasty was then transposed and sutured into place. At 2 months after suture removal, the patient's dorsal nose had a normal straight-line contour (Fig. 22.6F).

## RUNNING W-PLASTY

The running W-plasty and "geometric" broken lines closure are based on the concept that a long and continuous incision line is easily tracked by the human eye, and that a series of shorter and irregular crooked incision lines are more difficult to see. When performing the running W-plasty as a scar revision technique, the orientation of the triangular flaps should be parallel to the RSTL or slanted in their direction. The running W-plasty is made by creating a series of triangles (or Ws) that have apices of 60° and are 5–7 mm from the scar's edge.[6] A mirror image of the first side is then drawn on the opposite side of the scar (Fig. 22.7). The triangular flaps are aligned with dermal and epidermal sutures so that their tips interdigitate. Placement of half buried horizontal mattress sutures at each tip juncture optimizes the appearance of the running W-plasty and helps preserve the overall contour of the newly repaired skin. The multiple flaps and angles used in this type of closure may result in a pebbly surface.

One issue with the running W-plasty technique is that the resultant scar has a predictable regular pattern; this is more evident with a long scar. In contrast, use of a "geometric" broken lines closure results in an unpredictable irregular pattern to better camouflage a scar.[7] The "geometric" broken lines closure is similar to a running W-plasty, but uses geometric shapes (triangles, squares, and rectangles)

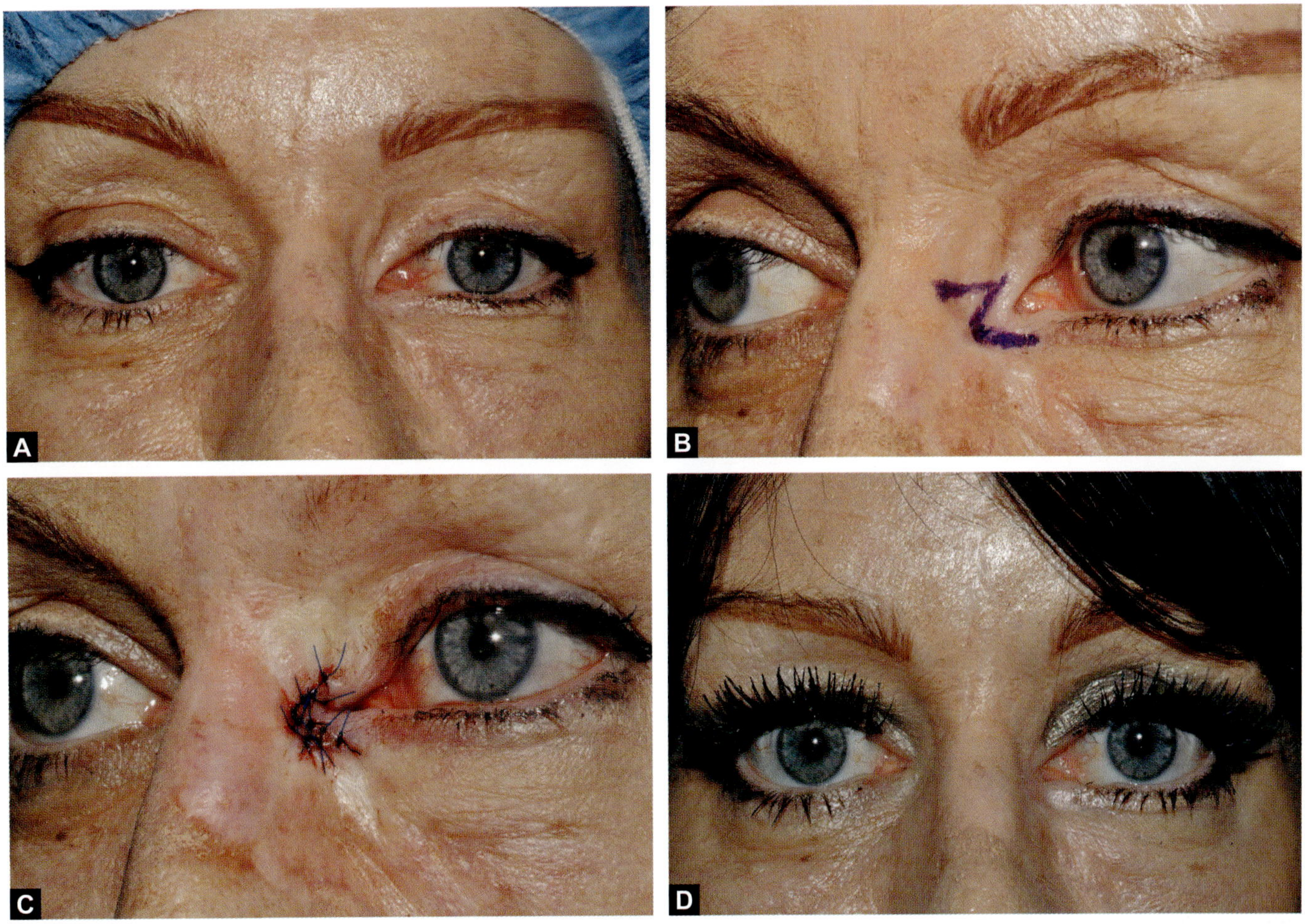

**Figs. 22.5A to D:** (A) Preoperative photo demonstrating inferior displacement of a patient's left medial canthus after a prior flap procedure to the left nose. (B) Z-plasty marked to elevate the inferiorly displaced left medial canthus. (C) Sutured wound after flap transposition. (D) Two months after suture removal showing corrected alignment of the patient's medial canthi.

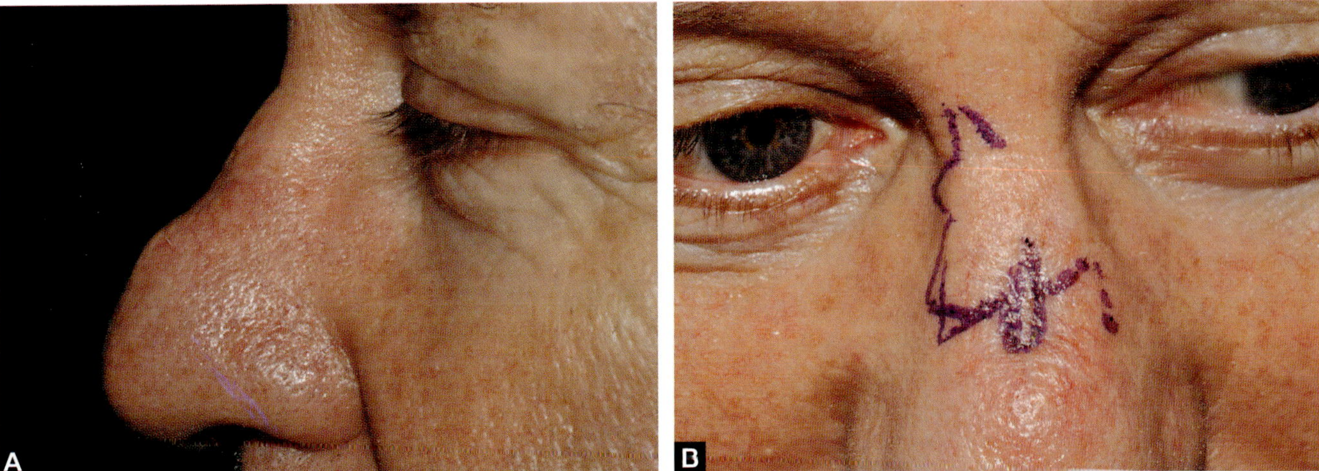


**Figs. 22.6A and B:** (A) Patient presented with a saddle-nose deformity after vertical linear closure on dorsal nose performed by another surgeon. (B) Marking of the dorsal nose indicating the proposed revisions. A rhombic flap with a double Z-plasty was performed on the patient's right side, while a Z-plasty was performed on the patient's left side.

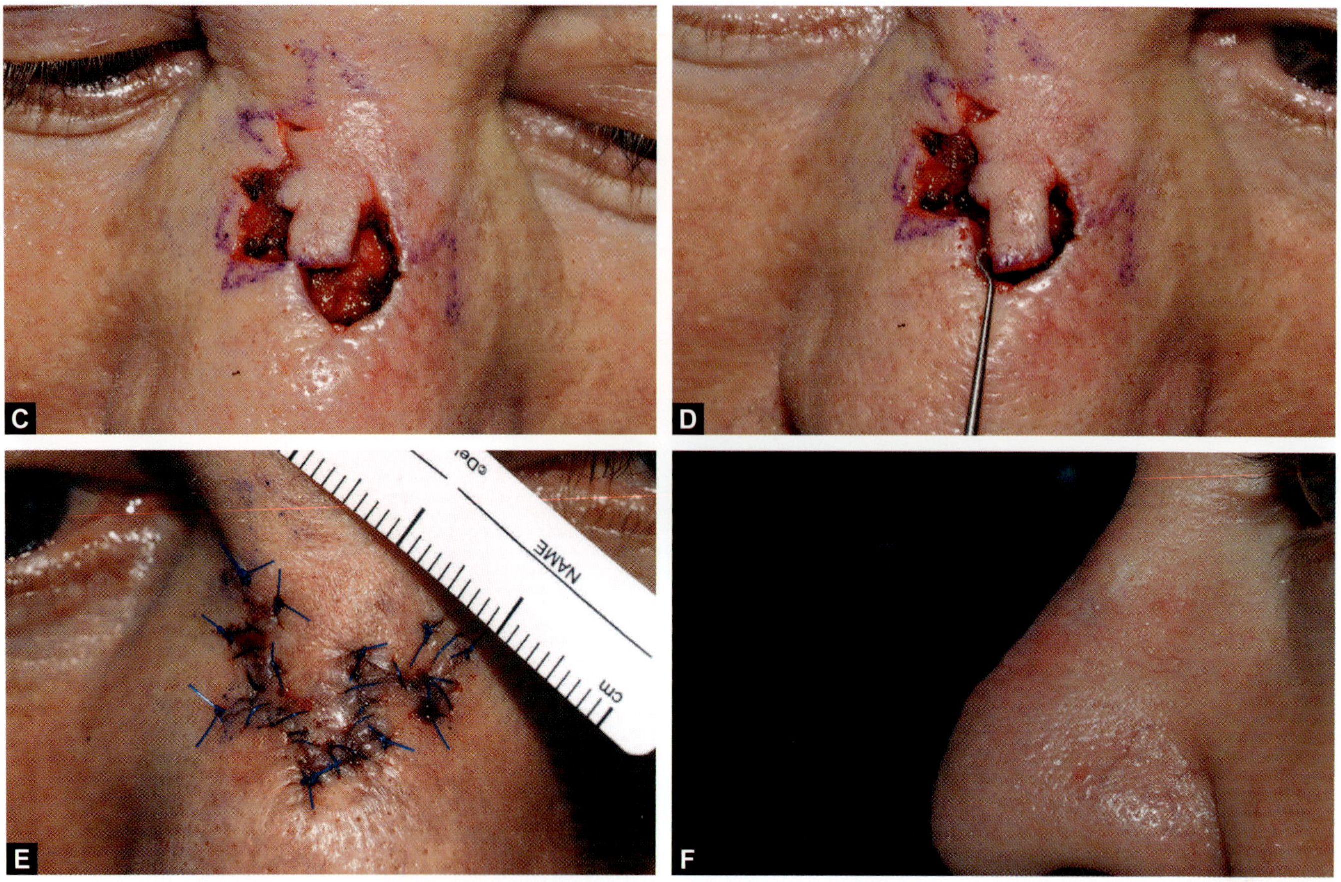

**Figs. 22.6C to F:** (C) Excision of the rhombic flap with double Z-plasty. (D) Transposition of the rhombic flap with double Z-plasty. (E) Sutured result. Note a second Z-plasty on the patient's left nose (marked in Fig. 22.6B) was also used to further lengthen the tissue across the dorsal nose. (F) Healed nose 2 months after surgery. Note the normal straight line contour compared to Fig. 22.6A.

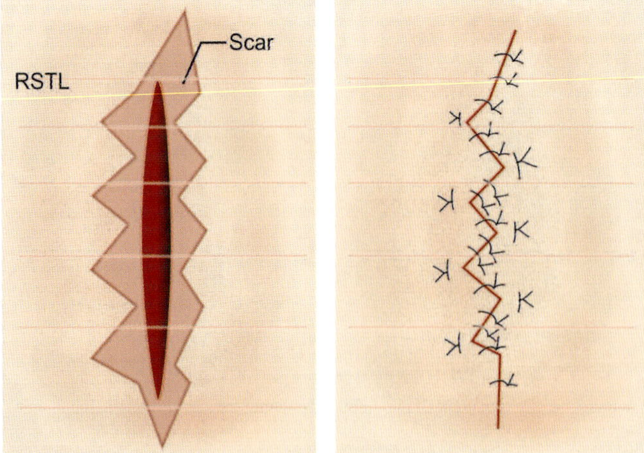


**Fig. 22.7:** Existing scar with running W-plasty marked. (RSTL: Relaxed skin tension lines).

rather than similar triangles. The various geometric shapes are cut along one border of the scar with their mirror images placed on the opposite side (Fig. 22.8). The random geometric shapes make the scar more difficult to track visually compared to the running W-plasty.

## V-TO-Y ADVANCEMENT FLAP

The V-to-Y advancement flap may lengthen a contracted scar or readjust a free margin that has been distorted by scar contracture. For a contracted scar, a V-shaped incision is initially made along one end of the contracted scar, with the prongs of the V on either side of the scar and the tip of the V at the scar end. After the region is widely undermined, the scar tissue from the V-shaped incision is advanced starting at the vertex. This converts the V-shaped incision into a Y-shaped configuration and advances the entire triangular flap region. In practice, however, converting a V to a Y scar minimally lengthens the contracted scar. The configuration change of the scar, however, may be beneficial to the surface contour of the skin.[8] Another use of the V-to-Y

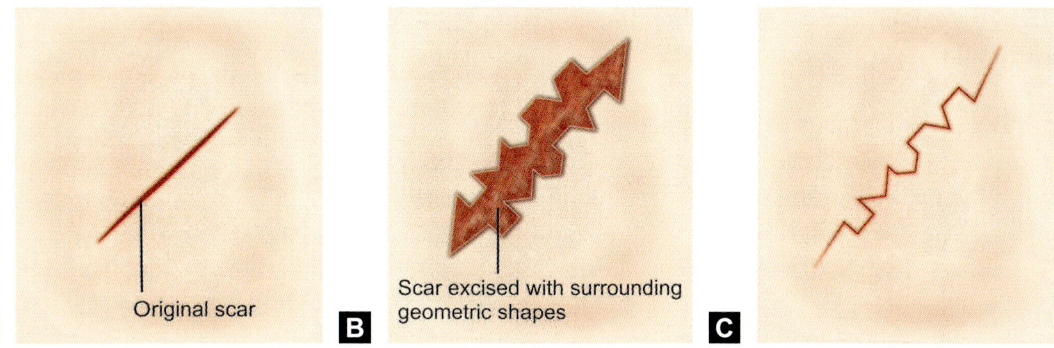


**Figs. 22.8A to C:** (A) Original scar. (B) Existing scar with "geometric" broken lines marked. (C) Final appearance of geometric scar.

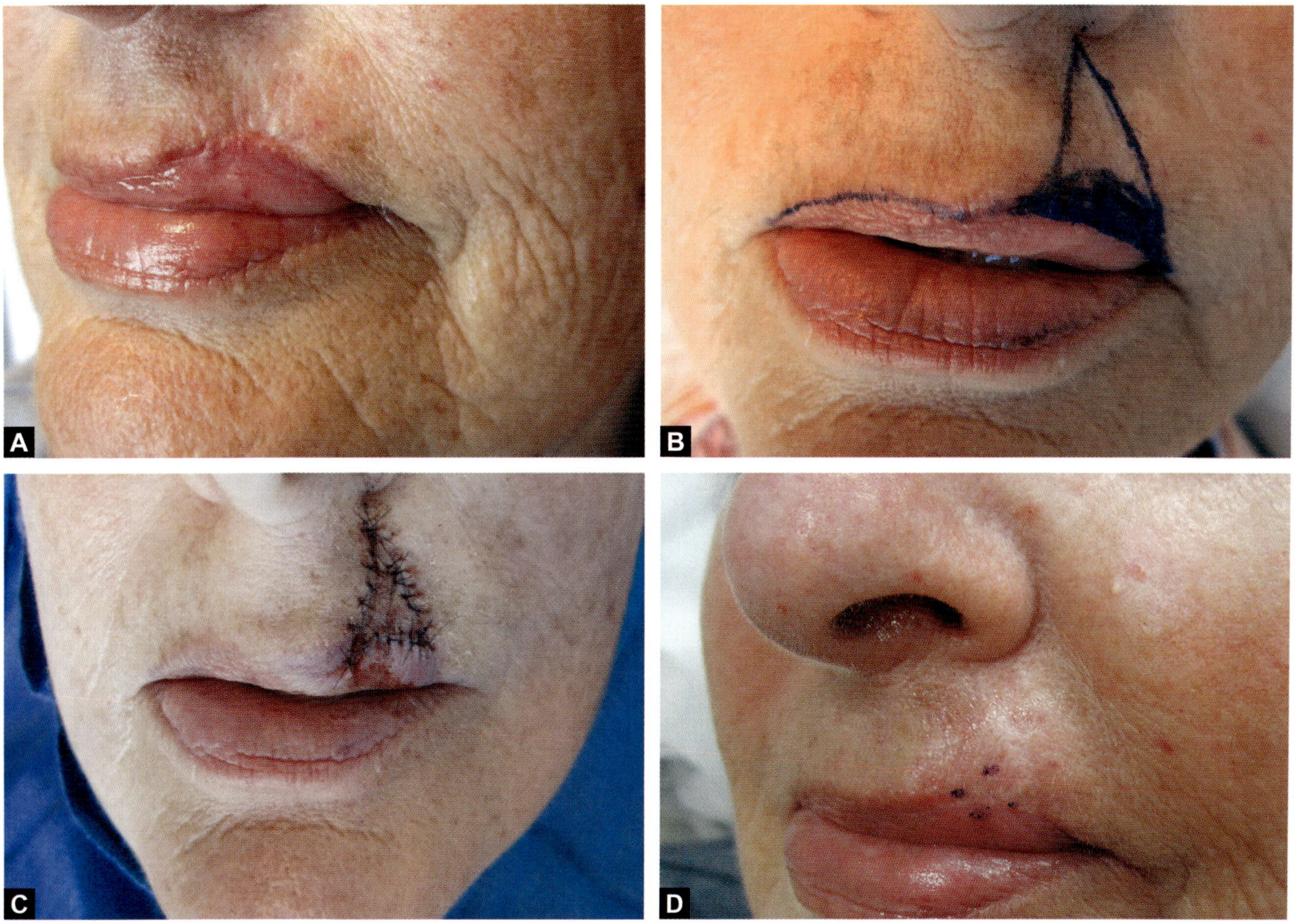

**Figs. 22.9A to D:** (A) A surgical scar that resulted in elevation of the vermilion border. (B) Marking of a V-to-Y repair. (C) Sutured wound after V-to-Y repair showing reapproximation of the upper lip. (D) Healed upper lip after repair showing improved position vermilion border. Note that the area demarcated with gentian violet was further refined with a punch biopsy.
*Courtesy*: S Brian Jiang, MD, San Diego, California, USA.

advancement flap is to readjust a distorted free edge, like the eyelid or lip after prior surgery or trauma (Figs. 22.9A to D). In this instance, the V is positioned with the open portion of the V directed toward the free edge. After the incision, the V-shaped piece of skin is advanced, resulting in a Y-shaped configuration to elevate the free edge. As seen in Figure 22.9D, this procedure is often suboptimal and may require an additional revision procedure.

Conversely, the Y-to-V advancement flap may shorten a wound. In this case, the prongs of a Y-shaped incision are directed toward the tissue to be shortened. After the Y-shaped incision is made, and the triangle between the prongs is undermined, the triangle is advanced into the stem of the Y. After suturing, the flap subsequently assumes a V configuration.

## CONCLUSION

All surgical incisions result in some sort of scar, and the various revision techniques trade a cosmetically unacceptable scar for one that is more acceptable to the patient. It is important for the reconstructive surgeon to have an understanding of the various scar revision technique principles, especially if the surgeon routinely performs advanced reconstructive procedures. Careful assessment of the existing scar allows the surgeon to decide which scar revision technique will ultimately be most beneficial for the patient.

## REFERENCES


1. Lee KK, Gorman AK, Swanson NA. Scar revision. In: Robinson JK, Hanke CW, Sengelmann RD, et al. (Eds). Surgery of the Skin: Procedural Dermatology. Philadelphia, PA: Mosby; 2005. pp. 401-9.
2. Borges AF. Z-plastic scar revision. In: Borges AF (Ed). Elective Incisions and Scar Revision. Boston, MA: Little, Brown and Company; 1973. p. 163.
3. Sharma M, Wakure A. Scar revision. Ind J Plast Surg. 2013; 46(2):408-18.
4. McGregor IA. Fundamental Techniques of Plastic Surgery, 2nd edition. Edinburgh: Livingstone; 1962.
5. Jankauskas S, Cohen IK, Grabb WC. Basic technique of plastic surgery. In: Smith JW, Aston SJ (Eds). Grabb and Smith's Plastic Surgery, 4th edition. Boston, MA: Little, Brown and Company; 1991. p. 74.
6. Leake DS, Baker SR. Scar revision and local flap refinement. In: Baker SR (Ed). Local Flaps in Facial Reconstruction, 2nd edition. St Louis, MO: Mosby; 2007. p. 734.
7. Garg S, Dahiya N, Gupta S. Surgical scar revision: an overview. J Cutan Aesthet Surg. 2014;7(1):3-13.
8. Schultz RC. Soft tissue injuries of the face. In: Smith JW, Aston ST (Eds). Grabb and Smith's Plastic Surgery, 4th edition. Boston, MA: Little, Brown and Company; 1991. p. 343.

# CHAPTER 23

# Scar Refinement

*Anne Marie Tremaine, Arisa E Ortiz, Mathew M Avram*

In addition to poor cosmesis, scarring can cause psychosocial distress and impact quality of life. Scars are not only unappealing but can also be painful, pruritic, and limit mobility causing significant discomfort for the patient. Surgical scars may take months to years to mature and can often show improvement without any intervention. Patients often focus on the appearance of the scar long after the surgery has been completed successfully. There are many invasive and noninvasive treatment options to improve scars. Despite the many treatment options, none are ideal. In fact, the management of scars can be quite challenging. Patients often require multiple treatments along with adjuvant treatments. Too often these treatments achieve, at best, partial success.

There are a wide spectrum of scars. Prior to intervention it is imperative to categorize the scar because different scars respond best to different treatments (Table 23.1). The types of scars include:

- *Hypertrophic scars*: Firm, raised scar within the margins of the original wound. This type of scar can improve spontaneously and often responds well to treatment.
- *Keloid scars*: Firm, raised scar that extends beyond the wound margins, often delayed in onset. Rarely resolves spontaneously and often resistant to treatment. Often recurs with re-excision.
- *Mature scars*: Quiescent, light colored, flat line scars.
- *Immature scar*: Red scar, often itchy or painful.

Other descriptive scar types include atrophic, depressed, icepick, boxcar, rolling, hypopigmented, and hyperpigmented. Additional concerns when treating scars include associated erythema, pain, and pruritus.

The Vancouver scar scale (Table 23.2) is the most commonly used scale to assess scars. It is mostly used to evaluate scar treatments in clinical trials rather than in daily clinical practice. The medical literature has numerous studies regarding scar treatments. In fact, there are several recent scar treatment consensus and guideline papers that are very useful.[1-3]

**Table 23.1:** Scar treatment options.

| | |
|---|---|
| Hypertrophic scars | Pulsed dye laser (PDL)<br>Fractionated photothermolysis<br>Intralesional treatment<br>Dermabrasion |
| Keloid scars | PDL<br>Intralesional treatment<br>Re-excision<br>Pressure<br>Radiation |
| Atrophic scars | PDL<br>Fractionated photothermolysis<br>Dermabrasion<br>Subcutaneous fillers |
| Tethered scars | Subcision<br>Subcutaneous fillers |
| Scar erythema | PDL |
| Scar symptoms: pruritus/pain | PDL<br>Intralesional treatment |

In addition to deciding what scar treatment to use, another important question is when to intervene. In most cases, it is best to treat the scar prior to its maturity. Early intervention, even as early as the time of suture removal, is often the best practice.

## PREVENTION

A surgeon must first try to prevent and minimize scar formation at the time of surgery. This is aided by proper surgical technique to decrease tension on the wound edges and reduce inflammation during the procedure.

**Table 23.2:** Vancouver scar scale.

| | |
|---|---|
| Pigmentation | |
| 0 | Normal color (resembles nearby skin) |
| 1 | Hypopigmentation |
| 2 | Hyperpigmentation |
| Vascularity | |
| 0 | Normal |
| 1 | Pink (slight increase in local blood supply) |
| 2 | Red (significant increase in local blood supply) |
| 3 | Purple (excessive local blood supply) |
| Pliability | |
| 0 | Normal |
| 1 | Supple (flexible with minimal resistance) |
| 2 | Yielding (giving way to pressure) |
| 3 | Firm (solid/inflexible, not easily moved, resistant to manual pressure) |
| 4 | Banding (rope-like, blanches with extension of scar, does not limit range of motion |
| 5 | Contracture (permanent shortening of scar producing deformity or distortion; limits range of motion) |
| Height (mm) | |
| 0 | Normal (flat) |
| 1 | $<2$ |
| 2 | $>2$ and $<5$ |
| 3 | $>5$ |

One can consider postsurgical taping, such as steri-strips, to decrease tension. Providing verbal and written instructions to patients to ensure proper wound care is imperative. Postprocedure hydration to the wound is critical. It should be kept moist with emollients. Ointments are most effective. Studies show, that after wound healing, water evaporates more rapidly through scar tissue compared to normal skin.[4]

Silicone gel or sheets have mixed reviews in the literature. The proposed mechanisms of action include increasing hydration; increasing temperature which may increase collagenase activity; and finally increasing oxygen tension which turns off the negative feedback loop of hypoxic tissue.[5] The evidence for both prevention and treatment of hypertrophic and keloid scarring is weak and unstandardized.[6] It is recommended to wait at least 1 month after the procedure before application of silicone. Silicone gel sheeting should be worn for a minimum of 12 hours a day in order to be effective.[2]

Several topical medications have been used for prevention of scar formation in the postoperative period. Imiquimod has been investigated for keloid prevention when applied after excision. Onion extract is in many antiscar products and has conflicting reports of success, but controlled studies show it was not effective in improving scar outcome. Topical verapamil at a concentration of 50 μM showed promising results from one study with improved scar cosmesis and decreased development of keloids and hypertrophic scars 3 months after abdominoplasty.[7]

Evidence for massage as an effective scar intervention is weak, with varied, unstandardized, anecdotal reports of success.[8] Notwithstanding, massage offers the patient some control over the scar. In general, the recommendation is to wait at least 10–14 days after the procedure to initiate massage.[8]

Finally, ultraviolet irradiation in the postoperative period has a negative impact on scar appearance.[9] Ultravoilet protection of the scar is not only imperative in the postoperative period, but should be an ongoing recommendation for patients. This can be particularly true for patients with more pigmented skin, who are more prone to dyspigmentation of their scar.

## LASER TREATMENTS

Lasers can improve the symptoms and appearance of scars. In order to understand laser therapy's mechanism of action, it is important to have a basic understanding of the theory of selective photothermolysis.[10] Essentially, it holds that successful laser therapy depends on the target chromophore of treatment (i.e. pigment and oxygenated hemoglobin), the fluence of the laser treatment, and the pulse duration of the laser irradiation (i.e. the length of time the laser fires at the target tissue). The wavelength and parameters chosen will depend on the scar type, patient skin type, and patient expectations.

### Vascular Lasers

The 595 nm pulsed dye laser (PDL) is a common laser employed in scar treatment and has long been considered the treatment of choice for red scars. The target chromophore is oxyhemoglobin, and the PDL is selectively absorbed by the vasculature of the scar with insignificant damage to surrounding tissue. Other laser and light-based energy treatments for scar erythema include the potassium titanyl phosphate (KTP) (532 nm) laser and intense pulsed light (polychromatic light source). The PDL had been shown to decrease scar erythema, improve scar thickness, pliability, and the texture of the scar.[10-14] In addition, PDL treatment can reduce associated pruritus. The reduction in erythema is based on the treatment of the vascularity of the scar, but it is unclear how the laser improves pliability and thickness.

Treatment with the PDL is quick, tolerable, and requires no anesthesia. It is important to remove all makeup or creams, which may interfere with the laser penetration, prior to the procedure. Potential side effects with the PDL include erythema, edema (lasting 2–3 days), purpura (lasting 7 days), and temporary hyper- or hypopigmentation. Dyspigmentation is a greater concern with darker skin types; the PDL is typically only used on skin types I–IV. Strict photoprotection and sun avoidance decrease the risk of hyperpigmentation.

There is some debate on what parameters are best for the treatment of red scars. Many advocate that purpuric settings result in quicker and increased improvement of scars compared to subpurpuric settings. This is especially thought to be true for older scars. Many patients, however, may prefer nonpurpuric treatments to avoid obvious post-procedure cosmetic side effects.

The timing of treatment is important. Early intervention may prevent onset of hypertrophic scar, but treatment of mature scars can also be effective. Many favor treatment on the day of suture removal and studies have shown that early intervention with the PDL is safe and effective. Studies have shown improvement in scars without any significant side effects.[15-21] Laser treatment in the early healing phases may have an effect on the type of scar a patient ultimately develops. The concern with early treatment is that it could aggravate the scar and stimulate further proliferation, but this has not been shown in the literature.

Suggested settings for hypertrophic erythematous scars vary depending on the source. Studies favor low fluences and short pulse durations. Suggested settings range from 10 mm spot, 4.0–5.5 J/cm$^2$, and 0.45–1.5 ms pulse duration; or 7 mm spot size, 7.0–8.0 J/cm$^2$, 0.45–1.5 ms pulse duration[3] using single pass, nonoverlapping pulses. Others have found success for fresh scars with a 7 mm spot, 3.5–4.0 J/cm$^2$, and 0.45–1.5 ms pulse duration. The endpoint will either be erythema or purpura depending on the settings (i.e. more purpura with shorter pulse durations and higher energies). Scars generally require multiple treatments performed at 4–8 week intervals. Older scars may require additional treatments compared to younger scars.[3] If initiating treatment at suture removal, an average of two to three treatments are needed to impact scar outcome. The PDL can be combined with many of the other treatment options discussed in this chapter. It is most commonly combined with intralesional triamcinolone acetonide to decrease scar thickness. Intralesional 5-fluorouracil can be effective as well. When combing these treatments, the PDL should be employed first followed by the intralesional injection to avoid altering the laser absorption characteristics.

Another treatment option to target red scars is the 532 nm KTP laser (Figs. 23.1 and 23.2). Studies have shown comparable efficacy with the PDL.[22] However, its depth of penetration is less than the PDL, and it may not sufficiently penetrate into a thickened scar. At 532 nm there is also increased absorption of melanin as compared with the PDL, thus increasing the risks of dyspigmentation in darker skin types (skin types III–VI). Intense pulsed light may also improve scar erythema through similar mechanisms.

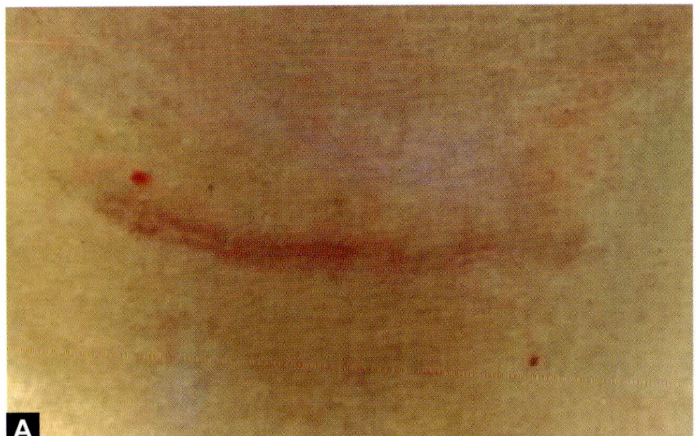

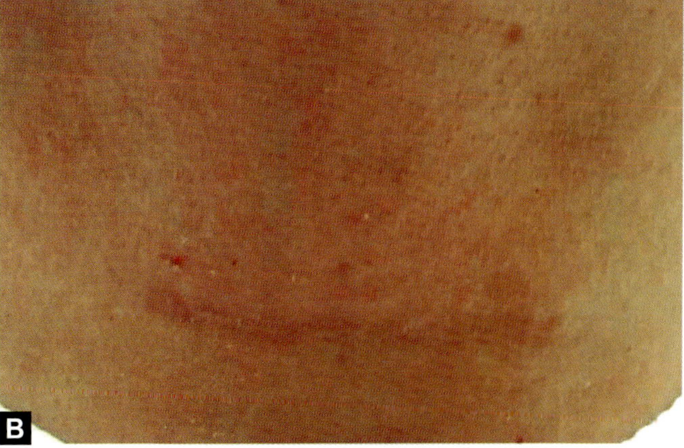


**Figs. 23.1A and B:** (A) Red thyroidectomy scar. (B) Improvement in erythema after 2 treatments with a 532 nm KTP (potassium titanyl phosphate) laser.

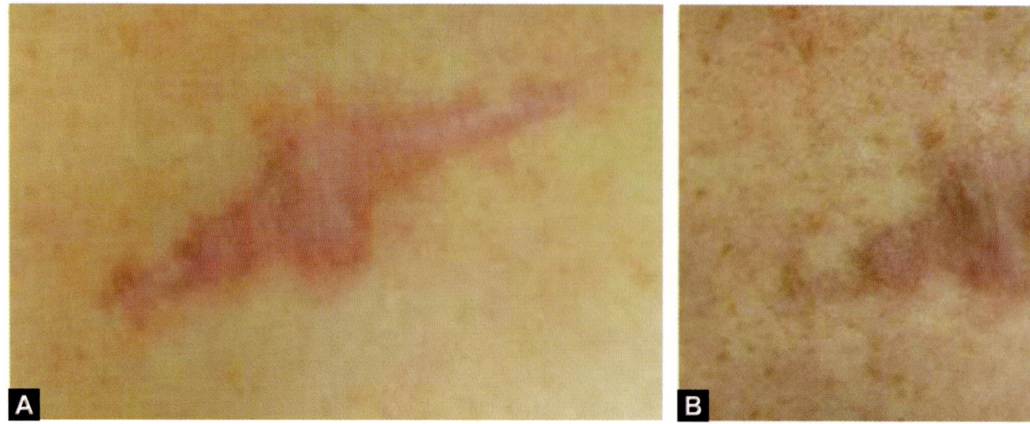

**Figs. 23.2A and B:** (A) Red surgical scar. (B) Improvement in erythema after three treatments with a 532 nm KTP (potassium titanyl phosphate) laser.

## Fractional Lasers

Fractionated ablative and nonablative photothermolysis (FP) resurfacing is an alternative, effective and commonly used treatment option for many types of scars. Both ablative and nonablative FP wavelengths target water as the chromophore. Fractional technology delivers columns of energy with sparing of the surrounding tissue to avoid excessive thermal damage and increase the safety of these treatments.

There are several ablative fractional resurfacing (AFR) options including the 10,600 nm carbon dioxide ($CO_2$) laser and the 2,940 nm erbium:yttrium aluminum garnet (Er:YAG) laser. There are multiple commercial devices that employ these technologies. Fractional ablative lasers vaporize and coagulate the tissue. Traditional resurfacing has been used in the past for ablation of keloid scars or resurfacing of atrophic scars. However, fully ablative traditional $CO_2$ or Er:YAG have fallen out of favor with the advent of fractionated technology due to excessive wound healing times and the greater risk of side effects such as scarring and depigmentation.

Nonablative fractional laser (NAFL) resurfacing includes wavelengths such as 1,440, 1,470, 1,540, and 1,550 nm. These technologies deliver microcolumns of heat creating cylinders of tissue coagulation to the dermis. Both methods stimulate a wound healing response with remodeling of collagen. Both ablative fractional laser (AFL) and NAFL require a series of treatments but NAFL has the benefit of a shorter recovery time.

While laser parameters can vary among various devices, the fluence is always proportional to depth of penetration. Thus, higher fluences will penetrate deeper into the tissue. This is important to consider when selecting appropriate parameters. The goal is to match the energy to the depth of the pathology that you are treating. Therefore, atrophic scars may require a lower fluence than a thickened hypertrophic scar.

Choosing the appropriate density is very important to scar outcomes. Low density is key when treating scars.[23] It is recommended to keep the density <15% and consider as low as 5% density with AFR in a hypertrophic scar. It is always a risk that fractionated lasers could worsen a scar. This can be prevented by using low densities, narrow beam diameters, short pulse widths, and a low number of passes to avoid excessive thermal damage.[3] It is crucially important to recognize the AFR lasers measure density differently. Some measure based upon the ablative channels only. Others measure the zone of ablation as well as its surrounding coagulated tissue. It is important to determine how these densities are calculated in different devices to reduce the risk of over or undertreatment.

Resurfacing generally requires local anesthesia via topicals, injections, and/or nerve blocks. Sedation can be used for more aggressive treatments, especially if they are undergoing other invasive surgical procedures. In terms of post-treatment side effects, patients should be counseled to expect transient erythema, edema, a sandpaper type skin texture, and mild peeling. In addition, patients will have pinpoint bleeding with ablative resurfacing procedures. More rare complications include prolonged erythema, postprocedure pain, itch, infection, and postinflammatory hyperpigmentation. Patients receiving AFL will require postoperative wound care instructions such as using dilute vinegar soaks and occlusive creams/

ointments. Prophylactic antibiotics and antivirals may be required, although are typically not indicated if treating a small area in anatomic locations that are at low risk of infection.

There is no consensus on the most effective and efficient laser technology to use. Treating scars usually requires multiple treatments. When comparing AFR and NAFL, AFR is more effective per treatment, thus requiring fewer treatments, but requires more downtime. Device choice often depends on patient preference of what better fits their lifestyle. Although some improvement can be seen with one treatment (Figs. 23.3 and 23.4), patients should be counseled to expect three treatments with AFL and likely four to six treatments with NAFL. Fractional lasers are more effective than PDL for improving the texture of scars,[3,24] but a combination of PDL and fractional resurfacing is often synergistic (Figs. 23.5A and B). Treatments may be administered every 1–3 months until reaching a therapeutic plateau or sufficient improvement. Similar to PDL, early intervention with fractionated treatments is key.[25,26] There is no need to let the scar mature, but consider using more conservative settings on an acute scar compared to a quiescent mature scar.

When using any laser device, laser safety is important for the patient and all those present in the room. Wavelength specific eyewear should be worn at all times. This

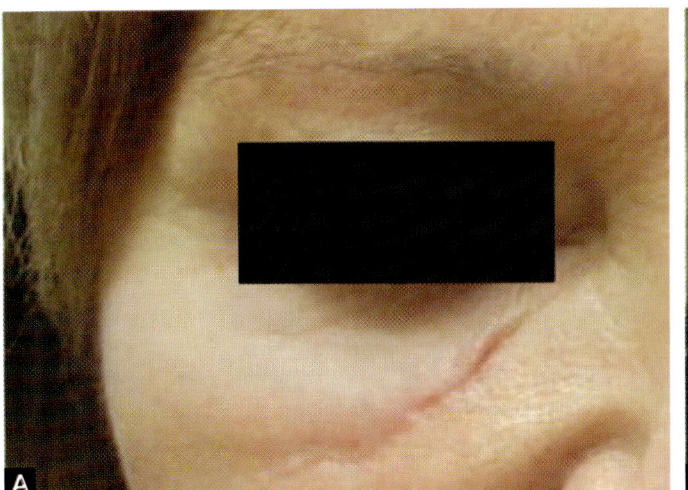


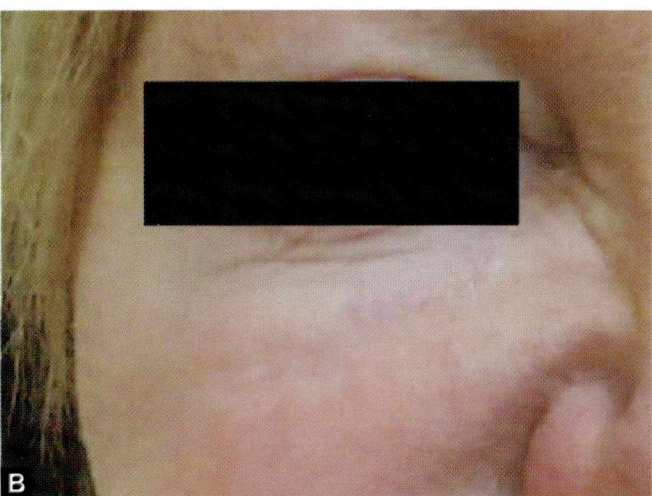


**Figs. 23.3A and B:** (A) Hypertrophic Mohs micrographic surgery scar on the right cheek. (B) Appearance of scar 1 month after one treatment with a hybrid 1,470 nm/2,940 nm nonablative and ablative laser.

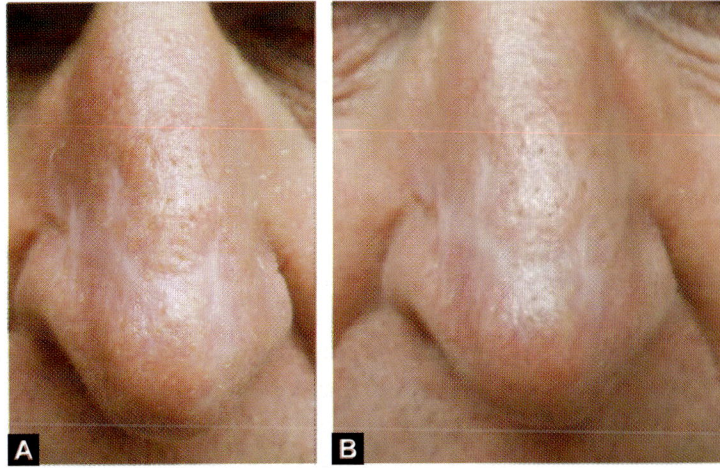


**Figs. 23.4A and B:** (A) Mohs micrographic surgery scar on the nose. (B) Appearance of scar 4 months after one treatment with a fractional $CO_2$ laser.

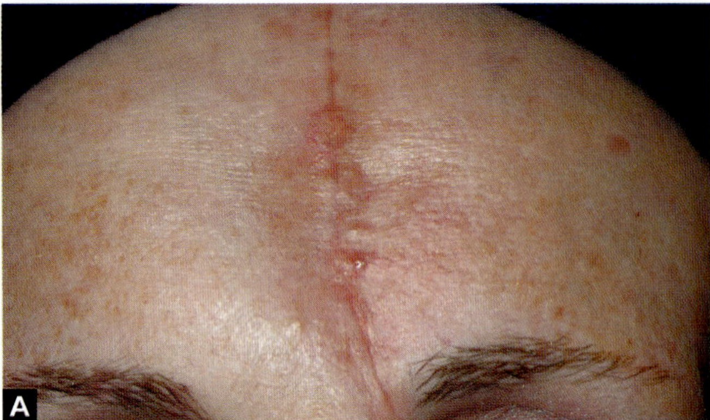


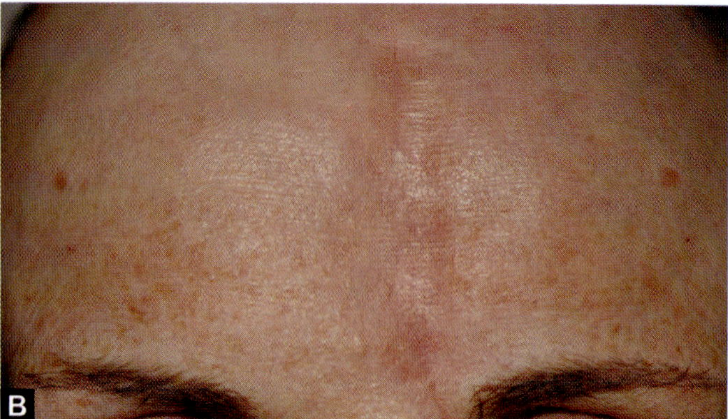


**Figs. 23.5A and B:** (A) Surgical scar on the mid-forehead prior to treatment. (B) Improvement in texture and erythema after three treatments with a pulsed dye laser and fractional $CO_2$ laser.

will ensure eye safety and avoid retinal and corneal damage. Another risk is that ablative lasers are a potential fire hazard and the use of flammable products, such as alcohol, should be avoided. In the operating room, exposed oxygen adds increased risk. It is recommended to apply wet gauze around the patient's airway to prevent a potential fire hazard.

Finally, with all laser treatments strict photoprotection and sun avoidance is important to avoid pigmentation issues. Patients must follow this rule before and after each treatment to decrease the risk of hyper- or hypopigmentation. If hyperpigmentation does ensue, treatments should be halted until hyperpigmentation improves. Hyperpigmentation usually improves with time but can also be improved with bleaching creams. Patients with a tan or recent sun exposure should not be treated until the tan has subsided.

## DERMABRASION

Dermabrasion is another technique that is useful for the treatment of scars.[27-31] Its efficacy does not reach that of the fractional lasers. Serious side effects can occur. Dermabrasion can be performed with a motorized, rotating abrasive surface or done manually. The power devices most commonly utilize a wire brush or a diamond fraise head. The wire brush is considered the most aggressive tool. The diamond fraise is easier to use and has a greater margin of safety. With either option, technique is of the greatest importance. Proper training and experience is key to treatment success and avoidance of side effects. One must understand the depth of penetration that is needed. Treating deeper than the lower papillary dermis or upper reticular dermis could result in further scarring. Pinpoint bleeding indicates entry into the papillary dermis. The appearance of a smooth and shiny white surface indicates entry into the reticular dermis.

Manual dermabrasion can be done with sterilized silicon carbide sandpaper or wallscreen. Some feel this technique is safer than a motorized tool, as it allows for more controlled depth of treatment and feathering of edges. The treatment progress and outcome depends on type of sandpaper used (fine, medium, or coarse), the force of application, and duration of the treatment.

Use of preoperative antibiotics or antivirals is left to the discretion of the physician. The patient should be counseled appropriately. Consider intralesional lidocaine, nerve blocks, and/or topical skin refrigerants for anesthesia. Proper technique includes keeping the skin taught during the treatment. Some surgeons apply dichlorotetrafluoroethane or other skin refrigerants to create a rigid surface for treatment. When using the manual technique, it is suggested to wrap the sandpaper around the barrel of a syringe or a rolled up gauze pad; keep the site hydrated with saline; use circular or back and forth technique. Make sure to wash off any paper particles after the treatment, which if left on the patient could develop into a tattoo.[32,33]

Common postoperative effects include bleeding, edema, serous drainage, discomfort, erythema, itching, milia formation, or pigmentary alteration.[34] Persistent or new onset pain after day 2 is concerning for an infection. Postoperative care includes hydrogen peroxide soaks, application of biosynthetic dressings, petrolatum ointment, or mupirocin under gauze occlusion for 5–7 days.

Early intervention at about 4–8 weeks after a surgical excision is optimal for increased efficacy in scar improvement, but improvement will be seen with intervention at any time point.[27]

## SUBCISION

Subcision, first described by Orentreich and Orentreich in 1995,[35] is a technique of subdermal undermining used to release the tethering of a depressed scar. Subcision is most useful for rolling acne scars but may have benefit in a tethered surgical scar. There are many different tools, but a tri-beveled hypodermic needle (16–30 gauge) or a subcision spatula are often used.[35] Many physicians prefer the 18-gauge Nokor needle as larger gauges may leave additional scars.

After ensuring adequate local anesthesia, several small punctures are made around the scar to permit access from different angles and allow full release of the scar. The needle should be positioned at the subdermis parallel to the skin. Back and forth or fan-like motions are made under the scar to release the fibrous attachments tethering the epidermis to the subcutis. It is common to hear an audible crunching and popping sound as the tissue releases. Care must be taken to remain superficial to deep vessels and the nerves.

Postprocedure excess blood should be evacuated to prevent a large hematoma, although a small hematoma may support further release of the scar.[36] Pressure dressings and ice are useful for hemostasis in the first 24 hours. Postoperative bruising and swelling should be expected for up to a week and palpable induration typically takes 3 months to resolve.[37]

## INTRALESIONAL INJECTIONS

Intralesional medications, such as triamcinolone acetonide, are regularly utilized for the management of scars.[38] Triamcinolone acetonide is thought to work by inhibiting fibroblasts, promoting collagen breakdown, and inhibiting TGF-beta.[39,40] Triamcinolone is injected into the scar at the dermal level, with the doses ranging between 10 and 40 mg/mL, every 4 weeks until the scar is flattened. Common side effects from corticosteroid injection include pain, atrophy, hypopigmentation, and telangiectasia formation. Atrophy is more common if injecting into the subcutis or using a high concentration. This treatment typically requires multiple sessions and can be more effective when combined with other injectables or lasers. The authors prefer using high concentrations in small doses for improvement of thickened scars.

Other less commonly used intradermal injections include 5-fluorouracil, bleomycin, and verapamil. 5-fluorouracil inhibits fibroblast proliferation and TGF-beta.[41,42] The typical concentration used is 50 mg/mL. Side effects include pain, ulceration, and hyperpigmentation. Contraindications to 5-FU include anemias, pregnancy, bone marrow depression, and active infections. Bleomycin is thought to decrease collagen synthesis.[43] It may be applied topically to the scar or introduced into the lesion with serial puncture.[44] Side effects of bleomycin include atrophy and hyperpigmentation. Verapamil is a calcium channel blocker that may also improve the appearance of scars. In case reports, physicians have used a 2.5 mg/mL intralesional dose of verapamil.[39]

Avotermin is an investigational recombinant, active, human transforming growth-factor beta 3 that is in Phase II studies for scar improvement.[45-48] This clinical drug is injected immediately after scar revision surgery and the results show improved scar outcomes compared to placebo or standard wound care. Other agents that have been studied include intralesional interferon alpha and gamma, mitomycin C, and tumor necrosis factor alpha.[38]

## PRESSURE

Pressure is a modality used to prevent keloid formation or recurrence.[49-51] It is most commonly used after re-excision of a keloid on the ear lobe. Pressure therapy can be accomplished using clips, buttons, or form-pressure garments. High-pressure devices are more effective than low pressure. Pressure may be effective by inducing hypoxia, which results in degeneration of fibroblasts[49] or decreased blood flow, which will prevent $\alpha$2-macroglobulin from entering the site and inhibiting collagenase.[51]

It is recommended to employ 8–24 hours of daily pressure, and the compression needs to be continued for 6–12 months to achieve the best results. With the lengthy treatment time, compliance is often an issue.[52]

## RADIATION

Low dose radiation has been used to decrease keloid recurrence. It is often used as an adjunct after excision of a keloid.[53-55] In one study, patients were treated between 1–12 days with a median cumulative dose of 28 Gy.[55] Others recommend from 15–20 Gy fractionated over five to six treatments.[56]

The main concern with radiation is therapy-induced malignancy. This is considered to be low risk, with only a few cases described.[57,58] It is important to keep thyroid, breast, or other surrounding tissues adequately shielded. Radiation is not indicated in children. The only other main side effect is pigmentary changes.

## RE-EXCISION

Surgical revision or re-excision of a scar is always a consideration with the goal to reduce tension and is addressed in further detail in Chapter 22. Surgical intervention is not recommended if the scar is still active.[2] At least 1 year is recommended to allow for scar maturation and remodeling. Surgical intervention options include simple re-excision, Z-plasty, W-plasty, S-plasty, flaps, and grafts. Scar recurrence is common and patients should be counseled prior to revision. Postexcision prophylaxis is especially important to decrease risk of scar recurrence, especially if treating a keloid scar. Post-treatment intralesional triamcinolone, silicone sheets, and pressure should be considered.

## OTHER MODALITIES

Medium-to-deep chemical peels are used for atrophic acne scars, ice pick acne, and chicken pox scars, but are not often used for isolated surgical scars.

Dermal fillers and fat transfer can be utilized in atrophic scars. Often the fillers will be used in combination with fractional lasers for atrophic scars or in combination with subcision for rolling scars.

## CONCLUSION

The treatment modalities discussed in this chapter are often used in combination or succession to get the best clinical outcome.[59] Various treatment modalities can be combined to address both the color and texture of scars. Often these procedures are performed on the same day. Scar refinement can require multiple treatments and setting patient expectations is crucial to the process.

## REFERENCES

1. Gold MH, Berman B, Clementoni MT, et al. Updated international clinical recommendations on scar management: part 1—evaluating the evidence. Dermatol Surg. 2014;40(8):817-24.
2. Gold MH, McGuire M, Mustoe TA, et al. Updated international clinical recommendations on scar management: part 2—algorithms for scar prevention and treatment. Dermatol Surg. 2014;40(8):825-31.
3. Anderson RR, Donelan MB, Hivnor C, et al. Laser treatment of traumatic scars with an emphasis on ablative fractional laser resurfacing: consensus report. JAMA Dermatol. 2014; 150(2):187-93.
4. Suetake T, Sasai S, Zhen YX, et al. Functional analyses of the stratum corneum in scars. Sequential studies after injury and comparison among keloids, hypertrophic scars, and atrophic scars. Arch Dermatol. 1996;132(12):1453-8.
5. Berman B, Perez OA, Konda S, et al. A review of the biologic effects, clinical efficacy, and safety of silicone elastomer sheeting for hypertrophic and keloid scar treatment and management. Dermatol Surg. 2007;33(11):1291-302; discussion 302-3.
6. O'Brien L, Jones DJ. Silicone gel sheeting for preventing and treating hypertrophic and keloid scars. Cochrane Database Syst Rev. 2013;9:CD003826.
7. Boggio RF, Boggio LF, Galvao BL, et al. Topical verapamil as a scar modulator. Aesthetic Plast Surg. 2014;38(5):968-75.
8. Shin TM, Bordeaux JS. The role of massage in scar management: a literature review. Dermatol Surg. 2012;38(3): 414-23.
9. Due E, Rossen K, Sorensen LT, et al. Effect of UV irradiation on cutaneous cicatrices: a randomized, controlled trial with clinical, skin reflectance, histological, immunohistochemical and biochemical evaluations. Acta Dermato-venereol. 2007;87(1):27-32.
10. Alster TS. Improvement of erythematous and hypertrophic scars by the 585-nm flashlamp-pumped pulsed dye laser. Ann Plast Surg. 1994;32(2):186-90.
11. Alster TS, McMeekin TO. Improvement of facial acne scars by the 585 nm flashlamp-pumped pulsed dye laser. J Am Acad Dermatol. 1996;35(1):79-81.
12. Alster TS, Nanni CA. Pulsed dye laser treatment of hypertrophic burn scars. Plast Reconstr Surg. 1998;102(6): 2190-5.
13. Alster TS, Williams CM. Treatment of keloid sternotomy scars with 585 nm flashlamp-pumped pulsed-dye laser. Lancet. 1995;345(8959):1198-200.
14. Dierickx C, Goldman MP, Fitzpatrick RE. Laser treatment of erythematous/hypertrophic and pigmented scars in 26 patients. Plastic and reconstructive surgery. 1995;95(1):84-90; discussion 1-2.
15. Alam M, Pon K, Van Laborde S, et al. Clinical effect of a single pulsed dye laser treatment of fresh surgical scars: randomized controlled trial. Dermatol Surg. 2006;32(1): 21-5.
16. Conologue TD, Norwood C. Treatment of surgical scars with the cryogen-cooled 595 nm pulsed dye laser starting on the day of suture removal. Dermatol Surg. 2006;32(1): 13-20.
17. Nouri K, Elsaie ML, Vejjabhinanta V, et al. Comparison of the effects of short- and long-pulse durations when using a 585-nm pulsed dye laser in the treatment of new surgical scars. Lasers Med Sci. 2010;25(1):121-6.
18. Nouri K, Jimenez GP, Harrison-Balestra C, et al. 585-nm pulsed dye laser in the treatment of surgical scars starting on the suture removal day. Dermatol Surg. 2003;29(1):65-73; discussion73.
19. Nouri K, Rivas MP, Stevens M, et al. Comparison of the effectiveness of the pulsed dye laser 585 nm versus 595

nm in the treatment of new surgical scars. Lasers Med Sci. 2009;24(5):801-10.
20. Gladsjo JA, Jiang SI. Treatment of surgical scars using a 595-nm pulsed dye laser using purpuric and nonpurpuric parameters: a comparative study. Dermatol Surg. 2014;40 (2):118-26.
21. McCraw JB, McCraw JA, McMellin A, et al. Prevention of unfavorable scars using early pulse dye laser treatments: a preliminary report. Ann Plast Surg. 1999;42(1):7-14.
22. Keaney TC, Tanzi E, Alster T. Comparison of 532 nm potassium titanyl phosphate laser and 595 nm pulsed dye laser in the treatment of erythematous surgical scars: a randomized, controlled, open-label study. Dermatol Surg. 2016;42(1):70-6.
23. Lin JY, Warger WC, Izikson L, et al. A prospective, randomized controlled trial on the efficacy of fractional photothermolysis on scar remodeling. Lasers Surg Med. 2011; 43(4):265-72.
24. Tierney E, Mahmoud BH, Srivastava D, et al. Treatment of surgical scars with nonablative fractional laser versus pulsed dye laser: a randomized controlled trial. Dermatol Surg. 2009;35(8):1172-80.
25. Sherling M, Friedman PM, Adrian R, et al. Consensus recommendations on the use of an erbium-doped 1,550-nm fractionated laser and its applications in dermatologic laser surgery. Dermatol Surg. 2010;36(4):461-9.
26. Oliaei S, Nelson JS, Fitzpatrick R, et al. Use of lasers in acute management of surgical and traumatic incisions on the face. Facial Plast SurgClin N Am. 2011;19(3):543-50.
27. Katz BE, Oca AG. A controlled study of the effectiveness of spot dermabrasion ('scarabrasion') on the appearance of surgical scars. J Am Acad Dermatol. 1991;24(3):462-6.
28. Farrior RT. Dermabrasion in facial surgery. Laryngoscope. 1985;95(5):534-45.
29. Yarborough JM Jr. Ablation of facial scars by programmed dermabrasion. J Dermatol Surg Oncol. 1988;14(3):292-4.
30. Roenigk HH Jr. Dermabrasion for miscellaneous cutaneous lesions (exclusive of scarring from acne). J Dermatol Surg Oncol. 1977;3(3):322-8.
31. Roenigk HH Jr. Dermabrasion: state of the art. J Dermatol Surg Oncol. 1985;11(3):306-14.
32. Monheit GD, Chastain MA. Chemical and mechanical skin resurfacing. In: Bolognia J, Jorizzo J, Schaffer J (Eds). Dermatology, 3rd edition. Elsevier; 2009. pp. 2493-508.
33. Alt TH. Facial dermabrasion: advantages of the diamond fraise technique. J Dermatol Surg Oncol. 1987;13(6):618-24.
34. Guidelines of care for dermabrasion. American academy of dermatology committee on guidelines of care. J Am Acad Dermatol. 1994;31(4):654-7.
35. Orentreich DS, Orentreich N. Subcutaneous incisionless (subcision) surgery for the correction of depressed scars and wrinkles. Dermatol Surg. 1995;21(6):543-9.
36. Chandrashekar B, Nandini A. Acne scar subcision. J Cutan Aesthet Surg. 2010;3(2):125-6.
37. Alam M, Omura N, Kaminer MS. Subcision for acne scarring: technique and outcomes in 40 patients. Dermatol Surg. 2005;31(3):310-7; discussion 7.
38. Ledon JA, Savas J, Franca K, et al. Intralesional treatment for keloids and hypertrophic scars: a review. Dermatol Surg. 2013;39(12):1745-57.
39. Xu SJ, Teng JY, Xie J, et al. Comparison of the mechanisms of intralesional steroid, interferon or verapamil injection in the treatment of proliferative scars. Zhonghua Zheng Xing Wai Ke Za Zhi [Chinese J Plast Surg]. 2009;25(1):37-40.
40. McCoy BJ, Diegelmann RF, Cohen IK. In vitro inhibition of cell growth, collagen synthesis, and prolyl hydroxylase activity by triamcinolone acetonide. Proc Soc Exp Biol Med. 1980;163(2):216-22.
41. Wendling J, Marchand A, Mauviel A, et al. 5-fluorouracil blocks transforming growth factor-beta-induced alpha 2 type I collagen gene (COL1A2) expression in human fibroblasts via c-Jun NH2-terminal kinase/activator protein-1 activation. Mol Pharmacol. 2003;64(3):707-13.
42. Huang L, Wong YP, Cai YJ, et al. Low-dose 5-fluorouracil induces cell cycle G2 arrest and apoptosis in keloid fibroblasts. Br J Dermatol. 2010;163(6):1181-5.
43. Hendricks T, Martens MF, Huyben CM, et al. Inhibition of basal and TGF beta-induced fibroblast collagen synthesis by antineoplastic agents. Implications for wound healing. Br J Cancer. 1993;67(3):545-50.
44. Naeini FF, Najafian J, Ahmadpour K. Bleomycin tattooing as a promising therapeutic modality in large keloids and hypertrophic scars. Dermatol Surg. 2006;32(8):1023-9; discussion 9-30.
45. Ferguson MW, Duncan J, Bond J, et al. Prophylactic administration of avotermin for improvement of skin scarring: three double-blind, placebo-controlled, phase I/II studies. Lancet. 2009;373(9671):1264-74.
46. Bush J, Duncan JA, Bond JS, et al. Scar-improving efficacy of avotermin administered into the wound margins of skin incisions as evaluated by a randomized, double-blind, placebo-controlled, phase II clinical trial. Plast Reconstr Surg. 2010;126(5):1604-15.
47. Bush J, So K, Mason T, et al. Therapies with emerging evidence of efficacy: avotermin for the improvement of scarring. Dermatol Res Pract. vol. 2010, 2010, http://dx.doi.org/10.1155/2010/690613. Accessed 29 April 2017.
48. So K, McGrouther DA, Bush JA, et al. Avotermin for scar improvement following scar revision surgery: a randomized, double-blind, within-patient, placebo-controlled, phase II clinical trial. Plast Reconstr Surg. 2011;128(1):163-72.
49. Kischer CW, Shetlar MR, Shetlar CL. Alteration of hypertrophic scars induced by mechanical pressure. Arch Dermatol. 1975;111(1):60-4.
50. Linares HA, Larson DL, Willis-Galstaun BA. Historical notes on the use of pressure in the treatment of hypertrophic scars or keloids. Burns. 1993;19(1):17-21.
51. Urioste SS, Arndt KA, Dover JS. Keloids and hypertrophic scars: review and treatment strategies. Semin Cutan Med Surg. 1999;18(2):159-71.
52. Wolfram D, Tzankov A, Pulzl P, et al. Hypertrophic scars and keloids—a review of their pathophysiology, risk factors, and therapeutic management. Dermatol Surg. 2009;35(2): 171-81.

53. Borok TL, Bray M, Sinclair I, et al. Role of ionizing irradiation for 393 keloids. Int J Radiat Oncol Biol Phys. 1988;15(4):865-70.
54. Craig RD, Pearson D. Early post-operative irradiation in the treatment of keloid scars. Br J Plast Surg. 1965;18(4):369-76.
55. Klumpar DI, Murray JC, Anscher M. Keloids treated with excision followed by radiation therapy. J Am Acad Dermatol. 1994;31(2 Pt 1):225-31.
56. Slemp AE, Kirschner RE. Keloids and scars: a review of keloids and scars, their pathogenesis, risk factors, and management. Curr Opin Pediatr. 2006;18(4):396-402.
57. Malaker K, Vijayraghavan K, Hodson I, et al. Retrospective analysis of treatment of unresectable keloids with primary radiation over 25 years. Clin Oncol (R Coll Radiol). 2004; 16(4):290-8.
58. Ogawa R, Yoshitatsu S, Yoshida K, et al. Is radiation therapy for keloids acceptable? The risk of radiation-induced carcinogenesis. Plast Reconstr Surg. 2009;124(4):1196-201.
59. Eilers RE Jr, Ross EV, Cohen JL, et al. A combination approach to surgical scars. Dermatol Surg. 2016;42(Suppl 2): S150-6.

# CHAPTER 24

# Complications

**_Brienne Cressey, Murad Alam, Kira Minkis_**

## INTRODUCTION

A complication in dermatologic surgery is defined as any deviation from the expected course of a surgical procedure. The favorable safety profile of dermatologic surgery is well established, with overall low morbidity and mortality. Although there is some paucity of data on the exact incidence of some specific complications within dermatologic surgery, in general, the existent data as well as most experts agree on low incidence of complications in cutaneous surgery. Studies have found complications rates to be 1.6–6.0%. These include minor complications such as minor bleeding, vasovagal syncope, local infection, and very rarely major complications such as major bleeding, anaphylaxis, and systemic infection.[1,2] These complications can be a direct result of surgery or related to a side effect of a medication prescribed in the preoperative or postoperative period.[3] Despite the low incidence of complications, the dermatologic surgeon should anticipate potential pitfalls before, during, and after surgery. The following chapter will focus on the complications of dermatologic surgery, ways to anticipate and mitigate them, and what to do when complications inevitably occur.

## COMPLICATIONS OF LOCAL ANESTHESIA: LIDOCAINE TOXICITY

Lidocaine toxicity, although rare, is a well-reported complication of dermatologic surgery. Problems may occur due to overdose of medication, an excessively rapid systemic uptake,[4,5] impaired hepatic metabolism,[6] due to drug interactions,[7] or inadvertent infiltration directly into the intravascular compartment.

Symptoms of lidocaine toxicity begin at serum lidocaine concentrations of about 1–5 μg/mL with subjective sensory alterations, starting with complaints of dizziness and lightheadedness, and followed by tinnitus, circumoral paresthesias, blurred vision, and metallic taste (Table 24.1). With higher serum concentrations of ~5–8 μg/mL, nystagmus, slurred speech, localized muscle twitching, and fine tremors may occur. At 8–12 μg/mL, focal seizure activity begins and may progress to tonic-clonic seizures, and at even higher concentrations, to respiratory depression, cardiac arrest, and coma.[8]

Absorption of anesthetic will occur more effectively over thin skin, such as eyelids and mucosa than on thicker areas. Local adverse effects of anesthesia infiltration can occur based on vascular compromise secondary to excessive volumes. Infiltration of large volumes of anesthesia into distal digits may lead to necrosis, although this is very unlikely to occur as a direct consequence of anesthesia itself.[9] It should also be noted that care needs to be exercised when using local and topical anesthetics on eyelid skin, as ocular damage including vision loss has been reported.[8,10-14] Caution must also be exercised when topical anesthetics are used over large surface areas as systemic absorption can occur. Cardiovascular collapse and even death have been reported secondary to application of topical anesthesia under occlusion to skin prior to laser treatment.[15-17] The mechanism of action of severe toxicity when large areas are treated with topical anesthesia under occlusion is believed to be methemoglobinemia, which may occur even more commonly in infants.[18-20] Staying within known, predetermined safe doses of anesthetic calculated on the basis of body weight is the first step in the prevention of toxicity. The maximum safe dose of lidocaine in an adult is 5 mg/kg without epinephrine and 7 mg/kg with epinephrine at standard lidocaine (1–2%) concentrations.[21] Additionally, concentrations of dilute (tumescent) lidocaine (0.05–0.1%) are safe for

**Table 24.1:** Symptoms and management of lidocaine toxicity.

| *Systemic lidocaine level* | *Symptoms of toxicity* | *Management* |
| --- | --- | --- |
| 1–6 μg /mL | Circumoral and digital paresthesias, restlessness, drowsiness, euphoria, lightheadedness | Observation |
| 6–9 μg /mL | Nausea, vomiting, muscle twitching, tremors, blurred vision, tinnitus, confusion, excitement, psychosis | Diazepam, airway maintenance |
| 9–12 μg /mL | Seizures, cardiopulmonary depression | Respiratory support |
| >12 μg /mL | Coma, cardiopulmonary arrest | Cardiopulmonary resuscitation and life support |

subcutaneous injection at 55 mg/kg.[21] In children, the maximum safe dose of lidocaine is determined by age and is adjusted downward as age decreases.[21] It is recommended that patients of > 7 years who weigh > 20 kg should have no more than 20 g of emla applied to their skin, with this covering no more than 200 cm$^2$ of surface area for 4 hours or less. Newborns of <3 months of age weighing <5 kg should have no more than 1 g of EMLA applied to an area no larger than 10 cm$^2$ and for < 1 hour.[22] Guidelines for other topical mixtures, such as lomefloxacin (LMX), are distinct and physicians should refer to manufacturer guidelines for specific recommendations.

The most important step in managing an overdose of anesthetic is the rapid recognition of the toxicity. The patient should be placed in the supine position if one begins to experience any of the signs and symptoms associated with lidocaine toxicity. Vital signs should be obtained, and supplemental oxygen administered, and emergency medical services (EMS) activated. If the patient has lost consciousness, it is important to maintain an airway and begin ventilation. Although outside the scope of the dermatologic practice, serum lidocaine concentration may be obtained and the patient may be given benzodiazepines to treat the central nervous system manifestations (e.g., midazolam in 1 mg doses, titrated to effect) or barbiturates (e.g., thiopental in 25 mg doses, titrated to effect).[23]

## BLEEDING/HEMORRHAGE COMPLICATIONS (FIG. 24.1)

Bleeding-associated complications are the most commonly occurring complications in dermatologic surgery.[24] Studies estimate that the incidence of bleeding complications is ~3% in all dermatologic surgical procedures, accounting for ~40–50% of all complications.[1,2] The vast majority of these are considered minor and nonlife-threatening. However, inability to achieve adequate hemostasis could result in hemorrhage, hematoma formation, and subsequently wound infection, dehiscence, and necrosis. These complications can, in turn, cause suboptimal scar formation, and in a cosmetically sensitive area—such as the face—significant patient anxiety and decreased quality of life can result as a consequence. A number of patient-specific and surgery-specific factors can affect the risk for bleeding complications. These include patient's age, comorbid conditions, medications, procedure type, and location, and patient's postoperative activity. Although bleeding complications in dermatologic surgery are infrequent and relatively minor, every physician performing skin surgery should be prepared to anticipate and treat this complication.

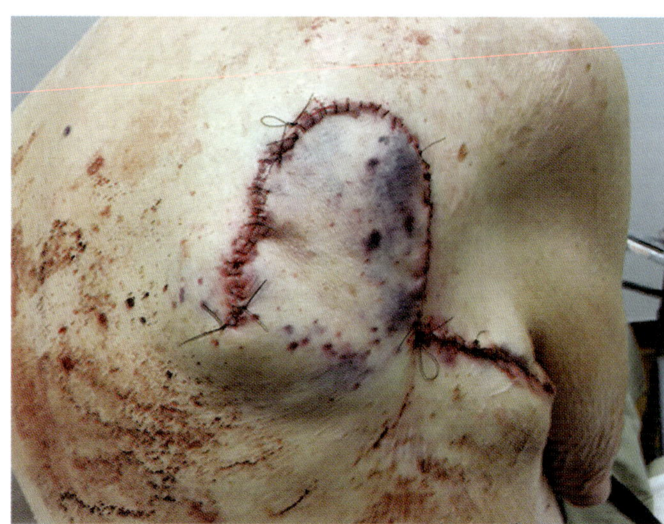

**Fig. 24.1:** Postoperative hematoma following a transposition flap of a large mohs surgery resection.

### Preoperative History and Physical Examination

Prior to beginning any surgical intervention, a detailed medical history and medication review should be performed to identify potential risk factors for bleeding com-

**Table 24.2:** Risk factors for bleeding.

| *Decreased vasoconstriction* | *Decreased platelet adhesion and aggregation* | *Decreased coagulation* | *Increased fibrinolysis* |
|---|---|---|---|
| Increasing age<br>Skin atrophy<br>Chronic steroid use<br>Ethanol<br>Ehlers–Danlos syndrome<br>Osler–Weber–Rendu syndrome | Platelet inhibiting drugs or supplements (aspirin, clopidogrel, vitamin E, gingko)<br>Ethanol<br>Von Willebrand disease<br>Osteogenesis imperfecta<br>Marfan's syndrome<br>Epstein's syndrome<br>Down's syndrome<br>Liver and kidney disease | Factor I–XIII deficiencies<br>Ethanol<br>Use of anticoagulant medications (warfarin, heparin, dabigatran, apixaban, rivaroxaban, argatroban) | Liver transplant<br>Disseminated intravascular coagulation<br>Inherited fibrinolytic abnormalities |

*Source*: Adapted from Peterson SR, Joseph AK. Inherited bleeding disorders in dermatologic surgery. Dermatol Surg. 2001; 27(10): 885-9.

plications. In regard to bleeding, the medical history should focus on underlying coagulopathies that may be congenital or acquired. A positive finding on preoperative history or physical examination suggestive of easy bruising should prompt the surgeon to consider ordering preoperative laboratory testing, including a complete blood count focusing on platelet count, prothrombin time, and partial thromboplastin time.

Disorders that may lead to defects in hemostasis can be divided into causes related to vascular constriction, decreased platelet function, decreased coagulation, or increased fibrinolysis (Table 24.2). Of the congenital coagulopathies, the three most common are von Willebrand's disease, factor VIII deficiency (hemophilia A), and factor IX deficiency (hemophilia B), collectively affecting ~1% of the general population.[25] In patients identified to have congenital coagulopathies, it is recommended that the surgeon take five steps to ensure a successful operation:

1. Close preoperative consultation with a hematologist
2. Factor replacement therapy as needed
3. Maintaining good operative technique
4. Considering reconstructive options that minimize undermining and potential bleeding without compromising aesthetic or functional repair
5. Close postoperative follow-up

The most significant social behavior that affects hemostasis is alcohol consumption. Alcohol is believed to moderate hemostasis by four major mechanisms: inhibition of platelet aggregation by decreasing platelet response to collagen and adenosine diphosphate; coagulation impairment by decreasing fibrinogen, von Willebrand factor, and factor VII; increasing fibrinolysis through activation of tissue plasminogen activator; and vasodilatation, which exacerbates all factors associated with bleeding.[24] Furthermore, chronic excessive alcohol consumption is associated with liver dysfunction and coagulation dysfunction.[26,27] While mild-to-moderate alcohol consumption is likely to have no significant effect on bleeding risk, excessive consumption has been associated with increased complications in elective intra-abdominal surgery.[28] Although there is a paucity of data in the dermatologic literature to support this practice, we endorse the cessation of alcohol consumption—in those not at risk for alcohol withdrawal—48 hours prior to surgery and for the immediate postoperative period.

## Antiplatelet and Anticoagulation Medications

Increased bleeding during the perioperative period is most commonly attributed to therapeutic anticoagulant, antiplatelet, and nonsteroidal anti-inflammatory drugs (NSAIDs).[29] The issue of how to manage medications during the perioperative period has long been debated by dermatologists. Previous studies offered conflicting evidence on whether or not aspirin, NSAID, or warfarin use significantly increased bleeding complications.[30-36] A more recent meta-analysis of 1,373 dermatologic surgery patients randomized to continuing or stopping existing anticoagulation or antiplatelet treatment found that severe complications occurred in 1.3% of aspirin users and 5.7% of warfarin users (severe complications defined as hematoma formation, graft or flap failure, bleeding presenting a significant threat to the wound or the patient, wound necrosis, wound dehiscence >2 mm, or bleeding requiring a procedure). Compared to controls, patients on warfarin were 6.7 times as likely to have a moderate-to-severe complication, and aspirin/NSAID users were 2 times as likely.[37] However, it remains to be said that given the overall low frequency of severe bleeding complications in dermato-

**Table 24.3:** Frequency of postoperative complications in anticoagulated patients.

| | *Mild (%)* | *Moderate (%)* | *Severe (%)* | *Total (%)* |
|---|---|---|---|---|
| Aspirin (NSAIDs) | 5.5 | 2.8 | 1.3 | 9.5 |
| Warfarin | 16.4 | 6.6 | 5.7 | 28.7 |
| Control | 4.5 | 1.5 | 0.5 | 6.5 |

*Source*: Adapted from Lewis KG, Dufresne RG Jr. A meta-analysis of complications attributed to anticoagulation among patients following cutaneous surgery. Dermatol Surg. 2008;34(2):160-4; discussion 164-5.

logic surgery, the absolute risk increase from warfarin is only 5.2% and that from aspirin is 0.8% (Table 24.3).

Patients on more than one anticoagulation medication have an additional increased bleeding risk, with combined warfarin and Plavix therapy associated with up to 40 times the bleeding risk compared to patients on no anticoagulation.[38] Again, the low incidence of complications in general makes this seemingly significant increase still relatively low in terms of absolute risk. However, to help mitigate the risk of complications, patients on warfarin should aim for an appropriate therapeutic internatioal normalized ratio (INR) between 2.0 and 3.5.[39,40] The safety of operating under supratherapeutic conditions has not been well studied and we would recommend avoiding surgery until coagulation levels are within the patient's targeted therapeutic range.

Life-threatening complications attributed to dermatologic surgery and anticoagulation use have not been seen in the literature. Therefore, compared to the potentially devastating complications (i.e., stroke, myocardial infarction, and thromboembolic events) that may occur with discontinuation of anticoagulation therapy, we recommend that all therapeutic anticoagulants be continued during the perioperative period. As with patients who have congenital coagulopathies, we recommend that extra intraoperative care be undertaken to minimize the risk of bleeding. These patients should be closely followed postoperatively, particularly if there was significant intraoperative hemorrhage or difficulty controlling bleeding.

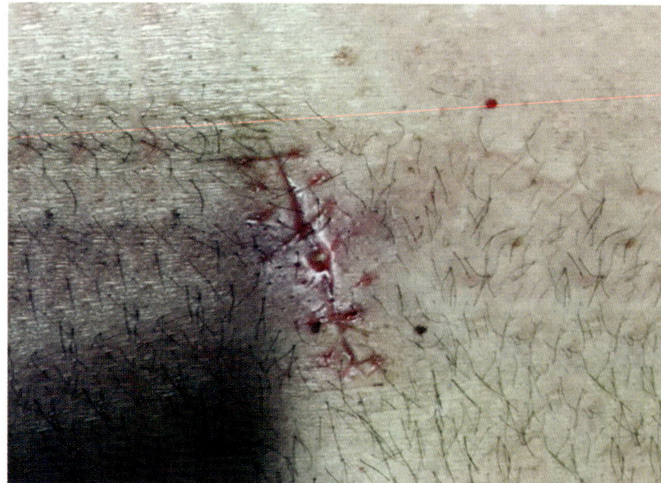

**Fig. 24.2:** Postoperative surgical site infection. Cultures grew Staph aureus. Note the focal area of dehiscence and central pustule.

## INFECTIOUS COMPLICATIONS

Infections resulting from dermatologic and Mohs micrographic surgery (MMS) are rare. Studies have shown that the overall incidence of infectious complications range from 1.32% to 2%.[2,41,42] The overwhelming majority of infections are localized to the incision site, and rarely result in systemic infection.[2] Despite a relatively low incidence of postsurgical infections, the ever-rising number of dermatologic procedures indicates that the number of infectious complications can be significant. Infectious complications are the second most common complication of dermatologic surgery following bleeding.[2]

Surgical site infections (SSIs) are identified through a combination of clinical and laboratory findings, and are classified as either incisional or organ/space; nearly all dermatologic surgery infections fall into the incisional category. Incisional SSIs are further subdivided into superficial and deep: superficial SSIs involve only the skin or subcutaneous tissue whereas deep incisional SSIs involve deeper tissues such as the fascial or muscle layers (Figs. 24.2 and 24.3). The Centers for Disease Control and Prevention (CDC) clearly defines guidelines for the diagnosis of SSIs.[43] Diagnosis of SSI is made if the infection involves the tissue surrounding the site of incision, occurs within the last 30 days of surgery, and includes at least one of the following:

- Purulent drainage
- Increasing pain or tenderness
- Localized swelling, redness, or heat

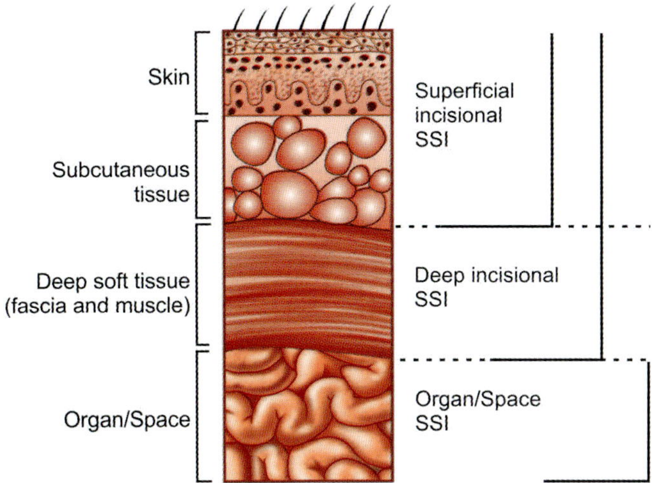


**Fig. 24.3:** Cross-section of an abdominal wall depicting CDC classifications of surgical site infection (SSI). CDC, Center for Disease Control and Prevention.

- Spontaneous wound dehiscence or the surgeon deliberately opens the wound (unless wound culture is negative)
- Abscess formation
- Isolation of organisms obtained aseptically from fluid or tissue at the surgical site

## Risk Factors

Studies on the risk factors for infectious complications in dermatologic surgeries are limited. This is due, in part, to the overall low incidence. Much of what we know about risks for infection is derived from the general surgery and orthopedic surgery literature. Risk factors for infectious complications can be divided into three categories:

1. Patient risk factors
2. Procedural risk factors
3. Wound classification

### *Patient Risk Factors*

Patient risk factors are often the most significant contributors to infection and the most difficult to control. The following patient risk factors have being associated with SSI: remote site infections, extremes of age, male sex, poor nutritional status, obesity, systemic steroid use, smoking, diabetes, and colonization with *Staphylococcus aureus.*[2,43-46]

Smoking has been cited as an independent risk factor for infection and wound dehiscence in patients undergoing cardiac surgery, general surgery, and oral surgery.[43,47,48] The link between smoking and infection after cutaneous surgery has been less clear. There is evidence to suggest that smoking increases flap necrosis and delays wound healing, but a concomitant increase in infections has not been found.[49] We suspect that these studies are limited by heterogeneity in how smoking is defined as well as in the amount that patients smoke. One study found a significant dose-dependent relationship between smoking and necrosis, with 1-pack-per-day (PPD) smokers having twice the risk for necrosis and 2-PPD smokers having six times the risk, and <1-PPD smokers having negligible risk.[50] We suspect a similar relationship exists between smoking and infections.

The association between diabetes and SSIs is similarly controversial.[43] Early studies of diabetic patients undergoing cutaneous surgery initially showed no association; however, a later multivariate analysis, when controlling for confounders, showed a statistically significant increased risk of infection.[51,52] Further studies are needed to elucidate the true association.

Nasal colonization with *S. aureus* has been suggested to be a risk for SSI in general and orthopedic surgery, and evidence suggests the same is true for MMS. Studies show the rate of infection in patients with confirmed nasal colonization is nearly four times that of noncarriers.[45] A Cochrane review of all-cause nosocomial infections found a significant decrease in infection rates after decolonization with nasal mupirocin.[53] A clinical trial of colonized patients undergoing MMS found that decolonization using a regimen of nasal mupirocin and chlorhexidine body wash significantly decreased SSI rates.[45] In a separate study of colonized patients comparing topical decolonization against prophylactic oral antibiotics, decolonized patients were significantly less likely to have a SSI.[54]

### *Procedural Risk Factors*

Certain procedural characteristics, such as procedure type, location, and closure type, are associated with higher risks of infection. Studies have found that smaller procedures (<2 cm) are significantly less likely to become infected when compared to larger incisions.[2] Similarly, the longer the duration of a procedure the greater the infection risk.[2,41] Patients with anesthetic or hemorrhagic complications—especially hematoma formation—during or after the procedure were also associated with increased infection risk.

**Table 24.4:** Wound classification.[41,57]

| Class | Skin condition | Body location/surgical technique | Infection risk (%) | Antibacterial recommendations |
|---|---|---|---|---|
| I | Clean | Sterile procedure on normal skin | <5 | No prophylaxis |
| II | Clean contaminated | Procedure on contaminated skin or moist areas such as the oral cavity, respiratory tract, nasal mucosa, perineum, and axillae | 10 | Prophylaxis if immunocompromised |
| III | Contaminated | Visibly inflamed skin without purulent discharge, traumatic wounds, nonsterile procedure | 20 | Therapeutic antibacterials |
| IV | Infected | Gross contamination, infected skin with purulent discharge, devitalized tissue, and foreign body | 30–40 | Therapeutic antibacterials |

Incisions located in the head and neck, as well as moist areas such as the groin, intertriginous areas, axillae, and oral mucosa, have been cited as areas with higher than average rates of infection approaching 5–12% compared to 1–2% in other areas.[2,46,51,55] Areas of highest risk in the face appear to be in the nasal and auricular areas, with SSI rates three to four times that found in the rest of the face. This is particularly true for skin flaps involving the nose. This is likely a consequence of *S. aureus* colonization in the nares and the high concentration of sebaceous glands in both the nares and the ears.[56]

Cancerous sites also appear to be at higher risk; one series found excision of cancerous lesions were 15 times more likely to have SSI complications when compared with excisions of benign lesions.[56] The lower extremities below the knee also appear to be an area of increased vulnerability. One study found an infection rate of nearly 7% in procedures below the knees compared to a background population SSI rate of 1.47%.[51]

### *Wound Classification*

Wounds are classified on the basis of the CDC guidelines for prevention of surgical wounds. This classification has been found to be a strong predictor of postsurgical infection rates.[43] Class I wounds are clean incisions made on an uninfected area with no visible signs of inflammation. Class II wounds are clean incisions made on uninfected areas with visible contamination or high likelihood of contamination such as the nasal mucosa, perineum, or axillae. The majority of wounds in dermatologic surgery will fall into these two categories. Class III incisions are nonsterile, contaminated wounds that show visible signs of inflammation such as traumatic wounds or nonsterile procedures. Class IV incisions are those made on grossly infected skin with or without purulent discharge, devitalized tissue, or foreign bodies. Each level has a corresponding increase in risk for infection (Table 24.4).

## Antibiotics Prophylaxis

Prophylactic antibiotics are recommended and routinely used in general surgery and orthopedic procedures. The American Academy of Dermatology (AAD) has issued an advisory statement regarding the appropriate use of prophylactic antibiotics, but acknowledges the ongoing controversy as there is a lack of high-quality randomized controlled trials.[43] At present, there does not appear to be any role for the routine use of prophylactic antibiotics except in a select high-risk population. This recommendation is supported by the relative low risk of SSIs when considering the potential adverse reactions of routine antibiotic usage. In general, the decision to give prophylactic antibiotics preoperatively should take into consideration the overall risk of infection and the severity of morbidity should an infectious complication arise. If the decision is made to give prophylactic antibiotics, we recommend it be given 30–60 minutes prior to the procedure.

### *Antibiotic Prophylaxis for Prevention of SSIs*

We recommend the use of prophylactic antibiotics in surgical procedures with an anticipated high infection rate (Table 24.5). These are sites that have been shown to have a higher than normal (>5%) rates of SSI. Infected surgical sites will tend to heal with poorer cosmesis and greater distortion of natural anatomy compared to uninfected sites. Furthermore, SSIs are a potential source for bacteremia, which could lead to hematogenous spread resulting in

**Table 24.5:** Sites associated with higher incidence (>5%) of infectious complications.*

| |
|---|
| Lower extremity below the knee |
| Wedge excisions of lip or ear |
| Groin or intertriginous areas |
| All skin grafts |
| Extensive inflammatory skin disease |
| Flaps on the nose |

**Adopted from reference 55.*

**Table 24.6:** High-risk cardiac conditions.*

| |
|---|
| Prosthetic cardiac valve |
| Previous infective endocarditis |
| Congenital heart defect (CHD) |
| Unrepaired cyanotic CHD, including palliative shunts and conduits |
| Completely repaired CHDs with prosthetic material or device during the first 6 months after procedure |
| Repaired CHD with residual defects at the site or adjacent to site of prosthetic patch or prosthetic device |
| Cardiac transplant recipients who develop cardiac valvulopathy |

**Adopted from reference 55.*

**Table 24.7:** Prophylactic antibiotics to prevent infective endocarditis or prosthetic joint infections.*

| *Anatomic site* | *Skin condition* | *Indication* | *Prophylaxis* |
|---|---|---|---|
| Oral mucosa | Any | High risk | Yes |
| All skin except oral mucosa | Infected | Low or high risk | Treat aggressively |
| All skin except oral mucosa | Noninfected | Low or high risk | No |

**Adopted from reference 55.*

endocarditis in patients with high-risk cardiac conditions, or total joint infections in those with high-risk orthopedic conditions.

### *Antibiotic Prophylaxis in High-Risk Patients*

The occurrence of infective endocarditis and total joint infection as a result of cutaneous infections has been documented in the literature.[58-60] The common mechanism for both is the hematogenous spread of bacteria from distant infected skin sites to vulnerable areas such as prosthetic heart valves and joints. Borrowing recommendations from the American Heart Association, the American Dental Association, and the American Academy of Orthopedic Surgeons, the AAD has made an advisory statement regarding the role of prophylactic antibiotics in patients at risk for endocarditis and total joint infections.

## Prevention of Endocarditis

Though rare, endocarditis after a dermatologic procedure on uninfected skin has been documented. The high morbidity and mortality associated with this complication highlight the importance of infection prevention in these patients. In a case series of four patients with endocarditis after a sterile dermatologic procedure, three of the patients died as a result of the complication.[61]

For patients with high risk for endocarditis (Table 24.6), perforating procedures that do not involve infected skin or the oral mucosa do not require prophylactic antibiotics. This is because the rates of bacteremia following clean surgical wounds (Class I) as detected by positive blood cultures appear to be equivalent to those of the general population performing normal daily activities (1.9% vs 2.1%).[55] Perforating procedures include any procedure that invades the epidermis or mucosa, such as excisions, MMS, biopsy, ablative laser, incision and drainage, and electrodessication and curettage. Nonperforating procedures include such therapies as cryotherapy and nonablative laser treatments.

For high-risk patients undergoing any procedure involving the oral mucosa, we recommend antibiotic prophylaxis since endocarditis is associated with a high risk of morbidity and mortality. If the procedure involves any contaminated (Class III) or infected (Class IV) skin areas, regardless of cardiac risk factors, we recommend aggressive therapeutic treatment with antibiotics prior to incision (Table 24.7).

## Prevention of Joint Infections

The AAD has similarly identified a group of patients at increased risk of prosthetic total joint infections secon-

| **Table 24.8:** High-risk orthopedic conditions.* |
|---|
| First 2 years following joint replacement |
| Previous prosthetic joint infections |
| Immunocompromised/immunosuppressed patients |
| Inflammatory arthropathies (rheumatoid arthritis, systemic lupus erythematosus) |
| Drug or radiation-induced immunosuppression |
| Insulin-dependent diabetes |
| Human immunodeficiency infection |
| Malignancy |
| Malnourishment |
| Hemophilia |

**Table 24.9:** Suggested antibiotic prophylaxis in patients at high risk for hematogenous infective endocarditis or total joint infections.*

| *Anatomic site* | *Medication restrictions* | *Antibiotic* | *Dose* |
|---|---|---|---|
| Nonoral | No penicillin allergy | Cephalexin | 2 g PO |
| | | Dicloxacillin | 2 g PO |
| Nonoral | Penicillin allergy | Clindamycin | 600 mg PO |
| | | Azithromycin | 500 mg PO |
| | | Clarithromycin | 500 mg PO |
| Nonoral | Unable to take PO | Cefazolin | 1 g IM/IV |
| | | Ceftriaxone | 1 g IM/IV |
| Nonoral | Unable to take PO with penicillin allergy | Clindamycin | 600 mg IM/IV |
| Oral | No penicillin allergy | Amoxicillin | 2 g PO |
| Oral | Penicillin allergy | Clindamycin | 600 mg PO |
| | | Azithromycin | 500 mg PO |
| | | Clarithromycin | 500 mg PO |
| Oral | Unable to take PO | Cefazolin | 1 g IM/IV |
| | | Ceftriaxone | 1 g IM/IV |
| | | Ampicillin | 2 g IM/IV |
| Oral | Unable to take PO with penicillin allergy | Clindamycin | 600 mg IM/IV |

(PO: Postoperative; IM: Intramuscular; IV: Intravenous).
**Adopted from reference 55.*

**Adopted from reference 55.*

dary to bacteremia (Table 24.8).[55] In accordance with the AAD advisory statement, we recommend prophylaxis in this group of high-risk orthopedic patients if they are to undergo procedures perforating the oral mucosa, a contaminated site at high risk for infection, or grossly infected skin. This recommendation is supported by evidence that the most common source for late-onset total joint prosthesis infection is skin infections.[59] Similar to recommendations for infective endocarditis, there is a limited role for the use of prophylactic antibiotics in orthopedic patients undergoing sterile perforating procedures of clean, uninfected skin, and antibiotics should not be used routinely in these low-risk patients. For prophylactic antibiotic regimens, we recommend selecting antibiotics with activity against *S. aureus* and β-hemolytic streptococci (Table 24.9). If a pathogen is known on an infected site from culture, targeted antibiotic therapy is recommended.

## Infectious Pathogens

The skin is host to a large flora of cutaneous bacterial pathogens. The normal skin flora consists of aerobic cocci, gram-negative bacteria, aerobic and anaerobic *Coryneform* bacteria, and yeast. In a nonpathologic state, this flora can act as a natural defense against skin infections by providing local ecologic competition. The predominant bacteria can vary depending on skin location and the availability of moisture and sebaceous lipids. The most important infectious bacterial pathogens identified in dermatologic surgery include S. aureus, coagulase-negative *Staphylococcus*, *Streptococcus*, and *Propionibacterium acnes*.[61] *Pseudomonas* and Enterobacteriaceae are also of concern in immunocompromised patients, those with diabetes, and hospitalized patients. In frequently hospitalized patients, there should be heightened awareness for methicillin-resistant *S. aureus* (MRSA), multidrug-resistant bacteria and vancomycin-resistant *Enterococcus*. In immunocompromised patients, opportunistic infections such as *Cryptococcus*, *Mucor*, *Aspergillus*, and atypical mycobacterium are of concern.

## Antibiotic Choice

Upon recognition of infection, empiric treatment with antibiotics needs to begin in the absence of wound culture information. Understanding the natural and pathologic flora (Table 24.10), based on the location of infection and underlying patient risk factors, is important in selecting the correct antibiotic agent.

In glabrous skin, the primary pathogens are *Streptococcus pyogenes* and *S. aureus*. First-generation cephalosporins such as cephalexin are an effective empiric antibiotic choice for infections of these skin areas (Table 24.11). Although these antibiotics offer antimicrobial activity

**Table 24.10:** Most common skin flora by anatomic site.*

| *Location* | *Normal skin flora* | *Pathogenic bacteria* |
|---|---|---|
| Glabrous skin | Aerobic cocci: *Staphylococcus aureus, Staphylococcus saprophyticus, Staphylococcus epidermidis, Micrococcus luteus, Micrococcus roseus, Micrococcus varians* | *S. aureus, Streptococcus pyogenes, S. epidermidis* (rare) |
| Oral or nasal mucosa | *S. aureus*, streptococci, lactobacilli, corynebacteria, anaerobes (bacteroides) | *Streptococcus viridans*, anaerobes *(Peptostreptococcus)* |
| Intertriginous areas (axillae, perineum, interdigital webs, antecubital fossa) | *Corynebacterium minutissimum, Corynebacterium lipophilicus, Corynebacterium xerosis, Corynebacterium jeikeium, Brevibacterium epidermidis, Acinetobacter, S. aureus* | *S. aureus, Escherichia coli, Enterococcus, Bacteroides, Pseudomonas aeruginosa, Corynebacterium, Candida* species, *Serratia* species |
| Sebaceous glands and follicles | *Propionibacterium acnes, Propionibacterium granulosum, Propionibacterium avidum, Yeast: Malassezia furfur* | *S. aureus*, streptococcus, anaerobic bacteria, *Pseudomonas aeruginosa*, gram-negative species |

**Adopted from reference 55.*

**Table 24.11:** Antibiotic choices.*

| *Location* | *Bacterial pathogen* | *Antibiotic* | *Dose* | *Notes* |
|---|---|---|---|---|
| Glabrous skin | *Staphylococcus aureus, Streptococcus Pyogenes* | Cephalexin | 500 mg PO QID | |
| | | Dicloxacillin | 125–500 mg PO QID | Pregnancy category B |
| | | Clindamycin | 150–300 mg PO TID or QID | If penicillin allergic offers strep, MSSA, and MRSA coverage |
| | | Azithromycin | 500 mg PO daily × 1 day, 250 mg PO daily × 4 days | If penicillin allergic |
| | | Clarithromycin | 250 mg PO BID | If penicillin allergic |
| | | Amoxicillin with clavulanic acid | 875 mg PO BID or 500 mg PO TID | Strep and MSSA coverage |
| | | Vancomycin | 15 mg/kg IV q12h | Treats MRSA |
| Oral or nasal mucosa | *Streptococcus viridans, anaerobes (Peptostreptococcus), Staphylococcus aureus, MRSA* | Amoxicillin ± clavulanic acid | 500 mg PO TID | |
| | | Clindamycin | 150–300 mg PO TID or QID | If penicillin allergic offers both MSSA and MRSA coverage |
| | | Azithromycin | 500 mg PO daily × 1 day, 250 mg PO daily × 4 days | If penicillin allergic |
| | | Clarithromycin | 250 mg PO BID | If penicillin allergic |
| Ear, groin, intertriginous areas, or lower extremities | *Pseudomonas, S. aureus, Escherichia coli, Enterococcus* | Ciprofloxacin | 500 mg PO BID | Treats pseudomonas |
| | | Cephalexin | 500 mg PO QID | |
| | | DS TMP-SMX | 1–2 tablets PO BID | Pregnancy category C in first two trimesters, category D in third trimester<br>Treats MRSA |
| | | Levofloxacin | 500 mg PO daily | Treats pseudomonas |

QID: Four times a day; TID: Three times a day; MSSA: Methicillin-sensitive Staphylococcus aureus; MRSA. Methicillin-resistant *Staphylococcus aureus*; BID: Two times a day; PO: postoperative; IV: Intravenous.
*Adapted from Wright TI, Baddour LM, Berbari EF, et al. Antibiotic prophylaxis in dermatologic surgery: advisory statement 2008. J Am Acad Dermatol. 2008;59(3):464-73.

against some gram-negative bacteria such as *Escherichia coli*, *Klebsiella*, and *Proteus*, they are not effective against Pseudomonas, *Staphylococcus epidermis*, or MRSA.[62]

Clindamycin shows excellent effectiveness against methicillin-sensitive *S. aureus* (MSSA) and is the ideal agent for patients with penicillin allergy. It also shows activity against MRSA; however, MRSA resistance to clindamycin is increasing. An alternative treatment regimen when MRSA is of concern is adding double strength trimethoprim-sulfamethoxazole with a first-generation cephalosporin.

The oral mucosa is colonized with a combination of streptococci, lactobacilli, staphylococci, corynebacteria, as well as anaerobic bacteria such as bacteroides. These bacteria are normally nonpathogenic, but with perforating procedures that violate the mucosal barrier infection can ensue. The most common pathogenic bacteria isolated from oral mucosal infections are *Streptococcus viridans* and *Peptostreptococcus*. Amoxicillin with or without clavulanic acid is often adequate for treatment of oral or mucosal pathogens; however, it is not effective against S. aureus.

In moist skin areas such as the groin, perineum, or intertriginous areas, *Enterococcus* and *E. coli* are the most common pathogens. These wounds are most likely to be infected by contamination owing to their proximity to the anus. Double strength Bactrim or cephalosporins are effective antibiotics for these pathogens. When *pseudomonas* is suspected, consider a quinolone such as ciprofloxacin and levofloxacin. The quinolones offer good gram-negative coverage, some gram-positive coverage, and show excellent activity against *pseudomonas*.

## WOUND FAILURE AND TISSUE ISCHEMIA COMPLICATIONS

### Wound Failure

Acute wound failure is a dreaded complication for all surgeons. Wound failure can contribute to increased healing time, increased risk of infection, poor cosmetic outcome, and patient anxiety. Understanding the stages of proper wound healing is essential to the prevention and management of wound failure. Reliable wound healing is the hallmark of any successful surgical closure. Healing depends on a time-dependent pattern of cellular, humoral, and molecular events. These events follow a predictable sequence beginning with the clearance of devitalized tissue and foreign bodies, followed by new tissue growth, and completed by rebuilding tissue integrity through remodeling. Acute wound failure occurs when there is a disruption in the degree or duration of the sequential components of tissue healing.[63]

### Wound Healing

Classically, wound healing is divided into four phases: hemostasis, inflammation, fibroproliferation, and scar remodeling. Hemostasis begins with vasoconstriction, which is initiated by platelet plug formation in the first 5–10 minutes after injury.[64] Fibrin production at the site of injury triggers a coagulation cascade that provides the substrate for the inflammatory phase. Platelet-derived growth factor and transforming growth factor β trigger the chemotaxis and proliferation of inflammatory cells into the extracellular matrix.[64,65]

The inflammatory phase occurs immediately following hemostasis. Production of histamine, prostaglandins, and vascular endothelial cell growth factor causes local vasodilation and increased endothelial permeability, increasing blood flow and migration of inflammatory cells. Polymorphonuclear leukocytes predominate in the wound during the first 24 hours, followed by macrophages in the next 48 to 72 hours. Together, they work in concert to clear the wound of devitalized tissue, clots, foreign material, and bacteria. Cytokines and growth factors released by macrophages induce fibroblast and endothelial cell proliferation, as well as contribute to the production of extracellular matrix.[63,65]

The fibroproliferation phase is characterized by formation of new connective tissue consisting of collagen, reticulum, elastin, and ground substance consisting of mucopolysaccharides, mucoproteins, and glycoproteins. The mechanical properties of this new tissue are supplied primarily by collagen, which comprises ~50% of this connective tissue. Fibroblasts produce procollagen, which forms a cable-like network of filaments. During this time, new capillaries are formed through neovascularization, induced by growth factors and proliferation of endothelial cells.[66]

Collagen production predominates for 2–3 weeks, after which the wound begins the remodeling phase. Until this time, tensile strength has increased moderately, achieving about 3–5% of the original tensile strength of unwounded skin. During remodeling, collagenases degrade the existing collagen network into a more organized network with increased intermolecular bonds, causing exponential increases in tensile strength across the wound. The wound reaches ~15–20% of its original strength by week 3, and

**Table 24.12:** Risk factors for wound dehiscence.

| *Systemic* | *Surgical complications* |
|---|---|
| Age >65 | Crush injury |
| Nutrition (zinc, vitamin C, protein deficiency, etc.) | Electrocautery |
| Obesity | Hematoma or seroma formation |
| Uremia | Local wound infection |
| Cushing's disease | Excessive tension |
| Thyroid disease | |
| Liver disease | *Medications* |
| Congestive heart failure | Anticoagulants |
| Pulmonary hypertension | Antiplatelets (e.g., aspirin and clopidogrel) |
| Ascites | Colchicines |
| Hyperalimentation | Systemic corticosteroids |
| Systemic infection | Penicillamine |
| Malignancy | Cyclosporine |
| Peripheral vascular disease | Metronidazole |
| Anemia | Cytotoxic and chemotherapeutic agents |
| Edema | β-aminopropionitrile |
| Diabetes | |
| Location | *Other* |
| Chest | Smoking |
| Back | Radiation |
| Extremities | Physical activity |
| Sebaceous regions of the face | Trauma |

*Source*: Adapted from Gloster HM. Complications in cutaneous surgery. New York, NY: Springer; 2008.

35% by week 4.[65,66] The exponential increase in wound strength begins to plateau around 2–3 months, at which point the wound has achieved ~70–80% of its original strength; however, the wound never regains strength of uninjured tissue. To avoid wound failure, the injured tissue must be allowed to progress sequentially through the stages of healing.

## Wound Necrosis and Dehiscence

Wound necrosis and dehiscence are caused by any disturbance in the normal trajectory of wound healing. Factors that increase the risk for wound failure can be divided into preprocedural, procedural, and postprocedural. Preprocedural factors include factors intrinsic to the patient such as age, underlying comorbidities, nutritional deficiencies, and adverse behaviors such as smoking. Nutritional deficiencies inhibit the natural wound healing process. Hypoalbuminemia, vitamin C, A, $B_6$ deficiency can adversely affect collagen crosslinking and wound tensile strength. Deficiencies in vitamins $B_1$ and $B_2$, zinc, and copper can retard the immune response, limit opsonization of bacteria and sterilization of the wound, and inhibit wound repair. Deficiencies in essential fatty acids—required for cell synthesis—can slow down cell turnover, essential in areas of wound repair.[63] Certain comorbid illnesses and behaviors impair oxygen delivery and tissue perfusion. These include age over 65 years, systemic infection, anemia, peripheral vascular disease, hypertension, diabetes, uremia, immunosuppression, hyperalimentation, malignancy, Cushing's disease, hypertension, and a history of smoking or alcohol abuse (Table 24.12).[67,68]

Oxygen is essential for the synthesis of reactive oxygen species during the inflammatory phase, proper collagen synthesis, angiogenesis, and cellular proliferation.[69] Chronic wounds have been shown to be relatively hypoxic compared to healthy tissue, with $PO_2$ levels in the range of 5–20 mm Hg compared to 35–50 mm Hg in healthy tissue.[70]

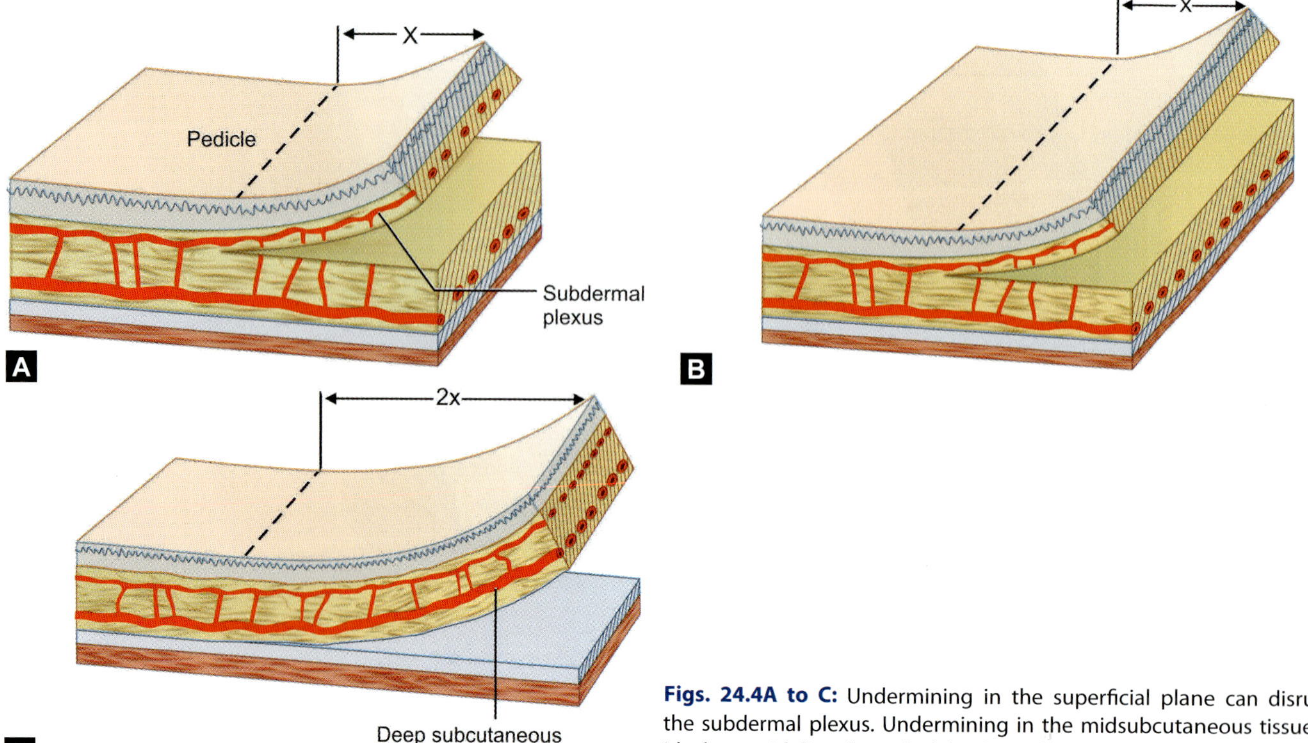


**Figs. 24.4A to C:** Undermining in the superficial plane can disrupt the subdermal plexus. Undermining in the midsubcutaneous tissue is ideal to avoid disturbing the blood supply.

Any disease that limits oxygen delivery such as chronic pulmonary disease, heart failure, or peripheral vascular disease can lead to increased risk of wound necrosis and dehiscence.

Review of patient medications is essential. Systemic steroid treatment, penicillamine, cyclosporine, metronidazole, and other cytotoxic agents have all been shown to impair wound healing.[71] Anticoagulant and antiplatelet medications increase the risk of intraoperative and postoperative bleeding, as well as hematoma formation. Hematoma and seroma formation increases the risk of dehiscence by increasing wound edge tension and necrosis by compressing on the surrounding microcirculation and impairing blood flow. Although we do not recommend routine discontinuation of anticoagulants or antiplatelet medications, the surgeon should be mindful of their effects especially since most patients on these medications have additional comorbidities that can contribute to a poor surgical outcome.

Intraoperative risk factors include the surgery location, flap design, and surgical technique. Body areas that are prone to high tension such as the back, chest, deltoids, and sebaceous areas of the face are at increased risk of wound dehiscence.[65] Areas that are at increased risk for infection are also at risk for wound failure.[72] Historically, it has been recommended not to use epinephrine in certain areas such as the ear, nose, digits, and penis; however, there is no evidence to suggest that injection of 0.5% lidocaine with epinephrine (1:200,000) increases the local risk for necrosis.[73] We recommend taking caution when using epinephrine in these areas, particularly in patients already at high risk for tissue ischemia and necrosis due to comorbid conditions.

Improper surgical technique is perhaps the most preventable risk factor to wound failure. Surgical technique refers to closure design, tissue handling, undermining, suture type, and suture placement. Cutaneous flaps are more vulnerable to ischemia than primary closures because flap perfusion relies solely on vasculature from the pedicle.[72] Rough handling of the tissue, particularly at the wound edges can impair wound healing. Skin hooks or toothed forceps should be used in place of serrated forceps as the latter can cause crush injury and ischemia to the epidermal margins.

Undermining is essential to decreasing excessive wound tension; however, excessive or improper undermining in the superficial plane can disrupt the superficial dermal plexus, the main blood supply to the flap (Figs. 24.4A to C).

The location of undermining can vary based on anatomic site, but should generally be performed in the midsubcutaneous tissue to avoid disturbing the blood supply.[72] Skin flaps should not exceed the 4:1 length-to-base ratio, as longer flaps decrease the perfusion pressure at the distal tip.[63] Flaps have a critical length beyond which these flaps are no longer adequately perfused regardless of the length-to-base ratio; therefore, widening the width of the pedicle further will not increase the distal perfusion pressure.[29]

The temptation to overcompensate tense closures by tying excessively tight sutures increases the risk of strangulation, necrosis, and dehiscence. Tense closures can also cause "railroad track" markings, particularly if postoperative edema develops. Sutures with higher elasticity, such as nylon and prolene, should be used for top sutures to allow for wound edema and expansion. This maintains the integrity of the closure without causing tissue strangulation. Layered closures using buried sutures can help decrease closure tension and eliminate the need for tight superficial sutures.[72]

Postoperatively, wound failure can be caused by hematoma and seroma formation, infection, excessive activity, and early suture removal. A sterile compressive dressing should be applied postoperatively to assist with hemostasis and provide a barrier to bacteria and foreign bodies. The CDC's guideline for the Prevention of Surgical Site Infection recommends the dressing remain for 24–48 hours postoperatively, during which the incision can epithelialize.[43] Petrolatum can be applied to the wound to increase epithelialization time and decrease scarring.

Early removal of sutures before adequate collagen production is a common cause of wound dehiscence. The recommended time for suture removal on the face is from 5 to 7 days, 10 to 14 days on the extremities and trunk, and at least 2 weeks in areas of movement and high tension. However, it is important to note during the first week of wound healing that the tensile strength of the wound is entirely reliant on suture material.[66] By the time most sutures are removed, tensile strength barely reaches 5% that of unwounded skin.[64]

Following surgery, the patient should be instructed to limit his/her activity to avoid putting excessive tension on the wound. This is particularly important when wounds are in areas of high mobility or tension such as the back, chest, and joints. Smokers should be encouraged to stop smoking for an additional 1–4 weeks postoperatively.[74] In diabetic patients, tight glycemic control is needed to optimize healing. The surgeon should also ensure that the patient has adequate analgesia upon returning home. Pain can trigger catecholamine surges that cause peripheral vasoconstriction and potentially impair perfusion at the wound site.[65,75]

## COMPLICATIONS BY ANATOMIC LOCATION

Certain complications during cutaneous surgery are specific to the anatomic location of surgery. In the periorbital area, one must take care to avoid nerve injuries to the infraorbital (less common), supraorbital, and supratrochlear nerves that can result in dysesthesias in their respective sensory distributions. Additionally, tension vectors that can cause downward tension on the free margin of the lower eyelid can cause ectropion of the eyelid and, therefore, need to be taken into consideration when planning reconstruction in the periocular region. Furthermore, actual injury to eyelid structures may lead to significant functional consequences including lacrimal duct obstruction, lagophthalmos, and vision compromise—either field obstruction or complete vision loss as the most severe complication. Nasal reconstruction should avoid injury to the nasal cartilaginous framework so as to minimize the risk of either functional or aesthetic compromise such as development of alar retraction, nasal valve collapse, saddle nose deformity, and nasal asymmetry. Perioral reconstruction should take care to avoid tension on the free margins of the lip, which can lead to eclabion.

## EMERGENCIES IN DERMATOLOGIC SURGERY

In general, the incidence of serious adverse events in the context of dermatologic surgery is exceedingly low, in large part because of the inherent safety of outpatient procedures under local anesthesia. Despite the numerous studies that have repeatedly demonstrated the remarkable safety profiles and minuscule serious adverse event rates associated with office-based dermatologic surgery, certain very rare but potentially serious complications can arise and will be reviewed briefly in this section. Retrobulbar hematoma (RBH) can occur as a complication of blepharoplasty or eyelid surgery/reconstruction. It represents a true ocular emergency that can result in permanent vision loss.[76] With prompt treatment, vision impairment is often reversible.[77,78] Although no reported cases have been described in dermatology, it is important to be aware

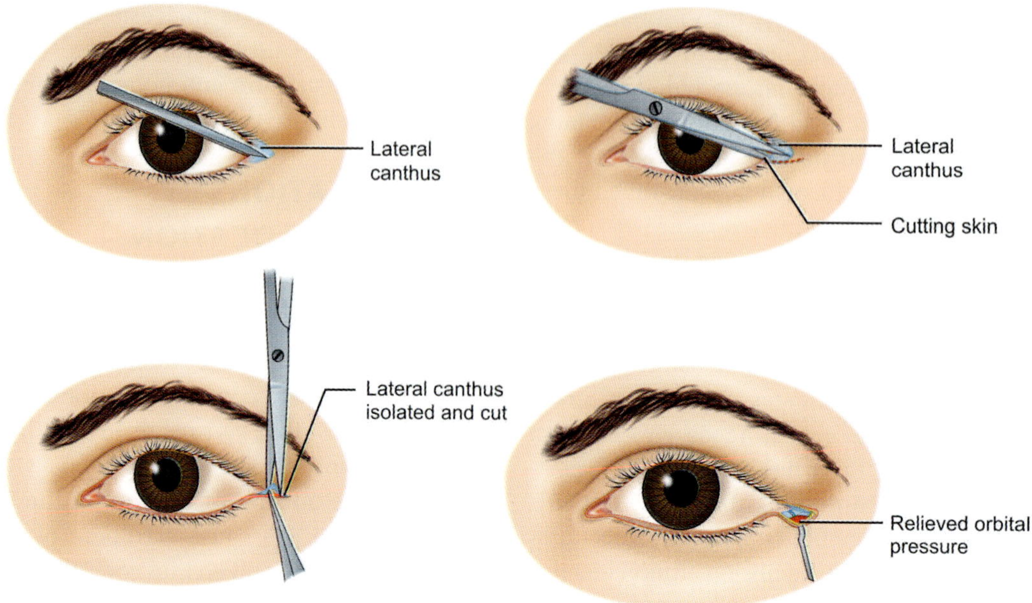


**Fig. 24.5:** A lateral canthotomy and inferior cantholysis can be performed for immediate decompression of the orbit.

of patient risk factors, clinical features, and treatment/management options in the event of occurrence.[76] Patient characteristics that have been found to increase the risk for postoperative RBH[79] including hypertension, vascular disease, glaucoma, coagulopathy, or courses of drugs such as aspirin or warfarin.[79] It appears that pressure induced on the neurovascular optic bundle by proximal hemorrhage can lead to permanent compromise of the essential structures and thus cause blindness. Visual loss occurs secondary to an increase in intraocular pressure due to the inflexible boundaries of the orbit, resulting in a compartment syndrome-like effect with decreased perfusion due to increased tissue pressures.[80,81]

Orbital hemorrhage is most common within the first 24 hours after surgery.[76] Signs and symptoms include pain, proptosis, chemosis, diplopia, subconjuctival ecchymosis, increased infraocular pressure, stony hard eyeball, mydriasis, pressure sensation, decreasing visual acuity, ophthalmoplegia, loss of direct papillary light reflex with preservation of consensual light reflex, loss of vision, diplopia, nausea, and vomiting.[76,80,82,83] Acute orbital hemorrhage is a medical and surgical emergency. The diagnosis can be made clinically, with tonometry or with ultrasound; however, confirmation may require computed tomography or magnetic resonance imaging to detect the so-called guitar-pick sign.[83] Prevention of RBH formation is essential by meticulous intraoperative hemostasis when performing eyelid surgery.[77,84] The mainstay of treatment is immediate surgical decompression of the affected orbit.[77,81,83,84] A lateral canthotomy and inferior cantholysis can be performed immediately under local anesthesia while waiting to bring the patient to the operating room for definitive treatment (Fig. 24.5).[77,81,83] If immediate symptomatic relief is not seen, further exploration of the orbit may be needed to find the bleeding source and evacuate the hematoma; thus, an ophthalmologic consultation is essential.[77,83]

## MOTOR NERVE TRANSECTION

Another potential dermatologic surgery emergency is transection of the facial nerve. The nerves at greatest risk for transection, trauma, ligation, or electrical injury during cutaneous surgery are the temporal branch of the facial nerve, which travels superiorly under the zygomatic arch and courses upward superficially under the skin; the marginal mandibular branch of the facial nerve where it crosses over the mandible;[85] and the spinal accessory nerve at Erb's point, the area in the posterior cervical triangle of the neck where it exits the posterior edge of the sternocleidomastoid muscle. The temporal branch of the facial nerve is most susceptible to transection at its most superficial course, superior to the zygomatic arch and lateral to the lateral eyebrow (Fig. 24.6).[86] Although nerve transection during cutaneous surgery has been reported in association with resection of large cutaneous

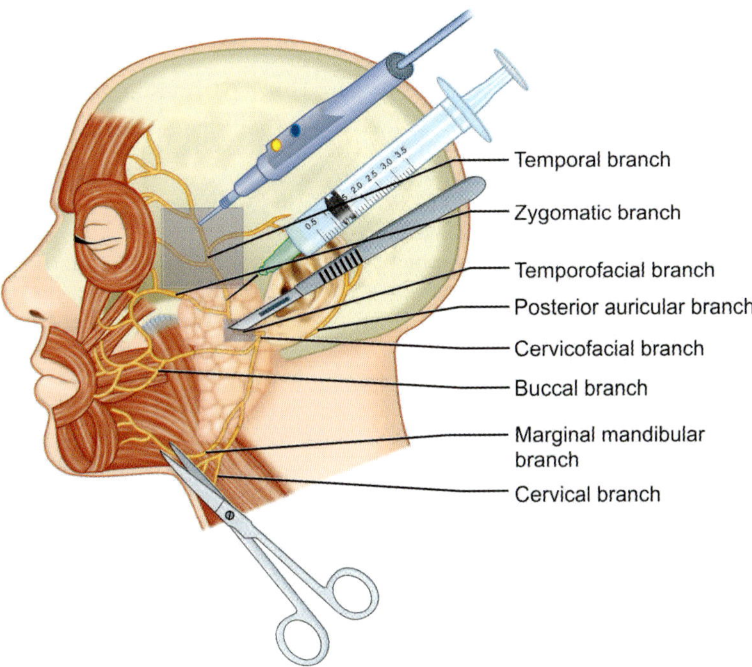


**Fig. 24.6:** Nerve injury danger zones.

tumors in this "danger zone,"[87] the highest incidence of paralysis is following rhytidectomy.[86] The marginal mandibular nerve is typically found 1–2 cm below the lower border of the mandible. However, in elderly patients with lax and atrophic tissue, the nerve may be present much lower in the neck.[86] Patients at greatest risk for nerve damage in this area are those with atrophy or hypoplasia of the platysma muscle and skin atrophy. The spinal accessory nerve is most susceptible to injury, as noted above, at Erb's point where the transverse cervical, lesser auricular, and spinal accessory nerves emerge from beneath the posterior border of the sternocleidomastoid muscle. Most commonly, inadvertent transection occurs during procedures in the posterior triangle of the neck, such as radical neck dissection, lymph node dissection, an extensive cervical lift, or tumor resection in the area.[88]

The presentation of temporal nerve transection is a flattened forehead, eyebrow ptosis, and an inability to raise the eyebrow. In addition to causing functional and cosmetic morbidity, the resultant eyebrow ptosis and redundant upper eyelid skin can cause upper visual field compromise.[89] Palsy of the marginal mandibular nerve results in inability to draw the lower lip downward and laterally or to evert the vermillion border on the affected side, which becomes evident on smiling. Injury to the spinal accessory nerve presents with shoulder pain and trapezius muscle palsy that subsequently results in a droop of the shoulder girdle inferiorly and laterally as well as flaring of the wing of the scapula and, commonly, loss of abduction of the arm.

Paralysis of the facial nerve postoperatively is typically transient with restoration of complete or partial motor function in about 80% of injuries, albeit over as long as 6 months to 2 years.[86,87] Treatment options for temporal nerve transection in cases without eventual return of function include microsurgical nerve reconstruction that includes either reapproximation of the severed nerve or placement of a nerve graft.[90] Flynn et al.[87] recommend marking the ends of the severed nerve with nonabsorbable colored suture in the event that a large facial nerve is severed. An alternative treatment option is surgical repair of the ptotic brow by unilateral brow lift on the affected side.[89] Treatment of marginal mandibular nerve and spinal accessory nerve transection entails conservative management including exercises, physiotherapy, or other noninvasive methods. Other very rare emergent situations can occur during the course of dermatologic office-based surgery, either as a result of surgery or as a coincidental complication. These include anaphylaxis, cardiac arrhythmias, stroke, anaphylaxis, hypertensive urgency, cardiac arrhythmias, etc. These are outside the scope of this chapter and can be best referenced elsewhere.

## REFERENCES


1. Cook JL, Perone JB. A prospective evaluation of the incidence of complications associated with Mohs micrographic surgery. Arch Dermatol. 2003;139(2):143-52.
2. Amici JM, Rogues AM, Lasheras A, et al. A prospective study of the incidence of complications associated with dermatological surgery. Br J Dermatol. 2005;153(5):967-71.
3. Kimyai-Asadi A, Goldberg LH, Peterson SR, et al. The incidence of major complications from Mohs micrographic surgery performed in office-based and hospital-based settings. J Am Acad Dermatol. 2005;53(4):628-34.
4. Covino BG. Systemic toxicity of local anesthetic agents. Anesth Analg. 1978;57(4):387-8.
5. Albright GA. Cardiac arrest following regional anesthesia with etidocaine or bupivacaine. Anesthesiology. 1979;51(4): 285-7.
6. Thomson PD, Melmon KL, Richardson JA, et al. Lidocaine pharmacokinetics in advanced heart failure, liver disease, and renal failure in humans. Ann Intern Med. 1973;78(4): 499-508.
7. Feely J, Wilkinson GR, McAllister CB, et al. Increased toxicity and reduced clearance of lidocaine by cimetidine. Ann Intern Med. 1982;96(5):592-4.
8. Sobanko JF, Miller CJ, Alster TS. Topical anesthetics for dermatologic procedures: a review. Dermatol Surg. 2012;38(5):709-21.
9. Denkler K. A comprehensive review of epinephrine in the finger: to do or not to do. Plast Reconstr Surg. 2001;108(1): 114-24.
10. Shiramizu KM, Kreiger AE, McCannel CA. Severe visual loss caused by ocular perforation during chalazion removal. Am J Ophthalmol. 2004;137(1):204-5.
11. Parikh M, Kwon YH. Vision loss after inadvertent corneal perforation during lid anesthesia. Ophthal Plast Reconstr Surg. 2011;27(5):e141-2.
12. Kim JH, Yang SM, Kim HM, et al. Inadvertent ocular perforation during lid anesthesia for hordeolum removal. Korean J Ophthalmol. 2006;20(3):199-200.
13. Eaglstein NF. Chemical injury to the eye from EMLA cream during erbium laser resurfacing. Dermatol Surg. 1999;25(7):590-1.
14. McKinlay JR, Hofmeister E, Ross EV, et al. EMLA cream-induced eye injury. Arch Dermatol. 1999;135(7):855-6.
15. Elsaie ML. Cardiovascular collapse developing after topical anesthesia. Dermatology. 2007;214(2):194.
16. Anaesthetic ointments: fatal overdose in adults. Prescrire Int. 2010;19(109):218.
17. Marra DE, Yip D, Fincher EF, et al. Systemic toxicity from topically applied lidocaine in conjunction with fractional photothermolysis. Arch Dermatol. 2006;142(8):1024-6.
18. Raso SM, Fernandez JB, Beobide EA, et al. Methemoglobinemia and CNS toxicity after topical application of EMLA to a 4-year-old girl with molluscum contagiosum. Pediatr Dermatol. 2006;23(6):592-3.
19. Touma S, Jackson JB. Lidocaine and prilocaine toxicity in a patient receiving treatment for mollusca contagiosa. J Am Acad Dermatol. 2001;44(2 Suppl):399-400.
20. Hahn IH, Hoffman RS, Nelson LS. EMLA-induced methemoglobinemia and systemic topical anesthetic toxicity. J Emerg Med. 2004;26(1):85-8.
21. Hruza GJ. Anesthesia, 3rd edition. Philadelphia, PA: Saunders; 2012.
22. [database online]. Gold Standard. (2013). [online] Available from http://clinicalpharmacology-ip.com.ezproxy.galter.northwestern.edu/Forms/Monograph/monograph.aspx?cpnum=1109&sec=monindi&t=1 [Accessed April, 2014].
23. Nouri K, Lubarsky DA, Harris EA: Complications of Anesthesia (Local, Topical, General). Complications in Dermatologics Surgery, Mosby Elsevier, 2008, Chapter 2:19-36..
24. Bunick CG, Aasi SZ. Hemorrhagic complications in dermatologic surgery. Dermatol Ther. 2011;24(6):537-50.
25. Peterson SR, Joseph AK. Inherited bleeding disorders in dermatologic surgery. Dermatol Surg. 2001;27(10):885-9.
26. Kamath PS, Wiesner RH, Malinchoc M, et al. A model to predict survival in patients with end-stage liver disease. Hepatology. 2001;33(2):464-70.
27. Orman ES, Odena G, Bataller R. Alcoholic liver disease: pathogenesis, management, and novel targets for therapy. J Gastroenterol Hepatol. 2013;28(Suppl 1):77-84.
28. Klotz HP, Candinas D, Largiader F. [Preoperative risk assessment in elective visceral surgery. Study design–results–perspectives]. Langenbecks Arch Chir. 1994;379(6): 341-6. [Article in German]
29. Baker SR. Local Flaps in Facial Reconstruction, 3rd edition. Philadelphia, PA: Saunders; 2014.
30. Otley CC, Fewkes JL, Frank W, et al. Complications of cutaneous surgery in patients who are taking warfarin, aspirin, or nonsteroidal anti-inflammatory drugs. Arch Dermatol. 1996;132(2):161-6.
31. Billingsley EM, Maloney ME. Intraoperative and postoperative bleeding problems in patients taking warfarin, aspirin, and nonsteroidal antiinflammatory agents. A prospective study. Dermatol Surg. 1997;23(5):381-3; discussion 384-5.
32. Kargi E, Babuccu O, Hosnuter M, et al. Complications of minor cutaneous surgery in patients under anticoagulant treatment. Aesthetic Plast Surg. 2002;26(6):483-5.
33. Dixon AJ, Dixon MP, Dixon JB. Bleeding complications in skin cancer surgery are associated with warfarin but not aspirin therapy. Br J Surg. 2007;94(11):1356-60.
34. Stables G, Lawrence CM. Management of patients taking anticoagulant, aspirin, non-steroidal anti-inflammatory and other anti-platelet drugs undergoing dermatological surgery. Clin Exp Dermatol. 2002;27(6):432-5.
35. Otley CC. Continuation of medically necessary aspirin and warfarin during cutaneous surgery. Mayo Clin Proc. 2003; 78(11):1392-6.
36. Alcalay J, Alkalay R. Controversies in perioperative management of blood thinners in dermatologic surgery: continue or discontinue? Dermatol Surg. 2004;30(8):1091-4; discussion 1094.
37. Lewis KG, Dufresne RG Jr. A meta-analysis of complications attributed to anticoagulation among patients following cutaneous surgery. Dermatol Surg. 2008;34(2):160-4; discussion 164-5.

38. Bordeaux JS, Martires KJ, Goldberg D, et al. Prospective evaluation of dermatologic surgery complications including patients on multiple antiplatelet and anticoagulant medications. J Am Acad Dermatol. 2011;65(3):576-83.
39. Ah-Weng A, Natarajan S, Velangi S, et al. Preoperative monitoring of warfarin in cutaneous surgery. Br J Dermatol. 2003;149(2):386-9.
40. Callahan S, Goldsberry A, Kim G, et al. The management of antithrombotic medication in skin surgery. Dermatol Surg. 2012;38(9):1417-26.
41. Wood LD, Warner NM, Billingsley EM. Infectious complications of dermatologic procedures. Dermatol Ther. 2011; 24(6):558-70.
42. O'Neill JL, Lee YS, Solomon JA, et al. Quantifying and characterizing adverse events in dermatologic surgery. Dermatol Surg. 2013;39(6):872-8.
43. Mangram AJ, Horan TC, Pearson ML, et al. Guideline for Prevention of Surgical Site Infection, 1999. Centers for Disease Control and Prevention (CDC) Hospital Infection Control Practices Advisory Committee. Am J Infect Control. 1999;27(2):97-132; quiz 133-4; discussion 196.
44. Rosengren H, Dixon A. Antibacterial prophylaxis in dermatologic surgery: an evidence-based review. Am J Clin Dermatol. 2010;11(1):35-44.
45. Tai YJ, Borchard KL, Gunson TH, et al. Nasal carriage of Staphylococcus aureus in patients undergoing Mohs micrographic surgery is an important risk factor for postoperative surgical site infection: a prospective randomised study. Australas J Dermatol. 2013;54(2):109-14.
46. Kulichova D, Geimer T, Muhlstadt M, et al. Surgical site infections in skin surgery: a single center experience. J Dermatol. 2013;40(10):779-85.
47. Nagachinta T, Stephens M, Reitz B, et al. Risk factors for surgical-wound infection following cardiac surgery. J Infect Dis. 1987;156(6):967-73.
48. Jones JK, Triplett RG. The relationship of cigarette smoking to impaired intraoral wound healing: a review of evidence and implications for patient care. J Oral Maxillofac Surg. 1992;50(3):237-9; discussion 239-40.
49. Dixon AJ, Dixon MP, Dixon JB, et al. Prospective study of skin surgery in smokers vs. nonsmokers. Br J Dermatol. 2009;160(2):365-7.
50. Goldminz D, Bennett RG. Cigarette smoking and flap and full-thickness graft necrosis. Arch Dermatol. 1991;127 (7):1012-5.
51. Dixon AJ, Dixon MP, Askew DA, et al. Prospective study of wound infections in dermatologic surgery in the absence of prophylactic antibiotics. Dermatol Surg. 2006;32(6):819-26; discussion 826-7.
52. Dixon AJ, Dixon MP, Dixon JB. Prospective study of skin surgery in patients with and without known diabetes. Dermatol Surg. 2009;35(7):1035-40.
53. van Rijen M, Bonten M, Wenzel R, et al. Mupirocin ointment for preventing Staphylococcus aureus infections in nasal carriers. Cochrane Database Syst Rev. 2008;(4):CD006216.
54. Cherian P, Gunson T, Borchard K, et al. Oral antibiotics versus topical decolonization to prevent surgical site infection after Mohs micrographic surgery—a randomized, controlled trial. Dermatol Surg. 2013;39(10):1486-93.
55. Wright TI, Baddour LM, Berbari EF, et al. Antibiotic prophylaxis in dermatologic surgery: advisory statement 2008. J Am Acad Dermatol. 2008;59(3):464-73.
56. Sylaidis P, Wood S, Murray DS. Postoperative infection following clean facial surgery. Ann Plast Surg. 1997;39 (4):342-6.
57. Levender MM, Davis SA, Kwatra SG, et al. Use of topical antibiotics as prophylaxis in clean dermatologic procedures. J Am Acad Dermatol. 2012;66(3):445-51.
58. Ainscow DA, Denham RA. The risk of haematogenous infection in total joint replacements. J Bone Joint Surg Br. 1984;66(4):580-2.
59. Maderazo EG, Judson S, Pasternak H. Late infections of total joint prostheses. A review and recommendations for prevention. Clin Orthop Relat Res. 1988(229):131-42.
60. Wagner RF Jr, Grande DJ, Feingold DS. Antibiotic prophylaxis against bacterial endocarditis in patients undergoing dermatologic surgery. Arch Dermatol. 1986;122(7):799-801.
61. Spelman DW, Weinmann A, Spicer WJ. Endocarditis following skin procedures. J Infect. 1993;26(2):185-9.
62. Rossi AM, Mariwalla K. Prophylactic and empiric use of antibiotics in dermatologic surgery: a review of the literature and practical considerations. Dermatol Surg. 2012;38 (12):1898-921.
63. Dubay DA, Franz MG. Acute wound healing: the biology of acute wound failure. Surg Clin North Am. 2003;83(3):463-81.
64. Steed DL. Wound-healing trajectories. Surg Clin North Am. 2003;83(3):547-55, vi-vii.
65. Gloster HM. Complications in Cutaneous Surgery. New York, NY: Springer; 2008.
66. Harris DR. Healing of the surgical wound. I. Basic considerations. J Am Acad Dermatol. 1979;1(3):197-207.
67. Riou JP, Cohen JR, Johnson H Jr. Factors influencing wound dehiscence. Am J Surg. 1992;163(3):324-30.
68. Craig S, Rees TD. The effects of smoking on experimental skin flaps in hamsters. Plast Reconstr Surg. 1985;75(6): 842-6.
69. Sen CK. Wound healing essentials: let there be oxygen. Wound Repair Regen. 2009;17(1):1-18.
70. Eisenbud DE. Oxygen in wound healing: nutrient, antibiotic, signaling molecule, and therapeutic agent. Clin Plast Surg. 2012;39(3):293-310.
71. Lawrence C. Drug management in skin surgery. Drugs. 1996;52(6):805-17.
72. Delaney A, Diamantis S, Marks VJ. Complications of tissue ischemia in dermatologic surgery. Dermatol Ther. 2011;24 (6):551-7.
73. Firoz B, Davis N, Goldberg LH. Local anesthesia using buffered 0.5% lidocaine with 1:200,000 epinephrine for tumors of the digits treated with Mohs micrographic surgery. J Am Acad Dermatol. 2009;61(4):639-43.
74. Wong LS, Martins-Green M. Firsthand cigarette smoke alters fibroblast migration and survival: implications for impaired healing. Wound Repair Regen. 2004;12(4):471-84.

75. Huskisson EC. Catecholamine excretion and pain. Br J Clin Pharmacol. 1974;1(1):80-2.
76. Hass AN, Penne RB, Stefanyszyn MA, et al. Incidence of postblepharoplasty orbital hemorrhage and associated visual loss. Ophthal Plast Reconstr Surg. 2004;20(6):426-32.
77. Klapper SR, Patrinely JR. Management of cosmetic eyelid surgery complications. Semin Plast Surg. 2007;21(1):80-93.
78. Hueston JT, Heinze JB. Successful early relief of blindness occurring after blepharoplasty. Case report. Plast Reconstr Surg. 1974;53(5):588-92.
79. Anderson RL. Bilateral visual loss after blepharoplasty. Arch Ophthalmol. 1981;99(12):2205.
80. Winterton JV, Patel K, Mizen KD. Review of management options for a retrobulbar hemorrhage. J Oral Maxillofac Surg. 2007;65(2):296-99.
81. Brucoli M, Arcuri F, Giarda M, et al. Surgical management of posttraumatic intraorbital hematoma. J Craniofac Surg. 2012;23(1):e58-61.
82. Allen M, Perry M, Burns F. When is a retrobulbar haemorrhage not a retrobulbar haemorrhage? Int J Oral Maxillofac Surg. 2010;39(11):1045-9.
83. Colletti G, Valassina D, Rabbiosi D, et al. Traumatic and Iatrogenic retrobulbar hemorrhage: an 8-patient series. J Oral Maxillofac Surg. 2012;70(8):e464-8.
84. Lelli GJ Jr, Lisman RD. Blepharoplasty complications. Plast Reconstr Surg. 2010;125(3):1007-17.
85. Moffat DA, Ramsden RT. The deformity produced by a palsy of the marginal mandibular branch of the facial nerve. J Laryngol Otol. 1977;91(5):401-6.
86. Baker DC, Conley J. Avoiding facial nerve injuries in rhytidectomy. Anatomical variations and pitfalls. Plast Reconstr Surg. 1979;64(6):781-95.
87. Flynn TC, Emmanouil P, Limmer B. Unilateral transient forehead paralysis following injury to the temporal branch of the facial nerve. Int J Dermatol. 1999;38(6):474-7.
88. Wiater JM, Bigliani LU. Spinal accessory nerve injury. Clin Orthop Relat Res. 1999(368):5-16.
89. Grabski WJ, Salasche SJ. Management of temporal nerve injuries. J Dermatol Surg Oncol. 1985;11(2):145-51.
90. Hausamen JE, Schmelzeisen R. Current principles in microsurgical nerve repair. Br J Oral Maxillofac Surg. 1996;34(2):143-57.

# Index

Page numbers followed by *f* refer to figure and *t* refer to table.

## C



## D

## E



## F

## G



## H



## I



## J



## K



## L

## O



## P



## Q



## R



## S

## T



## U



## V

## W



## Y



## Z